E. Bombardieri · G. Bonadonna · L. Gianni (Eds.)

Breast Cancer

Nuclear Medicine in Diagnosis and Therapeutic Options

With Contributions by

R. Agresti · A. Alessi · H. Bender · S. Bergomi · T. Beyer · H.-J. Biersack · E. Bombardieri
A. K. Buck · E. Brugola · J. R. Buscombe · I. Butti · V. Cappelletti · A. Carbone
M. L. Carcangiu · A. Coli · P. F. Conte · F. Crippa · M. G. Daidone · A. Fabbri · F. Fazio
L. Florimonte · R. Fonti · O. Gentilini · A. Gerali · L. Gianni · L. Gianolli · M. Gion
V. Guarneri · N. Harbeck · K. Hausegger · O. S. Hoekstra · I. Igerc · M. Intra · F. Iommelli
N. C. Krak · J. M. H. de Klerk · M. G. E. H. Lam · A. A. Lammertsma · C. Landoni · P. Lind
G. Lucignani · G. Madeddu · L. Maffioli · C. Di Maggio · C. L. Maini · S. Manoukian
P. Mariani · N. Mazzuca · C. Messa · A. J. Nordin · H. Palmedo · G. Paganelli · L. Pagani
F. Pallotti · A. Paradiso · R. Pasqualoni · F. Piacentini · M. Picchio · P. Reinprecht · S. N. Reske
P. P. van Rijk · I. Roca · M. Salvatore · O. Schillaci · M. Schmitt · R. Sciuto · E. Seregni
G. Serfini · A. Spanu · L. Strigari · F. Sweep · L. Tagliabue · G. Trecate · G. Trifirò
S. Del Vecchio · D. Vernaghi · U. Veronesi · G. Viale · B. Zangheri · A. Zannetti

With 72 Figures in 156 Separate Illustrations, 56 in Color and 30 Tables

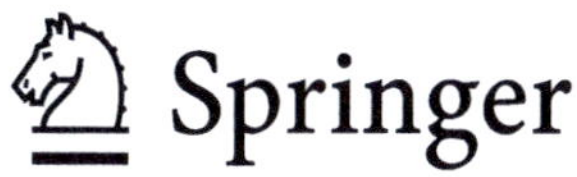

EMILIO BOMBARDIERI, MD
Division of Nuclear Medicine
Department of Diagnostic Imaging and Radiotherapy
Fondazione IRCCS
Istituto Nazionale dei Tumori
Via Venezian 1
20133 Milano
Italy

LUCA GIANNI, MD
Division of Medical Oncology
Fondazione IRCCS
Istituto Nazionale dei Tumori
Via Venezian 1
20133 Milano
Italy

GIANNI BONADONNA, MD
Chair, Perspective Clinical Trials
Fondazione IRCCS
Istituto Nazionale dei Tumori
Via Venezian 1
20133 Milano
Italy

Library of Congress Control Number: 2007933314

ISBN 978-3-540-36780-2 Springer Berlin Heidelberg New York

Springer is part of Springer Science+Business Media

http//www.springer.com

Medical Editor: Dr. Ute Heilmann, Heidelberg
Desk Editor: Ursula N. Davis, Heidelberg
Production Editor: Kurt Teichmann, Mauer
Typesetting: Verlagsservice Teichmann, Mauer
Cover-Design: Frido Steinen-Broo, eStudio Calamar, Spain

Printed on acid-free paper – 21/3180xq – 5 4 3 2 1 0

Foreword

Breast cancer is the most common malignant disease among Western women and represents a major public health problem, with more than 370,000 new cases and 130,000 deaths per year in women aged 35–64 years in Europe alone. It accounts for one third of the cancer-related deaths in women aged 35–55 years.

The efforts of modern oncology to deal with this clinical problem are focused on reaching a diagnosis at the earliest stage, when the disease is still limited, the tumour is resectable and it is still possible to treat with curative intent. Another essential goal of modern research is to characterise the tumour cells in order to categorise patients into different risk groups, identify responders versus nonresponders to therapy, and design adequate targeted therapies that are effective also in the adjuvant setting to eradicate breast cancer cells that might have already spread to distant sites at the time of diagnosis.

The great impact of nuclear medicine in oncology is due to its important progress in this field in recent years, and the effect of such progress has been particularly noticeable in breast cancer. Research into molecular imaging has led to the development of several radiopharmaceuticals that can explore the cellular metabolism and visualise, at the molecular and subcellular level, pathological processes specific to cancer. Advances in diagnostic equipment have made high-technology instruments available such as PET, which is capable of producing high-quality tomographic images. Such imaging has become of major value to physicians because it often reveals alterations and lesions not demonstrated by conventional morphological techniques such as X-rays, US, CT or MRI. Research into image fusion techniques has led to the design of software programmes capable of merging the molecular, functional and metabolic information of nuclear medicine with the morphological information provided by radiology into a single image. Hybrid instruments (PET/CT, SPECT/CT) are now available which allow the fusion of images of a patient in just one diagnostic session.

All these impressive achievements are going to produce important results not only for the diagnosis but also the treatment of cancer. Nuclear medicine explores the function and biology of cells and tissues, and can be considered an experimental area of drug development for individual tailored therapies. In fact, radiopharmaceuticals developed specifically to target and visualise malignant tumours can also be used, at high doses, for therapeutic purposes. Nuclear medicine therapeutics thus takes advantage of selective radiopharmaceuticals that have demonstrated anticancer efficacy in many types of tumours.

This book on the diagnostic and therapeutic applications of nuclear medicine in breast cancer aims to describe the state of the art and the current position of nuclear medicine in the light of these recent developments and in comparison with conventional radiological and nonradiological modalities. Some basic concepts regarding breast cancer are treated and discussed with the aim of providing a general overview on a disease that is the subject of continuous stimulating proposals for research and clinical investigation. The text is therefore intended as an update also for non-nuclear-medicine specialists working in senology and oncology. The new definition of nuclear medicine is 'molecular imaging' and 'targeted therapy' and its clinical impact is becoming increasingly important. We have no doubt that the diagnosis and treatment of breast cancer will benefit from the new horizons opened up by nuclear medicine.

Gianni Bonadonna
Emilio Bombardieri
Luca Gianni

Acknowledgements
The editors are grateful to Ms Anna Luisa De Simone Sorrentino for her precious help in compiling this manuscript.

Preface

The last three decades have witnessed tremendous advances in the understanding and treatment of breast cancer. As a result, starting shortly before the 1990s, a persistent decrease in breast cancer mortality has been documented, primarily in the United States and in several European countries. Breast cancer, however, remains an important health problem. In this book, which is mainly dedicated to nuclear medicine, experts have thoroughly reviewed the achievements made in the diagnosis, monitoring and treatment of this disease. There is no doubt that breast cancer has always been one of the most appealing areas of cancer research; the vast number of new clinical and preclinical studies published every day in the medical literature is an example.

More recently, the development of molecular biology techniques has allowed the identification and analysis of molecular factors that play an important role in normal cell growth and differentiation. Such factors have also been shown to influence the behavior of tumors in terms of cellular differentiation, growth rate, metastatic pattern and response to therapy. Furthermore, they will be instrumental in the development of new agents for targeted therapies. Using molecular tracers to characterize neoplastic tissues and to select, among the available effective regimens, the one with the highest probability of cure for the individual patient, is an appealing way to conduct new research. The ability to predict who will need medical therapy and who will or will not respond to a given drug or drug regimen will serve to guide clinical decision-making and treatment recommendations. Although predictive accuracy may not be an all-or-none phenomenon, patients can be spared treatments that are devoid of efficacy but are associated with toxicity instead. Besides this, delivering treatments that have a more pronounced activity against tumors with specific molecular features will lead to improved benefit for the patient, making the difference between cure and palliation.

In this area nuclear medicine follows the new developments in oncology: the modern term "molecular imaging" means to visualize a biological phenomenon at the molecular level according to the specificity and the specific biodistribution of a molecular probe. Cancer can be imaged through metabolic pathways (such as glucose and amino-acid transport, DNA precursor incorporation, hormone receptors, angiogenesis, hypoxia, antigen expression) targeted by radioactive tracers. This makes it possible to supplement the morphological description of a tumor with a considerable amount of biological information. Nuclear medicine images may provide prognostic indications, predict the response to different treatments, and detect the presence and activity of viable cancer cells in already treated patients. The same radiopharmaceuticals that target neoplasia and are used in diagnostic imaging can carry high amounts of radioactivity to cancer cells and thus selectively deliver a lethal irradiation dose to a tumor. For all these reasons nuclear medicine techniques have acquired an important role in the study and management of breast cancer, and are becoming more and more integrated in the new developments of molecular biology, pharmacology, diagnostic imaging and therapy.

Gianni Bonadonna

Contents

List of Contributors

Roberto Agresti
Unit of Surgical Oncology
Fondazione IRCCS
Istituto Nazionale dei Tumori
Milan, Italy

Alessandra Alessi
PET Unit, Nuclear Medicine Division
Fondazione IRCCS
Istituto Nazionale dei Tumori
Milan, Italy

Hans Bender
Department of Nuclear Medicine
University Hospital Bonn
Bonn, Germany

Serenella Bergomi
Nuclear Medicine Department
Regina Elena National Cancer Instiute
Rome, Italy

Thomas Beyer
Department of Nuclear Medicine
University Hospital
Essen, Germany

Hans-Jürgen Biersack
Department of Nuclear Medicine
University Hospital Bonn
Bonn, Germany

Emilio Bombardieri
Division of Nuclear Medicine
Department of Diagnostic Imaging and Radiotherapy
Fondazione IRCCS
Istituto Nazionale dei Tumori
Milano, Italy

Andreas K. Buck
Department of Nuclear Medicine
University Hospital Ulm,
Ulm, Germany

Elisabetta Brugola
Institute of Radiological Sciences
University of Milan
Unit of Nuclear Medicine
Hospital San Paolo
Milan, Italy

John R. Buscombe
Department of Nuclear Medicine
Royal Free Hospital
London, United Kingdom

Ivana Butti
Division of Health Physics
Ospedale A. Manzoni
Lecco, Italy

Vera Cappelletti
Research Unit 10
Department of Experimental Oncology
Fondazione IRCCS
Istituto Nazionale dei Tumori
Milan, Italy

Antonino Carbone
Department of Pathological Anatomy
Fondazione IRCCS
Istituto Nazionale dei Tumori
Milan, Italy

Maria Luisa Carcangiu
Department of Pathological Anatomy
Fondazione IRCCS
Istituto Nazionale dei Tumori
Milan, Italy

Antonio Coli
Nuclear Medicine Unit
Ospedale S. Andrea
La Spezia, Italy

Pier Franco Conte
Department of Oncology and Hematology
University of Modena and Reggio Emilia
Modena, Italy

Flavio Crippa
PET Unit - Nuclear Medicine Division
Fondazione IRCCS
Istituto Nazionale dei Tumori
Milan, Italy

Maria Grazia Daidone
Research Unit 10
Department of Experimental Oncology
Fondazione IRCCS
Istituto Nazionale dei Tumori
Milan, Italy

Alessandra Fabbri
Department of Pathological Anatomy
Fondazione IRCCS
Istituto Nazionale dei Tumori
Milan, Italy

Ferruccio Fazio
Department of Nuclear Medicine
Scientific Institute San Raffaele
IBFM-CNR
University of Milano-Bicocca
Milan, Italy

Luigia Florimonte
Department of Nuclear Medicine
Fondazione IRCCS
Ospedale Maggiore Policlinico
Mangiagalli Regina Elena
Milan, Italy

Rosa Fonti
Institute of Biostructures and Bioimages
of the National Research Council (CNR)
Naples, Italy

Oreste Gentilini
Division of Senology
European Institute of Oncology
Milan, Italy

Alberto Gerali
PET Unit – Nuclear Medicine Division
Fondazione IRCCS
Istituto Nazionale dei Tumori
Milan, Italy

Luca Gianni
Division of Medical Oncology
Fondazione IRCCS
Istituto Nazionale dei Tumori
Milan, Italy

Luigi Gianolli
Department of Nuclear Medicine
Scientific Institute San Raffaele
Milan, Italy

Massimo Gion
Centro Regionale Indicatori Biochimici di Tumore
Ospedale Civile
Venice, Italy

Valentina Guarneri
Department of Oncology and Haematology
University of Modena and Reggio Emilia
Modena, Italy

Nadia Harbeck
Clinical Research Unit
Department of Obstetrics and Gynecology
Technical University of Munich
Munich, Germany

Klaus Hausegger
Department of Radiology
Klagenfurt, Austria

Otto S. Hoekstra
Department of Nuclear Medicine and PET Research
VU University Medical Centre
Amsterdam, The Netherlands

Isabel Igerc
Landeskrankenhaus-Klagenfurt
PET/CT Center Klagenfurt
Klagenfurt, Austria

Matti Intra
Division of Senology
European Institute of Oncology
Milan, Italy

Francesca Iommelli
Department of Biomorphological and
Functional Sciences
Naples, Italy

Nanda C. Krak
Department of Nuclear Medicine and PET Research
VU University Medical Centre
Amsterdam, The Netherlands

John M.H. de Klerk
Department of Nuclear Medicine
University Medical Center Utrecht
Utrecht, The Netherlands

Marnix G.E.H. Lam
Department of Nuclear Medicine
University Medical Center Utrecht
Utrecht, The Netherlands

Adriaan A. Lammertsma
Department of Nuclear Medicine and PET Research
VU University Medical Centre
Amsterdam, The Netherlands

Claudio Landoni
Department of Nuclear Medicine
Scientific Institute San Raffaele
University of Milano Bicocca
Milan, Italy

Peter Lind
Department of Nuclear Medicine and Endocrinology
Landeskrankenhaus-Klagenfurt
PET/CT Center
Klagenfurt, Austria

Giovanni Lucignani
Institute of Radiological Sciences
University of Milan
Unit of Nuclear Medicine
Hospital San Paolo
Milan, Italy

Giuseppe Madeddu
Department of Nuclear Medicine
University of Sassari
Sassari, Italy

Lorenzo Maffioli
Division of Nuclear Medicine
Ospedale Civile di Legnano
Legnano, Italy

Cosimo Di Maggio
Diagnostic Breast Unit
University of Padua
Padua, Italy

Carlo L. Maini
Nuclear Medicine Department
Regina Elena National Cancer Instiute
Rome, Italy

Siranoush Manoukian
Department of Experiomental Oncology-Medical Gnetics
Fondazione IRCCS
Istituto Nazionale dei Tumori
Milan, Italy

Paola Mariani
Division of Medical Oncology
Fondazione IRCCS
Istituto Nazionale dei Tumori
Milan, Italy

Nicola Mazzuca
Nuclear Medicine Division
Ospedale Misericordia
Grosseto, Italy

Cristina Messa
Department of Nuclear Medicine
Scientific Institute San Raffaele
IBFM-CNR
University of Milano Bicocca
Milan, Italy

Abdul Jalil Nordin
Department of Radiology
University Putra
Putra, Malysia

Holger Palmedo
Department of Nuclear Medicine
University Hospital Bonn
Bonn, Germany

Giovanni Paganelli
Division of Nuclear Medicine
European Institute of Oncology
Milan, Italy

Luca Pagani
Division of Nuclear Medicine
Ospedale A. Manzoni
Lecco, Italy

Frederica Pallotti
Nuclear Medicine Division
Fondazione IRCCS
Istituto Nazionale dei Tumori
Milan, Italy

Angelo Paradiso
Department of Experimental Oncology
Istituto Oncologico
Bari, Italy

Rosella Pasqualoni
Nuclear Medicine Department
Regina Elena National Cancer Institute
Rome, Italy

Frederico Piacentini
Department of Oncology and Hematology
University of Modena and Reggio Emilia
Modena, Italy

Maria Picchio
Department of Nuclear Medicine
Scientific Institute San Raffaele
Milan, Italy

Peter Reinprecht
Landeskrankenhaus-Klagenfurt
Department of Radiology
Klagenfurt, Austria

Sven N. Reske
Department of Nuclear Medicine
University Hospital Ulm
Ulm, Germany

Peter P. van Rijk
Department of Nuclear Medicine
University Medical Center Utrecht
Utrecht, The Netherlands

Isabel Roca
Division of Nuclear Medicine
Hospital Universitari Vall Hebron
Barcelona, Spain

Marco Salvatore
Department of Biomorphological and Functional Sciences
University of Naples
Naples, Italy

Orazio Schillaci
Department of Biopathology and Diagnostic Imaging
University Tor Vergata
Rome, Italy

Manfred Schmitt
Department of Chemical Endocrinology
University Medical Center Nijmegen
Nijmegen, The Netherlands

Rosa Sciuto
Nuclear Medicine Department
Regina Elena National Cancer Instiute
Rome, Italy

Ettore Seregni
Radioisotopes Laboratory
Nuclear Medicine Division
Fondazione IRCCS
Istituto Nazionale dei Tumori
Milan, Italy

Gianluca Serafini
Division of Nuclear Medicine
Fondazione IRCCS
Istituto Nazionale dei Tumori
Milan, Italy

Angela Spanu
Department of Nuclear Medicine
University of Sassari
Sassari, Italy

Lidia Strigari
Physical Department
Regina Elena National Cancer Instiute
Rome, Italy

Fred Sweep
Department of Chemical Endocrinology
University Medical Center Nijmegen
Nijmegen, The Netherlands

Luca Tagliabue
Institute of Radiological Sciences
University of Milan
Unit of Nuclear Medicine
Hospital San Paolo
Milan, Italy

Giovanna Trecate
Department of Diagnostic Imaging and Radiotherapy
Unit of Diagnostic Radiology 1
Fondazione IRCCS
Istituto Nazionale dei Tumori
Milan , Italy

Giuseppe Trifirò
Division of Nuclear Medicne
European Institute of Oncology
Milan, Italy

Silvana Del Vecchio
Department of Biomorphological and Functional Sciences
Naples, Italy

Daniele Vernaghi
Department of Diagnostic Imaging and Radiotherapy
Unit of Diagnostic Radiology 1
Fondazione IRCCS
Istituto Nazionale dei Tumori
Milan , Italy

Umberto Veronesi
Scientific Direction
European Institute of Oncology
Milan, Italy

Giuseppe Viale
Division of Pathology
European Institute of Oncology
Milan, Italy

Barbara Zangheri
Department of Nuclear Medicine
Scientific Institute San Raffaele
Milan, Italy

Antonella Zannetti
Institute of Biostructures and Bioimages
of the National Research Council (CNR)
Naples, Italy

Introduction

1

The Editors

This book is a multidisciplinary textbook dealing with the diagnosis of breast cancer and at the same time considering the most important modalities to study breast tumours. Besides the different options among the imaging modalities, other aspects are overviewed including the biology and histology of breast cancer as well as the available laboratory tests and treatments. One chapter is dedicated to the histological classification of breast cancer and another to biomolecular features of clinical relevance. The routine use of tumour marker assays is discussed, with a critical evaluation of their clinical usefulness, interpretation criteria and diagnostic limits. The most important nuclear medicine procedures are described and the most remarkable results published in the recent literature are analysed. A number of chapters focus on nuclear medicine procedures: scintimammography, sentinel lymph node biopsy after lymphoscintigraphy, bone scintigraphy with ^{99m}Tc-labelled phosphonates and positron-emission tomography (PET) with ^{18}F-fluorodeoxyglucose (FDG). The place of these nuclear medicine modalities and other radiological tools in the diagnostic workup of breast cancer patients is examined and their relevance in patient management is stressed. Particular characteristics of these diagnostic modalities are discussed, such as the biological value of the information deriving from PET, the role of PET in axillary staging, the added value of the combined use of PET with tumour markers in detecting relapse and metastases, the importance of FDG-PET in staging and follow-up and the role of PET in monitoring and predicting the response to therapy. The technological developments that provided a new hybrid system, PET/CT, combining metabolic (PET) and morphological (CT) imaging, are described in a dedicated chapter that analyses the added value of image fusion. Radiological methods including mammography, ultrasonography and magnetic resonance imaging are treated in two different sections that highlight the state of the art of diagnostic radiology in the detection, staging and characterisation of breast cancer. Two chapters pay attention to the use of osteotropic radiopharmaceuticals labelled with ^{186}Re (rhenium) and ^{153}Sm (samarium), which are successful in the palliative treatment of patients with skeletal metastases. A general chapter on medical therapy for breast cancer patients provides an update on the state of the art of medical oncology, with a discussion of how cancer can be cured and how advanced disease can be treated today.

This book deals mostly with molecular imaging issues, but since nuclear medicine has a wide range of applications today, also other breast cancer-related areas are covered. The emphasis is on the integration of various diagnostic methods, different techniques for tumour characterisation and different treatment approaches. The information is highly diversified and therefore interesting not only to nuclear medicine physicians and radiologists, but also to oncologists, senologists and surgeons who wish to update their knowledge of a rapidly developing field.

Histological Classification of Breast Cancer

2

Alessandra Fabbri, Maria Luisa Carcangiu, and Antonino Carbone

CONTENTS

Abstract

Cancer of the breast is one of the most common human neoplasms, accounting for one quarter of all cancers in females. It is associated with the western life style. Risk factors include early menarche and late childbirth. Breast cancer is further characterized by a marked genetic susceptibility. The typing of invasive breast cancer, its histological variants and their grading systems are well established. More difficult is the classification of the pre-invasive breast lesions that are now increasingly detected by mammography.

2.1 Epidemiology and Risk Factors

Breast cancer is the most common cancer of women worldwide (Parkin et al. 1984). There have been sustained increases in the incidence of this cancer in developing countries in recent years. Breast cancer accounts for 22% of all female cancers, which is more than twice the occurrence of cancer in women at any other site (Parkin et al. 2001). Male breast cancer is rare compared with female breast cancer. Female: male incidence ratios vary from 70 to 130 around the world.

Breast cancer incidence, as with most epithelial tumours, increases rapidly with age. The curves show a characteristic shape, rising steeply up to menopausal age and less rapidly or not at all afterwards. Around the 1990s, breast cancer incidence varied 10-fold worldwide, indicating important differences in the distribution of the underlying causes (Parkin et al. 2001). There is substantial variation in breast cancer rates among different countries. Rates are some six times higher in the USA, Canada and northern Europe than in Asia or among black populations in Africa. These international differences in breast cancer rates do not appear to be determined primarily by variation in genetic susceptibility. Studies of populations migrating from low- to high-risk areas, which show that migrant populations approach the risk of the host country in one or two generations (Balzi et al. 2003; Kliewer and Sith 1995; Ziegler et al. 1993; Buell 1973; Prentice et al. 1988), clearly suggest an important role of environmental factors in the aetiology of the disease.

The aetiology of breast cancer is multifactorial and involves diet, reproductive factors and related hormonal imbalances. The known risk factors for breast cancer (Table 2.1) can be understood as measures of the cumulative exposure of the breast to oestrogen and, perhaps, progesterone. The actions of these ovarian hormones (and the hormones used in combination oral contraceptives and hormone replacement therapy) on the breast do not appear to be genotoxic, but they do affect the rate of cell division. Their effects on breast cancer rates are manifest in their effects on proliferation of the breast epithelial cell. The activation of oncogenes and inactivation of tumour-suppressor genes (e.g. BRCA1, TP53) produce a sequence of genetic changes that lead to a malignant phenotype.

As endogenous hormones directly affect the risk of breast cancer, there is reason for concern about the effects on breast cancer risk if the same or closely related hormones are administered for therapeutic purposes. Specific environmental exposure operative in the development of breast cancer (e.g., radiation, alcohol, exogenous hormones) have been identified, but carry a lower risk.

More than most other human neoplasms, breast cancer often shows familiar clustering. Two high-penetrance genes have been identified (BRCA 1/2) that greatly increase the breast cancer risk. Table 2.1 shows the events of reproductive life that have been considered to be risk factors for breast cancer in women. Breast cancer occurs more frequently among women who have an early menarche, remain nulliparous or, if parous, have few children with a late age at first delivery. Finally, late age at menopause also increases the risk (Kelsey et al. 1993).

Table 2.1. Breast cancer risk factors

Early menarche
Late menopause
Obesity (postmenopausal women)
Oestrogen replacement therapy
Older age at first full-tem birth
Nulliparity
Oral contraceptives

2.2 Histological Classification

The most significant effort in the classification of tumours of the breast was that produced by the World Health Organization (Tavassoli and Devilee 2003). Other identified subentities have been listed in the classification reported in the last edition (third series) of the fascicle "Tumors of the mammary gland" issued by the US Armed Forces Institute of Pathology (Rosen and Oberman 1992).

All carcinomas of the breast, both invasive and non-invasive, are classified on the basis of the histological and/or cytological appearance. Irrespective of the type of carcinoma, a number of gross findings should always be recorded including site, size, shape, consistency, colour, gross appearance of margins, relationship to adjacent mammary (skin, nipple) and extramammary structures (fascia, muscle), and the number of foci that appear malignant.

2.2.1 Grading

In situ ductal carcinoma and all invasive tumours are routinely graded. Among the various grading systems that have been proposed, the combined grading method of Elston and colleagues from Nottingham, England, which is a modification of the grading system originally elaborated by Scarff, Bloom and Richardson, is currently the most widely used in Europe (Bloom et al. 1957; Robins et al. 1995; Elston and Ellis 1991). In this system three parameters are evaluated: tubule formation, nuclear polymorphism and mitotic rate. A numerical scoring system of 1–3 is used to ensure that each factor is assessed individually.

The three values are added together to produces scores of 3 to 9, to which the grade is assigned:

- Point total 5: grade 1, well differentiated;
- Point total 6–7: grade 2, moderately differentiated;
- Point total 8–9: grade 3, poorly differentiated.

2.2.2 TNM

Breast cancer staging is useful because of its ability to estimate prognosis. It also provides valuable information about appropriate treatment options for each cancer stage (Sobin and Wittekind 2002).

The principal changes incorporated into the recently revised staging system for breast cancer (Tables 2.2 and 2.3) are related to the size (micrometastases and isolate tumour cells), number, location and methods of detection of metastases to the regional lymph nodes (IHC staining and molecular techniques such as reverse-transcriptase polymerase chain reaction, RT-PCR).

Table 2.2. Recently revised staging system for breast cancer

Classification	Definition
Primary tumour (T)	
TX	Primary tumour cannot be assessed
T0	No evidence of primary tumour
Tis	Carcinoma in situ
Tis (DCIS)	Ductal carcinoma in situ
Tis (LCIS)	Lobular carcinoma in situ
Tis(Paget)	Paget's disease of the nipple with no tumour (Paget's disease associated with a tumour is classified according to the size of the tumour)
T1	Tumour ≤2 cm in greatest dimension
T1mic	Microinvasion ≤0.1 cm in greatest dimension
T1a	Tumour >0.1 cm but ≤0.5 cm in greatest dimension
T1b	Tumour >0.5 cm but ≤1 cm in greatest dimension
T1c	Tumour >1 cm but ≤2 cm in greatest dimension
T2	Tumour >2 cm but ≤5 cm in greatest dimension
T3	Tumour >5 cm in greatest dimension
T4	Tumour of any size with direct extension to chest wall or skin, only as described below
T4a	Extension to chest wall, not including pectoralis muscle
T4b	Oedema (including peau d'orange) or ulceration of the skin of the breast, or satellite skin nodules confined to the same breast
T4c	Both T4a and T4b
T4d	Inflammatory carcinoma
Regional lymph node	
NX	Regional lymph nodes cannot be assessed (e.g., previously removed)
N0	No regional lymph node metastasis
N1	Metastasis in movable ipsilateral axillary lymph node(s)
N2	Metastases in ipsilateral axillary lymph nodes fixed or matted, or in clinically apparent* ipsilater internal mammary nodes in the absence of clinically evident axillary lymph-node metastases
N2a	Metastasis in ipsilateral axillary lymph nodes fixed to one another (matted) or to other structures
N2b	Metastasis only in clinically apparent* ipsilateral internal mammary nodes and in the absence of clinically evident axillary lymph-node metastasis
N3	Metastasis in ipsilateral infraclavicular lymph node(s), or in clinically apparent* ipsilateral internal mammary lymph node(s), and in the presence of clinically evident axillary lymph-node metastasis, or metastasis in ipsilateral supraclavicular lymph node(s) with or without axillary or internal mammary lymph-node involvement
N3a	Metastasis in ipsilateral infraclavicular lymph node(s) and axillary lymph node(s)
N3b	Metastasis in ipsilateral internal mammary lymph node(s) and axillary lymph node(s)
N3c	Metastasis in ipsilateral supraclavicular lymph node(s)

Classification	Definition
Regional lymph nodes (pN)†	
pNX	Regional lymph nodes cannot be assessed (e.g., previously removed or not removed for pathologic study)
pN0	No regional lymph node metastasis histologically, no additional examination for isolated tumour cells‡
pN0 (i-)	No regional lymph node metastasis histologically, negative immunohistochemical staining
pN0 (i+)	Isolated tumour cells identified histologically or by positive immunohistochemical staining, no cluster >0.2 mm§
pN0 (mol-)	No regional lymph-node metastasis histologically, negative molecular findings (RT-PCR)†††
pN0 (mol+)	No regional lymph-node metastasis histologically, positive molecular findings (RT-PCR)†††
pN1	Metastasis in one to three axillary lymph nodes, and/or in internal mammary nodes with microscopic disease detected by sentinel lymph node dissection but not clinically apparent*
pN1mi	Micrometastasis (>2 mm, none >2.0 mm)
pN1a	Metastasis in one to three axillary lymph nodes
pN1b	Metastasis in internal mammary nodes with microscopic disease detected by sentinel lymph-node dissection but not clinically apparent*
pN1c	Metastasis in one to three axillary lymph nodes** and in internal mammary lymph nodes with microscopic disease detected by sentinel lymph-node dissection but not clinically apparent*
pN2	Metastasis in four to nine axillary lymph nodes, or in clinically apparent* internal mammary lymph nodes in the absence of axillary lymph-node metastasis

Adapted from Greene et al, with permission from Springer Publishing

*Clinically apparent is defined as detected by imaging studies (excluding lymphoscintigraphy) or by clinical examination.

†Classification is based on axillary lymph node dissection with or without sentinel lymph-node dissection. Classification based solely on sentinel lymph-node dissection without subsequent axillary lymph node dissection is designated (sn) for "sentinel node", such as pN0(i+)(sn).

‡Isolated tumour cells are defined as single tumour cells or small cell clusters ≤0.2 mm, usually detected only by immunohistochemical or molecular methods, but which may be verified on haematoxylin and eosin stains. Isolated tumour cells do not usually show evidence of metastatic activity (e.g., proliferation or stromal reaction).

§Definition of (i+) was adapted in 2003 in order to be consistent with the updated International Union against Cancer (UICC) classification.

†††RT-PCR: reverse transcriptase/polymerase chain reaction.

**If associated with more than three positive axillary lymph nodes, the internal mammary nodes are classified as pN3b to reflect increased tumour burden.

2.2.3 Carcinoma in Situ

Carcinoma in situ is a proliferation of malignant epithelial cells within the ductulo-lobular system of the breast that on light microscopy shows no evidence of breaching the basement membrane to invade the adjacent stroma. There are two forms: ductal and lobular. Lobular intraepithelial neoplasia (LIN) is located within the terminal duct-lobular unit, often accompanied by pagetoid involvement of the adjacent terminal ducts (Fig. 2.1). These are markedly distended by a proliferation of monomorphous cells that have effaced the lumen (Bratthauer and Tavassoli 2002). The nuclei are round, regular and evenly spaced. Intracellular lumens are often present. The stroma is thinned. No necrosis or microcalcifications are usually present.

LIN is usually found during the perimenopausal period, is unapparent clinically and is usually detected incidentally in biopsies that were done because of other lesions. It is associated with an increase in the risk of developing invasive breast cancer of any type, in either breast, and usually many years later.

Ductal carcinoma in situ (DCIS), on the other hand, is a heterogeneous group of pre-malignant lesions that

Table 2.3. Recently revised staging system for breast cancer

	Fifth Edition	Sixth Edition
Size of regional lymph-node metastases	Micrometastases were defined as tumour deposits not larger than 2.0 mm and classified as pN1a	Micrometastases are distinguished from isolated tumour cells on the basis of size
	No quantitative distinction was made between micrometastases and isolated tumour cells	Micrometastases are defined as tumour deposits larger than 0.2 mm, but not larger than 2.0 mm and classified as pN1mi. Isolated tumour cells are defined as tumour deposits not larger than 0.2 mm identified by either standard histology or by immunohistochemical staining. They are classified as pN0(i+)
Number of regional lymph- node metastases	The number of affected axillary lymph nodes was considered only in subcategories of pN1	Major classification of lymph node status are defined by the number of affected axillary lymph nodes
Location of regional lymph-node metastases	Metastases in infraclavicular lymph nodes (axillary level III) were considered equivalent to metastases in other axillary lymph nodes	Metastases in the infraclavicular lymph nodes are classified as N3, because of their association with extremely poor prognosis
	Metastases to the internal mammary nodes were classified as N3/pN3	Metastases to the internal mammary nodes are classified as N1, N2 or N3, based on the size of the lesion and the presence or absence of concurrent axillary nodal involvement
	Metastases to the supraclavicular lymph nodes were classifies as M1	Metastases to the supraclavicular lymph nodes are classified as N3
The use of descriptors to indicate size and method of detection of nodal metastases	No descriptors were used	The descriptor (i+) is used to indicate the presence of isolated tumour cells not larger than 0.2 mm by either standard histology or by immunohistochemical staining. The descriptor (i-) means no detectable tumour cells by either histology or immunohistochemical staining. The descriptor sn is used to indicate that the staging classification was based solely on sentinel lymph node dissection. The descriptor (mol+)/(mol-) is used to designate cases that are negative by standard histological staining for regional lymph node metastasis and in which reverse transcriptase-polymerase chain reaction was used to assess the node for tumour cells

are usually asymptomatic and impalpable, but may be identifiable on mammography as foci of microcalcification (Holland et al. 1994). The classification of DCIS is based primarily on cytonuclear differentiation and, secondarily, on architectural differentiation (cellular polarisation). Three categories are defined:

Poorly differentiated DCIS is composed of cells with markedly pleomorphic nuclei, evidence of individual cell necrosis and autophagocytosis. Mitoses and central necrosis are often present. The growth pattern may be solid, pseudo-cribriform or micropapillary. This sub-type has the highest risk of stromal invasion (Fig. 2.2).

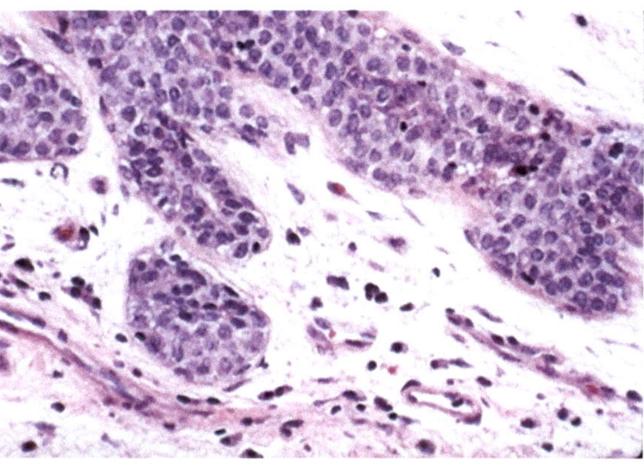

Fig. 2.1. Lobular intraepithelial neoplasia

Intermediately differentiated DCIS is composed of cells showing some pleomorphism, but not so marked as in the poorly differentiated group. There is always evidence of some architectural differentiation, whereas necrosis and calcification are variable.

Well-differentiated DCIS consists of cells with monomorphic nuclei. Architectural differentiation is pronounced, and the growth pattern may be cribriform, micropapillary and clinging. Necrosis is not present (Fig. 2.3).

Lesions in the poorly differentiated group are usually Neu (c-erbB-2) positive and are less frequently oestrogen and progesterone receptor positive, conversely to those in the well-differentiated group. The treatment of DCIS depends on the size and distribution of the lesion. The status of excision margins around the tumour remains the most important factor in terms of risk of local recurrence. Microinvasive carcinoma (size limit of 1 mm) is rare and occurs mostly in association with in situ carcinoma, usually of the poorly differentiated type (Rosen 1997).

2.2.4 Invasive Breast Cancer

Invasive breast cancer is a group of malignant epithelial tumours characterized by invasion of adjacent tissue and a marked tendency to metastasize to distant sites. Breast cancer arises from the mammary epithelium, most frequently from the cells of the terminal duct lobular unit. The vast majority of these tumours are adenocarcinomas. They exhibit a wide range of morphological phenotypes and specific histological types. The typing of invasive breast cancer and its histological variants is well established in the WHO Classification (Tavassoli and Devilee 2003) (Table 2.4).

2.2.5 Invasive Ductal Carcinoma (Not Otherwise Specified, NOS)

This is a heterogeneous group, which represents the most common type of invasive carcinoma, comprising between 40% and 75% in the published series (Elston and Ellis 1991; Elston and Ellis 1998). Ductal NOS tumours, like all other major forms of breast cancer, are less common below the age of 40 (Kollias et al. 1997). These tumours have no specific macroscopic features. There is marked variation in size; they can have an irregular, stellate outline or nodular configuration. They are firm, and the cut surface is usually grey-white with yellows streaks (Fig. 2.4).

Architecturally, the tumour cells may be arranged in cords, clusters and trabeculae, but the predominantly invasive pattern is solid with occasionally glandular differentiation. The stromal component is extremely variable. There may be a highly cellular fibroblastic proliferation, a scanty connective tissue or marked hyalinization with elastosis. Tumour cells have a variable appearance, with cytoplasm often abundant and eosinophilic. Nuclei may be regular or pleomorphic with prominent nucleoli. Mitotic activity may be increased in the poorly differentiated form.

Invasive carcinoma is often associated with high grade ductal carcinoma in situ, but all other patterns

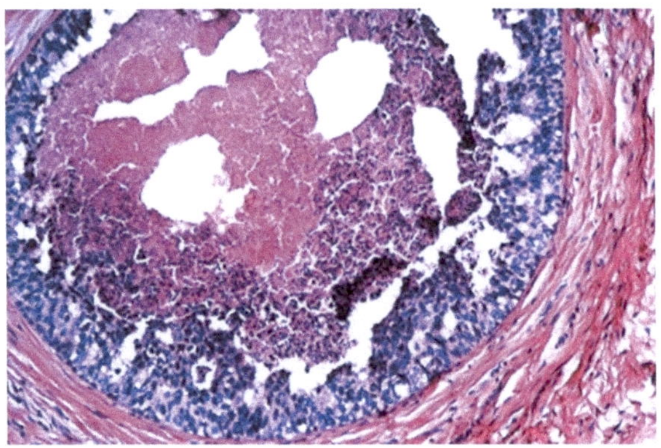

Fig. 2.2. Poorly differentiated ductal carcinoma in situ

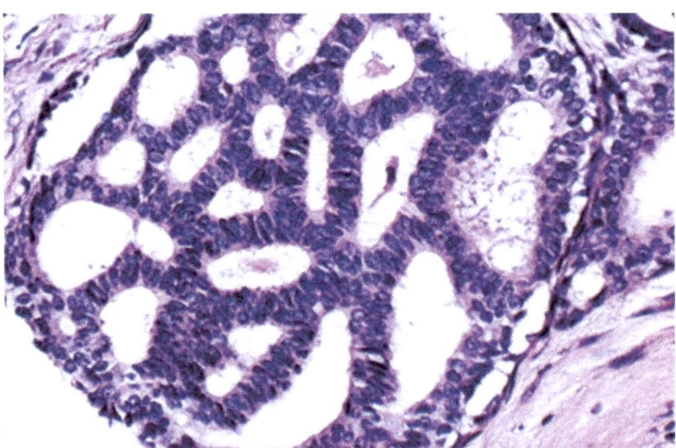

Fig. 2.3. Well-differentiated ductal carcinoma in situ with a cribriform pattern of growth

Table 2.4. Histological classification of carcinoma of breast [adapted from WHO (Tassavoli and Devilee 2003)]

Invasive ductal carcinoma, not otherwise specified (NOS)	8500/3
Mixed type carcinoma	
Pleomorphic carcinoma	8022/3
Carcinoma with osteoclastic giant cells	8035/3
Invasive lobular carcinoma	8520/3
Tubular carcinoma	8211/3
Invasive cribriform carcinoma	8201/3
Medullary carcinoma	8510/3
Mucinous carcinoma and other tumours with abundant mucin	
Mucinous carcinoma	8480/3
Cystadenocarcinoma and columnar cell mucinous carcinoma	8480/3
Signet ring cell carcinoma	8490/3
Invasive papillary carcinoma	8503/3
Invasive micropapillary carcinoma	8507/3
Apocrine carcinoma	8401/3
Metaplastic carcinomas	8575/3
Pure epithelial metaplastic carcinomas	8575/3
Mixed epithelial/mesenchymal metaplastic carcinomas	8575/3
Lipid-rich carcinoma	8314/3
Adenoid cystic carcinoma	8200/3
Acinic cell carcinoma	8550/3
Glycogen-rich clear cell carcinoma	8315/3
Inflammatory carcinoma	8530/3
Lobular carcinoma in situ	8520/2
Ductal carcinoma in situ	8500/2
Microinvasive carcinoma	

may be seen (Fig. 2.5). If a ductal carcinoma NOS is accompanied by a second distinct morphologic pattern (lobular), the cancer is defined as mixed. There are several variants of ductal carcinoma NOS: pleomorphic (a high grade cancer characterized by proliferation of pleomorpic and bizarre tumour giant cells) (Silver and Tavassoli 2000); with osteoclastic giant cells (Gupta 1996); with choriocarcinomatous features (Horne et al. 1976). Approximately 70–80% of ductal NOS breast cancers are oestrogen receptor positive, and between 15–30% of cases are ERBB2 positive.

2.2.6 Invasive Lobular Carcinoma

Invasive lobular carcinoma represents 5–15% of invasive breast tumours and is frequently multifocal and bilateral (Winchester et al. 1998). It is character-

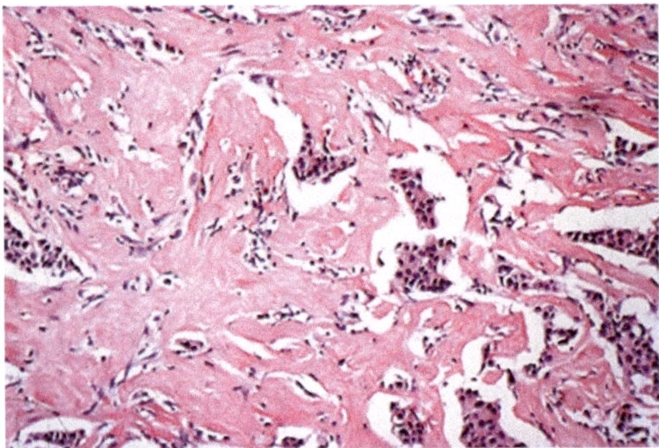

Fig. 2.4. Invasive ductal carcinoma (NOS)

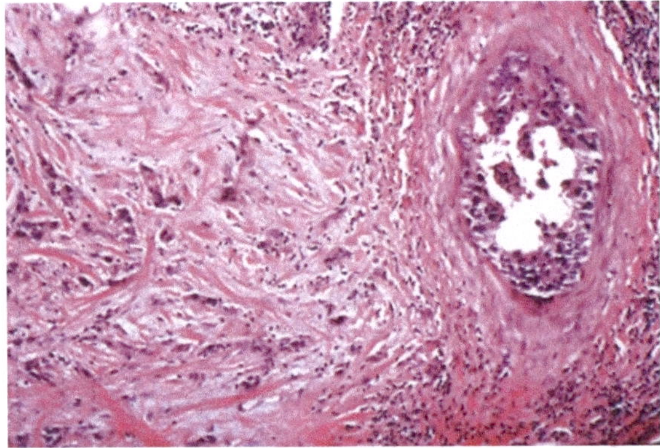

Fig. 2.5. Invasive ductal carcinoma associated with high grade ductal carcinoma in situ

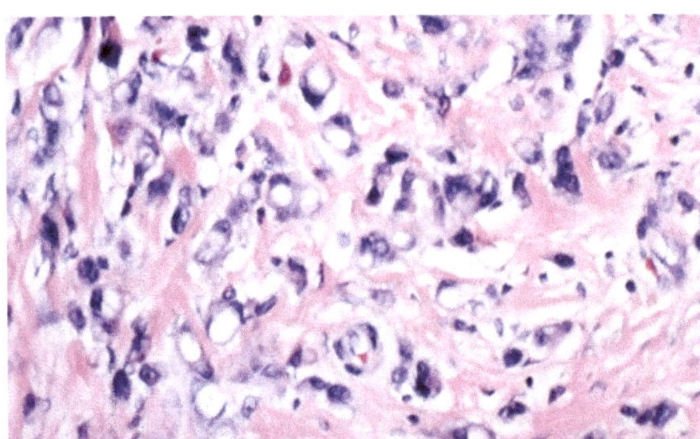

Fig. 2.6. Invasive lobular carcinoma

ized by indistinct tumour margins. This neoplasm is composed of non-cohesive cells individually dispersed or arranged in single file linear pattern (Indian file) in a fibrous stroma. The neoplastic cells have round or notched ovoid nuclei and a thin rim of cytoplasm with an occasional intracytoplasmic lumen (signet ring cells) (Fig. 2.6).

There are different patterns: classical (Martinez and Azzopardi 1979), solid (Fechner 1975), alveolar (Shousha et al. 1986), pleomorphic, (Weidner and Semple 1992) and mixed (Martinez and Azzopardi 1979). The admixture of a tubular growth pattern and small uniform cells arranged in a linear pattern defines the variant known as tubulo-lobular carcinoma (Fisher et al. 1977). All of these patterns are associated with lobular carcinoma in situ.

About 70–95% of lobular carcinomas are ER positive and 60–70% are PR positive (Sastre-Garau et al. 1996). Overexpression of ERBB2 is lower than in invasive ductal carcinoma, with the exception of the pleomorphic pattern (Soomro et al 1991).

2.2.7 Tubular Carcinoma

This is a special type of carcinoma with favourable prognosis that accounts for under 2% of invasive breast cancer in most series. It consists of a haphazard distribution of rounded and angulated tubules with open lumens, lined by only a single layer of epithelial cells separated by abundant reactive fibroblastic stroma. The cancer cells are small and regular, with little nuclear pleomorphism and scanty mitotic figures (Patchefsky et al. 1977). Ductal carcinoma in situ (usually of low grade) is found in association; occasionally the in situ component is of lobular type. Oestrogen and progesterone receptors are always positive and ERBB2 is negative (Papadatos et al. 2001).

2.2.8 Invasive Cribriform Carcinoma

This is a carcinoma with an excellent prognosis that accounts for 0.8–3.5% of breast cancers (Venable et al. 1990). The tumour cells are small and show a low to moderate degree of nuclear pleomorphism. The tumour is arranged as invasive islands (often angulated), within which well-defined spaces are formed by arches of cells. Mitoses are rare. Associated intraductal carcinoma, generally of the cribriform type, is observed in as many as 80% of cases. Oestrogen and progesterone receptors are positive in 100% and 69% of the cases, respectively (Venable et al. 1990).

2.2.9 Medullary Carcinoma

This is a carcinoma with a good prognosis, which represents between 1 and 7% of all breast cancers. A high frequency of this tumour type has been reported in patients with BRCA1 germ line mutations (Wargotz and Silverberg 1988; Marcus et al. 1996). It is composed of poorly differentiated cells arranged in large sheets, with no glandular structures, scant stroma and a prominent lymphoplasmacytic infiltrate. Classically, five morphological criteria have been said to characterize medullary carcinoma: syncytial growth pattern in over 75% of the tumour; absence of glandular structures, diffuse lymphoplasmacytic stromal infiltrate, lymphoid follicles and/or epithelioid granuloma, marked nuclear pleomorphism and complete histological circumscription. Tumours showing the association of a predominantly syncytial architecture with only two or three of the other criteria are usually designated as atypical medullary carcinoma (Ridolfi et al. 1997). Medullary carcinoma lacks oestrogen receptor expression (Ponsky et al. 1984).

2.2.10 Mucinous Carcinoma

Pure mucinous carcinoma accounts for about 2% of all breast cancer in patients over 60 years and has a favourable prognosis (Scopsi et al. 1994). Macroscopically, the tumour appears as a glistening gelatinous nodule with pushing margins. Microscopically, it is characterized by proliferation of clusters of generally uniform round cells with a thin rim of eosinophilic cytoplasm floating in lakes of mucus (Fig. 2.7). These lesions are further subdivided into cellular and hypocellular variants. Grimelius stain and chromogranin and synaptophysin immunostain demonstrate in a high proportion of cases neuroendocrine differentiation (Feyrter and Hartmann 1963). Mucinous carcinoma is oestrogen receptor positive (Shousha et al. 1989).

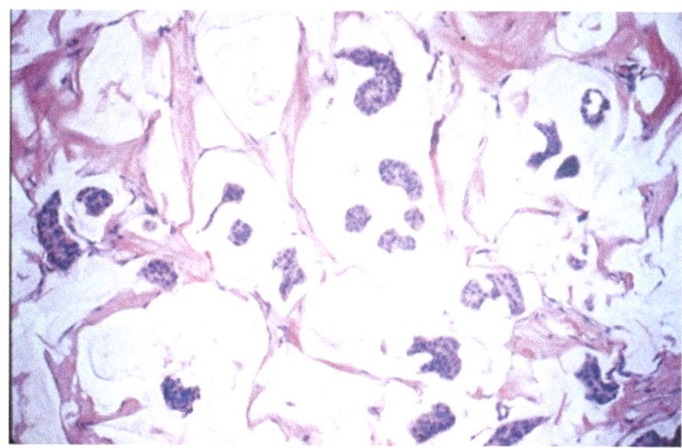

Fig. 2.7. Mucinous carcinoma, hypocellular variant

2.2.11 Invasive Papillary Carcinoma

This tumour type comprises less than 1–2% of all breast cancers and is characterized by a relatively good prognosis (Schneider 1989). It represents a papillary intraductal carcinoma located within a large cystic duct and characterized by thin fibrovascular stalks with a myoepithelial cell layer and a neoplastic cell population with areas of infiltrating duct carcinoma (Leal et al. 1998).

2.2.12 Invasive Micropapillary Carcinoma

This is a carcinoma composed of small clusters of tumour cells lying within clear stromal spaces resembling dilatated vascular spaces. This growth pattern accounts for less than 2% of all invasive breast cancers and often is associated with the presence of vascular invasion and axillary lymph node metastases (Paterakos et al. 1999).

2.2.13 Apocrine Carcinoma

This is a rare cancer (0.3–4%) in which the tumour cells show cytological and immunohistochemical features of apocrine cells in 90% or more of the tumour (Frable and Kays 1968). Apocrine cells have abundant eosinophilic cytoplasm and vesicular nuclei with prominent nucleoli, and are typically GCDFP15 positive. It should be noted, however, that expression of GCDFP15 is a feature common to many variants of breast carcinoma (Mazoujian 1983).

2.2.14 Metaplastic Carcinoma

This tumour accounts for less than 1% of all invasive cancers (Huvos 1973). These are a heterogeneous group of neoplasms generally characterized by an admixture of adenocarcinoma with dominant areas of spindle cell, squamous and /or mesenchymal differentiation. There are two forms: purely epithelial and mixed epithelial/mesenchymal (Wargotz and Norris 1990; Kaufman et al. 1984). Oestrogen and progesterone receptors are always negative.

2.2.15 Glycogen-Rich Clear Cell Carcinoma

This is a rare cancer (1–3%) in which more than 90% of the neoplastic cells have abundant clear cytoplasm containing glycogen (Hull and Warkel 1986). The hormone receptor status is similar to that of ductal carcinoma NOS.

2.2.16 Lipid-Rich Carcinoma

This is a breast cancer in which approximately 90% of the neoplastic cells contain abundant cytoplasmic neutral lipids (Dina and Eusebi 1997).

2.2.17 Adenoid Cystic Carcinoma and Acinic Cell Carcinoma

These neoplasms are the breast counterpart of the homonymous tumours that occur in the salivary gland (Lamovec et al. 1989).

2.2.18 Paget's Disease of the Nipple

This term is applied to the presence of malignant glandular epithelial cells within the squamous epithelium of the nipple, almost always in association with an underlying intraductal or infiltrating carcinoma. In general, the Paget cells have the same immunophenotype as the underlying carcinoma (Cohen et al. 1993)

2.2.19 Inflammatory Carcinoma

This is a form of advanced breast carcinoma with prominent dermal lymphatic infiltration by tumour and a lymphoplasmacytic infiltrate (Rosen 2001).

Acknowledgements

The authors thank Maria Morelli for her help in the preparation of this manuscript and for her editorial assistance.

References

Balzi D, Buiatti E, Geddes M, Khlat M, Masuyer E, Parkin DM (2003) Summary of the results by site. In: Cancer in Italian migrant populations, IARC Scientific Publication, International Agency for Research on Cancer: Lyon, 123: 193–292

Bratthauer GL, Tavassoli FA (2002) Lobular neoplasia: previously unexplored aspects assessed in 775 cases and their clinical Implication. Virchows Arch 440: 134–138

Bloom HJ, Richardson WW (1957) Histological grading and prognosis in breast cancer. Br J Cancer 11: 359–377

Buell P (1973) Changing incidence of breast cancer in Japanese-American women. J Natl Cancer Inst 51: 1479–1483

Cohen C, Guarner J, DeRose PB (1993) Mammary Paget's disease and associated carcinoma. An immunohistochemical study. Arch Pathol Lab Med 117: 291–294

Dina R, Eusebi V (1997) Clear cell tumors of the breast. Semin Diagn Pathol 14: 175–182

Elston CW, Ellis IO (1991) Pathological prognostic factors in breast cancer. The value of histological grade in breast cancer: Experience from a large study with long-term follow-up. Histopathology 19: 403–410

Elston CW, Ellis IO (1998) Classification of malignant breast disease. In: The breast systemic pathology. Edinburgh, Churchill Livingstone, pp 239–247

Fechner RE (1975) Histologic variants of infiltrating lobular carcinoma of the breast. Hum Pathol 6: 373–378

Feyrter F, Hartmann G (1963) Uber die carcinoide Wuchsform des Carcinoma mammae, insbesondere das Carcinoma solidum (gelatinosum) mamma. Fradf Z Pathol 73: 24–30

Fisher ER, Gregorio RM, Redmond C, Fisher B (1977) Tubulolobular invasive breast cancer: a variant of lobular invasive cancer. Hum Pathol 8: 679–683

Frable WJ, Kays S (1968) Carcinoma of the breast. Histologic and clinical features of apocrine tumors. Cancers 21:756–763

Gupta RK (1996) Aspiration cytodiagnosis of a rare carcinoma of breast with bizarre malignant giant cells. Diagn Cytopathol 15: 66–69

Holland R, Peterse JL, Mills RR, Eusebi V, Faverly D, van de Vijver MJ, Zafrani B (1994) Ductal carcinoma in situ:

a proposal for a new classification. Sem Diagn Pathol 3:167–180

Horne CH, Reid IN, Milne GD (1976) Prognostic significance of inappropriate production of pregnancy proteins by breast cancers. Lancet 2: 2769–282

Hull MT, Warkel KA (1986) Glyocogen-rich clear cell carcinomas of the breast. A clinicopathologic and ultrastructural study. Am J Surg Pathol 10: 553–559

Huvos AG, Lucas JC Jr, Foote FW Jr (1973) Metaplastic breast carcinoma. Rare form of mammary cancer. N Y State J Med 73: 1078–1082

Kaufman MW, Marti JR, Gallager HS, Hoehn JL (1984) Carcinoma of the breast with pseudosarcomatous metaplasia. Cancer 53: 1908–1917

Kelsey JL, Gammon MD, John EM (1993) Reproductive factors and breast cancer. Epidemiol Rev 15: 36–47

Kliewer EV, Sith KE (1995) Breast cancer mortality among immigrants in Australia and Canada. J Natl Cancer Inst 87: 1154–1161

Kollias J, Elston CW, Ellis IO, Robertson JF, Blamey RW (1997) Early-onset breast cancer-histopathological and prognostic considerations. Br J Cancer 75: 1318–1323

Lamovec J, Us-Krasovec M, Zidar A, Kljun A (1989) Adenoid cystic carcinoma of the breast: a histologic, cytologic, and immunohistochemical study. Semin Diagn Pathol 6: 153–164

Leal C, Costa I, Fonseca D, Lopes P, Bento MJ, Lopes C (1998) Intracystic (encysted) papillary carcinoma of the breast: a clinical, pathological, and immunohistochemical study. Hum Pathol 29: 1097–1104

Marcus JN, Watson P, Page DL, Narod SA, Lenoir GM, Tonin P, Linder-Stepherson L, Salerno G, Conway TA, Lynch HT (1996) Hereditary breast cancer: pathobiology, prognosis, and BRCA1 and BRCA2 gene linkage. Cancer 77: 697–709

Martinez V, Azzopardi JG (1979) Invasive lobular carcinoma of the breast: incidence and variants. Histopathology 3: 467–488

Mazoujian G, Pinkus GS, Davis S, Haagensen DE Jr (1983) Immunohistochemistry of a gross cystic disease fluid protein (GCDFP-15) of the breast. A marker of apocrine epithelium and breast carcinomas with apocrine features. Am J Pathol 110: 105–112

Papadatos, g, Rangan AM, Psarianos T, Ung O, Taylor R, Boyages J (2001) Probability of axillary node involvement in patients with tubular carcinoma of the breast. Br J Surg 88: 860–864

Parkin DM, Stjernsward J, Muir CS (1984) Estimates of worldwide frequency of 12 major cancers. Bull World Health Org 62: 163–182

Parkin DM, Bra F, Ferlay J, Pisani P (2001) Estimating the world cancer burden. Globocan 2000. Int J Cancer 94: 153–156

Parkin DM, Whelan SL, Ferlay J Raymond L, Young J (2001) Cancer incidence in five continents, Vol VII (IARC Scientific Publication n. 143). Lyon, Fance, International Agency for Research on Cancer: Lyon, France

Patchefsky AS, Shaber GS, Schwartz GF, Feig SA, Nerlinger RE (1977) The pathology of breast cancer detected by mass population screening. Cancer 40: 1659–1670

Paterakos M, Watkin WG, Edgerton SM, Moore DH, Thor AD (1999) Invasive micropapillary carcinoma of the breast. A prognostic study. Hum Pathol 30: 1459–1463

Ponsky JL, Gliga L, Reynolds S (1984) Medullary carcinoma of the breast: an association with negative hormonal receptors. J Surg Oncol 25: 76–78

Prentice RL, Kakar F, Hursting S, Sheppard L, Klein R, Kushi LH (1988) Aspects of the rationale for the women's health trial. J Natl Cancer Inst 80: 802–814

Ridolfi RL, Rosen PP, Port A, Kinne D, Mike V (1977) Medullary carcinoma of the breast: a clinicopathologic study with 10 year follow-up. Cancer 40: 1365–1385

Robbins P, Pinder S, de Klerk N, Dawkins H, Harvey J, Sterret G, Ellis I, Elston C (1995) Histological grading of breast carcinomas: a study of interobserver agreement. Hum Pathol 26: 873–879

Rosen PP, Oberman HA (1992) Tumors of the mammary gland. In: Atlas of tumor pathology, AFIP

Rosen PP (1997) Rosen's breast pathology. Lippincott-Raven, Philadelphia

Rosen PP (2001) Rosen's breast pathology. Lippincott William and Wilkins, Philadelphia

Sastre-Garau X, Jouve M, Asselain T, Durand JC, Fourquet A, Pouillart P (1996) Infiltrating lobular carcinoma of the breast. Clinicopathologic analysis of 975 cases with reference to data on conservative therapy and metastatic patterns. Cancer 77: 113–120

Schneider JA (1989) Invasive papillary breast carcinoma: mammographic and sonographic appearance. Radiology 171: 377–379

Scopsi L, Andreola S, Pilotti S, Bufalino R, Baldini MT, Testori A, Rilke F (1994) Mucinous carcinoma of the breast. A clinicopathologic, histochemical, and immunocytochemical study with special reference to neuroendocrine differentiation. Am J Surg Pathol 18: 702–711

Shousha S, Backhous Cm, Alaghband-Zadeh J, Burn I (1986) Alveolar variant of invasive lobular carcinoma of the breast. A tumor rich in estrogen receptors. Am J Clin Pathol 85: 1–5

Shousha S, Coady AT, Stamp T, James KR, Alaghbadn-Zadeh J (2989). Oestrogen receptors in mucinouc carcinoma of the breast: an immunohistochemical study using paraffin wax sections. J Clin Pathol 42: 902–905

Silver SA, Tavassoli FA (2000) Pleomorphic carcinoma of the breast: clinicopathological analysis of 26 cases of an unusual high-grade phenotype of ductal carcinoma. Histopathology 36: 505–514

Singletary SE, Connolly JL (2006) Breast cancer staging: Working with the 6th edition of the AJCC cancer staging manual. CA Cancer J Clin 56: 37–47

Sobin LH, Witekind CH (2002) TNM, classification of malignant tumours. Uicc, Wiley-Liss, New York

Soomro S, Shousha S, Taylor P, Shepard HM, Feldmann M (1991) c-erbB-2 expression in different histological types of invasive breast carcinoma. J Clin Pathol 44: 211–214

Tavassoli FA, Devilee P (2003) Pathology and genetics. Tumours of the breast and female genital organs: In: World Health Organization classification of tumours 2001, Lyon

Venable JG, Schwartz AM, Silverberg SG (1990) Infiltrating cribiform carcinoma of the breast: a distinctive clinicopathologic entity. Hum Pathol 21: 333–338

Wargotz ES, Norris HJ (1990) Metaplastic carcinoma of ductal origin. Cancer 65: 272–276

Wargotz ES, Silverberg SG (1988) Medullary carcinoma of the breast: a clinicopathologic study with appraisal of current diagnostic criteria. Hum Pathol 19: 1340–1346

Weidner N, Semple JP (1992) Pleomorphic variant of invasive lobular carcinoma of the breast. Hum Pathol 23: 1167–1171

Winchester DJ, Chang HR, Gravies Ta, Menck HR, Bland KL, Winchester DP (1998) A comparative analysis of lobular and ductal carcinoma of the breast: presentation, treatment, and outcomes. J Am Coll Surg 186: 416–422

Ziegler RG, Hoover RN, Pike MC, Hildesheim A, Nomura AMM, West DW, Wu-Williams AH, Koloner LN, Horn-Ross PL, Rosentahal JF, Hyer MB (1993) Migration patterns and breast cancer risk in Asian-American women. J Natl Cancer Inst 85: 1819–1827

Biomarkers for Breast Cancer: Towards the Proposition of Clinically Relevant Tools*

3

Maria Grazia Daidone, Vera Cappelletti, Angelo Paradiso, Massimo Gion, Nadia Harbeck, Fred Sweep, and Manfred Schmitt

CONTENTS

Abstract

Breast cancer heterogeneity represents a major hurdle to improve patient survival. Notwithstanding its potential curability due to the availability of treatment modalities that are effective in the presence of favourable clinical or patho-biologic features, there is still a great deal of controversy in its clinical management. In the last decades, tumour biomarkers that are indicative of or related to cell traits characterising malignancy, such as self-sufficiency in proliferative growth signals, insensitivity to growth inhibitory signals, evasion of apoptosis, limitless replicative potential, activation of pathways leading to neo-angiogenesis, invasion and metastasis, have provided information that have proved to be associated with disease progression. However, when singly analysed, their prognostic relevance was modest, and the only clinically useful biomarkers that remained are cell proliferation and plasminogen activation-related factors for prognosis, steroid hormone receptors and HER2/neu for prediction of response to hormonal or to the novel targeted anti-HER2/neu therapy, respectively. It therefore remains necessary to reduce the intrinsic complexity of breast cancer in order to improve its clinical outcome. One way to achieve this objective derives directly from the concept that cancer is a genetic disease at the somatic level and from the recent availability of high-throughput post-genomic analytical tools such as gene and protein expression techniques for global gene expression analysis. The knowledge derived from gene expression-profiling studies is impressive and challenges currently used breast cancer classification and existing theories about metastatic progression and breast cancer biology. Several studies employing this technology have been consistent in reproducing a molecular classification for breast cancer in which: (1) oestrogen receptor status and tumour grade are the most important discriminators of gene expression subgroups; (2) tumours can be grouped into at least four subsets according to steroid receptor and HER2/neu status; (3) each subset of tumours has a distinct clinical outcome and may therefore respond differentially to various treatments. Additionally, prognostic gene expression signatures have been proposed that outperform traditional clinical risk classification systems, suggesting the possibility to reduce over-treatment in early breast cancer, notwithstanding that the identification of high-risk patients still needs to be improved. A number of recent studies have been directed to answer different clinical and biological questions. However, despite initial enthusiasm doubts have

*On behalf of the PathoBiology Group of the European Organization for Research and Treatment of Cancer (PBG-EORTC)

been raised recently regarding the reliability of gene expression profiling for clinical applications, and the outcome of these novel studies still needs to be validated with the cooperation of different specialists and the integration between all the different skills involved in translational research in oncology.

3.1 Background

Breast cancer is a heterogeneous disease, and its consequent high complexity is a major challenge for physicians and biologists. The application of adjuvant systemic therapies in women with operable tumours has markedly improved the clinical outcome of patients with high-risk carcinoma of the breast as defined by clinico-pathologic features, and continuum improvements and refinements of these treatment modalities have been outstanding. However, the empirical approach of risk definition has the inherent limitation of delivering the same therapy to all patients, including those who are potentially cured by a locoregional modality and those who have residual tumour resistant to the planned therapy. This scenario underscores the need for designing treatments tailored to the actual characteristics of the primary tumour and to the clinical needs of the individual patient.

The majority of human tumours develop as a result of the accumulation of genetic and epigenetic alterations that may translate into a wide range of alterations in cell morphology, structure and functions. These hallmarks of cancer, summarised by Hanahan and Weinberg (2000), include self-sufficiency in proliferative growth signals, insensitivity to growth inhibitory signals, evasion of apoptosis, limitless replicative potential, activation of pathways leading to neo-angiogenesis, invasion and metastasis. They are involved in tumorigenesis and, in breast cancer, are exemplified by genetic lesions and/or functional alterations that proved to play a significant role also on the clinical outcome of patients (Fitzgibbons et al. 1999). Breast cancer, even at an early stage, is a heterogeneous disease in which the presence of alterations in molecular mechanisms affecting tumour growth, progression and metastatic potential limits the prognostic value of a purely histopathological assessment such as the TNM classification. However, in contrast to other malignancies, breast cancer is a potentially curable disease owing to very effective treatment modalities and to the presence of favourable clinical or pathobiological tumour features. Thus, the major challenge for clinical and preclinical investigators involved in translational studies lies in increasing our knowledge and trying to reduce the intrinsic clinico-biological complexity of the neoplasm in order to improve disease outcome with the final aim to accurately assess individual patient risk profiles at the initial diagnosis (prognostic assessment) and to identify optimal loco-regional and systemic treatment modalities accordingly (prediction of treatment response).

The identification of patients at low risk of relapse, potentially curable with local-regional therapy only, and of those at high-risk, who need aggressive treatments, and the selection of systemic adjuvant therapy are based on prognostic and predictive factors. For breast cancer, at present, accepted prognostic and predictive factors are few and include *patient characteristics that are disease-independent* such as age, *disease-related characteristics* such as tumour size and axillary lymph node status, *standardized histological grade* and *biological tumour features*. Among these biological tumour features, several tissue markers related to different cell functions, such as proliferation, apoptosis, hormonal dependence, neoangiogenesis, invasion and metastasis, have been investigated as prognostic factors during the last 3 decades using gene-by-gene or protein-by-protein approaches. However, even now, we are unable to determine whether any of the investigated markers could actually be important and useful in clinical patient management in a reliable and reproducible way. The only exceptions are cell proliferation measurement (Daidone and Silvestrini 2001) and plasminogen activation-related factors (Thomssen et al. 2003) for prognosis and steroid hormone receptors and the oncogene HER2/neu for prediction of response to hormonal or to the novel targeted anti-HER2/neu therapy (Bast et al. 2000). In addition, for the majority of the biological variables up to now singly investigated as a function of disease outcome, presence or expression levels associated with unfavourable prognosis correspond to a really moderate difference in the risk of disease recurrence, with the hazard of developing unfavourable events generally 1.5–2.5 times higher compared to the putatively favourable prognosis subset.

It therefore remains necessary to reduce the intrinsic complexity of breast cancer in order to improve its clinical outcome. One way to achieve this objective derives directly from the recent availability of high-throughput array-based technologies and the sequencing of the human genome, which made it possible to perform a comprehensive analysis of the transcriptional variation at the genomic level. High-throughput technologies presently available, which allow investigation of the gene and/or protein-altered profiles through comprehensive molecular approaches, and bioinformatics tools, which allow interpretation of millions of data and elicitation of biologically and clinically relevant pathways, represent the ideal instruments to accomplish such a goal and are rapidly changing our understanding of cancer biology. The knowledge derived from these gene expression-profiling studies is already impressive in terms of challenging the currently used classification of breast cancer and the existing theories about metastatic progression and breast cancer biology. Following these novel approaches, a number of recent studies have produced gene expression profiles in breast cancer markedly associated to disease progression and directed to answer different clinical and biological questions. Still, the outcome of these novel studies needs to be validated with the cooperation of different specialists and the integration among all the different skills involved in translational research in oncology.

In parallel with these studies, the experience acquired in terms of standardisation and reproducibility assessment, ethical issues for human cancer research, decision criteria and clinical trial methodology for marker utilisation and validation in the clinic, which have always been a priority for the European Organisation for Research and Treatment of Cancer (EORTC), and in particular for the Receptor and Biomarker Group (RBG, that recently merged with the Pathology Group into the Patho-Biology Group, PBG), will represent an added value of the past years of translational cancer research.

In the present paper we discuss the relevance of novel putative prognostic/predictive biomarkers classified in terms of structural and functional features acquired by tumour cells (Hanahan and Weinberg 2000), the clinical utility of using laboratory information in association with pathobiological features to plan risk-adapted individualised therapy decisions and future directions driven by the application of results obtained from comprehensive molecular analyses of breast cancer.

3.2 Biological Markers Providing Clinically Relevant Information

Cancer can be considered as a genetic disease at a somatic level, and its development requires coordinated interaction of gene products and signal pathways in the genetically deranged cancer cells and heterotypic signalling among the different cell types, transformed and normal, coexisting within the tumour, which is comparable to a complex tissue. In recent years, extensive studies of the molecular pathogenesis of cancer elicited novel regulatory pathways and networks that allowed us to identify those genes and proteins whose altered expression parallels oncogenic transformation and translates into morphological and histological cell modifications. Cell signatures may change during cancer development, and such changes are detectable through biological markers, or biomarkers, i.e., measurable alterations of cell products/functions characterising the different stages of the disease.

In breast cancer, cell traits characterising malignancy, which are self-sufficiency in proliferative growth signals (as indicated by alterations involving oncogene products, such as ras, c-myc, hormone and growth factor receptors as members of the HER/erbB family), insensitivity to growth inhibitory signals [i.e., deregulated expression of cyclins, cyclin-dependent kinases (CDK), and CDK inhibitors (CDKIs)], evasion of apoptosis, limitless replicative potential (sustained also by telomerase reactivation), activation of pathways leading to neo-angiogenesis, invasion and metastasis, are exemplified by biomarkers that proved to be associated with disease progression. However, some of them, when considered as a single marker, failed to provide clinically relevant information. There is a direct or indirect association among presence/expression of biomarkers, which are related to malignancy and clinical outcome (Fig. 3.1). Such an association concurs to identify a gradient in the risk profile. In fact, absence of steroid hormone receptors is frequently (although not exclusively) associated with other unfavourable factors, such as rapid proliferation, expression of cyclins and down-regulation of cyclin-dependent kinase inhibitors (CDKI), aneuploid DNA content, weak or absent bcl-2 expression as an indication of dedifferentiation, p53 accumulation, HER2/neu amplification/

overexpression, high levels of vascular endothelial growth factor (VEGF) and invasion factors [urokinase-type plasminogen activator (uPA) and its main inhibitor PAI-1]. Conversely, the presence of steroid hormone receptors is more frequently associated with favourable biological variables (low proliferative activity and cyclin expression, CDKIs and bcl-2 overexpression, lack of p53 accumulation and HER2/neu amplification/overexpression, low levels of VEGF and invasion factors), and corresponds to a more favourable profile, characterised by occurrence of smaller tumours of lobular histotype, generally in women at a more advanced age. When considered in association, ER, PgR, tumour rate of proliferation, p53 and bcl-2 expression concur to define a biological risk profile that also parallels clinico-pathologic risk factors, such as tumour size or patient age. In fact, the number of tumours co-expressing high-risk biomarkers (i.e., absence of steroid receptors, fast proliferative rate, overexpression of p53 and absent/low expression of bcl-2) increased as a function of tumour size (Fig. 3.2a), while decreased as a function of patient age (Fig. 3.2b).

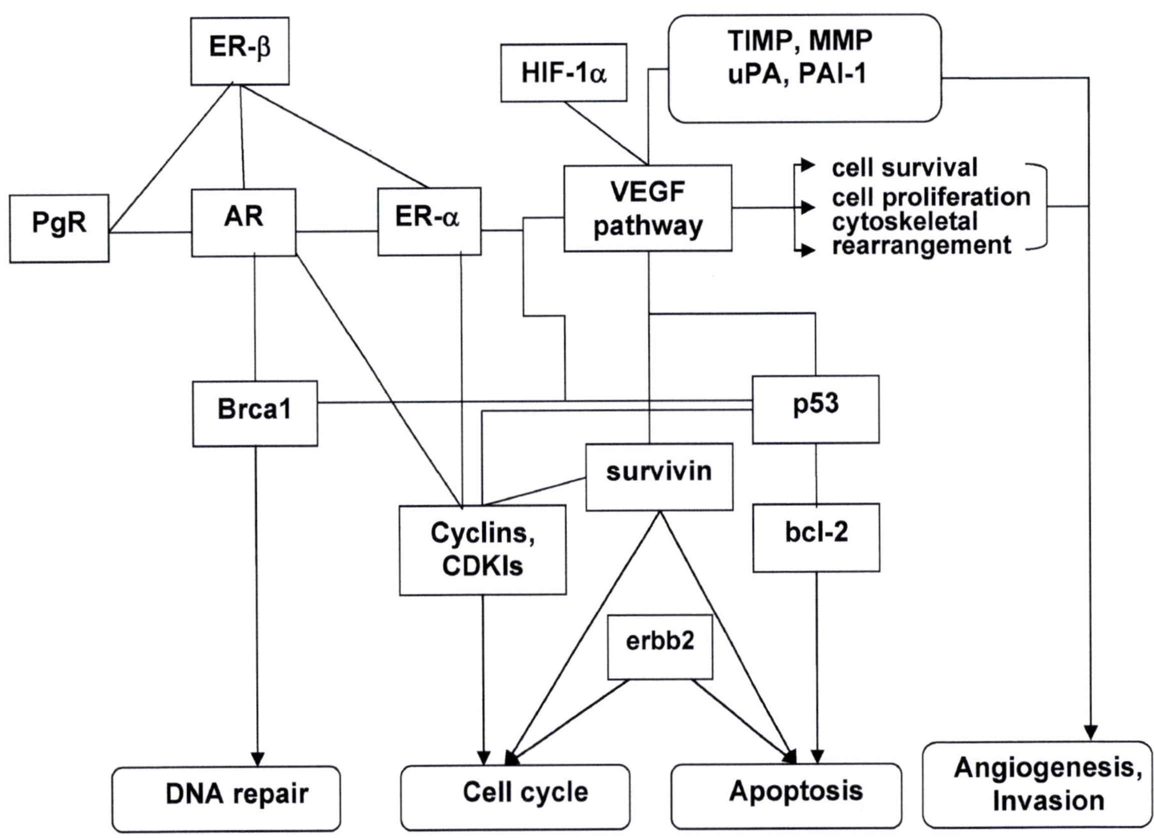

Fig. 3.1. Schematic representation of interactions existing among the most common tumour-associated biomarkers in breast cancer [modified from (Arciero et al. 2004)]. *AR* androgen receptor; CDKI, cyclin-dependent kinase inhibitor; *ER* estrogen receptor; *HIF* hypoxia inducible factor; *MMP*, matrix metalloproteases; *PAI-1*, plasminogen activator inhibitor-1; *PgR* progesterone receptor; *TIMP* tissue inhibitor of metalloproteases; *uPA* urokinase-type plasminogen activator; *VEGF* vascular endothelial growth factor

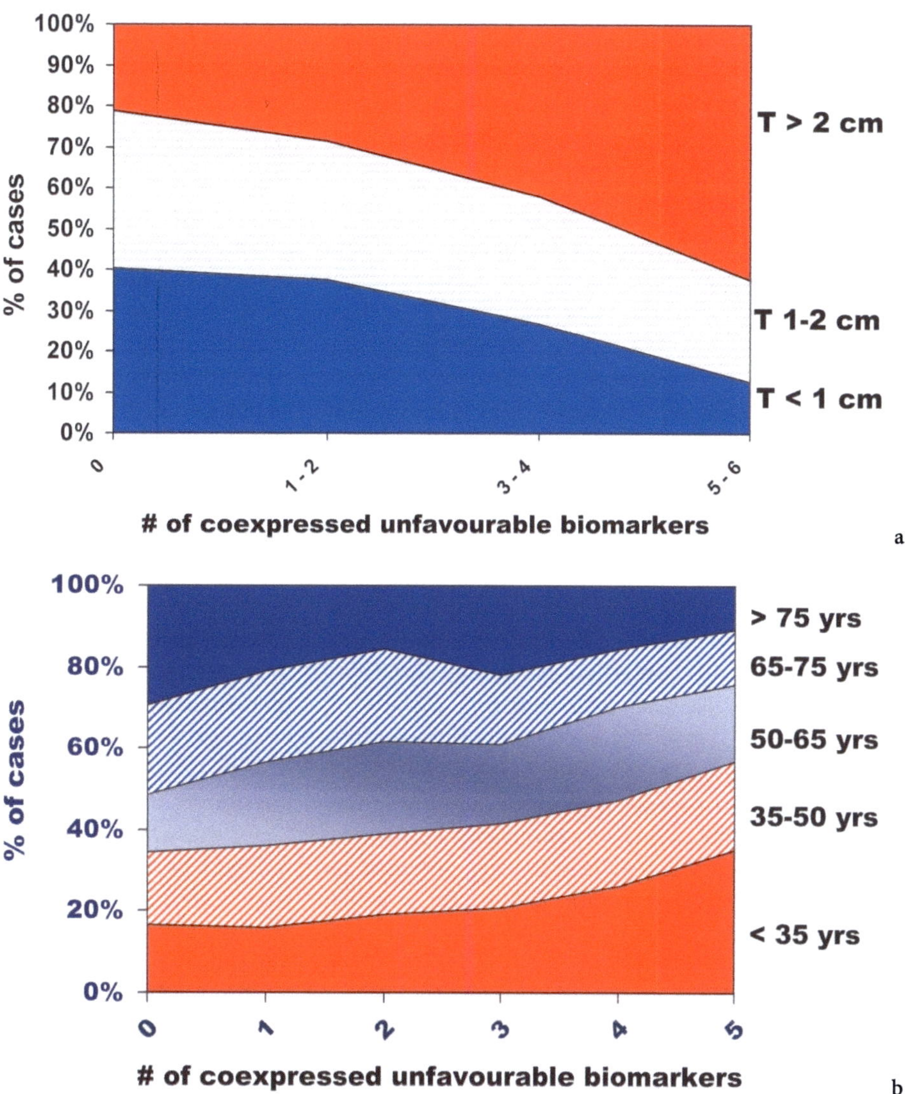

Fig. 3.2a,b. The number of tumours co-expressing high-risk biomarkers (i.e., absence of steroid receptors, fast proliferative rate, overexpression of p53 and absent/low expression of bcl-2) increased as a function of tumour size (**a**), while decreased as a function of patient age (**b**)

3.2.1 Proliferation-Related Markers

Cell proliferative activity represents one of the biological processes most thoroughly investigated for its association with tumour progression, and in the past years many laboratories have set up and challenged different approaches to measure the proliferation of tumour cells for clinical use. At present, in breast cancer the contribution of the different cell proliferation indices [mitotic figure count, measurement of S-phase cell fraction by flow-cytometry (FCM-SPF) or nucleic acid precursors incorporation (thymidine or bromodeoxyuridine, as assessed by TLI or BrdULI, respectively) and Ki67/MIB-1] was defined in retrospective studies for the identification of patients at high risk of relapse or death (who thus will need aggressive treatments) and of patients with an indolent disease (who are potentially curable by local-regional treatment alone). In fact, the majority of published articles indicate a direct association between high proliferation indices and the probability of relapse, mainly at distant sites (but also locally or in the local-regional area), and death as shown in multivariate analysis (Daidone and Silvestrini 2001). This association held true in patients subjected to only local-regional therapy until relapse and in those subjected to some kind of adjuvant systemic treatments after radical or conservative surgery and was shown regardless of the proliferative index adopted and the criteria used to classify tumours as slowly or rapidly proliferating. These studies represent phase I and II exploratory investigations [providing level of evidence (LOE) 3, since they include large studies, even within therapeutic trials, for which a variable number of samples are available or selected without any a priori study design or planning] (Hayes et al. 1996). The association between high proliferation and poor outcome was generally maintained in all the studies, also in the presence of features related to the patient (age and menopausal status), the disease (tumour size, regional lymph nodal status and histologic/cytologic findings) or the biology of the tumour (markers associated with differentiation, hormone-responsiveness, neo-angiogenesis and genomic alterations). In particular, phase-specific proliferation indices, also including counts of mitotic figures, maintained their predictivity for disease-, event- or relapse-free survival and for overall or cancer-specific survival even in the presence of information provided by histological or nuclear grade, despite the fact that all grading systems already included information on proliferation, provided by mitotic index.

From a molecular point of view, the growth of a cell population represents the result of a complex network of positive and negative mediators. Most of the negative feedback loops modulate cyclin function to control cell cycle progression and altered expression of cyclins (A, B, D, E), CDKs or CDKIs are frequently found in malignancy. As expected, also in breast cancer proteins involved in driving cell proliferation are frequently overexpressed, whereas those that restrain cell proliferation, such as the classes of CDKI belonging to KIP/CIP family (p21, p27, p57) as well as those comprised in the INK4 family (p15, p16, p18 and p19) are frequently inactivated. Cyclin overexpression and/or CDKI underexpression are generally, although not univocally, associated with poor prognosis and aggressive phenotype. However, translational studies involving such a new generation of proliferation-related proteins are extremely complex. The absolute number of positive and negative modulators of cell cycle checkpoints, the presence of complex interaction among them and, most importantly, the possibility that cancer cells could partially compensate for the deregulated expression of one of these proteins raise some doubts about the possibility to understand the network of alterations determining an abnormal regulation of the cell cycle and to investigate their absolute role on tumour progression by studying individual factors in clinical specimens. Alternatively, conflicting results may also indicate that cyclins and CDKIs are not the only cell cycle-related molecules involved in breast cancer invasion and metastasis.

Cyclins A and E (Rudolph et al. 2003; Bukholm et al. 2001; Michalides et al. 2002; Han et al. 2003; Kühling et al. 2003; Foulkes et al. 2004; Porter et al. 1997; Lindahl et al. 2004; Keyomarsi et al. 2002; Porter et al. 2006), the former synthesised during S-phase and G2/M transition and the latter induced in the late G1-phase and regulating the G1/S transition, more consistently than other cyclins provided information to identify patients at risk of relapse and death, also in the presence of information provided by histological grade or by other conventional proliferation indices. However, the case series under investigation were generally heterogeneous in terms of clinico-pathological stage and treatment, and the possibility that treatment may be a confounding factor that affects the identification of patients with indolent or aggressive disease should be taken in consideration in validating and/or translating these results into clinical practice. In fact, cyclin E does not appear to be a pure prognostic factor, but also a predictor of response to endocrine treatment (Span et al. 2003). The strongest prognostic association with survival in either node-negative or node-positive cases has been recently reported (Keyomarsi et al. 2002) using reagents able to detect both full-length and low-molecular-weight isoforms of cyclin E by Western blot analysis. In addition to the association with cell proliferation and to a causative role in chromosomal instability and polyploidization, it is likely that cyclin E, and in particular the expression of its low-molecular-weight isoforms, might also be indicative of other proliferation-related cellular processes, reflecting upstream gene alterations such as protease activation or loss of ubiquitin ligation (Borg et al. 2003). However, these results, very interesting and promising, still need to be challenged in terms of predictivity performance and reproducibility, since reagents able to detect cyclin E isoforms as well as Western blotting have not yet been validated for routine use. Moreover, the clinical case series in which these results are validated need to be carefully defined.

The most promising prognostic marker among CDKIs (Michalides et al. 2002; Han et al. 2003; Foulkes et al. 2004; Porter et al. 1997; Porter et al. 2006; Leivonen et al. 2001; Nohara et al. 2001; Barbareschi et al. 2000; Gillett et al. 1999; Dublin et al. 1998; Gohring et al. 2001; Thor et al. 2000; Volpi et al. 2000; Barnes et al. 2003; Wu et al. 1999; Chappuis et al. 2000; Catzavelos et al. 1997; Tan et al. 1997; Chu et al. 1999) appears to be $p27^{Kip1}$, which acts at the G1→S boundary and is strongly indicative of the proliferative activity of the tumour cell population since it plays major negative regulatory roles both in quiescent and in G1 cells by inhibiting cyclin-CDK complexes. Overall, the role of $p27^{Kip1}$ expression as a prognostic factor is controversial. In fact, on the one hand, it does not emerge from multivariate analyses carried out on case series subjected only to local-regional treatment (Volpi et al. 2000; Barnes et al. 2003) and seems to be associated with short- rather than with long-term follow-up (Leivonen et al. 2001). On the other hand, it proves to be inversely associated with a favourable clinical outcome in case series subjected to some forms of systemic treatments (Foulkes et al. 2004; Porter et al. 1997; Nohara et al. 2001; Wu et al. 1999; Chappuis et al. 2000; Catzavelos et al. 1997; Tan et al. 1997; Chu et al. 1999) and within specific subsets [Ashkenazi Jewish women (Foulkes et al. 2004; Chappuis et al. 2000), patients very young (Porter et al. 1997), at a high risk according to ER, histological grade and tumour proliferative rate (Han et al. 2003), but also at a low risk since presenting with very small tumours (Tan et al. 1997)].

Overall, discrepancies in the findings of the different studies may reflect technical differences (including use of different antibodies and scoring systems) or patient selection criteria (in terms of node-negative versus node-positive disease and local-regional treatment versus different types of adjuvant systemic treatment). However, it should be also considered that the prognostic role of $p27^{Kip1}$ more frequently emerged from multivariate analyses in which the traditional proliferation indices (TLI, or FCM-SPF or Ki67) were not considered as covariates. Therefore, $p27^{Kip1}$ might provide prognostic information that is not statistically independent of that already provided by conventional proliferation indices.

A *proliferation signature* emerged as a common feature across more than 40 distinct tumour data sets, comparing low-grade with high-grade tumours. In breast cancer, results obtained with array-based technologies consistently showed that: (1) the biggest difference between normal tissue and tumour samples consists in the expression level of genes that control cell proliferation due to a differential expression of genes that are involved in the fundamental process of cell proliferation (Whitfield et al. 2006) and that includes genes whose expression correlates with mitotic activity, cell-cycle progression and replication time and that (2) proliferation-related genes appear to be a common finding of several existing prognostic gene expression signatures, are consistently differentially expressed between low-grade and high-grade breast cancers, outperform the prognostic relevance of ER status, providing clinical information more relevant for ER-positive than ER-negative cases (Desmedt and Sotiriou 2006). These findings, which confirm previous results obtained by single marker analyses, highlight the importance of proliferation genes in breast cancer biology.

3.2.2 Apoptosis-Related Markers

Apoptosis-related proteins, and in particular those involved in mitochondrial membrane disruption such as bcl-2 (anti-apoptotic) and bax (pro-apoptotic), have been extensively studied in breast cancer as both prognostic and predictive markers. Differently from other tumour types, in breast cancer bcl-2 expression is associated with low-risk features (ER positivity, low proliferative activity and differentiated tumour grade) and with a favourable prognosis. However, if the prognostic value of bcl-2 alone (Chang et al. 2003) or expressed as bcl-2/bax ratio (Schiller et al. 2002) appears quite consolidated, its predictive role is more debated notwithstanding recent findings (Yang et al. 2001) indicating that bcl-2 expression is positively associated with treatment benefit following chemotherapy plus endocrine therapy, and thus indicative of a favourable prognosis.

Survivin, the smallest member of the inhibitor of apoptosis protein (IAP) gene family, is strongly expressed in embryonic and foetal organs and in many types of human cancers, where it represents one of the most tumour-specific genes so far identified in the human genome. It is, however, undetectable in most terminally differentiated normal tissues, thus suggesting that reactivation of its expression may be a common event in tumorigenesis (Altieri 2001). Survivin exists in different forms, which behave differently at the cellular and molecular level, and accumulating evidence supports the existence of a non-redundant, multifunctional survivin pathway positioned at the interface between mitotic progression and apoptosis inhibition and required to preserve the viability of proliferating tumour cells. Being functionally located at the crossroad between cell death and cell division and being associated with clinical progression, survivin can be considered among the most promising tumour molecular targets to be exploited for diagnosis and contrasted for anticancer activity (Altieri 2003). Multiple and different factors proved to affect or to be involved in the survivin pathway, including host- (hormonal milieu, hypoxia and viral infection) and tumour-related alterations (APC/ß-catenin signalling, COX-2 and VEGF overexpression). In clinical tumours survivin expression correlates with reduced tumour cell apoptosis in vivo and with unfavourable clinical outcome, either in terms of increased relapse rate or shortened patient survival, or increased resistance to treatments. Its expression proved to contribute either to the "poor prognosis signature" genes by array-based gene profiling studies in breast and colorectal cancers and in non-Hodgkin's lymphoma (Altieri 2003) or to the recurrence score recently developed on the basis of selected gene expression profiles obtained in paraffin-embedded specimens (Paik et al. 2004) that reliably predict the likelihood of distant recurrence in individual patients with ER+ tumours subjected to adjuvant tamoxifen treatment and also to chemotherapy, in the adjuvant (Paik et al. 2006) and neoadjuvant settings (Gianni et al. 2005), where it also correlates with complete response.

However, in breast cancer the few available results dealing with survivin expression as a single marker are not univocal. In fact, survivin, detected at cytoplasmic or nuclear levels in about 80% (Daidone et al. 2002) and 60% (Kennedy et al. 2003) of cases, respectively, appears to be either directly (Daidone et al. 2002) or inversely (Kennedy et al. 2003) associated with unfavourable clinical outcome. Further studies are needed to elucidate its role when expressed in different cellular areas and to assess its impact on breast cancer progression.

3.2.3 Angiogenesis- and Invasion-Related Markers

Similarly to other solid tumours, invasion and metastasis of breast cancer depend on activation of neo-angiogenesis and on modifications of the extracellular matrix. In recent years many papers have been published on these topics, reporting data suggestive of a significant association between overexpression of markers related or indicative of these functions and disease progression. In particular, hypervascularization and surrogate markers related to the formation of new blood vessels, such as CD31 and VEGF, proved to be associated with new disease manifestation either in node-negative or in node-positive patients (Arora et al. 2002; Coradini et al. 2001; Coradini et al. 2003). However, recent preclinical studies provided novel information on hypoxia, the main patho-physiological factor responsible for angiogenesis activation, and on early hypoxia-related factors: hypoxia-inducible factor 1 (HIF-1) and tumour-associated transmembrane carbonic anhydrase (CA) IX and XII.

High HIF-1α (the inducible subunit of the factor) levels are correlated with tumour progression, and more recent findings (Bos et al. 2003) indicate that increased HIF-1α levels are associated with a short survival in patients with lymph node-negative breast cancer. However, since the majority of neoplasms, including breast cancers, constitutively expressed high HIF-1α levels, the value of this factor as a prognosticator appears quite weak compared to the opportunity to use it as a molecular target to inhibit the cascade of events activated by hypoxia.

CA XII is an enzyme catalysing the reversible hydration of carbon dioxide to carbonic acid, which provides a potential link between metabolism and pH regulation. It is frequently expressed in invasive breast cancers and strongly associated with several favourable prognostic parameters including low tumour grade, ER-positive status, EGFR-negative status and absence of necrosis. For this reason patients whose tumour overexpresses CA XII had a better prognosis (Watson et al. 2003).

Proteases and their inhibitors determine the extracellular matrix (ECM) turnover in normal and pathological processes. In cancer, proteolysis is abnormally regulated, favouring ECM degradation and, subsequently, tumour invasion and metastasis. A variety of proteases putatively involved in metastasis have been investigated, and several have been shown to be promising as prognostic indicators and to provide clinically useful information. Among the latter there is the urokinase-plasminogen activation system, including the serine protease uPA, its specific receptor (uPAR) and its inhibitors (PAI-1, and PAI-2), which participate in the proteolytic processes that take place in tissue remodelling, cell migration and angiogenesis, as well as in invasion and metastasis in several tumour types (Harbeck et al. 2004). Consistent with their role in tumour progression, several groups have independently shown that high uPA and PAI-1 concentrations in primary breast cancers correlate with the occurrence of unfavourable events, such as distant metastasis and death (Look et al. 2002; Foekens et al. 1992; 1994), particularly in the node-negative group, alone or in association with other prognostic factors such as HER2 (Zemzoum et al. 2003) or angiogenic factors (Dazzi et al. 2003; Hansen et al. 2003). In addition, patients with high uPA/PAI-1 levels appear to markedly benefit from adjuvant chemotherapy (Harbeck et al. 2002) or be resistant to palliative endocrine therapy (Foekens et al. 1995; Manders et al. 2004). The prognostic relevance of uPA/PAI-1 also emerged from LOE 2 studies (investigations companion to therapeutic clinical trials, not specifically designed to test marker utility, but in which the determination of the marker was a priori planned) (Janicke et al. 1994) and was mainly strengthened by a pooled analysis (Look et al. 2002) carried out on 8,377 breast cancer patients (among whom node-negative tumours accounted for 42% of the cases, and about one third of the overall cases received only local-regional treatment until relapse), with a median follow-up of 6.5 years. Eighteen prospective and retrospective studies carried out in nine European countries on behalf of the EORTC were included in the pooled analysis, which represents, at present, a unique effort in translational studies to validate published data from lower LOE studies. uPA and PAI-1 proved to be the strongest predictors of clinical outcome after nodal involvement and the strongest ones in node-negative cases.

Other biomarkers involved in tumour invasion, such as tenascin and fibronectin (Ioachim et al. 2002), soluble adhesion molecules (E-selectin, ICAM-1, VCAM-1) (O'Hanlon et al. 2002) or maspin (Umekita et al. 2002) at present failed to provide strong evidence of a prognostic impact.

3.3 Clinical Utility

In breast cancer, most of the tissue markers investigated in the last decades and related to cell proliferation, apoptosis, hormonal dependence, neoangiogenesis, invasion and metastasis proved to be associated with disease progression and patient outcome. However, few of them at present could be considered useful for clinical patient management since they: (1) are sensitive and selective enough to identify low- and high-risk patients with clinically relevant differences in the outcome; (2) provide information not achievable by using other more established biomarkers; (3) are potentially able to allow selection of different therapeutic options within subsets of patients already defined according to other clinicopathologic features (i.e., axillary nodal involvement); (4) are useful in the majority of breast cancers. Moreover, in addition to clinico-biologic effectiveness and usefulness, also laboratory effectiveness (in terms of robustness of the assays, long-term performance and availability of quality assurance programs) should be considered to promote the transferability of these measurements from the research laboratories to general practice. Taking all these factors into consideration, besides steroid hormone receptors and HER2/neu oncogene, only uPA/PAI-1 and some of the proliferation-related markers whose relation with prognosis is discussed in this paper do fulfil the criteria required to translate laboratory results from the bench to the bedside (Table 3.1).

3.3.1 Prospective Trials

All previous findings demonstrated that tumour cell proliferation (with a variable level of sensitivity, specificity and feasibility for the different proliferation indices) and increased levels of uPA/PAI-1 could provide information to identify patients: (1) at a minimal risk of relapse or, conversely, (2) destined to relapse and progression regardless of treatment. Preliminary data also support the hypothesis that they could also provide information to identify patients likely responding or developing resistance to a specific treatment. Moreover, proliferation indices seem to provide information on treatment schedules, since in a randomized treatment protocol comparing sequential versus alternating regimens of doxorubicin and CMF in node-positive breast cancer patients, the benefit of sequential administration was mainly evident in patients with tumours with low to intermediate proliferation rates (LOE 2 study) (Silvestrini et al. 2000). However, findings relating biomarker expression to treatment response should be further investigated on independent adjuvant settings and analysed with techniques appropriately developed to test the biomarker's clinical utility.

Table 3.1. Evaluation profile of tissue biomarkers as prognostic factors

	Studies with LOE[1]:			Characteristics:			
				identification of:			
	1	2	3	patients with distinct outcome	a significant % of study population	Reproducibility	Feasibility
Proliferation-related markers[2]							
TLI, BrdULI	√	√	√	Yes	Yes	Assessed with QCPs[3]	Intermediate Prospective determination (based on an active incorporation of nucleotide precursors): fresh tissue and specific procedures required
FCM-SPF	√	√	√	Yes	Yes	Assessed with QCPs problems with data interpretation	Intermediate-low Better results obtained from fresh or frozen tissue; specific procedures/devices required
KI67, MIB-1		√	√	Yes	Yes	Not yet assessed	High IHC[4] on formalin-fixed paraffin-embedded sections
MI, MAI, M/V	√	√	√	Yes	Yes	Assessed with QCPs	High Routinely determined during diagnosis
Cyclin E			√	Yes	Yes	Not yet assessed	Intermediate Better results obtained by techniques requiring frozen tissue and specific procedures
p27			√	Yes	Yes	Not yet assessed	High IHC on formalin-fixed paraffin-embedded sections
Invasion-related markers[5]							
uPA/PAI-1	√	√	√	Yes	Yes	Assessed with QCPs	Intermediate: Fresh or frozen tissue required

[1]Level of evidence. [2]BrdULI, bromodeoxyuridine labelling index; TLI, ^{3}H-thymidine labelling index; FCM-SPF, flow-cytometric S-phase cell fraction; MI, mitotic index; MAI, mitotic activity index; M/V, volume/corrected mitotic index. [3]Quality control program. [4]Immunohistochemistry. [5]Urokinase-type plasminogen activator and its main inhibitor PAI-1

Recently the prognostic relevance of proliferation- and invasion-related markers has been challenged by comparing their clinical usefulness with that of other pathobiological information. In fact, the outcome of the first therapeutic clinical trials in which the determination of proliferation indices and uPA/PAI-1 was a priori planned, even with the consequent consideration in the statistical sizing of the study, became available in the last years and provided initial information about the actual utility of their determination in the presence of a risk profile already identified by other clinico-pathological and biological factors.

In particular, for proliferation indices LOE 2 studies, companion to therapeutic clinical trials, provided evidence in favour of:

1. a contribution of cell proliferation (evaluated as FCM-SPF) to define, in association to patient age, PgR status and tumour size, a broad spectrum of clinico-patho-biological categories with different 10-year risks for developing distant metastasis within a subset of 800 node-negative ER-positive cancers given adjuvant tamoxifen (Bryant et al. 1998). Patients' risk probabilities range from 70% (for patients younger than 35 years with large, PgR-negative tumours and a very high FCM-SPF) to 20% (for patients 50 years old with PgR-positive 1-cm tumours and a negligible proliferative activity). On a total of 1,118 women with node-negative invasive breast cancer up to 5 cm in size in which KI67/MIB1 was considered in addition to FCM-SPF, proliferation also provided information on:
2. a favourable prognosis for women with slowly proliferating tumours, regardless of the adjuvant treatment received after surgery (with superimposable disease-free survival rates for women who received only surgery versus those who received tamoxifen alone versus those who were administered doxorubicin and cyclophosphamide) (Jones et al. 2001);
3. a survival advantage for those with rapidly proliferating tumours who received postoperative adjuvant chemotherapy with doxorubicin and cyclophosphamide, whose disease-free survival rate was superimposable to that of patients with slowly proliferating tumours (Jones et al. 2002).

Such information provides an accurate assessment of the individual patient prognosis and could suggest an aggressive therapy only for some of the women with node-negative tumours, i.e., for those presenting with rapidly proliferating cancers. This suggestion is concordant with findings provided by the U.S. Intergroup prospective randomized clinical trial (LOE 1), in which FCM-SPF was able to identify within the "uncertain" risk subset (ER or PgR positive tumours less than or equal to 2 cm) patients at a low or at a high risk of relapse (Hutchins et al. 1998).

The successive step of prospective translational studies was to investigate whether node-negative breast cancer patients defined at a high risk on the basis of the tumour-related biomarkers could benefit from adjuvant polychemotherapy. For cell proliferation, three mono- or multicenter phase III randomized trials using TLI (Amadori et al. 2000; Paradiso et al. 2001) or mitotic figure count (Baak et al. 1993) have been activated in Europe, and in all the studies the prognostic factor hypothesis has been combined with a treatment hypothesis. Patients with node-negative breast cancer have been stratified into low- and high-risk groups based on the proliferation index of their primary tumour. Those with slowly proliferating tumours were not treated with systemic therapy following radical or conservative surgery plus radiotherapy. Patients with rapidly proliferating tumours were randomised to receive adjuvant chemotherapy (CMF or FAC) or to be followed without systemic therapy. Activation of those studies, as well as that of similar studies applying the determination of proliferation indices, was paralleled by promotion and maintenance of quality control programs for analytical and pre-analytical phases of cell kinetic determinations. Results are currently available from the study by Amadori et al. (2000) performed between 1989–1993 and from that by Paradiso et al. (2001) performed between 1989–1994. These two studies randomised to receive chemotherapy or no further treatment a total of 278 and 248 patients, respectively, with node-negative tumours histologically assessed. Survival curves showed a disease-free survival benefit in CMF or FAC-treated vs. untreated patients [83% vs. 72% (Amadori et al. 2000) and 81% vs. 69% (Paradiso et al. 2001), with a reduction in both local-regional and distant relapses, and a benefit of systemic treatment mostly evident for the cases with the highest TLI values (Amadori et al. 2000). Results are now available also from the nationwide Multicenter Mammary Carcinoma Project prospectively carried out in 516 lymph node-negative breast cancer patients younger than 55 years with the collaboration of Pathologists and Medical Oncologists from Dutch, Norwegian and Belgian Cancer Centres (Baak et al. 2005). In this program, in which much effort has been devoted to the reproducibility of the quantitative assessment of morphometric parameters and to an adequate training of personnel, a strong and independent prognostic relevance of the mitotic activity index has been demonstrated for distant metastasis.

Proliferation indices can be considered markers of clinical utility. In fact, in node-negative breast cancers the usefulness of the different proliferation indices to identify subsets at a very low risk of relapse has been assessed in large retrospective studies and validated in prospective studies (Jones et al. 2001; Hutchins et al. 1998). Moreover, the benefit from chemotherapy regimens including antimetabolites has been suggested from retrospective analyses in companion studies of randomised treatment protocols and assessed in phase III prospective confirmatory studies (Jones et al. 2002; Amadori et al. 2000; Paradiso et al. 2001; Andre et al. 2005). All these findings contributed to the ranking of mitotic figure count as a category I prognostic factor by the College of American Pathologists (Fitzgibbons et al. 1999), i.e., as a factor proven to be of prognostic importance and usefulness in clinical patient management. Mitotic figure count is the oldest measurement of cell proliferation, represents an integral part of histological grade and is feasible and routinely assessable on histological section/cytological smears used for diagnosis, without additional processing or staining procedures. These advantages over the other proliferation indices probably convinced panellists of the last NIH Consensus Development Conference to support its consideration in the clinical practice, alone or in association with the other components of grading systems (National Institutes of Health 2001). However, if mitotic figure count is used in the clinical routine, an assessment of the assay performance, including within- and between-laboratory variation, is mandatory. Recent studies would indicate a role for proliferation-related indices as pharmacodynamic intermediate markers of the effectiveness of medical therapies, even though such findings are not univocal and should be carefully interpreted in relation to the type of treatment and timing of biological monitoring (Urriticoechea et al. 2005; Burcombe et al. 2006; Dowsett et al. 2006).

A prospective randomised multicentre therapeutic trial (Chemo N0) was conducted from 1993 to 1998 in Germany and Slovenia, with the participation of 14 different institutions including 689 patients with node-negative breast cancer who were stratified into low- and high-risk groups based on uPA/PAI-1 tumour antigen levels. Patients presenting at diagnosis with high uPA and/or PAI-1 tumours were randomised to receive adjuvant CMF or to be followed without systemic therapy, while low uPA and PAI-1 tumours were not treated with systemic therapy following radical or conservative surgery plus radiotherapy (Janicke et al. 2001). This LOE 1 prospective study: (1) confirmed that the risk of distant metastasis was twice as high in high-risk compared to low-risk patients; (2) demonstrated that administration of adjuvant CMF significantly reduced the risk of relapse in the high risk group. The 10-year follow-up information of the Chemo N0 trial demonstrated that risk assessment by the biomarkers uPA/PAI-1 is able to outperform that by a mathematical modelling algorithm based on epidemiological data (AdjuvantOnline!), which is frequently used in the clinic (Euler et al. 2006). A follow-up trial (NNBC-3) is currently comparing clinico-pathological criteria and uPA/PAI-1 regarding their usefulness for clinical risk assessment in node-negative breast cancer. Moreover, in high-risk patients, the question of optimal chemotherapy is also addressed in this trial, which is conducted together with the German AGO (Working Group for Gynecological Oncology), GBG (German Breast Group) and EORTC PBG.

Studies based on TLI or uPA/PAI-1 stratification of patients in low- or high-risk subgroups represent a novel strategy to combine a prognostic factor hypothesis with a treatment hypothesis. They can either prospectively and definitively assess tumour-related biomarkers as prognostic factors comparing low- and high-risk subgroups or address therapy-related questions in the high-risk subset.

3.3.2 Quality Assessment and Quality Assurance Programs

In recent years, efforts have been devoted to standardise reagents, methodologies and interpretation criteria to improve reliability, accuracy and reproducibility of assay results within and among the different laboratories by promoting and maintaining quality control programs in order to provide clinicians networks of qualified laboratories for promising tumour-related markers to be used for therapy decisions. This area of investigation represents a priority for the RBG, now PBG-EORTC, whose activity started in 1980 with measurement of ER and PgR (EORTC 1980; Guerts-Moespot 2000). The group then significantly contributed to the positive results obtained by uPA/PAI-1 in recent years (Sweep et al. 1998), and is now dealing also with quality, performance and reproducibility of molecular assays.

It is worth mentioning that all the phase-III randomised prospective trials that have been activated in the last decade to test the clinical utility of identifying high-risk node-negative breast cancer patients on the basis of invasion markers or tumour cell proliferation (by mitotic figure count, TLI or FCM-SPF) and of randomising them to observation or chemotherapy have been preceded by quality control programs to address analytical and also pre-analytical phases of the determinations (Paradiso et al. 2002; Collan et al. 1996; Baldetorp et al. 1995).

3.4 Future Directions: Global Profiling of Tumour Markers

During the last years, we have faced a change of attitude probably destined to profoundly affect cancer research with the utilisation of information emerging from genomic research and high-throughput technologies for a novel disease approach in terms of diagnosis, prevention and treatment. In the near future, we will probably witness the long-time demanded integration between the different disciplines of cancer research. As a consequence, traditional clinico-pathological assessment of tumour stage is now put together with results of gene and protein expression profiling. Together they will aid to identify molecular signatures associated with prognosis and treatment response and molecular alterations likely responsible for initiating, maintaining neoplastic conditions and/or driving clinical progression, thus representing targets for new molecular therapeutic agents with a potential for improved efficacy and selectivity against cancer cells.

Currently, the knowledge of the sequence of the human genome and the availability of novel technologies to investigate simultaneously the expression level of thousands of genes from a limited amount of mRNA obtained from clinical tumour specimens and to analyze the massive data that are being produced are providing an extraordinary opportunity to identify the molecular changes that occur during cancer development and to complement the current tumour classification based on morphologic features with classification schemes based on cancer molecular alterations. In particular, in breast cancer the knowledge derived from gene expression-profiling studies is impressive and challenges currently used breast cancer classification and existing theories about metastatic progression and breast cancer biology. Several studies employing this technology have been remarkably consistent in reproducing a similar molecular classification for breast cancer (Sorlie et al. 2001, Sotiriou et al. 2003). Overall, the conclusions are that: (1) oestrogen receptor (ER) status and tumour grade are the most important discriminates of expression subgroups; (2) tumours carrying mutations in the BRCA1 gene exhibit a molecular signature distinct from BRCA2-positive or sporadic tumours; (3) breast tumours can be grouped according to at least four individual subgroups: the "basal-like", which is mainly ER-negative, PgR-negative and ERBB2-negative (often referred to as triple negative), the ERBB2-like subtype, characterised by high expression of several genes of the erbb2 amplicon, and at least two luminal subgroups (luminal A and luminal B) being predominantly ER-positive; (4) each subgroup has a distinct clinical outcome and may therefore respond differentially to various therapeutics (Rouzier et al. 2005); (5) gene signatures associated to metastatisation in specific distant sites have already been proposed and validated (Minn et al. 2005, 2005; Smid et al. 2006). Surprisingly, other clinically relevant variables such as menopausal status, tumour size and nodal status were not associated with very dissimilar gene expression patterns, suggesting that these important clinico-pathological prognostic variables capture essentially information about the disease stage rather than intrinsic biological properties of the tumour. Moreover, such a comprehensive molecular approach, applied by different research groups using different technological platforms, has already identified expression profiles that differentiate node-negative breast cancer patients with distinct prognosis that otherwise may have been indistinguishable (van't Veer et al. 2002, van de Vijer et al. 2002, Wang et al. 2005). The 70 and the 76 gene signatures developed by the Amsterdam and Rotterdam groups, respectively, are examples of such an approach (van de Vijer et al. 2002, Wang et al. 2005). These *poor prognosis signatures* proposed for breast cancer by gene expression profiling identify a subset of patients with a five- to ten-fold risk of distant metastasis and includes genes involved in cell cycle, invasion and metastatisation, neo-angiogenesis and signal transduction, which already proved to be clinically relevant when singly analysed, but with a limited predictive power likely due to their consideration with a gene-by-gene approach. Their prognostic refinement may surpass the prognostic accuracy of classification criteria developed according to the guidelines proposed by NIH-NCI (2001) or St. Gallen Consensus Conferences (Goldhirsch et al. 2005) based on tumour size, patient age, grade of differentiation and oestrogen or progesterone receptors. A common feature of both signatures is that when their performance in stratifying patients according to risk classification results is compared with the traditional clinical risk classification systems, they were consistently superior in correctly identifying the low-risk patients, suggesting a potential for reducing over treatment in early breast cancer. However, the identification of high-risk patients could still be improved, since half of these patients did not have a disease recurrence.

Gene expression profile research has been until recently limited by the requirement of fresh/frozen tissue for sample preparation and labelling. This has hampered many studies and biased patients' cohorts in retrospective studies. However, formalin-fixed paraffin-embedded (FFPE) tissues are widely available and have the advantage of a known patient outcome and drug response history. Unfortunately, RNA derived from such samples is often badly degraded and hardly can be used for conventional microarray studies. New methods have however been developed that allow working with partially degraded RNA samples (Perou et al. 2004) ranging between 100–50 nucleotides using very small RNA quantities like those that can be extracted from a 5-μm tissue section (1–2 μg). Furthermore, the possibility now exists to lincarly amplify tiny RNA quantities without affecting further gene expression results. The first results using FFPE tissues were reported by Paik et al. (2004) using RT PCR, but also new approaches like the DASL (cDNA mediated, annealing, selection, extension and ligation) have been developed allowing work with partially degraded RNA (Bibikova et al. 2004).

Despite the initial enthusiasm, however, several doubts have been raised regarding the reliability of this new tool in clinical applications such as disease diagnostics, staging, prognostication and treatment prediction, as several microarray studies that investigated the same clinical problem (prediction of prognosis or treatment response in similar clinical situations) generated different gene expression classifiers with only a small number of overlapping genes. From this perspective, several independent validation studies have been or are currently carried out in Europe (Buyse et al. 2006) and in US.

Moreover, the enormous power of the novel high-throughtput approaches, which already succeeded in reinforcing the notion that breast cancer is a heterogeneous disease, has to be used without forgetting lessons learned from the past single gene/single marker prognostic studies and cannot be pursued without planning a validation on prospectively collected samples. Validation represents a major challenge, partially addressed by the majority of already published studies, that can only be faced with the cooperation of different specialists and the integration between the different skills involved in translational research. Patient cohorts in which these novel high-throughput approaches are being validated have to be carefully selected in order to avoid biases due to treatment heterogeneity. For example, molecular patterns that are associated with disease aggressiveness in the absence of adjuvant systemic therapy may be quite distinct from patterns that predict disease progression in patients who received chemo- and/or endocrine therapy. Moreover, technology is reaching a high level of complexity, and method standardization is a mandatory step before any conclusion is reached concerning the possible translation of a tumour biomarker into clinical practice. To this purpose, the PBG of EORTC will play a major role in validating and fostering the clinical implementation of the outcome of present and future translational research.

3.5 Conclusions

The gap between the ever-growing knowledge about the genome sequence and the bio-functional role of this enormous amount of genes is filling quickly. Several signatures able to predict disease outcome have been developed through different approaches, but al least four of the most popular overlap in prediction despite the absence overlapping genes (Fan et al. 2006). The consequence is that to obtain a better accuracy in prediction it is important to 'expand' the information of actual signatures (Massague 2007). As demonstrated by the intrinsic gene signature (Sorlie et al. 2001), molecular classification of tumours has clear implications on prognosis, which due to their nature itself, are independent from the specific patient series and not affected by case series overfitting. Interestingly, new signatures have been developed with a different concept in mind, aiming at identifying gene sets associated with a single cancer-cell property. Such signatures, developed mostly in pre-clinical models have the unexpected property of being not cancer-type specific, as they predict prognosis in more than one histology. An excellent example is the hypoxia signature (Chi et al. 2006), which is associated with poor outcome in breast and ovarian cancer. Similarly, the death-from-cancer signature predicting the clinical outcome in patients with multiple types of cancer, epithelial and non-epithelial (Glinsky et al. 2005), and the so-called 186-genes' invasiveness signature, recently developed by comparing tumorigenic breast cancer cells with normal epithelial cells (Liu et al. 2007), predict metastases-free survival in breast cancer, but also in lung, prostate and medulloblastoma. In the case of breast cancer, its prognostic power increases when combined with the wound response signature (Chang et al. 2004). Other signatures, of the same type, addressing specific oncogenic pathways have been developed (Bild et al. 2006) and are likely to increase prediction accuracy when combined with earlier signatures developed and validated in clinical breast cancer.

Therefore, at this time, integration of clinical and pre-clinical results seems to be a must in the development of tailored treatments, and not only for breast cancer.

References

Altieri DC (2001) The molecular basis and potential role of survivin in cancer diagnosis and therapy. Trends Molecular Med 7:542–547

Altieri DC (2003) Survivin, versatile modulation of cell division and apoptosis in cancer. Oncogene 22:8581–8589

Amadori D, Nanni O, Marangolo M et al (2000) Disease-free survival advantage of adjuvant cyclophosphamide, methotrexate and fluorouracil in patients with node-negative rapidly proliferating breast cancer: a randomized multicenter study. J Clin Oncol 18:3125–3134

Andre F, Khalil A, Slimane K, Massard C, Mathieu MC, Vignot S, Assi H, Delaloge S, Spielmann M (2005) Mitotic index and benefit of adjuvant anthracycline-based chemotherapy in patients with early breast cancer. J Clin Oncol 23:2996–3000

Arciero C, Somiari SB, Shriver CD, Brzeski H, Jordan R, Hu H, Ellsworth DL, Somiari RI (2004) Functional relationship and gene ontology classification of breast cancer biomarkers. Int J Biol Markers 18:241–272

Arora R, Joshi K, Nijhawan R et al (2002) Angiogenesis as an independent prognostic indicator in node-negative breast cancer. Anal Quant Cytol Histol 24:228–233

Baak JP, van Diest PJ, Benraadt T et al (1993) The Multi-Center Morphometric Mammary Carcinoma Project (MMMCP) in the Netherlands; value of morphometrically assessed proliferation and differentiation. J Cell Biochem [Suppl] 17G:220–225

Baak JPA, van Diest PJ, Voorhorst FJ, van der Wall E, Beek LVAM, Vermorken JB, Janssen EAM (2005) Prospective multicentri calidation of the independent prognostic value of the mitotic activity index in lymph node-negative breast cancer patients younger than 55 years. J Clin Oncol 23:5993–6001

Baldetorp B, Bendahl PO, Ferno M et al (1995) Reproducibility in DNA flow cytometric analysis of breast cancer: comparison of 12 laboratories' results for 67 sample homogenates. Cytometry 22:115–127

Bast RC, Ravdin P, Hayes DF et al (2001) 2000 Update of recommendations for the use of tumor markers in breast and colorectal cancer: clinical practice guidelines of the American Society of Clinical Oncology. J Clin Oncol 19:1865–1878

Barbareschi M, van Tinteren H, Mauri FA, Veronese S, Peterse H, Maisonneuve P, Caffo O, Scaioli M, Doglioni C, Galligioni E, Dalla Palma P, Michalides R (2000) p27Kipl expression in breast carcinomas: an immunohistochemical study on 512 patients with long-term follow-up. Int J Cancer (Pred Oncol) 89:236–241

Barnes A, Pinder SE, Bell JA, Paish EC, Wencyk PM, Robertson JFR, Elston CW, llis IO (2003) Expressoin of p27kipl in breast cancer and its prognostic significance. J Pathol 201:451–459

Bibikova M, Yeakley JM, Chudin E, Chen J, Wickham E, Wang-Rodriguez J, Fan JB (2004) Gene expression profiles in formalin-fixed, paraffin-embedded tissues obtained with a novel assay for microarray analysis. Clin Chem 50:2384–2386

Bibikova M, Talantov D, Chudin E, Yeakley JM,Chen J, Doucet D, Wickham E, Atkins D, Barker D, Chee M, Wang Y, Fan JB (2004) Quantitative gene expression profiling in formalin-fixed, paraffin-embedded tissues using universal bead arrays. Am J Pathol 2004; 165:1799–1807

Bild AH, Yao G, Chang JT, Wang Q, Potti A, Chasse D, Joshi MB, Harpole D, Lancaster JM, Berchuck A, Olson JA Jr, Marks JR, Dressman HK, West M, Nevins JR (2006) Oncogenic pathway signatures in human cancers as a guide to targeted therapies. Nature 439:353–357

Borg A, Fernö M, Peterson C (2003) Predicting the future of breast cancer. Nature medicine 9:16–18

Bos R, van der Groep P, Greijer AE et al (2003) Levels of hypoxia-inducible factor-lalpha independently predict prognosis inpatients with lymph node negative breast carcinoma. Cancer 97:1573–1581

Bryant J, Fisher B, Gunduz N, Costantino JP, Emir B (1998) S-phase fraction combined with other patient and tumor characteristics for the prognosis of node-negative, estrogen-receptor-positive breast cancer. Breast Cancer Res Treat 51:239–253

Bukholm IR, Bukholm G, Nesland JM (2001) Over-expression of cyclin A is highly associated with early relapse and reduced survival in patients with primary breast carcinomas. Int J Cancer 3:283–287

Burcombe R, Wilson GD, Dowsett M, Khan I, Richman PI, Daley F, Detre S, Makris A (2006) Evaluation of Ki-67 proliferation and apoptotic index before, during and after neoadjuvant chemotherapy for primary breast cancer. Breast Cancer Res 8:R31

Buyse M, Loi S, van't Veer L, Viale G, Delorenzi M, Glas AM, d'Assignies MS, Bergh J, Lidereau R, Ellis P, Harris A, Bogaerts J, Therasse P, Floore A, Amakrane M, Piette F, Rutgers E, Sotiriou C, Cardoso F, Piccart MJ; TRANSBIG Consortium (2006) Validation and clinical utility of a 70-gene prognostic signature for women with node-negative breast cancer. J Natl Cancer Inst 98:1183–1192

Catzavelos C, Bhattacharya N, Ung YC, Wilson JA, Roncari L, Sandhu C, Shaw P, Yeger H, Morava-Protzner I, Kapusta L, Franssen E, Pritchard KI, Slingerland JM (1997) Decreased levels of the cell-cycle inhibitor p27Kipl protein: prognostic implications in primary breast cancer. Nat Med 3:227–230

Chang J, Clark GM, Allred D et al (2003) Survival of patients with metastatic breast cancer: importance of prognostic markers of the primary tumor. Cancer 97:545–553

Chang HY, Sneddon JB, Alizadeh AA, Sood R, West RB, Montgomery K, Chi JT, van de Rijn M, Botstein D, Brown PO (2004) Gene expression signature of fibroblast serum response predicts human cancer progression: similarities between tumors and wounds. PLoS Biol 2:E7

Chappuis PO, Kapusta L, Begin LR, Wong N, Brunet J-S, Narod SA, Slingerland J, Foulkes WD (2000) Germline BRCA1/2 mutaions and p27Kip1 protein levels independently predict outcome after breast cancer. J Clin Oncol 18:4045–4052

Chi JT, Wang Z, Nuyten DS, Rodriguez EH, Schaner ME, Salim A, Wang Y, Kristensen GB, Helland A, Borresen-Dale AL, Giaccia A, Longaker MT, Hastie T, Yang GP, van de Vijver MJ, Brown PO (2006) Gene expression programs in response to hypoxia: cell type specificity and prognostic significance in human cancers. PLoS Med 3:e47

Chu JS, Huang CS, Chang KJ (1999) p27 expression as a prognostic factor of breast cancer in Taiwan. Cancer Letter 141:123–130

Collan YU, Kuopio T, Baak JP et al (1996) Standardized mitotic counts in breast cancer. Evaluation of the method. Pathol Res Pract 192:931–941

Coradini D, Boracchi P, Daidone MG, Pellizzaro C, Miodini P, Ammatuna M, Tomasic G, Biganzoli E (2001) Prognostic contribution of vascular endothelial growth factor to the Nottingham prognostic index in node-negative breast cancer. Br J Cancer 85: 795–797

Coradini D, Biganzoli E, Pellizzaro C et al (2003) Vascular endothelial growth factor in node-positive breast cancer patients treated with adjuvant tamoxifen. Br J Cancer 89:268–270

Daidone MG, Silvestrini R (2001) Prognostic and predictive role of proliferation indices in adjuvant therapy of breast cancer. J Natl Cancer Inst Monogr 30: 27–35

Daidone MG, Della Porta C, Pilotti S, Zaffaroni N (2002) Coexpression of survivin and hTERT in soft tissue sarcoma. Lancet 360:877

Dazzi C, Cariello A, Maioli P et al (2003) A high cytosol value of urokinase-type plasminogen activator (uPA) may be predictive of early relapse in primary breast cancer. Cancer Invest 21:208–216

Desmedt C, Sotiriou C (2006) Proliferation. The most prominent predictor of clinical outcome in breast cancer. Cell Cycle 5:2198–2202

Dowsett M, Smith IE, Ebbs SR, Dixon JM, Skene A, Griffith C, Boeddinghaus I, Salter J, Detre S, Hills M, Ashley S, Francis S, Walsh G, A'Hern R (2006) Proliferation and apoptosis as markers of benefit in neoadjuvant endocrine therapy of breast cancer. Clin Cancer Res 12:1024s–1030s

Dublin EA, Patel NK, Gillett CE, Smith P, Peters G, Barnes DM (1998) Retinoblastoma and p16 proteins in mammary carcinoma: their relationship to cyclin D1 and histopahological parameters. Int J Cancer (Pred Oncol) 79:71–75

EORTC Breast Cancer Cooperative Group (1980) Revision of the standard for the assessment of hormone receptors in human breast cancer. Eur J Cancer 16:1513–1515

Euler U, Meisner C, Friedel C, Schmidt M, Untch M, Lisboa B, Jaenicke F, Schmitt M, Thomssen C, Harbeck N (2006) Comparison of outcome prediction in node-negative breast cancer based on biomarkers uPA/PAI-1 or Adjuvant Online™ using the 10-year follow-up of the randomized multicenter Chemo N0 trial. ASCO Proceedings

Fan C, Oh DS, Wessels L, Weigelt B, Nuyten DS, Nobel AB, van't Veer LJ, Perou CM (2006) Concordance among gene-expression-based predictors for breast cancer. N Engl J Med 355:560–569

Fitzgibbons PL, Page DL, Weaver D et al (2000) Prognostic factors in breast cancer. College of American Pathologists Consensus Statement 1999. Arch Pathol Lab Med 124:966–978

Foekens JA, Schmitt M, van Putten WLJ, Peters HA, Bontenbal M, Jänicke F, Klijn JGM (1992) Prognostic value of urokinase-type plasminogen activator in 671 primary breast cancer patients. Cancer Res 52: 6101–6105

Foekens JA, Schmitt M, van Putten WLJ, Peters HA, Kramer MD, Jänicke F, Klijn JGM (1994) Plasminogen activator inhibitor-1 and prognosis in primary breast cancer. J Clin Oncol 12: 1648–1658

Foekens JA, Look MP, Peters HA, van Putten WLJ, Portengen H, Klijn JGM (1995) Urokinase-type plasminogen activator (uPA) and its inhibitor PAI-1 predict poor response to tamoxifen therapy in recurrent breast cancer. J Natl Cancer Inst87: 751–756

Foulkes WD, Brunet J-S, Stefansson IM, Straume O, Chappuis PO, Begin LR, Hamel N, Goffin JR, Wong N, Trudel M, Kapusta L, Porter P, Akslen LA (2004) The prognostic implication of the basal-like (cyclin Ehigh/ p27low/ p53+/ glomeruloid-microvascular-proliferation+) phenotype of BRCA1-related breast cancer. Cancer Res 64:830–835

Geurts-Moespot J, Leake R, Benraad TJ, Sweep CG (2000) Twenty years of experience with the steroid receptor external quality assessment program–the paradigm for tumour biomarker EQA studies. On behalf of the EORTC Receptor and Biomarker Study Group. Int J Oncol 17:13–22

Gianni L, Zambetti M, Clark K et al (2005) Gene expression profiules in paraffin-embedded core biopsy tissue predict response to chemotherapy in women with locally advanced breast cancer. J Clin Oncol 23:7265–7277

Gillett CE, Smith P, Peters G, Lu X, Barnes DM (1999) Cyclin-dependent kinase inhibitor p27Kip1 expression and interaction with other cell cycle-associated proteins in mammary carcinoma. J Pathol 187:200–206

Glinsky GV, Berezovska O, Glinskii AB (2005) Microarray analysis identifies a death-from-cancer signature predicting therapy failure in patients with multiple types of cancer. J Clin Invest 115:1503–1521

Gohring UJ, Bersch A, Becker M, Neuhaus W, Schondorf T (2001) p21(waf) correlates with DANN replication but not with prognosis in invasive breast cancer. J Clin Pathol 54:866–870

Goldhirsch A, Glick JH, Gelber RD, Coates AS, Thurlimann B, Senn HJ (2005) Panel members. Meeting highlights: international expert consensus on the primary therapy of early breast cancer 2005. Ann Oncol 16:1569–1583

Han S, Park K, Bae B-N, Kim KH, Kim H-J, Kim Y-D, Kim H-Y (2003) Prognostic implications of cyclin E expression and its relationship with cyclin D1 and p27Kip1 expression on tissue microarrays of node negative breast cancer. J Surg Oncol 83: 241–247

Hanahan D, Weinberg RA (2000) The hallmarks of cancer. Cell 100:57–70

Hansen S, Overgaard J, Rose C et al (2003) Independent prognostic value of angiogenesis and the level of plasminogen activator inhibitor type 1 in breast cancer patients. Br J Cancer 88:102–108

Harbeck N, Kates RE, Look MP et al (2002) Enhanced benefit from adjuvant chemotherapy in breast cancer patients classified high-risk according to urokinase-type plasminogen activator (uPA) and plasminogen activator inhibitor type 1 (n=3,424). Cancer Res 62:4617–4622

Harbeck N, Kates RE, Gauger K, Willems A, Kiechle M, Magdolen V, Schmitt M (2004) Urokinase-type plasminogen activator (uPA) and its inhibitor PAI-1 : novel tumor-derived factors with a high prognostic and predictive impact in breast cancer. Thromb Haemost 91:450–456

Hayes DF, Bast RC, Desch CE, Fritsche H Jr, Kemeny NE, Jessup JM, Locker GY, Macdonald JS, Mennel R G, Norton L, Ravdin P, Taube S, Winn RJ (1996) Tumor marker utility grading system: a framework to evaluate clinical utility of tumor markers. J Natl Cancer Inst 88:1456–1466

Hutchins L, Green S, Ravdin P, Lew D, Martino S, Abeloff M (1998) CMF versus CAF with and without tamoxifen in high-risk node-negative breast cancer patients and a natural history follow-up study in low-risk node-negative patients: first results of Intergroup trial INT 0102. Proceedings of the 34th Annual Meeting of the American Association of Cancer Research. Abstract # 2

Ioachim E, Charchanti A, Briasoulis E et al (2002) Immunohistochemical expression of extracellular matrix components tenascin, fibronectin, collagen type IV and laminin in breast cancer: their prognostic value and role in tumour invasion and progression. Eur J Cancer 38:2362–2370

Janicke F, Pache L, Schmitt M, Ulm K, Thomssen C, Prechtl A, Graeff H (1994) Both the cytosols and detergent extracts of breast cancer tissues are suited to evaluate the prognostic impact of the urokinase-type plasminogen activator and its inhibitor, plasminogen activator inhibitor type 1. Cancer Res 54:2527–2530

Janicke F, Prechtl A, Thomssen C et al (2001) Randomized adjuvant chemotherapy trial in high-risk, lymph node-negative breast cancer patients identified by urokinase-type plasminogen activator and plasminogen activator inhibitor type. J Natl Cancer Inst 93:913–920

Jones S, Clark G, Koleszar S, Ethington G, Mennel R, Paulson E et al (2001) Low proliferative rate of invasive node-negative breast cancer predicts for a favorable outcome: a prospective evaluation of 669 patients. Clin Breast Cancer 1:310–314

Jones S, Clark G, Koleszar S, Ethington G, Mennel R, Paulson E et al (2002) Adjuvant chemotherapy with doxorubicin and cyclophosphamide in women with rapidly proliferating node-negative breast cancer. Clin Breast Cancer 3:147–152

Kennedy SM, O'Driscoll L, Purcell R et al (2003) Prognostic importance of survivin in breast cancer. Br J Cancer 88:1077–1083

Keyomarsi K, Tucker SL, Buchholz TA, Callister M, Ding Y, Hortobagyi GN, Bedrosian I, Knickerbocker C, Toyofuku W, Lowe M, Herliczek TW, Bacus SS (2002) Cyclin E and survival in patients with breast cancer. N Engl J Med 347:1566–1575

Kühling H, Alm P, Olsson H, Ferno M, Baldetorp B, Parwaresch R, Rudolph P (2003) Expression of cyclins E, A, and B, and prognosis in lymph node-negative breast cancer. J Pathol 199:424–431

Leivonen M, Nordling S, Lundin J, von Boguslawski K, Haglund C (2001) p27 expression correlates with short-term, but not with long-term prognosis in breast cancer. Breast Cancer Res Treat 67:15–22

Lindahl T, Landberg G, Ahlgren J, Nordgren H, Norberg T, Klaar S, Holmberg L, Bergh J (2004) Overexpression of cyclin E protein is associated with specific mutation types in the p53 gene and poor survival in human breast cancer. Carcinogenesis 25:375–380

Liu R, Wang X, Chen GY, Dalerba P, Gurney A, Hoey T, Sherlock G, Lewicki J, Shedden K, Clarke MF (2007) The prognostic role of a gene signature from tumorigenic breast-cancer cells. N Engl J Med 356:217–226

Look MP, van Putten WLJ, Duffy MJ, Harbeck N, Christensen IJ, Thomssen C, Kates R, Spyratos F, Fernö M, Eppenberger-Castori S, Sweep CG, Ulm K, Peyrat JP, Martin PM, Magdelénat H, Brünner N, Duggan C, Lisboa BW, Bendahl PO, Quillien V, Daver A, Ricolleau G, Meijer-van Gelder ME, Manders P, Fiets WE, Blankenstein MA, Broët P, Romain S, Daxenbichler G, Windbichler G, Cufer T, Borstnar S, Küng W, Beex LVAM, Klijn JGM, O'Higgins N, Eppenberger U, Jänicke F, Schmitt M, Foekens JA (2002) Pooled analysis of prognostic impact of urokinase-type plasminogen activator and its inhibitor PAI-1 in 8,377 breast cancer patients. J Natl Cancer Inst 94:116–128

Manders P, Tjan-Heijnen VC, Span PN, Grebenchtchikov N, Foekens JA, Beex LV, Sweep CG (2004) Predictive impact of urokinase-type plasminogen activator: plasminogen activator inhibitor type-1 complex on the efficacy of adjuvant systemic therapy in primary breast cancer. Cancer Res 64:659–664

Massague J (2007) Sorting out breast-cancer gene signatures. N Engl J Med 356:294–297

Michalides R, van Tinteren H, Balkenende A, Vermorken JB, Benraadt, Huldij J, van Diest P (2002) Cyclin A is a prognostic indicator in early stage breast cancer with and without tamoxifen treatment. Br J Cancer 86:402–404

Minn AJ, Gupta GP, Siegel PM, Bos PD, Shu W, Giri DD, Viale A, Olshen AB, Gerald WL, Massague J (2005) Genes that mediate breast cancer metastasis to lung. Nature 436:518–524

Minn AJ, Kang Y, Serganova I, Gupta GP, Giri DD, Doubrovin M, Ponomarev V, Gerald WL, Blasberg R, Massague J (2005) Distinct organ-specific metastatic potential of individual breast cancer cells and primary tumors. J Clin Invest 115:44–55

National Institutes of Health Consensus Development Conference Statement (2001) Adjuvant Therapy for Breast Cancer, November 1–3, 2000. J Natl Cancer Inst 93:979–989

Nohara T, Ryo T, Iwamoto S, Gon G, Tanigawa N (2001) Expression of cell-cycle regulator p27 is correlated to the prognosis and ER expression in breast carcinoma patients. Oncology 60:94–100

O'Hanlon DM, Fitzsimons H, Lynch J et al (2002) Soluble adhesion molecules (E-selectin, ICAM-1 and VCAM-1) in breast carcinoma. Eur J Cancer 38:2252–2257

Paik S, Shak S, Tang G, Kim C, Baker J, Cronin M, Baehner FL, Walker MG, Watson D, Park T, Hiller W, Fisher ER, Wickerham DL, Bryant J, Wolmark N (2004) A multigene assay to predict recurrence of tamoxifen-treated, node-negative breast cancer. N Engl J Med 351:2817–2826

Paik S, Tang G, Kim C, Baker J, Kim W, Cronin M, Baehner FL, Watson D, Bryant J, Costantino JP, Geyer CE, Wickerham DL, Wolmark N (2006) Gene expression and benefit of chemotherapy in women with node-negative, estrogen receptor-positive breast cancer. J Clin Oncol 23:3726–3734

Paradiso A, Schittulli F, Cellamare G, Mangia A, Marzullo F, Lorusso V, De Lena M (2001) Randomized clinical trial of adjuvant fluorouracil, epirubicin, and cyclophosphamide chemotherapy for patients with fast-proliferating, node-negative breast cancer. J Clin Oncol 19:3929–3937

Paradiso A, Volpe S, Iacobacci A, Marubini E, Verderio P, Costa A et al (2002) Quality control for biomarker determination in oncology: the experience of the Italian Network for Quality Assessment of Tumour Biomarkers (INQAT). Int J Biol Markers 2002; 17:201–214

Perou CM, Sorlie T, Eisen MB et al (2000) Molecular portraits of human breast tumours. Nature 406:747–752

Porter PL, Malone KE, Heagerty PJ, Alexander GM, Gatti LA, Firpo EJ, Daling JR, Roberts JM (1997) Expression of cell-cycle regulators p27Kip1 and cyclin E, alone and in combination, correlate with survival in young breast cancer patients. Nat Med 3:222–225

Porter PL, Barlow WE, Yeh IT, Lin MG, Yuan XP, Donato E, Sledge GW, Shapiro CL, Ingle JN, Haskell CM, Albain KS, Roberts JM, Livingston RB, Hayes DF (2006) p27(Kip1) and cyclin E expression and breast cancer survival after treatment with adjuvant chemotherapy. J Natl Cancer Inst. 98:1723–1731

Rouzier R, Perou CM, Symmans WF, Ibrahim N, Cristofanilli M, Anderson K, Hess KR, Stec J, Ayers M, Wagner P, Morandi P, Fan C, Rabiul I, Ross JS, Hortobagyi GN, Pusztai L (2005) Breast cancer molecular subtypes respond differently to preoperative chemotherapy. Clin Cancer Res 11:5678–5685

Rudolph P, Kuhling H, Alm P, Ferno M, Baldetorp B, Olsson H, Parwaresch R (2003) Differential prognostic impact of the cyclins E and B in premenopausal and postmenopausal women with lymph node-negative breast cancer. Int J Cancer 105:674–680

Schiller AB, Clark WS, Cotsonis G, et al. Image cytometric bcl-2:bax and bcl-2:bcl-x ratios in invasive breast carcinoma: correlation with prognosis. Cytometry 2002; 50:203–209

Silvestrini R, Luisi A, Zambetti M, Cipriani S, Valagussa P, Bonadonna G, et al. Cell proliferation and outcome following doxorubicin plus CMF regimens in node-positive breast cancer. Int J Cancer 2000; 87:405–411

Smid M, Wang Y, Klijn JG, Sieuwerts AM, Zhang Y, Atkins D, Martens JW, Foekens JA (2006) Genes associated with breast cancer metastatic to bone. J Clin Oncol 24:2261–2267

Sorlie T, Perou CM, Tibshirani R, Aas T, Geisler S, Johnsen H, Hastie T, Eisen MB, van de Rijn M, Jeffrey SS, Thorsen T, Quist H, Matese JC, Brown PO, Botstein D, Eystein Lonning P, Borresen-Dale AL (2001) Gene expression patterns of breast carcinomas distinguish tumor subclasses with clinical implications. Proc Natl Acad Sci USA 98:10869–10874

Sotiriou C, Neo SY, McShane LM, Korn EL, Long PM, Jazaeri A, Martiat P, Fox SB, Harris AL, Liu ET (2003) Breast cancer classification and prognosis based on gene expression profiles from a population-based study. Proc Natl Acad Sci USA 100:10393–10398

Span PN, Tjan-Heijnen VCG, Manders P, Beex LVAM, Sweep CGJ (2003) Cyclin-E is a strong predictor of endocrine therapy failure in human breast cancer. Oncogene 22:4898–4904

Sweep CGJ, Geurts-Moespot J, Grebenschikov N, de Witte JH, Heuvel JJTM, Schmitt M, Duffy MJ, Jänicke F, Kramer MD, Foekens JA, Brünner N, Brugal G, Pedersen AN, Benraad TJ (1998) External quality assessment of trans-European multicentre antigen determinations (ELISA) of urokinase-type plasminogen activator (uPA) and its type-1 inhibitor (PAI-1) in human breast cancer tissue extracts. Br J Cancer 78:1434–1441

Tan P, Cady B, Wanner M, Worland P, Cukor B, Magi-Galluzzi C, Lavin P, Draetta G, Pagano M, Loda M (1997) The cell cycle inhibitor p27 is an independent prognostic marker in small (T1a,b) invasive breast carcinomas. Cancer Res 57:1259–1263

Thomssen C, Janicke F, Harbeck N (2003) Clinical relevance of prognostic factors in axillary node-negative breast cancer. Onkologie 26:438–445

Thor AD, Liu S, Moore II DH, Shi Q, Edgerton SM (2000) P21WAF1/CIP1 expression in breast cancer: associations with p53 and outcome. Breast Cancer Res Treat 61:33–43

Umekita Y, Ohi Y, Sagara Y, Yoshida H (2002) Expression of maspin predicts poor prognosis in breast cancer patients. Int J Cancer 100:452–455

Urriticoechea A, Smith IE, Dowsett M (2005) Proliferation marker Ki-67 in early breast cancer. J Clin Oncol 23:7212–7220

Volpi A, De Paola F, Nanni O, Granato AM, Bajorko P, Becciolini A, Scarpi E, Riccobon A, Balzi M, Amadori D (2000) Prognostic significance of biologic markers in node-negative breast cancer patients: a prospective study. Breast Cancer Res Treat 63:181–192

van't Veer LJ, Dai H, van de Vijver MJ et al (2002) Gene expression profiling predicts clinical outcome of breast cancer. Nature 415:530–536

van de Vijer MJ, He YD, van't Veer LJ et al (2002) A gene-expression signature as a predictor of survival in breast cancer. N Engl J Med 347:1999–2009

Wang Y, Klijn JG, Zhang Y, Sieuwerts AM, Look MP, Yang F, Talantov D, Timmermans M, Meijer-van Gelder ME, Yu J, Jatkoe T, Berns EM, Atkins D, Foekens JA (2005) Gene-expression profiles to predict distant metastasis of lymph-node-negative primary breast cancer. Lancet 365:671–679

Watson PH, Chia SK, Wykoff CC et al (2003) Carbonic anhydrase XII is a marker of good prognosis in invasive breast carcinoma. Br J Cancer 88:1065–1070

Whitfield ML, George LK, Grant GD, Perou CM (2006) Common markers of proliferation. Nature Reviews Cancer 6:99–106

Wu Z, Shen Z-Z, Lu J-S, Jiang M, Han Q-X, Fontana JA, Barsky SH, Shao Z-M (1999) Prognostic role of p27Kip1 and apoptosis in human breast cancer. Br J Cancer 79:1572–1578

Yang Q, Sakurai T, Yoshimura G et al (2003) Prognostic value of bcl-2 in invasive breast cancer receiving chemotherapy and endocrine therapy. Oncol Rep 10:121–125

Zemzoum I, Kates RE, Ross JS et al (2003) Invasion factors uPA/PAI-1 and HER2 status provide independent and complementary information on patient outcome in node-negative breast cancer. J Clin Oncol 21:1022–1028

Circulating Tumour Markers in Breast Cancer

4

Ettore Seregni, Antonio Coli, and Nicola Mazzuca

CONTENTS

Abstract

A large number of markers have been proposed for breast cancer, but among them only CA 15.3, CEA and cytokeratins (i.e. TPA, TPS and Cyfra 21.1) are currently used in clinical practice. Serum marker levels reflect tumour burden, and for this reason they are not sensitive enough to be used for screening and early diagnosis of primary breast cancer. By contrast, the role of tumour markers is established in the diagnosis of recurrent disease and in the evaluation of response to treatment. In the former case, however, prospective randomised studies are required to demonstrate any survival benefit when earlier therapeutic interventions are instituted upon elevation of serum markers. In the second case, tumour marker evaluation represents a simple, objective method for monitoring of therapeutic response that seems to offer significant advantages over conventional imaging methods (e.g., objectivity and modifications in tumour biology). Furthermore, research studies are ongoing to identify and validate new biochemical parameters that can be of use not only in advanced disease, but also in other stages of the diagnostic workup of breast cancer.

4.1 Introduction

Circulating tumour markers in patients affected by breast cancer have been known for several years. In contrast to markers detected in the primary tumour, they offer dynamic information regarding the clinical evolution of the neoplastic process. The major role of current blood markers is in the diagnosis of metastases and in evaluation of response to treatment. A large number of blood tumour markers have been proposed for breast cancer, but CA 15.3 and CEA or cytokeratins (i.e., TPA, TPS or Cyfra 21.1) are the most commonly used in clinical practice. The present review considers the basic principles in tumour marker detection, i.e., biological significance of the marker and measurement methodology, and the practice guidelines for tumour marker use in the clinic. Some thoughts on future perspectives will also be offered.

4.2 Breast Cancer Tumour Markers

4.2.1 MUC1

Different tests measure the serum levels of MUC1; the most widely used are CA 15.3, mucin-like associated antigen (MCA), CA 27.29 and CA 549. The differences among these tests derive from the immunoreagents, i.e., the monoclonal antibodies, used to detect epitopes on the MUC1 molecule. MUC1, also known as polymorphic epithelial mucin (PEM), is a large glycoprotein well expressed on the apical surface of most polarised epithelial cells of different organs including breast, stomach, pancreas, bladder and respiratory tract (Price and Tendler 1993; von Mensdorff-Pouilly et al. 2000). In normal breast tissue MUC1 is expressed in the ducts and acini from where it is released into the milk in soluble form or bound to milk fat globules. Neoplastic transformation is associated with disruption of normal cell polarisation and tissue architecture leading to MUC1 shedding in the bloodstream, where it can be measured by means of immunoassays. Biochemically, MUC1 is a high-molecular weight (from 250 to 1,000 kDa) glycoprotein consisting of a core protein moiety (apomucin) where a number of carbohydrate chains are attached to serines and threonines by O-glycosidic bonds. On a mass basis, O-linked carbohydrates form up to 80% of the molecule, and the length of the glucidic side chains varies from 1 to more then 20 residues. Structural analysis reveals the presence of three different domains: a large, high-glicosylated extracellular domain varying in length between 1,000 and 2,000 amino acids, a short transmembrane region and a cytoplasmic tail of 69 amino acids. The extracellular domain is composed of a variable number of multiple repeats of a 20-amino acid sequence referred to as the variable number tandem repeat (VNTR) domain. The number of repeats varies with the population studied and reflects the inherited polymorphism that is characteristic of the MUC1 gene. The fact that the extracellular domain protrudes much further into the pericellular space than most cell surface components suggests that the molecule might play an anti-adhesive role. By blocking the access to other membrane structures, MUC1 overexpression could, for instance, allow the neoplastic cell to escape detection by the immune system (Ligtemberg et al. 1992; Ogata et al. 1992). This could explain the negative prognostic significance of MUC1 overexpression often observed in breast cancer. In addition, other clues about the biological significance of MUC1 have been reported (Hudson et al. 2001; Schreiber et al. 2000). These studies indicate that MUC1 can activate membrane receptors for growth factors, reduce E-cadherin-mediated cell adhesion, thereby promoting cell migration, and reduce the cellular apoptotic response to oxidative stress (Quin and McGuckin 2000; Schroeder et al. 2001; Li et al. 2001; Yin et al. 2003).

Circulating MUC1 displays a high degree of heterogeneity both in normal subjects and, even more so, in neoplastic patients. This heterogeneity is due either to the proteic (polymorphism of VNTR domain) or the glucidic portion of the molecule. In tumours, polysaccharide side chains are generally shorter and less branched than those on the normally expressed molecule. Furthermore, aberrant glycosylation can occur and the actual glycosylation pattern of circulating MUC1 is largely unpredictable (Kirnarsky et al. 2000). A large series of monoclonal antibodies against MUC1 have been raised, and most of them react with the core protein, and particularly with the hydrophilic sequence PDTRPAP (Norum et al. 2001; Rye and McGuckin 2001). However, carbohydrates may represent the target of individual antibodies and, in any case, they are able to interfere with the monoclonal antibody reactivity with proteic epitopes. The heterogeneity of MUC1 glycosylation explains how different tests directed to detect circulating MUC1 can give discordant results. CA 15.3 is the most widely used test to assay MUC1 and can be considered the gold standard. CA 15.3 is a sandwich capture assay that uses the monoclonal antibodies 115D8 (raised against human milk fat globule membranes) and DF3 (against a membrane-enriched fraction of metastatic human breast carcinoma) (Hayes et al. 1985, 1986). As mentioned before, several tests are now available to detect circulating MUC1 in patients affected by breast cancer, including MCA, CA 549, breast cancer mucin (BCM), EMCA, M26 and M29. In 1998, CA 27.29 was approved by the FDA for clinical use in the detection of recurrent breast cancer in patients with stage II or III disease. CA 27.29 is measured using a solid-phase competitive immunoassay in which the monoclonal antibody B27.29

is used either as a "catcher" or as a "tracer". This monoclonal antibody recognises the same proteic epitope on the MUC1 core sequence as is recognised by the monoclonal DF3, but the binding of B27.29 does not seem to be influenced by the presence of glucidic residues (i.e., sialic acid) (Reddish et al. 1992). This property could offer advantages in terms of the diagnostic accuracy of CA 27.29 in comparison with the "classic" CA 15.3.

4.2.2 Carcinoembryonic Antigen (CEA)

CEA is one of the first tumour markers to be identified and characterised (Gold and Freedman 1965). Since its discovery, CEA has been investigated in a wide range of malignancies, including breast cancer. CEA is a single-chain glycoprotein of 641 amino acids with a molecular mass of 150–300 kDa containing 45%–55% carbohydrate. Immunobiological and biochemical studies have revealed that CEA consists of a large family of at least 30 closely related cell-surface glycoproteins encoded by about 10 genes located on chromosome 19 (Berling et al. 1990; Benchimol et al. 1989). The domain structure of CEA proteins and γ heavy chain of the immunoglobulin IgG are very similar, indicating that CEA is part of the immunoglobulin gene "superfamily". This finding suggests that CEA proteins may be involved in the intercellular or cellular-matrix recognition mechanisms. CEA can be measured by a number of commercially available immunoassays using either a radioisotope or a non-radioactive (i.e., enzyme or chemiluminescent) label.

4.2.3 Cytokeratins

Several widely used tumour markers such as TPA, TPS and Cyfra 21.1 are molecules that structurally belong to the family of cytokeratins (CKs). CKs constitute one of the seven classes of intermediates filaments that, together with microtubules and actin microfilaments, make up the cytoskeleton of most eukaryotic cells (Steiner and Roop 1988; Nagle 1988). Human CKs comprise 20 related polypeptides (CKs 1–20), which, on the basis of sequence homologies, can be separated into two subfamilies. CKs 9–20 are the more acidic, type-I CKs, while CKs 1–8 form the neutral/basic type-II group of proteins. The most interesting feature of CK expression is that different epithelial cells express a characteristic, differentiation-dependent combination of two or more CKs, with type-I and type II polypeptides always occurring in stechiometric amounts (i.e., as "pairs"). In simple epithelial cells from many tissues, the combinations CK8/CK18 and CK8/CK19 are very often expressed. These pairs of CKs are also very commonly found in the vast majority of epithelial carcinomas comprising breast cancer (Moll 1994; Bodenmuller et al. 1994; Sundrstrom and Stigbrand 1994). Different tumour marker assays measuring CK8, CK18 and CK19 fragments have been developed. The most widely used among them are TPA, TPS and Cyfra 21.1. The TPA test recognises all three CKs (CK8, CK18 and CK19), TPS measures CK8 and CK18, and Cyfra 21.1 detects CK8 and CK19.

4.3 Guidelines for Tumour Marker Use in Breast Cancer

Appropriate clinical guidelines or protocols can help physicians in adopting an evidence-based approach to medicine. Several international and national expert groups have worked to develop practice guidelines that include recommendations for the appropriate use of serum tumour markers in breast cancer. The guidelines formulated by the American Society of Clinical Oncology (ASCO) in 1996 (updated in 1997, 1998 and in 2000) (American Society of Clinical Oncology 1996, 1997; Bast et al. 2001;, Smith et al. 1999), by the National Federation of French Cancer Centres in 2000 (Basuyau et al. 2003) and by the European Group of Tumour Markers (EGTM) in 1999 (updated in 2005) (Molina et al. 2005) have all been widely employed. In the following section the appropriate applications of tumour markers in the diagnostic work-up of patients affected by breast cancer will be discussed, with reference to the above-mentioned guidelines, literature reports and the experience of our Institute (Molina and Gion 1998; Stearns et al. 1998; Cheung et al. 2000; Duffy 2001; Sturgeon 2002). Table 4.1 shows the established and potential roles of tumour markers in breast cancer management.

Table 4.1. Role of tumour markers in breast cancer management

Role	Comment
Determining risk	Not established. In evaluation for hormonal markers
Screening	No role
Early diagnosis	No role
Prognosis	Established. In evaluation the independent role of tumour markers in respect to other prognostic factors
Diagnosis of recurrences	Established. In evaluation the clinical utility in decreasing mortality
Predict response to therapy	Not established. In evaluation the role of HER-2 in predicting resistance to hormonal and chemical therapy
Monitor therapy	Established. In evaluation the efficacy in respect to imaging techniques

4.3.1 Screening and Early Diagnosis

Currently, no tumour marker exists that can be used for either screening or the early diagnosis of breast cancer. In fact, the diagnostic accuracy of tumour marker evaluation is limited by low sensitivity in early stage disease and by lack of specificity. Regarding CA 15.3, for instance, different studies have demonstrated that the diagnostic sensitivity of the test is about 10–15%, 20–25% and 30–45% in patients with stage I, stage II and stage III, respectively. Furthermore, increased levels of CA 15.3 can be observed in several non-neoplastic conditions including benign breast pathology, chronic liver disorders and immunological diseases. Recent reports indicate that CA 27.29 is a more sensitive test than CA 15.3; however, despite this diagnostic improvement low levels of CA 27.29 in patients suspected of having breast cancer do not exclude the presence of malignancy, at either primary or loco-regional sites (Gion et al. 2001).

4.3.2 Prognosis

Different studies have demonstrated that the pre-surgery CA 15.3 level is a prognostic factor, with both disease-free survival (DFS) and overall survival (OS) being shorter in patients with a high value for this marker (Duffy et al. 2000; Ebeling et al. 2002). However, it has not been proven that CA 15.3 is an independent prognostic factor. Some reports indicate that an initially elevated CA 15.3 level is a marker of enhanced risk of recurrence and mortality in both the early and late stage of breast cancer. In a study by Gion et al. (2002), the prognostic role of CA 15.3 was investigated in 362 node-negative breast cancer patients. Use of an interesting statistical approach revealed a continuous relationship between CA 15.3 and relapse-free survival, with increasing risk starting from a marker level of approximately 10 U/ml. Data about the ability of CEA to predict prognosis are much more conflicting. Reports have been published suggesting worse, unaffected or even better prognosis when CEA elevation is present at the time of diagnosis (Gaglia et al. 1988; Jong-Bakker et al. 1981; Cantwell et al. 1980; Wang et al. 1975). For these reasons CEA determination is of limited clinical utility. Very few studies have been published regarding the prognostic role of cytokeratin markers in breast cancer. In one study performed in 86 primary breast cancer patients, it was observed that serum Cyfra 21.1 levels were an independent indicator of prognosis. Patients with serum Cyfra 21.1 titer >3.5 ng/ml had a significantly shorter OS and DFS than those with lower serum titers (Nakata et al. 2000). The results of this study are very encouraging; however, before the adoption of Cyfra 21.1 as a prognosticator, they need to be confirmed by more extensive evaluations.

4.3.3 Early Diagnosis of Locoregional and/or Metastatic Recurrence

Blood tumour marker measurements have a minimal role in diagnosing loco-regional recurrence since the diagnosis can generally easily be made clinically or radiologically. By contrast, serial tumour marker determinations can be useful tools in the diagnosis of metastatic breast cancer. In the presence of distant metastases, the clinical sensitivity of CA 15.3 in different studies has ranged from 50% to 90% depending on the anatomical site (e.g., liver metastases are associated with the highest sensitivity, followed by skeletal and lung metastases) and the number or size of metastatic foci. Combining the results from seven different studies, it was shown by the Expert Panel of ASCO that about two thirds of patients (235 out of 352 patients) had CA 15.3 elevations either before or at the time of recurrence, with a lead time ranging from 2 to 9 months (American Society of Clinical Oncology 1996; Safi et al. 1989; Colomer et al. 1989; Nicolini et al. 1991; Repetto et al. 1993; Al-Jarallah et al. 1993; Soletormos et al. 1993; Markopoulos et al. 1994). In the same meta-analysis, 1,320 patients out of 1,435 without evidence of recurrence had normal CA 15.3 levels (diagnostic specificity of 92%). More recently, however, less positive results were obtained by Kokko et al. (2002) in a prospective study carried out on 243 patients. During 5 years of follow-up, 59 patients relapsed and CA 15.3 was elevated in only 21 (36%) of them. The test failed to detect locoregional relapses but, interestingly, also pulmonary-only recurrences and half of bone-only metastases were also associated with low levels of CA 15.3. The conclusions of this study are similar to those of our investigations published in the early 1990s (Crippa et al. 1992; Bombardieri et al. 1992). In those studies we found that locoregional lymph node or cutaneous metastases were generally CA 15.3 negative and that single metastastic skeletal lesions gave elevated serum levels only in a small number of patients. CA 27.29 seems to be more effective in detecting tumour relapse. In one prospective multicenter study, 193 patients with primary breast cancer were considered for the follow-up and among them there were 26 recurrences. Of these, 15 showed CA 27.29 positivity (sensitivity of 57.7%), with a median lead time from the first marker elevation of 5.3 months (Chan et al. 1997). Three patients with marker elevation had no evidence of recurrence and were considered as false positives (specificity 98%).

Despite the results obtained with MUC1 markers in predicting the diagnosis of metastatic disease, several points are still controversial. The first is that tumour markers are not sensitive enough to detect micrometastatic disease and that marker elevation during the postoperative follow-up is generally associated with a large tumour burden. The second point is related to the fact that effective and reliable therapeutic opportunities for advanced breast cancer are still lacking, and this makes the need of "early" detection of recurrence questionable. In an attempt to address these points, only two small-scale pilot studies have been carried out. In a preliminary randomised study by Jager et al. (1994), it has been shown that treatment of recurrences based only on increased CEA and CA 15.3 reduce the risk of developing metastasis from 88% to 39% at 12 months and prolong the DFS. In a retrospective, non-randomised study of 384 patients, Nicolini et al. (1997) evaluated the role of early therapeutic intervention based on the tumour markers CA 15.3, CEA and TPA. Among relapsed patients, 28 patients were treated on the basis of tumour marker elevations, while 22 patients were treated after instrumental diagnosis of metastases. An improvement of OS was observed when patients were treated as a consequence of only marker elevation (42.9% versus 22.7% at 72 months). Large prospective, randomised trials are now necessary to confirm these preliminary results.

CEA is still a widely used test for the surveillance of breast cancer patients and, frequently, this marker is assessed in combination with CA 15.3. Nevertheless, the individual role of CEA in breast cancer monitoring has been recently discussed. In this regard, the conclusions of the study of Guadagni et al. (2001) seem of outstanding interest. In a large prospective longitudinal study, CEA was evaluated in comparison to CA 15.3, during post-surgical follow-up of 549 patients. CEA was elevated in 38% and CA 15.3 in 70% of patients with recurrence. The combination of CEA and CA 15.3 increased the overall sensitivity by only 1.4%. The authors conclude that in their experience CEA should be considered as an expensive and inefficient method of follow-up, providing no additional value when used in combination with CA 15.3.

Cytokeratins, including TPA, TPS and Cyfra 21.1, have been reported to be useful in monitoring breast cancer. However, insufficient data are available to recommend the routine use of cytokeratin markers during the follow-up of breast cancer patients. Further prospective studies are necessary to validate the role of cytokeratins in breast neoplasms.

4.3.4 Therapy Monitoring

The use of tumour markers in the monitoring of therapeutic response in patients with metastatic breast cancer has been well investigated. CA 15.3 was found to be superior to the other "conventional" markers. This marker has been shown to be useful in the monitoring of response to either endocrine therapy or cytotoxic tharapy. Summarising the results of 11 studies, the ASCO Panel, however, found that in patients with responsive disease CA 15.3 serum levels decreased in about two thirds of cases; 73% of those with stable disease had no significant changes in marker concentrations, and 80% with progressive disease showed increased CA 15.3 levels (American Society of Clinical Oncology 1996). The risk of removing a patient from effective therapy due to the marker misclassification led the panel to conclude that "a marker cannot, in any situation, stand alone to define response to treatment". Nevertheless, Robertson et al. retrospectively derived and prospectively validated a biochemical score index using three markers, i.e., CA 15.3, CEA and erythrocyte sedimentation rate (ESR) (Robertson et al. 1999). In their experience this score system not only correlates with conventional UICC imaging criteria in the monitoring of therapeutic response, but seems to offer advantages in terms of reproducibility, diagnostic accuracy and cost savings. Furthermore, tumour markers represent the easiest way to evaluate response to systemic therapy for neoplastic disease that cannot be assessed by UICC criteria, e.g., pleural and peritoneal effusions, irradiated lesions, bone marrow infiltration and bone metastases. At least two points need to be borne in mind in order to interpret marker results correctly. First, the magnitude of variation ("critical difference") between successive marker levels that constitutes a clinically significant change is not well defined. This "critical difference" depends on both the analytical imprecision of the assay and the normal intra-individual biological variation. For CA 15.3, it has been estimated that at least a 30% change is required before successive marker concentrations can be regarded as significantly altered (Soletormos et al. 1993). Another point to be considered is the occurrence of "tumour marker spike" (Hayes et al. 1988; Yasaever et al. 1997). This is a paradoxical increase in tumour marker levels following initiation of chemotherapy due to massive neoplastic cell necrosis induced by cytotoxic agents. The phenomenon can be observed in up to 30% of patients who show a response to therapy. The peak usually occurs within 30 days from the commencement of therapy, but marker levels can remain elevated for as long as 3 months.

4.4 Perspectives

While the diagnostic relevance of conventional tumour marker is well established in breast cancer patients with metastatic disease, different laboratory and clinical studies are now ongoing to identify and validate new biochemical parameters that will be of use not only in advanced disease, but also in other stages of the diagnostic work up of breast cancer. In this section, the most promising and relevant aspects of this research will be briefly summarised.

4.4.1 Risk Assessment

Different studies have demonstrated that the "hormonal milieu" can be considered an important factor predisposing to breast cancer. High circulating levels of different hormones have been found to represent a risk factor for breast cancer development. Elevated concentrations of prolactin, insulin, insulin-like growth factor type I (IGF-I) and androgens (i.e., testosterone and adrenal androgens) are frequently detectable in subjects who finally develop malignant breast neoplasms. The causal role and the associated risk of individual hormones, however, remain largely to be defined.

4.4.2 Prognostic Markers

In recent years several circulating molecules have been revealed to be associated with patient outcome. These potential prognostic markers are involved in different processes of neoplastic transformation and progression, e.g., cell proliferation and its control, angiogenesis and metastatic spread (Arciero et al. 2003; Heer et al. 2001). Among them, cyclines and p53 (cell cycle controllers), matrix metalloproteases, urokinase plasminogen activator (uPA) and its inhibitor PA1-1, cathepsins (involved in local invasion and metastases) and vascular endothelial growth factors (angiogenesis) deserve particular mention. Although these form a very promising group of markers, the real impact of their application in clinical practice is currently unknown.

4.4.3 Predicting Response Markers

This group includes markers able to predict response or resistance to a specific therapy. Circulating HER-2 is the most representative example. HER-2 (also known as c-erbB2) oncoprotein is a 185 kD transmembrane glycoprotein showing structural and functional homology with the epidermal growth factor receptor. HER-2 overexpression, present in 20–30% of primary breast cancer, is associated with poor prognosis, short survival and recurrences. Like many cell surface transmembrane receptors, HER-2 can be proteolytically cleaved, and its ectodomain can be released as soluble molecules of about 105 kDa into the circulation. Circulating HER-2 ectodomain can be detected in about 80% of patients with tumour overexpressing HER-2 compared to 3% of those with tumours not overexpressing the oncoprotein. The negative prognostic effect of high circulating levels of HER-2 ectodomain seems to be related to the resistance to chemotherapy (Pegram et al. 1998; Mehta et al. 1998). This has been demonstrated in patients with metastatic disease before application of first-line chemotherapy with a combination of paclitaxel and doxorubicin. In a prospective pilot study it was found that the probability of obtaining a complete response and the duration of response were significantly lower and shorter in patients with elevated HER-2 ectodomain than in patients with low levels of the marker (0% and 7.5 months versus 26% and 11 months, respectively) (Colomer et al. 2000). Furthermore, the evaluation of circulating HER-2 ectodomain can be employed, as a surrogate marker, in identification of patients who will be benefit from trastuzumab treatment and, perhaps, to monitor this "target therapy" (Wu 2002).

4.4.4 Markers of Bone Metabolism

In addition to the traditional parameters such as serum alkaline phosphatase and urinary calcium and hydroxyproline, different circulating biochemical markers have recently gained clinical attention because of their accuracy in assessing the dynamic changes in bone remodelling (Seregni et al. 2001). Bone-specific alkaline phosphatase (BAP), osteocalcin and procollagen peptides, e.g., procollagen type I carboxyterminal propeptide (PICP) and procollagen type I aminoterminal propeptide (PINP), have been proposed as markers of bone formation, while amino or carboxy-telopeptides of type I collagen (NTX, CTx), tartrate-resistant acid phosphatase (TRAP) are markers of bone resorption. Different studies have demonstrated that these markers are not sensitive enough to be adopted in the early diagnosis of bone metastases (Bombardieri et al. 1997). By contrast the evaluation of bone metabolic markers can offer useful information in the monitoring of antineoplastic therapy of patients with skeletal metastases or in the evaluation of treatment-induced osteoporosis (Martinetti et al. 1997).

4.4.5 Proteomic Approach for the Identification of New Markers

Recent advances in mass spectrometry (MS) technology, such as surface-enhanced laser desorption/ionization time of flight (SELDI-TOF) MS, are opening up a new scenario in the discovery of disease-associated proteins in complex biological fluids such as serum or plasma. Adopting these technologies, serum samples can be rapidly visualized as a proteomic fingerprint in which it will be possible identify tumour-specific proteins (Wulfkuhle et al. 2003). Among the array of existing proteins in a patient's serum (serum proteoma), of particular interest is having those of low molecular weight (<20 kDa) (serum peptidoma), which can represent biomarker fragments generated by specific enzymatic activity of tumour cells (Liotta and Petricoin 2006). Preliminary results seem to indicate the great potential of this diagnostic approach in early detection of breast cancer (Li et al. 2005).

4.4.6 Circulating Tumour Cell

The development of distant metastases in breast cancer patients is based on the fact that tumour cells dissociating from primary cancer access to circulation either directly into blood vessels or through the lymphatic system. Thus, the detection of such cells in patients with primary breast cancer can be predictive of future distant metastases. Various detection techniques have been used for the identification of tumour cells in the peripheral blood of breast cancer patients, and among them immunocytochemistry (ICC) and reverse-trancriptase polymerase chain reaction (RT-PCR) are the most used (Braun and Naume 2005; Zach and Lutz 2006). Epithelial cytokeratins and mammoglobin mainly represent the target proteins or the marker gene expression. Different authors have demonstrated that the detection of tumour cells in peripheral blood is more frequently observed in the advanced than in the early stage and is significantly related to the lymph node status and presence of metastases at diagnosis (Zehentner et al. 2004; Taubert et al. 2004). In few studies the presence of circulating tumour cells was found to have prognostic relevance, being associated to shorter disease-free survival (Stathopoulos et al. 2005). Tumor cell detection in peripheral blood represents an interesting approach in cancer diagnosis; however, different limitations, such as technical difficulties, lack of reproducibility, controversial results, choice of target genes or proteins, led to us to consider this approach as still experimental, and it cannot yet be taken into account for clinical decisions.

4.5 Conclusion

Measurement of circulating tumour marker levels in breast cancer is most established in advanced disease. In this situation, its clinical role is to detect recurrences in asymptomatic patients and to monitor antineoplastic treatments. In both cases the potential diagnostic and clinical utility of tumour markers has not yet been fully explored. This is of relevance when we consider the current important advances in imaging techniques and therapeutic modalities. Furthermore, intensive efforts have been made in basic and translational laboratory research in order to refine the measurement of existing markers, to develop better marker assays and to discover new markers with the ultimate goal of exploiting their use in the screening and early diagnosis of primary breast cancer.

References

Al-Jarallah MA et al (1993) Serum CA 15-3 and CEA patterns in postsurgical follow-up and in monitoring clinical course of metastatic cancer in patients with breast carcinoma. Eur J Surg Oncol 19:74–79

American Society of Clinical Oncology (1996) Clinical practice guidelines for the use of tumor markers in breast and colorectal cancer. J Clin Oncol 14:2843–2877

American Society of Clinical Oncology (1998) 1997 update of recommendations for the use of tumor markers in breast and colorectal cancer. J Clin Oncol 16:793–795

Arciero C et al (2003) Functional relationship and gene ontology classification of breast cancer biomarkers. Int J Biol Markers 18:241–272

Bast RC et al for the American Society of Clinical Oncology Tumor Markers Expert Panel (2001) Recommendations for the use of tumor markers in breast and colorectal cancer. J Clin Oncol 19:1865–1878

Basuyau JP et al (2003) Summary report of the standards, options and recommendations for the use of serum tumour markers on breast cancer: 2000. Br J Cancer 89:532–534

Benchimol S et al (1989) Carcinoembryonic antigen, a human tumor marker, functions as a intercellular adhesion molecule. Cell 57:327–334

Berling B et al (1990) Molecular cloning of a carcinoembryonic antigen (CEA)-gene family-member expressed in leukocytes of chronic myeloid leukemia patients and bone marrow. Cancer Res 50:6534–6539

Bodenmuller H et al (1994) The tumor markers TPA, TPS, TPAcyk and CYFRA 21-1 react differently with the keratins 8, 18 and 19. Int J Biol Markers 9:70–74

Bombardieri E et al (1992) CA 15.3 determination in patients with breast cancer: clinical utility for the detection of distant metastases. Eur J Cancer 294:144–146

Bombardieri E et al (1997) Can bone metabolism markers be adopted as an alternative to scintigraphic imaging in monitoring bone metastases from breast cancer? Eur J Nucl Med 24:1349–1355

Braun S, Naume B (2005) Circulating and disseminated tumor cells. J Clin Oncol 23:1623–1626

Cantwell B et al (1980) Carcino-embryonic antigen assay as a guide to tumour bulk, response to therapy and prognosis in human breast cancer. J Med Sci 149: 469–474

Chan DW et al (1997) Use of truquant BR radioimmunoassay for early detection of breast cancer recurrence in patients with stage II and stage III disease. J Clin Oncol 15: 2322–2328

Cheung KL et al (2000) Tumour marker measurements in the diagnosis and monitoring of breast cancer. Cancer Treat Rev 26:91–102

Colomer R et al (1989) Circulating CA 15-3 levels in the postsurgical follow-up of breast cancer patients and in nonmalignant diseases. Breast Cancer Res Treat 13: 123–133

Colomer R et al (2000) Circulating HER2 extracellular domain and resistance to chemotherapy in advanced breast cancer. Clin Cancer Res 6:2356–2362

Crippa F et al (1992) Single determination of CA 15 and bone scintigraphy in the diagnosis of skeletal metastases of breast cancer. J Nucl Biol Med 36:115–116

Duffy MJ et al (2000) CA 15.3: a prognostic marker in breast cancer. Int J Biol Marker 15:330–333

Duffy MJ (2001) Biochemical markers in breast cancer: which ones are clinically useful? Clin Biochem 34:347–352
Ebeling FG et al (2002) Serum CEA and CA 15-3 as prognostic factors in primary breast cancer. Br J Cancer 86:1217–1222
Gaglia P et al (1988) Prognostic value of CEA and ferritin assay in breast cancer: a multivariate analysis. Eur J Cancer Clin Oncol 24:1151–1155
Gion M et al (2001) CA 27.29: a valuable marker for breast cancer management. A confirmatory multicentric study on 603 cases. Eur J Cancer 37:355–363
Gion M et al (2002) Prognostic role of serum CA 15.3 in 362 node-negative breast cancers: An old player for a new game. Eur J Cancer 38:1181–1188
Gold P, Freedman SO (1965) Demonstration of tumor-specific antigens in human colonic carcinoma by immunological tolerance and absorption techniques. J Exp Med 121:439–562
Guadagni F et al (2001) A re-evaluation of carcinoembryonic antigen (CEA) as a serum marker for breast cancer: a prospective longitudinal study. Clin Cancer Res 7:2357–2362
Hayes DF et al (1985) Use of murine monoclonal antibody for detection of circulating plasma DF3 antigen levels in breast cancer patients. J Clin Invest 75:1671–1678
Hayes DF et al (1986) Comparison of circulating CA 15.3 and carcinoembryonic antigen levels in patients with breast cancer. J Clin Oncol 10:1542–1550
Hayes DF et al (1988) CA 15.3 and CEA spikes during chemotherapy for metastatic breast cancer. Proc Am Soc Clin Oncol 7:38a
Heer K et al (2001) Serum vascular endothelial growth factor in breast cancer: its relation with cancer type and estrogen receptor status. Clin Cancer Res 7:3491–3494
Hudson MJ et al (2001) Human MUC1 mucin: a potent glandular morphogen. J Pathol 194:373–383
Jäger W et al (1994) Increasing serum tumour markers as decision criteria for hormone-therapy of metastatic breast cancer. Tumor Biol 12:60–66
Jong-Bakker MD et al (1981) Prognostic significance of CEA in breast cancer: a statistical study. Eur J Cancer Clin Oncol 17:1307–1313
Kirnarsky L et al (2000) Structural effects of O-glycosylation on a 15-residue peptide from the mucin (MUC1) core protein. Biochemistry 39:12076–12082
Kokko R et al (2002) CA 15-3 in the follow-up of localised breast cancer: a prospective study. Eur J Cancer 38:1189–1193
Li J et al (2005) Indipendent validation of candidate breast cancer serum biomarkers identified by mass spectrometry. Clin Chem 51:2229–2235
Li Y et al (2001) The c-Src tyrosine kinase regulated signaling of the human DF3/MUC1 carcinoma-associated antigen with GSK3ß and ß-catenin. J Biol Chemistry 276:6061–6064
Ligtemberg MJL et al (1992) Suppression of cellular aggregation by high levels of episialin. Cancer Res 52: 2318–2324
Liotta LA, Petricoin EF (2006) Serum peptidome for cancer detection: spinning biologic trash into diagnostic gold. J Clin Invest 116:26–30
Markopoulos CJ et al (1994) CA 15-3 in the prediction of recurrence of breast cancer. Breast Dis 7:1–5
Martinetti A et al (1997) Serum markers of bone metastases in post-menopausal breast cancer patients treated with Formestane. Tumor Biol 18:197–205
Mehta RR et al (1998) Plasma c-erbB-2 levels in breast cancer patients: prognostic significance in predicting response to chemotherapy. J Clin Oncol 16:2409–2416
Molina R, Gion M (1998) Use of blood tumour markers in the detection of recurrent breast cancer. Breast 7:187–189
Molina R et al (2005) Tumor markers in breast cancer-European Group on Tumor Markers recommendation. Tumor Biol 26:281–293
Moll R (1994) Cytokeratins in the histological diagnosis of malignant tumors. Int J Biol Markers 9:63–69
Nagle R (1988) Intermediate filaments: a review of the basic biology. Am J Surg Pathol 12:4–16
Nakata B et al (2000) Serum CYFRA 21-1 is one of the most reliable tumor markers for breast carcinoma. Cancer 89:1285–1290
Nicolini A et al (1991) Evaluation of serum CA 15-3 determination with CEA and TPA in the post-operative follow-up of breast cancer patients. Br J Cancer 64:154–158
Nicolini A et al (1997) Prolonged survival by "early" salvage treatment of breast cancer for patients: a retrospective 6-year study. Brit J Cancer 76:1106–1111
Norum LF et al (2001) New immunoassays for MUC1 breast cancer. Tumor Biol 22:216–222
Ogata S et al (1992) Mucins bearing the cancer-associated sialosyl-Tn antigen mediate inhibition of natural killer cell cytotoxicity. Cancer Res 52:4741–4764
Pegram MD et al (1998) Her-2/neu as a predictive marker of response to breast cancer therapy. Breast Cancer Res Treat 52:65–77
Price MR, Tendler JB (1993) Polymorphic epithelial mucins (PEM): molecular characteristic and association with breast cancer. Breast 2:3–7
Quin RJ, McGuckin A (2000). Phosphorylation of the cytoplasmic domain of the MUC1 mucin correlates with changes in cell-cell adhesion. Int J Cancer 87:499–506
Reddish MA et al (1992) Epitope mapping of Mab B27.29 within the protein core of the malignant breast carcinoma-associated mucin antigen MUC1. J Tumor Marker Oncol 7:19–27
Repetto L et al (1993) Serum CEA, CA 15-3 and MCA in breast cancer patients: a clinical evaluation. Cancer Detect Prev 17:411–415
Robertson JFR et al (1999) The objective measurement of remission and progression in metastatic breast cancer by use of serum tumour markers. Eur J Cancer 35:47–53
Rye PD, McGuckin MA (2001) MUC1: antibodies and immunoassays. Tumor Biol 22:269–272
Safi F et al (1989) Comparison of CA 15-3 and CEA in diagnosis and monitoring of breast cancer. Int J Biol Markers 4:207–214
Schreiber J et al (2000) Binding of tumor antigen mucin (MUC1) derived peptides to the heat shock protein DnaK. Anticancer Res 20:3093–3098
Schroeder JA et al (2001) Transgenic MUC1 interacts with epidemal growth factor receptor and correlates with mitogen-activated protein kinase activation in the mouse mammary gland. J Biol Chem 276:13057–13064
Seregni E et al (2001) Clinical utility of biochemical markers of bone remodelling in patients with bone metastases of solid tumors. QJ Nucl Med 45:7–17

Smith TJ et al for the American Society of Clinical Oncology Breast Cancer Surveillance Expert Panel (1999) American Society of Clinical Oncology 1998 update of recommended breast cancer surveillance guidelines. J Clin Oncol 17:1080–1082

Soletormos G et al (1993) A novel method for monitoring high-risk breast cancer with tumor markers: CA 15-3 compared to CEA and TPA. Ann Oncol 4:861–869

Soletormos G et al (1993) Interpretation of results for tumor markers on the basis of analytical imprecision and biological variation. Clin Chem 39:2077–2083

Stathopoulos EN et al (2005) Detection of CK-19 mRNA positive cells in peripheral blood of breast cancer patients with histologically and immunohistochemically negative axillary lymph nodes. Ann Oncol 16:240–246

Stearns V et al (1998) Circulating tumor markers in breast cancer: accepted utilities and novel prospects. Breast Cancer Res Treat 52:239–259

Steiner PM, Roop DR (1988) Molecular and cellular biology of intermediate filaments. Ann Rev Biochem 57:593–625

Sturgeon C (2002) Practice guidelines for tumor marker use in the clinic. Clin Chem 48:1151–1159

Sundrstrom BE, Stigbrand TI (1994) Cytokeratins and tissue polypepitde antigen. Int J Biol Markers 9:102–108

Taubert H et al (2004) Detection of disseminated tumor cells in peripheral blood of patients with breast cancer: correlation to nodal status and occurrence of metastases. Gyn Oncol 92:256–261

von Mensdorff-Pouilly S et al (2000) Human MUC1 mucin: a multifaceted glycoprotein. Int J Biol Markers 15:343–356

Wang DY et al (1975) Relationship between plasma carcinoembryonic antigen and prognosis in women with breast cancer. Eur J Cancer 11:615–618

Wu JT (2002) c-erbB2 oncoprotein and its soluble ectodomain: a new potential tumor marker for prognosis, early detection and monitoring patients undergoing Herceptin treatment. Clin Chim Acta 322:11–19

Wulfkuhle JD et al (2003) Proteomic application for the early detection of cancer. Nat Rev Cancer 3:267–275

Yasaever V et al (1997) Utility of CA 15.3 in monitoring breast cancer patients with bone metastases: special emphasis on "spiking" phenomenon. Clin Biochem 30:53–56

Yin L et al (2003) Human MUC1 carcinoma antigen regulates intracellular oxidant levels and the apoptotic response to oxidative stress. J Biol Chem 278:35458–35464

Zach O, Lutz D (2006) Tumor cell detection in peripheral blood and bone marrow. Curr Opin Oncol 18:48–56

Zehentner BK et al (2004) Mammoglobin as a novel breast cancer biomarker: multigen reverse transcription-PCR assay and sandwich ELISA. Clin Chem 50:2069–2076

Axillary Lymph Node Status Evaluation in Breast Cancer Patients: Role of SPECT and Pinhole SPECT with Cationic Lipophilic Radiotracers

5

Giuseppe Madeddu and Angela Spanu

CONTENTS

Abstract

The correct assessment of axillary lymph node status represents the most important goal in the preoperative phase of breast cancer patients since the presence of lymph node metastases together with primary tumor size can be considered, in the absence of distant metastatic localizations, the single most significant parameter to guide the therapeutic strategy and to better determine disease prognosis as well as serving as an indicator of the tumor ability to spread (Carter et al. 1989). In particular, the number of axillary metastatic nodes when it exceeds three is associated with a worse prognosis (Fisher et al. 1983; Carter et al. 1989; Saez et al. 1989). To date, the procedure of choice for pathological axillary status evaluation is represented by axillary lymph node dissection (ALND), which has a routine use in patients with newly ascertained invasive breast cancer in spite of its invasiveness and morbidity. However, ALND may not be necessary in many cases, in particular in early stage carcinomas with tumor size <10 mm and even more so when axillary clinical examination is negative, since in this case the percentage of lymph node metastases is very low. Moreover, even when axillary lymph node metastases are present, ALND may not affect the choice of adjuvant therapy and, apart from this, a change of treatment may give only a small survival benefit. Eventual complications and the costs of the procedure also have to be considered when the indication is equivocal. Thus, at present, the routine use of ALND is questionable.

5.1 Introduction

Non-invasive imaging procedures have been employed in the preoperative evaluation of axillary lymph nodes in breast cancer in order to avoid an unnecessary ALND. Mammography has not proved accurate for this purpose (Walsh et al. 1997) and neither has ultrasonography (Yang et al. 2000), which, although more sensitive than mammography, also presents limitations, in particular in the detection of non-palpable axillary metastatic lymph nodes. MRI has also been indicated, but has shown low sensitivity in small metastatic node identification (Yoshimura et al. 1999). Both mini-invasive and non-invasive nuclear medicine methods have also been employed as diagnostic tools. Among the former, radioisotopic lymphatic mapping combined with the radio-guided biopsy of sentinel lymph node (SN) procedure (RG-SLNB) has been proposed (Giuliano et al. 1994; Albertini et al. 1996; Pijpers et al. 1997; Krag et al. 1998; Gulec et al. 1998; Flett et al. 1998; Haigh et al. 2000; Boolbol et al. 2001) in order to avoid unnecessary ALND, such as in cases with early stage carcinomas and clinically negative axillae in which the probability of metastases is very low; this procedure has proved very effective to identify SN and highly accurate to predict lymph node status, also permitting the identification of micrometastatic foci in SN (Veronesi et al. 1997; Pijpers et al. 1997; Krag et al. 1998; Cox et al. 1998; Borgstein et al. 1998). According to the results obtained with this method, ALND could be avoided when SN is negative for metastasis, while it would be recommended when positive, though only in selected patients (Cox et al. 1998; Keshtgar et al. 2002). However, even if in a very low number of cases, the SN may not always be detected or may be false negative at histology; moreover, in other cases SN may be the only metastatic site, with the other axillary lymph nodes negative, and ALND, to which patients should be submitted according to conventional protocol, could be avoided. These considerations suggest that a further more accurate patient selection for ALND should be made; thus, in selected patients, other noninvasive diagnostic procedures could be employed, in combination with RGSLNB, as well as playing a useful role, even when RGSLNB is not indicated. For this purpose, there has been great interest in non-invasive nuclear medicine procedures, such as positron emission tomography (PET) with 2[^{18}F]fluoro-2-deoxy-glucose (FDG), which has shown a very high per-patient sensitivity and specificity in axillary metastatic node detection (Utech et al. 1996; Adler et al. 1997; Smith et al. 1998; Hubner et al. 2000; Greco et al. 2001), sometimes even without false-negative findings (Utech et al. 1996; Hubner et al. 2000). However, these data have not been confirmed by others (Ivancevic et al. 2000; Yutani et al. 2000; Guller et al. 2002; van der Hoeven et al. 2002), in particular in patients with small and few axillary lymph node metastases, even in very large casuistries (Wahl et al. 2004) and in the an early stage of the disease (Danforth et al. 2002; Barranger et al. 2003). Moreover, the data are still limited, and besides this, no result on the FDG-PET performance in defining the exact number of lymph nodes has been reported. Scintimammography with different gamma-emitting tumor-seeking radiotracers has also been employed in lymph node status evaluation in breast cancer patients. ^{201}Tl is a potassium analogue, and its uptake in tumor cells depends on the ATPase sodium-potassium transport system (Sehweil et al. 1989). Most studies have shown a high sensitivity value for 201Tl scintigraphy in patients with primary breast cancer, but low sensitivity in axillary lymph node metastasis detection (Sehweil et al. 1990; Waxman et al. 1993; Takahashi et al. 1994; Cimitan et al. 1995). The somatostatin analogue [^{111}In-DTPA-D-Phe1]-octreotide has also been used in some patients with breast cancer since in vitro studies have indicated that somatostatin receptors are present in this type of cancer (Bootsma et al. 1993). High sensitivity values in primary breast cancer detection have been reported by planar scintigraphy, while this procedure has proved less reliable in axillary lymph node status evaluation (van Eijck et al. 1994; Skanberg et al. 2002). Scintimammography with the cationic lipophilic radiotracers ^{99m}Tc-tetrofosmin and ^{99m}Tc-methoxyisobutylisonitrile (MIBI) have more recently had wider application in breast cancer axillary staging. Both radiotracers are routinely used for perfusion myocardial scintigraphy, but they have proved also to possess oncotropic properties. The uptake mechanism of these cationic lipophilic complexes in malignant cells is not yet well known, but in vitro studies have demonstrated that the uptake of these two radiotracers is favored by increased blood flow, capillary permeability and cellular elevated metabolic activity (Rodrigues et al. 2000) and that it is strictly dependent on cell membrane and mitochondrial potentials (Arbab et al. 1996; Bernard et al. 1998). However, a mechanism partially related to the Na^+/K^+ pump and N^+/H^+ antiport system has also been hypothesized for tetrofosmin (Arbab et al. 1997). ^{99m}Tc-tetrofosmin predominantly accumulates in the cytosol with only a small fraction in the mitochondria, while ^{99m}Tc-MIBI accumulates only in the mitochondria.

Both ^{99m}Tc-tetrofosmin and ^{99m}Tc-MIBI have proved in in-vivo studies to accumulate in many types of tumors (Caner et al. 1991; O'Tuama et al. 1990; Kao et al. 1993; Lind et al. 1997; Schillaci et al. 1999; Choi et al. 2000; Lee et al. 2001; Schillaci et al. 2003; Alonso et al. 2003; Spanu et al. 2003) including breast carcinoma (Khalkhali et al. 1994; Khalkhali et al. 1995; Palmedo et al. 1996; Waxman et al. 1997; Ortapamuk et al. 1999, Khalkhali et al. 2000; Nishiyama et al. 2001; Spanu et al. 2001) and its axillary lymph node metastases (Palmedo et al. 1996; Ortapamuk et al. 1999; Nishiyama et al. 2001; Spanu et al. 2001) and distant metastases (Cwikla et al. 1998; Yildiz et al. 2001; Spanu et al. 2003). An inverse correlation has been demonstrated between the uptake of these two radiotracers and the expression of p-glycoprotein, the latter being related to the multi-drug resistance of tumor cells; both ^{99m}Tc-tetrofosmin and ^{99m}Tc-MIBI have the property of being a substrate for p-glycoprotein (Ballinger et al. 1996; Kostakoglu et al. 1998; Tabuenca et al. 1998).

However, using the conventional planar acquisition method, scintimammography, with these gamma-emitting agents has revealed very low sensitivity in the identification of both non-palpable and small (<10 mm) primary carcinomas (Mekhmandarov et al. 1998; Howart et al. 1999; Khalkhali et al. 2000; Spanu et al. 2001) and of non-palpable, small size and low number axillary lymph node metastases (Spanu et al. 2001; Schillaci et al. 2002; Spanu et al. 2003). These findings suggest that the planar procedure cannot play a significant role in these conditions.

More recently, single photon emission computed tomography (SPECT) has been employed, since this tomographic procedure is recognized as having a higher contrast resolution than bi-dimensional planar imaging as well as a higher intrinsic sensitivity.

5.2 Single Photon Emission Computed Tomography (SPECT)

SPECT acquisition in scintimammography in patients with breast cancer has been employed most frequently using the cationic lipophilic radiotracers ^{99m}Tc-tetrofosmin and ^{99m}Tc-MIBI, given their more favorable physical properties in respect of other tumor-seeking agents, as previously observed in the detection of both primary tumors and axillary lymph node metastases when using planar scintimammography. An increasing number of SPECT studies have been reported in primary breast cancer detection in comparison with planar scintimammography (Aziz et al. 1999; Obwegeser et al. 1999; Spanu et al. 2001; Spanu et al. 2002; Myslivecek et al. 2004; Madeddu and Spanu 2004; Mathieu et al. 2005; Spanu et al. 2005). The accuracy of SPECT has proved higher than planar, in particular in small lesion detection with very encouraging results in T1b carcinomas (Spanu et al. 2002). However, the data reported on axillary lymph node metastasis detection are still limited; moreover, only a few studies have focused on the preoperative evaluation of axillary lymph node status, although some of these included a large number of patients (Spanu et al. 2001; Schillaci et al. 2002). Different clinical comparative studies with cationic lipophilic radiotracers have indicated in most cases a better performance of SPECT in respect of planar, as shown in Table 5.1, which illustrates the results of some of these studies. However, using prone ^{99m}Tc-MIBI SPECT 360° in some casuistries, which also included a small number of involved axillae from metastases, the sensitivity was identical (Palmedo et al. 1996) or slightly higher for SPECT (Tiling et al. 1998). In particular, Palmedo et al. (1996) obtained identical sensitivity values (81.8%) for prone SPECT (180° rotation, 6° steps, 30 s/step, 64×64 matrix) and for planar (prone lateral and anterior views) in a series of 24 breast cancer patients with 11 metastatic axillae, all of whom resulted positive for >3 axillary lymph node metastases, while both procedures were false negative in 2 patients with ascertained <3 metastatic nodes; moreover, a higher resolution of SPECT than planar was observed in focal areas of tracer accumulation in some concordant cases. Tiling et al. (1998) in 59 breast cancer patients with 17 metastatic axillae observed that prone SPECT (180 projec-

Table 5.1. Summary of studies reporting the diagnostic performance of SPECT with cationic lipophilic radiotracers, compared to planar scintimammography in breast cancer (BC) axillary lymph node metastasis detection

Study	Tracer	BC patient number	N+/N0 axillae	Sensitivity		Specificity	
				SPECT	Planar	SPECT	Planar
Palmedo et al. (1996)	MIBI	24	11/13	81.8% (9/11)	81.8% (9/11)	84.6% (12/13)	100% (13/13)
Schillaci et al. (1997)	MIBI	49	21/28	81% (17/21)	62% (13/21)	93% (26/28)	96% (27/28)
Tiling et al. (1998)	MIBI	59	17/42	64.7% (11/17)	41.2% (7/17)	90.5% (38/42)	95.2% (40/42)
Spanu et al. (2001)	Tetrofosmin	175	86/90	93% (80/86)	52.3% (45/86)	91 % (82/90)	100% (90/90)
Schillaci et al. (2002)	Tetrofosmin	85	56/31	94.6% (53/56)	92.9% (52/56)	61.3% (19/31)	87.1% (27/31)
Myslivececk et al. (2004)	MIBI	81	35/50	66% (23/35)	54% (19/35)	76% (38/50)	89% (43/50)

N+ = axillae with metastatic nodes at histology; N0 = axillae without metastatic nodes at histology

tions over 360°, 20 s/step, 128×128 matrix) slightly increased planar scintimammography (prone lateral and anterior views) sensitivity values from 41.2% to 64%, but only when using the iterative reconstruction (ISA) and not the filtered back projection (FBP) method, with SPECT yielding, however, more false-positive results than planar scintimammography. On the other hand, with conventional SPECT in supine position, high values of sensitivity and accuracy in predicting lymph node status have been reported, significantly improving planar data. Schillaci et al. (1997) in a large series of 49 breast cancer patients with axillary lymph node metastases reported a higher sensitivity value (81%) for ^{99m}Tc-MIBI supine SPECT (64 steps over 360°, 20 s/step, 64×64 matrix) in respect of planar (62%) performed in multiple anterior and lateral views; the sensitivity was higher for SPECT in both patients with >3 metastatic nodes (93.3% vs. 80%) and in those with ≤3 nodes (50% vs. 16.7%). Moreover, accuracy was also higher for SPECT (83.3% vs. 76.2%). Spanu et al. (2001), in a very large series of 175 breast cancer patients with 86 metastatic axillae, using ^{99m}Tc-tetrofosmin supine SPECT (60 steps over 360°, 30 s/step, 64×64 matrix) with the body contouring system during acquisition in order to ensure the minimum distance between the patient and the collimator and with image reconstruction by the filtered back projection method (FBP), showed a significantly higher sensitivity (93%) and accuracy (92%) in respect of planar (52.3% and 76.7%, respectively) acquired in supine anterior and lateral views. In particular, a significant increase in sensitivity as compared to planar imaging was observed in the detection of both palpable (100% vs. 82.6%) and non palpable (90.5% vs. 41.3%) metastatic nodes, as well as when the nodes were >3 (93.2% vs. 68.2%) and even more so when ≤3 (92.8% vs. 35.7%); one of these cases is illustrated in Figure 5.1. The difference in sensitivity was statistically significant except in the detection of palpable nodes. Moreover, all lymph nodes false negative at SPECT were in most cases non-palpable and <10 mm in size (range 3–6 mm) with partial metastatic involvement or with micrometastasis. Thus, these latter conditions can affect SPECT sensitivity, whereas planar imaging is also affected by axillary clinical status and node number. Furthermore, the very high negative predictive values obtained by SPECT (93.2%), but not by planar (68.7%) suggest that only the former procedure can be useful for a better selection of breast cancer patients to submit to ALND. These data were also confirmed by Schillaci et al. (2002) in a series

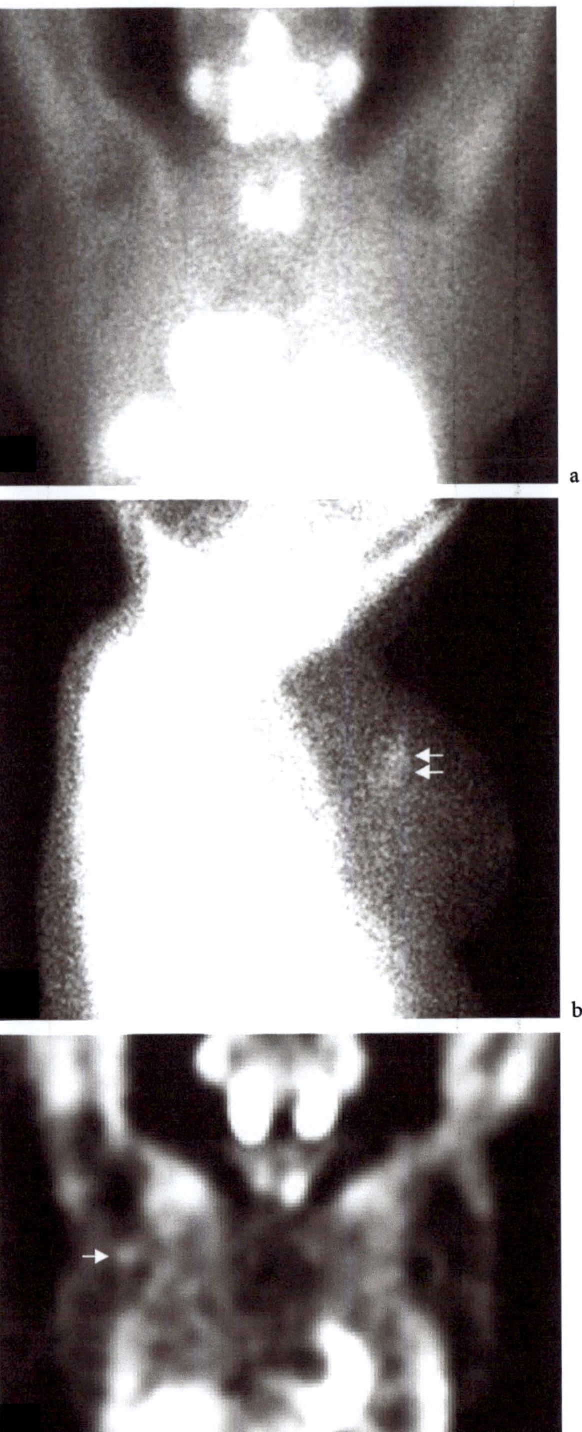

Fig. 5.1a-c. Patient with a T1c infiltrating ductal carcinoma in the right breast. The tumor was visible at planar scintimammography (**a,b**) only in the lateral view (**b**), but not in anterior view (**a**), and is identified by *double arrows*. Two metastatic nodes in the ipsilateral axilla were ascertained at histology; the latter were not evidenced at planar imaging, while SPECT (**c**) was true positive and showed a focal area of increased uptake (*single arrow*) in the involved axilla

of 85 breast cancer patients using ^{99m}Tc-tetrofosmin supine SPECT (64 projections over 360°, 20 s/step, 64×64 matrix) in comparison with planar (prone lateral and supine anterior views). This study also emphasized the high positive predictive values of SPECT (85.7%) in palpable metastatic lymph nodes, which could also have clinical importance in convincing the surgeon to perform ALND in selected patients despite conditions not considered optimal for surgery (e.g., patient age, obesity, systemic diseases). More recently, other authors (Myslivecek et al. 2004) in a comparative study between ^{99m}Tc-MIBI scintimammography supine SPECT (360° rotation, 3° angular step, 30 s/step, 64×64 matrix) and planar (supine anterior and prone lateral views) carried out on a series of 81 breast cancer patients with 85 metastatic axillae globally reported quite low sensitivity values for the two procedures in metastatic lymph node detection, with a slightly higher value for SPECT (66%) in respect of planar (54%), with specificity values more elevated for the latter (86% vs. 76%). However, the authors did not specify in detail the clinical status of the lymph nodes, their size or number.

5.3 Single Photon Emission Computed Tomography with Pinhole Collimator (Pinhole SPECT)

Notwithstanding its high per axilla sensitivity and accuracy values in the detection of lymph node metastases, in particular when non-palpable and in small number, conventional SPECT, like planar, is not able to determine the exact number of nodes, thus missing important information for disease prognosis, which can also contribute to a more correct selection of patients for adjuvant chemotherapy following surgical treatment of the primary lesion. This goal could be partially achieved by a high-resolution tomographic procedure, such as SPECT with pinhole collimator (pinhole SPECT) since it is recognized as having a better spatial resolution than planar and conventional SPECT with large field of view parallel-hole collimators, given the more favorable geometric properties of the cone beam collimator (Weber et al. 1994). Pinhole-SPECT has proved a powerful and widely available tool for the in vivo investigation of regional radiotracer distribution in mice and rats. The narrow aperture of the pinhole collimator, combined with short imaging distances and appropriate image reconstruction software, gives a spatial resolution two to three times higher than that of SPECT and comparable to that achieved by dedicated small-animal PET scanners (Yukihiro et al. 1996; Acton et al. 2002; Booij et al. 2002; Scherfler et al. 2002; Wu et al. 2003; Bennink et al. 2004). Pinhole SPECT has also proved useful in clinical settings to evaluate small structures such as the thyroid. In this context pinhole SPECT has demonstrated increased sensitivity in comparison with conventional planar thyroid scintigraphy in the detection of small nodules, improving the definition of tracer uptake and thus guiding the physician more accurately in fine-needle aspiration of the cold areas (Wanet et al. 1996; Krausz et al. 1997). Pinhole SPECT has also proved useful in the high-resolution imaging of both normal and morbid bones and joints and in the detection of ankle diseases, portraying many anatomical landmarks and pathological signs in useful detail (Bahk et al. 1998). Spanu et al. were the first to employ pinhole SPECT with ^{99m}Tc-tetrofosmin as tumor-seeking agent in large series of patients with malignant and benign tumors, and clinical applications have regarded: the detection of neck metastases from differentiated thyroid carcinoma in patients previously submitted to thyroidectomy and radioiodine therapy, the procedure demonstrating a higher per-lesion sensitivity than the planar method and than conventional SPECT with parallel-hole collimator (Spanu et al. 1998; Spanu et al. 2004); the identification of neck lymph node metastases from Kaposi sarcoma with higher sensitivity also than ultrasonography (Spanu et al. 2003); the identification of hyperfunctioning glands in both primary and secondary hyperparathyroidism, significantly increasing the sensitivity of conventional planar parathyroid scintigraphy (Spanu et al. 2003; Spanu et al. 2004). Moreover, Spanu et al. (2000) were the first to employ pinhole SPECT with ^{99m}Tc-tetrofosmin for the detection of breast cancer axillary lymph node metastases, adapting to the study of the axillary region an acquisition/processing software implemented on an SPX computer that was originally developed for the tomographic study of the thyroid. Clinical use of the procedure was preceded by evaluation in a phantom experimental model by the same authors (Chiaramida et al. 1998), with the first data on a large series of patients being published in 2000. In this first study comparing axillary pinhole SPECT lymph node metastasis detection with conventional SPECT and planar scintimammography, the authors used a circular single-head high-resolution gamma camera with a pinhole collimator (pinhole insert: 4.45 mm) in 112 patients with suspected breast lesions, in 100 of whom breast cancer was ascertained. After 740 MBq of ^{99m}Tc-tetrofosmin i.v. injection, with the patients in supine anterior position and the arm corresponding to the involved axilla raised over the head, images of axilla ipsilateral to the involved breast were acquired over 180°, using a matrix size of 128×128 and a zoom factor of 2 as fixed by the software acquisition protocol, an angular step of 3° and an acquisition time of 30 s/step. The images, which were pre-processed with a cone beam algorithm and then processed by the FBP method, always gave a clearer topographical portrayal of each axilla and important landmarks as well as better visualization of single or multiple metastases as compared to both conventional SPECT and planar images. Pinhole SPECT showed a slightly higher per-axilla sensitivity than conventional SPECT (100% vs. 96.2%) and the same specificity (93.6%); the sensitivity and specificity of planar scintimammography were 56.6% and 100%, respectively (Table 5.2). Moreover, pinhole SPECT identified a markedly higher number of nodes within the axillary cavities than SPECT and even more so than planar, and it was also the only method to determine the exact number of nodes in many patients with multiple lymph node metastases (Fig. 5.2); it correctly classified 89% of patients as having ≤3 or >3 metastatic lymph nodes, thereby providing additional useful prognostic data. In a subsequent comparative study of ^{99m}Tc-tetrofosmin pinhole SPECT, conventional SPECT and planar, the same authors (Spanu et al. 2003) focused on a large series of breast cancer patients, all with non-palpable lymph node metastases, known to be more frequent than palpable metastases and the most difficult to identify with conventional imaging methods, such as ultrasonography and MRI. The authors enrolled 188 consecutive patients with suspicious breast lesions, 176 of whom had cancer (bilateral in three cases), all submitted to ALND for a definitive diagnosis. In 74/179 axillae lymph node metastases were ascertained: 1 node in 29 cases, including 5 with micrometastasis, 2 to 3 nodes in 20 cases and >3 nodes in 25 cases. Pinhole SPECT showed significantly higher per-axilla sensitivity (93.2%) than both SPECT (85.1%; $P<0.05$) and planar imaging (36.5%; $P<0.0005$); the difference was also significant ($P<0.0005$) when SPECT was compared to planar. The only five pinhole SPECT false-negative cases had one metastatic node each, four of which were micrometastatic, while the remaining macrometastatic node had only partial involvement; SPECT and planar procedures were also false negative in these 5 cases and in 6 and 42 further cases,

Table 5.2. Summary of studies reporting the diagnostic performance of ^{99m}Tc-tetrofosmin pinhole SPECT in comparison with SPECT and planar scintigraphy in breast cancer (BC) axillary lymph node status evaluation

Study	BC patient number	N+/N0 axillae	Scan	Sensitivity	Specificity	Accuracy	NPV	PPV
Spanu et al. (2000)	100	(53/47)	Pinhole SPECT	100% (53/53)	93.6% (44/47)	97%	100%	94.6%
			SPECT	96.2% (51/53)	93.6% (44/47)	95%	95.6%	94.4%
			Planar	56.6% (30/53)	100% (47/47)	77%	67.1%	100%
Spanu et al. (2003)	176*	(74/105)	Pinhole SPECT	93.2% (69/74)	92.4% (97/105)	92.7%	95%	89.6%
			SPECT	85.1% (63/74)	94.3% (99/105)	90.5%	90%	91.3%
			Planar	36.5% (27/74)	99% (104/105)	73.2%	68.9%	96.4%

N+ = axillae with metastatic nodes at histology; N0 = axillae without metastatic nodes at histology; NPV= negative predictive value; PPV= positive predictive value; *all patients with non-palpable lymph node metastases

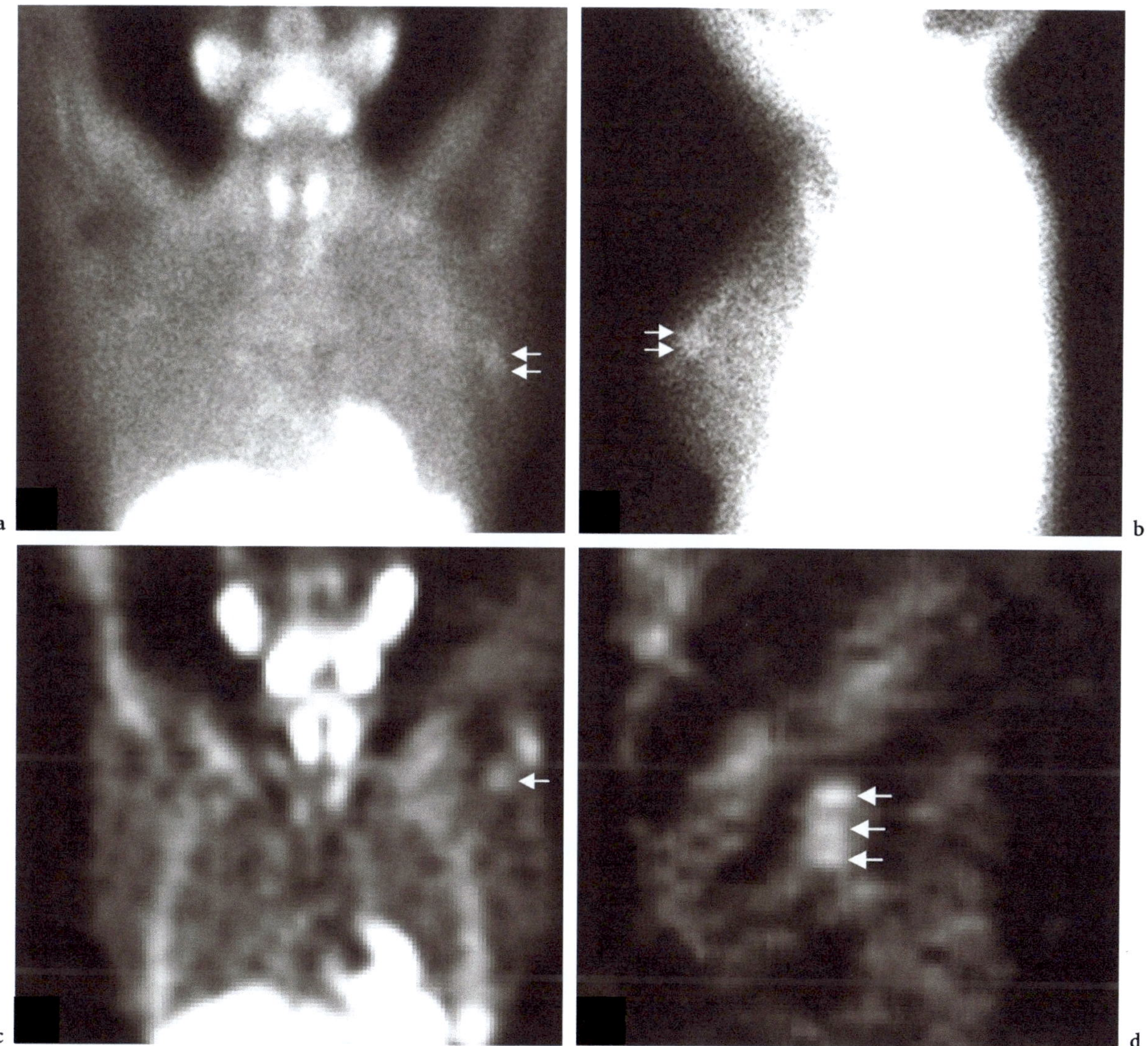

Fig. 5.2a–d. Patient with a T1c infiltrating ductal carcinoma in the left breast. The tumor was visible at planar scintimammography (**a**,**b**) in both the anterior (**a**) and the lateral view (**b**) and is identified by *double arrows*. Three metastatic nodes in the ipsilateral axilla were ascertained at histology. These nodes were not ascertained at planar imaging (**a**,**b**). Both SPECT (**c**) and pinhole SPECT (**d**) were positive in the left axilla (*single arrow*), but only pinhole SPECT determined the exact number of involved nodes, showing three focal areas of increased uptake

respectively. Except for the above five false-negative cases, Pinhole SPECT correctly detected 100% of the other cases with single nodes distinguishing single from multiple metastatic lymph nodes, while SPECT did so in 87.5% and planar in 16.6%. However, specificity values were slightly lower for pinhole SPECT (92.4%) than for SPECT (94.3%) and planar (99%), although accuracy was higher (92.7% vs. 90.5% and 73.2%, respectively). Thus, pinhole SPECT gave a better performance in respect of SPECT in this selected series with non-palpable lymph node metastases, also significantly improving both the quality and the resolution of the images with a better visualization of the axillary cavity as distinct from the surrounding muscle-skeletal structures and clearer evidence of the focal areas corresponding to lymph node metastases within the axilla. The negative predictive value was also higher for pinhole SPECT (95%) than for SPECT (90%) and planar scintimammography

(68.9%); this result could suggest a wider use of pinhole SPECT to better select breast cancer patients to submit to ALND, contributing to avoiding this invasive procedure in unnecessary cases, although the 7% false-negative rate obtained in this study is still too high to consider pinhole SPECT as a single diagnostic method for this purpose. Moreover, while SPECT also achieved a high accuracy and negative predictive value, only pinhole-SPECT gave information on the number of involved nodes and the correct patient classification for prognostic purposes differentiating in this series of patients with ≤3 nodes from those >3 in 89.8% of cases. The latter information has not been reported preoperatively with other non-invasive diagnostic imaging methods, including FDG-PET, but only by ALND during surgery. Therefore, axillary pinhole SPECT should be preferred to conventional SPECT in axillary metastasis detection in breast cancer patients and even more so for planar, which has proved an unreliable method. Furthermore, in these two studies the approximate Feldkamp algorithm and the FBP method were used for the image reconstruction of pinhole SPECT, as with most other authors who have employed this method for both experimental (Tornai et al. 2003) and clinical purposes (Wanet et al. 1996, Krausz et al. 1997, Bahk et al. 1998). However, an iterative reconstruction of 180° orbit pinhole SPECT with ordered subset expectation maximization (PH OS-EM) has been employed by others in phantom studies (Vanhove et al. 2000), and this procedure obtained a global gain in overall image quality, resolution and uniformity when compared with BPF reconstruction. Therefore, the iterative method improves pinhole SPECT in in-vivo performance in small-size axillary lymph node detection and further reduces false-negative cases, which, however, were very few in the series reported in the two studies described above (Spanu et al. 2000; Spanu et al. 2003) and were due to a single micrometastasis (≤2 mm) in most cases or to partial tumor involvement. It should be underlined that, apart from small size, biological tumor factors could also be responsible for a low radiotracer uptake, thus reducing the possibility of visualizing lymph nodes. However, to date, clinical application of this iterative reconstruction pinhole-SPECT method has not yet been reported. Nevertheless, it is unlikely that either this iterative method or FBP can make the identification of micrometastasis easy, the detection limit being probably intrinsic to the Anger camera revelation system. It should be noted that lymph node micrometastasis also represents a very important limitation factor for other imaging methods proposed for breast cancer axillary lymph node metastasis detection such as FDG-PET (Keleman et al. 2002; Barranger et al. 2003). Possibly in the future, a pinhole SPECT system employed with a dedicated small field of view very high resolution gamma camera could attempt to further improve the identification of a single micrometastasis, the presence of which should be taken into account, even if its clinical significance, and in particular its impact on overall survival in breast cancer patients, has not yet been established. Moreover, pinhole SPECT has also been proposed in primary breast cancer patients since the data reported with two pinhole SPECT procedures, incomplete (180°) circular orbit SPECT (Scarfone et al. 1997; Tornai et al. 2003) and emission-tuned aperture computed tomography (Fahey et al. 2001), have appeared very encouraging, these procedures proving their potential in detecting small size (<10 mm) spherical simulated lesions in breast phantom studies; however, up to date no clinical data have been reported with pinhole-SPECT in primary breast cancer.

RGSLNB with an accurate multi-sectioning histopathological examination of the nodes has recently emerged as a mini-invasive method that offers an alternative to ALND in the axillary staging of selected patients with breast cancer; moreover, it is also a reliable method to detect micrometastasis. However, in some cases RGSLNB gives false-negative results and when positive may not predict the status of the other axillary lymph nodes; furthermore, in a few cases the procedure does not identify the SLN. On the basis of the previous very encouraging results obtained with ^{99m}Tc-tetrofosmin pinhole SPECT in the detection of axillary metastatic lymph nodes, Spanu et al. (2001) used this method comparatively with RGSLNB in a large series of 101 T1/T2 breast cancer patients scheduled to be submitted to ALND; all the patients were without clinical evidence of axillary lymph node metastases or a previous history of excision biopsy. The SLN was identified in 97/101 cases (96%) and examined at histology by both hematoxylin and eosin staining and immunohistochemistry. SLN was not detected in four patients with primary cancer >15 mm by either lymphoscintigraphy or gamma probe; in these cases pinhole SPECT, which was always performed some days before RGSLNB, correctly determined the axillary lymph node status, compensating for

RGSLNB failure. In the 97 patients in whom SLN biopsy and pinhole SPECT could be compared, the correct prediction of axillary lymph node status was obtained by RGSLNB in 94.8% of cases and by pinhole SPECT in 93.8%, while the latter had a higher negative predictive value (95.2% vs. 92.5%), although the difference was not significant. RGSLNB was false negative in five patients with metastases, all of whom were true positive at pinhole SPECT, but it was true negative and true positive, respectively, in three false-positive and three false-negative cases at pinhole SPECT (two of the latter cases had a micrometastasis in the SNL). The combined use of the two procedures achieved 100% overall accuracy, thus suggesting their complementary use in particular in patients with primary carcinomas >15 mm, since in the cases observed in this study tumor size did not affect pinhole SPECT performance; however, 100% accuracy was also reached by RGSLNB alone in patients in whom primary breast cancer was <15 mm, also detecting micrometastases, which represent a diagnostic limitation of pinhole SPECT. This result demonstrates that RGSLNB seems to be indicated particularly in selected patients with small primary breast cancer at an early stage, and could be useful to avoid ALND when the SLN is negative for metastasis, given the low risk of metastatic lymph nodes in this situation. Nevertheless, in larger carcinomas the combined use of the two methods could be more useful for the better selection of patients for ALND, since tumor size does not affect pinhole SPECT performance. These data were confirmed by the same authors (Spanu et al. 2003; Spanu and Madeddu 2004) in a larger number of cases than in their first study, approximately 200 cases, as shown in Table 5.3, thus suggesting a management algorithm for the selection of patients for ALND described in more detail in the first study (Spanu et al. 2001) and also reported in later papers by the same group (Madeddu and Spanu 2004; Spanu et al. 2005). When both RGSLNB and ^{99m}Tc-tetrofosmin pinhole SPECT are negative, ALND should be excluded; when the two procedures are positive pinhole SPECT for more than one metastasis, ALND is indicated. However, ALND may also be indicated when SLN biopsy is negative, but pinhole SPECT is positive for more than one metastasis, since this condition was never associated with false-positive results in the above study; on the other hand, ALND might be avoided when SLN biopsy is positive, but pinhole SPECT is negative or positive for only one metastasis, histology excluding further metastatic nodes in this condition. However, in proposing these suggestions, the authors were aware that confirmation in further larger studies is necessary. The same authors, in the description of their large number of cases, also emphasized that SLN micrometastasis represents a diagnostic limitation of pinhole SPECT. This assumes major importance when a micrometastasis is present in the only metastatic lesion, although the clinical importance and management of micrometastasis is still under discussion, given the conflicting results reported to date in the literature regarding the influence of micrometastasis on disease prognosis. However, SLN micrometastasis can also be associated with macrometastases in other axillary nodes only ascertained at ALND; in these cases the combined use of pinhole SPECT with RGSLNB could be very useful to guide the most appropriate therapeutic decision. Moreover, the authors also observed that pinhole SPECT, unlike RGSLNB, provided important prognostic information, correctly differentiating patients with ≤3 nodes from those with >3 nodes in 93.75% of cases.

Table 5.3. Summary of studies reporting the diagnostic performance of ^{99m}Tc-tetrofosmin axillary pinhole SPECT compared to radio-guided sentinel node biopsy (RGSLNB) in the prediction of axillary lymph node status in breast cancer patients

Study	BC patient number	Scan	Sensitivity	Specificity	Accuracy	NPV	PPV
Spanu et al. (2001)	101	RGBLSB pinhole SPECT	85.7% 91.4%	100% 95.2%	94.8% 93.8%	92.5% 95.2%	100% 91.4%
Spanu et al. (2003)	148	RGBLSB pinhole SPECT	86.8% 92.5%	100% 93%	95% 92.8%	92.5% 95%	100% 89%
Spanu and Madeddu (2004)	194	RGBLSB pinhole SPECT	89.7% 91.2%	100% 94.8%	96.2% 93.5%	94.3% 94.8%	100% 91.2%

NPV= negative predictive value; PPV= positive predictive value

5.4 Conclusion

ALND still represents the method of choice to define axillary lymph node status in breast cancer patients in order to obtain prognostic information and to plan the most appropriate therapy; however, this surgical procedure is characterized by invasiveness, morbidity, high cost and, moreover, often proves unnecessary and could be avoided. Thus, the number of ALND should be reduced in particular in those cases without clinically apparent axillary lymph node involvement and even more so when primary cancer is at an early stage with a low incidence of lymph node metastases. A series of non-invasive diagnostic procedures have been proposed for the preoperative evaluation of axillary lymph node status. Scintimammography represents one of the most widely available diagnostic tools, particularly with cationic lipophilic ^{99m}Tc-tetrofosmin and ^{99m}Tc-MIBI as tumor-seeking agents; these radiotracers offer more favorable physical properties than the other gamma-emitting radiopharmaceuticals used for this purpose. The best performance of scintimammography with cationic lipophilc agents in the study of the axilla has been obtained with SPECT acquisition which, in comparative studies, has shown significantly higher sensitivity and accuracy than the conventional planar method, in particular when the lymph nodes are non-palpable, small and limited in number; in these conditions the role of planar is negligible, and SPECT should be preferred. SPECT, like planar scintimammography, can also simultaneously provide images of both breasts and axillary regions, and it is a simple method readily available in nuclear medicine centers. Moreover, it is time saving when multi-head gamma cameras are employed, thereby permitting its routine use. Thus, SPECT should be more extensively used in those patients without clinical suspicion of axillary involvement, given its high negative predictive value, although some false-negative results have been described, probably due to the small size of the lymph node and/or to partial or micrometastatic involvement. Furthermore, comparative studies in breast cancer patients have shown that the performance of conventional SPECT in the study of the axillary region is improved when a pinhole collimator is used for acquisition (pinhole SPECT). The data obtained in these studies, which, however, need to be confirmed in larger series, have shown higher sensitivity and accuracy values as well as higher negative predictive values for pinhole SPECT in respect of SPECT. Pinhole SPECT, with its very high intrinsic spatial resolution, seems to have the potentiality to improve the trade-off between sensitivity and resolution for small organ or structure imaging, such as the axillary cavity, more than other radioisotopic procedures; thus, it could represent one of the non-invasive diagnostic tools of choice in the prediction of axillary lymph node status in breast cancer, using cationic lipophilic radiotracers, in particular ^{99m}Tc-tetrofosmin, as a suitable oncotropic agent, on the basis of the results of literature. The contribution of this procedure is even more significant in non-palpable and small-size metastatic node detection, and its sensitivity is independent of primary tumor size; however, the detection of micrometastases represents a limitation for pinhole SPECT, as it also does for all other diagnostic imaging procedures. Moreover, pinhole SPECT, even more than SPECT, could find a useful application in combination with RGSLNB, which is now favored for selecting patients who should undergo ALND owing to its very high negative predictive value, as reported in numerous studies. Pinhole SPECT could predict axillary lymph node status in the few cases in which RGSLNB failed to detect SLN; moreover, it could provide useful information when SLN is either negative or positive for micrometastasis at RGSLNB, but metastases are present in the other axillary lymph nodes, or when SLN is positive at biopsy, but represents the only metastatic site. Pinhole SPECT has proved useful in increasing the accuracy of RGSLNB, permitting a more appropriate selection of breast cancer in whom ALND could be avoided. Moreover, the higher spatial resolution of pinhole SPECT also permits a better determination of the number of involved nodes, correctly differentiating the patients with >3 nodes from those with <3 nodes and thus providing important prognostic information; these latter results have not been reported for other non-invasive imaging procedures, including FDG-PET, but only for ALND. Pinhole SPECT seems to have great potential as a non-invasive diagnostic procedure in the preoperative evaluation of axillary lymph node status in breast cancer patients, but large prospective clinical trials are necessary to validate its usefulness before assigning to this procedure a definitive role in breast cancer axillary lymph node staging. On the other hand, pinhole SPECT only requires a conventional rotating single head gamma camera equipped with a pinhole collimator and a specific software for processing the data; it is easy to perform and to interpret after adequate training, time saving and well tolerated. Therefore, pinhole SPECT could be routinely applied in all nuclear medicine centers and could even represent a valid alternative to FDG-PET in respect of which it offers the advantage of being less expensive and widely available.

References

Acton PD, Choi SR, Plössl K et al (2002) Quantification of dopamine transporters in the mouse brain using ultra-high resolution single-photon emission tomography. Eur J Nucl Med 29:691–698

Adler LP, Faulhaber PF, Schnur KC et al (1997) Axillary lymph node metastases: screening with [F-18] 2-deoxy-2-fluoro-D-glucose (FDG) PET. Radiology 203:323–327

Albertini JJ, Lyman GH, Cox C et al (1996) Lymphatic mapping and sentinel node biopsy in the patient with breast cancer. JAMA 276:1818–1822

Alonso O, Martinez M, Delgado L et al (2003) Staging of regional lymph nodes in melanoma patients by means of ^{99m}Tc-MIBI scintigraphy. J Nucl Med 44: 1561–1565

Arbab AS, Koizumi K, Toyama K et al (1996) Uptake of technetium-99m-tetrofosmin, technetium-99m-MIBI and thallium-201 in tumor cell lines. J Nucl Med 37:1551–1556

Arbab AS, Koizumi K, Toyama K et al (1997) Ion transport systems in the uptake of 99Tcm-tetrofosmin, 99Tcm-MIBI and 201Tl in a tumor cell line. Nucl Med Commun 18:235–240

Aziz A, Hashmi R, Ogawa Y et al (1999) Tc-99m-MIBI scintimammography; SPECT versus planar imaging Cancer Biother Radiopharm 14:495–500

Bahk YW, Chung SK, Park YH et al (1998) Pinhole SPECT imaging in normal and morbid ankles. J Nucl Med 39:130–139

Ballinger JR, Bannerman J, Boxen I et al (1996) Technetium-99m-tetrofosmin as a substrate for P-glycoprotein: in vitro studies in multidrug-resistant breast tumor cells. J Nucl Med 37:1578–1582

Barranger E, Grahek D, Antoine M et al (2003) Evaluation of fluorodeoxyglucose positron emission tomography in the detection of axillary lymph node metastases in patients with early-stage breast cancer. Ann Surg Oncol 10:622–627

Bennink RJ, van Montfrans C, de Jong WJ et al (2004) Imaging of intestinal lymphocyte homing by means of pinhole SPECT in a TNBS colitis mouse model. Eur J Nucl Med Mol Imaging 31: 93–101

Bernard BF, Krenning EP, Breeman WA et al (1998) ^{99m}Tc-MIBI, ^{99m}Tc-tetrofosmin and ^{99m}Tc-Q12 in vitro and in vivo. Nucl Med Biol 25:233–240

Boolbol SK, Fey JV, Borgen PI et al (2001) Intradermal isotope injection: a highly accurate method of lymphatic mapping in breast carcinoma. Ann Surg Oncol 8:20–24

Booij J, de Bruin K, Habraken JBA et al (2002) Imaging of dopamine transporters in rats using high-resolution pinhole single-photon emission tomography. Eur J Nucl Med 29:1221–1224

Bootsma AH, van Eijck C, Shouten KK et al (1993) Somatostatin receptor-positive primary breast tumors: genetic, patient and tumor characteristic. Int J Cancer 28:357–362

Borgstein PJ, Pijpers R, Comans EF et al (1998) Sentinel lymph node biopsy in breast cancer: guidelines and pitfalls of lymphoscintigraphy and gamma probe detection. J Am Coll Surg 186:275–283

Caner B, Kitapci M, Aras T et al (1991) Increased accumulation of hexakis (2-methoxyisobutylisonitrile) technetium (I) in osteosarcoma and its metastatic lymph nodes. J Nucl Med 32:1977–1978

Carter C, Allen C, Henson D (1989) Relation of tumor size, lymph node status, and survival in 24,740 breast cancer cases. Cancer 63:181–187

Chiaramida P, Spanu A, Madeddu G (1998) 180° Pinhole (P) SPECT and 360° (C) SPECT spatial resolution. An experimental model. Q J Nucl Med 42 (Suppl 1): 11

Choi JY, Kim SE, Shin HJ et al (2000) Brain tumor imaging with ^{99m}Tc-tetrofosmin: comparison with 201Tl, ^{99m}Tc-MIBI, and ^{18}F-fluorodeoxyglucose. J Neurooncol 46:63–70

Cimitan M, Volpe R, Candiani E et al (1995) The use of thallium-201 in the preoperative detection of breast cancer: an adjunct to mammography and ultrasonography. Eur J Nucl Med 22:1110–1117

Cox CE, Pendas S, Cox JM et al (1998) Guidelines for sentinel node biopsy and lymphatic mapping of patients with breast cancer. Ann Surg 226:645–653

Cwikla JB, Buscombe JR, Parbhoo SP et al (1998) Use of 99Tcm-MIBI in the assessment of patients with suspected recurrent breast cancer. Nucl Med Commun 19:649–655

Danforth DN Jr, Aloj L, Carrasquillo JA et al (2002) The role of ^{18}F-FDG-PET in the local/regional evaluation of women with breast cancer. Breast Cancer Res Treat 75: 135–146

Fahey FH, Grow KL, Webber RL et al (2001) Emission tuned-aperture computed tomography: a novel approach to scintimammography. J Nucl Med 42: 1121–1127

Fisher B, Bauer M, Wickerham DL et al (1983) Relation of number of positive axillary nodes to the prognosis of patients with primary breast cancer: an NSABP update. Cancer 52:1551–1557

Flett MM, Going JJ, Stanton PD et al (1998) Sentinel node localization in patient with breast cancer. Br J Surg 85:991–993

Giuliano AE, Kirgan DM, Guenther JM et al (1994) Lymphatic mapping and sentinel lymphadenectomy for breast cancer. Ann Surg 220:391–398

Greco M, Crippa F, Agresti R et al (2001) Axillary lymph node staging in breast cancer by 2-fluoro-2-deoxy-D-glucose-positron emission tomography: clinical evaluation and alternative management. J Natl Cancer Inst 93:630–635

Gulec SA, Moffat FL, Carrol RG et al (1998) Sentinel node localization in early breast cancer. J Nucl Med 39:1388–1393

Guller U, Nitzsche EU, Schirp U et al (2002) Selective axillary surgery in breast cancer patients based on positron emission tomography with ^{18}F-fluoro-2-deoxy-D-glucose: not yet! Breast Cancer Res Treat 71:171–173

Haigh PI, Hansen NM, Giuliano AE et al (2000) Factors affecting sentinel node localization during preoperative breast lymphoscintigraphy. J Nucl Med 41:1682–1688

Howart D, Sillar R, Clark D et al (1999) Technetium-99m sestamibi scintimammography: the influence of histopatological characteristics, lesion size and the presence of carcinoma in situ in the detection of breast carcinoma. Eur J Nucl Med 26:1475–1481

Hubner KF, Smith GT, Thie JA et al (2000) The potential of F-18-FDG PET in breast cancer. Detection of primary lesions, axillary lymph node metastases, or distant metastases. Clin Positron Imaging 3:197–205

Ivancevic VV, Wolter A, Winzer K et al (2000) Intraindividual comparison of F-18-fluorodeoxyglucose and Tc-99m-tetrofosmin in planar scintimammography and SPECT. Clin Positron Imaging 3:17–29

Kao CH, Wang SJ, Lin WY et al (1993) Differentiation of single solid lesions in the lungs by means of single-photon emission tomography with technetium methoxyisobutylisonitrile. Eur J Nucl Med 20:249–254

Keleman PR, Lowe V, Phillips N (2002) Positron emission tomography and sentinel lymph node dissection in breast cancer. Clin Breast Cancer 3: 73–77

Khalkhali I, Mena I, Diggles L (1994) Review of imaging tecniques for the diagnosis of breast cancer: a new role of prone scintimammography using technetium-99m sestamibi. Eur J Nucl Med 21:357–362

Khalkhali I, Cutrone J, Mena I et al (1995) Technetium-99m-sestamibi scintimammography of breast lesions: clinical and pathological follow-up. J Nucl Med 36:1784–1789

Khalkhali I, Villanueva-Meyer J, Edell SL et al (2000) Diagnostic accuracy of ^{99m}Tc-seatamibi breast imaging: multicenter trial results. J Nucl Med 41:1973–1979

Keshtgar MRS and Ell PJ (2002) Clinical role of sentinel-lymph-node biopsy in breast cancer. Lancet Oncol 3:105–110

Kostakoglu L, Ruacan S, Ergun EL et al (1998) Influence of the heterogeneity of P-glycoprotein expression on technetium-99m-MIBI uptake in breast cancer. J Nucl Med 39:1021–1026

Krag DN, Weaver DL, Ashikaga T et al (1998) The sentinel node in breast cancer. A multicenter validation study. N Engl J Med 339:941–946

Krausz Y, Wilk M, Saliman F et al (1997) Role of high-resolution pinhole tomography in the evaluation of thyroid abnormalities. Thyroid 7:847–852

Lee JK, Tsai SC, Ho YJ et al (2001) Technetium-99m tetrofosmin scintigraphy for detecting malignant lymphomas. Anticancer Res 21:1509–1513

Lind P, Gallowitsch HJ, Langsteger W et al (1997) Technetium-99m-tetrofosmin whole-body scintigraphy in the follow-up of differentiated thyroid carcinoma. J Nucl Med 38:348–352

Madeddu G, Spanu A (2004) Use of tomographic nuclear medicine procedures, SPECT and pinhole SPECT, with cationic lipophilic radiotracers for the evaluation of axillary lymph node status in breast cancer patients. Eur J Nucl Med Mol Imaging 31 (Suppl 1):S23

Mathieu I, Mazy S, Willemart B et al (2005) Inconclusive triple diagnosis in breast cancer imaging. Is there a place for scintimammography? J Nucl Med 46: 1574–1581

Mekhmandarov S, Sandbank J, Cohen M et al (1998) Technetium-99m-MIBI scintimammography in palpable and non-palpable breast lesions. J Nucl Med 39:86–91

Myslivecek M, Koranda P, Kaminek M et al (2004) Technetium-99m-MIBI scintimammography by planar and SPECT imaging in the diagnosis of breast carcinoma and axillary lymph node involvement. Nucl Med Rev Cent East Eur 7:151–155

Nishiyama Y, Yamamoto Y, Ono Y et al (2001) Comparative evaluation of ^{99m}Tc-MIBI and ^{99m}Tc-HMDP scintimammography for the diagnosis of breast cancer and its axillary metastases. Eur J Nucl Med 28:522–528

Obwegeser R, Berghammer P, Rodrigues M et al (1999) A head-to-head comparison between technetium-99m-tetrofosmin and technetium-99m-MIBI scintigraphy to evaluate suspicious breast lesions. Eur J Nucl Med 26:1553–1559

Ortapamuk H, Ozmen MM, Ibis S et al (1999) Role of technetium tetrofosmin scintimammography in the diagnosis of malignant breast masses and axillary lymph node involvement: a comparative study with mammography and histopathology. Eur J Surg 165:1147–1153

O'Tuama LA, Packard AB, Treves ST (1990) SPECT imaging of pediatric brain tumor with hesakis (methoxyisobutylisonitrile) technetium (I). J Nucl Med 31:2040–2041

Palmedo H, Schomburg A, Grunwald F et al (1996) Technetium-99m-MIBI scintimammography for suspicious breast lesions. J Nucl Med 37:626–630

Pijpers R, Meijer S, Hoekstra OS et al (1997) Impact of lymphoscintigraphy on sentinel node identification with Technetium-99m-colloidal albumin in breast cancer. J Nucl Med 38:366–368

Rodrigues M, Chehne F, Kalinowska W et al (2000) Uptake of ^{99m}Tc-MIBI and ^{99m}Tc-tetrofosmin into malignant versus nonmalignant breast cell lines. J Nucl Med 41:1495–1499

Saez RA, McGuire WL, Clark GM (1989) Prognostic factors in breast cancer. Semin Surg Oncol 5:102–110

Scarfone C, Jaszczak RJ, Li J et al (1997) Breast tumour imaging using incomplete circular orbit pinhole SPET: a phantom study. Nucl Med Commun 18: 1077–1086

Scherfler C, Donnemiller E, Schocke M et al (2002) Evaluation of striatal dopamine transporter function in rats by in vivo ß-[123I]CIT pinhole SPECT. NeuroImage 17:128–141

Schillaci O, Scopinaro F, Danieli R et al (1997) Technetium-99m sestamibi imaging in the detection of axillary lymph node involvement in patients with breast cancer. Anticancer Res 17:1607–1610

Schillaci O, Monteleone F, D'Andrea N et al (1999) Technetium-99 tetrofosmin single photon emission computer tomography in the evaluation of suspected lung cancer. Cancer Biother Radiopharm 14:129–134

Schillaci O, Scopinaro F, Spanu A et al (2002) Detection of axillary lymph node metastases in breast cancer with Tc-99m tetrofosmin scintigraphy. Int J Oncol 20:483–487

Schillaci O, Spanu A, Scopinaro F et al (2003) Technetium-99m tetrofosmin scintigraphy in pediatric osteogenic sarcoma. Oncol Rep 10:605–608

Sehweil AM, McKillop JH, Milroy R et al (1989) Mechanism of 201Tl uptake in tumours. Eur J Nucl Med 15:376–379

Sehweil AM, McHillop JH, Milroy R et al (1990) Tl-201 scintigraphy in staging of lung cancer, breast cancer and lymphoma. Nucl Med Commun 11:263–269

Skanberg J, Ahlman H, Benjegard SA et al (2002) Indium-111-octreotide scintigraphy, intraoperative gamma-detector localization and somatostatin receptor expression in primary human breast cancer. Breast Cancer Res Treat 74:101–111

Smith IC, Ogston KN, Whitford P et al (1998) Staging of the axilla in breast cancer: accurate in vivo assessment using positron emission tomography with 2-(fluorine-18)-fluoro-2-deoxy-D-glucose. Ann Surg 228:220–227

Spanu A, Madeddu G (2004) Axillary lymph node status prediction in breast cancer (BC) patients: ^{99m}Tc-tetrofosmin axillary pinhole-SPECT (P-SPECT) imaging vs radioguided sentinel lymph node (RSLN) biopsy. Int J Mol Med 14 (Suppl 1):76

Spanu A, Solinas ME, Chiaramida P et al (1998) Tc-99m tetrofosmin (T) pinhole (P) SPECT in neck metastases from differentiated thyroid carcinoma. Eur J Nucl Med 25 (suppl): 934

Spanu A, Dettori G, Chiaramida P et al (2000) The role of ^{99m}Tc-tetrofosmin Pinhole-SPECT in breast cancer axillary lymph node staging. Cancer Biother Radiopharm 15:81–91

Spanu A, Dettori G, Nuvoli S et al (2001) ^{99m}Tc-tetrofosmin SPET in the detection of both primary breast cancer and axillary lymph node metastasis. Eur J Nucl Med 28:1781–1794

Spanu A, Dettori G, Chessa F et al (2001) ^{99m}Tc-Tetrofosmin pinhole-SPECT (P-SPECT) and radioguided sentinel node (SN) biopsy and in breast cancer axillary lymph node staging. Cancer Biother Radiopharm 16:501–513

Spanu A, Schillaci O, Meloni GB et al (2002) The usefulness of ^{99m}Tc-tetrofosmin SPECT scintimammography in the detection of small size primary breast carcinomas. Int J Oncol 21:831–840

Spanu A, Ginesu F, Pirina P et al (2003) The usefulness of ^{99m}Tc-tetrofosmin SPECT in the detection of intrathoracic malignant lesions. Int J Oncol 22:639–649

Spanu A, Farris A, Schillaci O et al (2003) The usefulness of ^{99m}Tc tetrofosmin scintigraphy in patients with breast cancer recurrences. Nucl Med Commun 24:145–154

Spanu A, Tanda F, Dettori G et al (2003) The role of $^{(99m)}$Tc-tetrofosmin pinhole-SPECT in breast cancer non palpable axillary lymph node metastases detection. Q J Nucl Med 47:116–128

Spanu A, Madeddu G, Cottoni F et al (2003) Usefulness of ^{99m}Tc-tetrofosmin scintigraphy in different variants of Kaposi's sarcoma. Oncology 65:295–305

Spanu A, Migaleddu V, Manca A et al (2003) The usefulness of single photon emission computerized tomography with pinhole collimator (P-SPECT) in preoperative localization of hyperfunctioning parathyroid glands in patients with secondary hyperparathyroidism. Radiol Med 106:399–412

Spanu A, Dettori G, Chessa F et al (2003) Radioguided sentinel node (SN) biopsy vs ^{99m}Tc-tetrofosmin axillary pinhole-SPECT (P-SPECT) in the prediction of breast cancer (BC) axillary lymph node status. 2nd Congress of the World Society of Breast Health. Budapest. Abstract book: p 47

Spanu A, Solinas ME, Migaleddu V et al (2004) The role of ^{99m}Tc-tetrofosmin neck pinhole (P)-SPECT in the follow up of patients with differentiated thyroid carcinoma (DTC). Eur J Nucl Med Molecular Imaging 31 (Suppl 2):S426

Spanu A, Falchi A, Manca A et al (2004) The usefulness of neck Pinhole SPECT as a complementary tool to planar scintigraphy in primary and secondary hyperparathyroidism. J Nucl Med 45:40–48

Spanu A, Schillaci O, Madeddu G (2005) ^{99m}Tc labelled cationic lipophilic complexes in malignant and benign tumors: the role of SPET and pinhole-SPET in breast cancer, differentiated thyroid carcinoma and hyperparathyroidism. Q J Nucl Med Mol Imaging 49:145

Tabuenca MJ, Vargas JA, Varela A et al (1998) Technetium-99m-tetrofosmin scintigraphy, P-glycoprotein and lung cancer. J Nucl Med 39:1830–1831

Takahashi T, Moriya E, Miyamoto Y et al (1994) The usefulness of 201TlCl scintigraphy for the diagnosis of breast tumor. Nippon Igaku Hoshasen Gakkai Zasshi 54:644–649

Tiling R, Tatsch K, Sommer H et al (1998) Technetium-99m-sestamibi scintimammography for the detection of breast carcinoma: comparison between planar and SPECT imaging. J Nucl Med 39:849–856

Tornai MP, Bowsher JE, Jaszczak RJ et al (2003) Mammotomography with pinhole incomplete circular orbit SPET. J Nucl Med 44: 583–593

Utech CI, Young CS, Winter PF (1996) Prospective evaluation of fluorine-18 fluorodeoxyglucose positron emission tomography in breast cancer for staging of the axilla related to surgery and immunocytochemistry. Eur J Nucl Med 23:1588–1593

van der Hoeven JJ, Hoekstra OS, Comans EF et al (2002) Determinants of diagnostic performance of [F-18]fluorodeoxyglucose positron emission tomography for axillary staging in breast cancer. Ann Surg 236:619–624

van Eijck CH, Krenning EP, Bootsma A et al (1994) Somatostatin-receptor scintigraphy in primary breast cancer. Lancet 343:640–643

Vanhove C, Defrise M, Franken PR et al (2000) Interest of the ordered subsets expectation maximization (OS-EM) algorithm in pinhole single-photon emission tomography reconstruction: a phantom study. Eur J Nucl Med 27: 140–146

Veronesi U, Paganelli G, Galimberti V et al (1997) Sentinel node biopsy to avoid axillary dissection in breast cancer with clinically negative lymph nodes. Lancet 349:1864–1887

Wahl RL, Siegel BA, Coleman RE et al (2004) Prospective multicenter study of axillary nodal staging by positron emission tomography in breast cancer: a report of the staging breast cancer with PET Study Group. J Clin Oncol 22:277–285

Walsh R, Kornguth PJ, Soo MS et al (1997) Axillary lymph nodes: mammographic, pathologic and clinical correlations. Am J Roentgenol 168:33–38

Wanet PM, Sand A, Abramovici J (1996) Physical and clinical evaluation of high-resolution thyroid pinhole tomography. J Nucl Med 37:2017–2020

Waxman AD, Ramanna L, Memsic LD et al (1993) Thallium scintigraphy in evaluation of mass abnormalities of the breast. J Nucl Med 34:18–23

Waxman AD (1997) The role of $^{(99m)}$Tc methoxyisobutylisonitrile in imaging breast cancer. Semin Nucl Med 27:40–54

Weber DA, Ivanovic M, Franceschi D et al (1994) Pinhole SPECT: an approach to in vivo high resolution SPECT imaging in small laboratory animals. J Nucl Med 35:342–348

Wu MC, Gao DW, Sievers RE et al (2003) Pinhole single-photon emission computed tomography for myocardial perfusion imaging of mice. JACC 42:576–582

Yang WT, Chang J, Metreweli C (2000) Patients with breast cancer: differences in color Doppler flow and gray-scale US features of benign and malignant axillary lymph nodes. Radiology 215:568–573

Yildiz A, Garipagaoglu M, Gungor F et al (2001) The role of technetium-99m methoxyisobutil isonitrile scintigraphy in suspected recurrent breast cancer. Cancer Biother Radiopharm 16:163–169

Yoshimura G, Sakurai T, Oura S et al (1999) Evaluation of axillary lymph node status in breast cancer with MRI. Breast Cancer 25:249–258

Yukihiro M, Inoue T, Iwasaki T et al (1996) Myocardial infarction in rats: high-resolution single-photon emission tomographic imaging with a pinhole collimator. Eur J Nucl Med 23:896–900

Yutani K, Shiba E, Kusuoka H et al (2000) Comparison of FDG-PET with MIBI-SPECT in the detection of breast cancer and axillary lymph node metastasis. J Comput Assist Tomogr 24:274–280

Breast Imaging with Scintimammography

6

Orazio Schillaci and John R. Buscombe

CONTENTS

Abstract

Carcinoma of the breast is the commonest form of cancer in women in most western countries: in the USA, it represents 32% of all invasive tumours in the female population. It is the second leading cause of death for women following lung cancer, accounting for 15% of all cancer deaths among women in the USA. In 2005, the American Cancer Society estimated 211,240 new cases and 40,410 female deaths from this disease (Jemal et al. 2005). Trends in incidence and mortality show that there has been a small, but steady annual increase in breast cancer (BC) incidence over the last 30 years, whereas the mortality rate has declined steadily since the beginning of the 1990s (Jemal et al. 2005).

Early diagnosis is of the utmost importance to improve prognosis. Mammography (MM) is currently the best imaging modality for early detection of BC, and the results of several trials have demonstrated that mammographic screening can decrease the death rate due to BC (Daniel and Kopans 2004; Tabar et al. 2001). Nevertheless, this technique has some limitations that reduce its accuracy (Berlin 2001): not all BCs are evident on mammograms, especially in dense or dysplastic breasts (Birdwell et al. 2001), even palpable cancer may not be seen mammographically (Holland et al. 1983), it lacks of adequate specificity in differentiating between malignant and benign lesions (Kopans 1992; Monusturi et al. 1991) and sometimes deciding which lesions require a biopsy may represent a challenge (Adler and Whal 1995).

Excisional biopsy is the most effective method to determine the nature of breast abnormalities; however, the high number of biopsies in patients with benign breast lesions is a result of the low positive predictive value of MM (Kopans 1992). Breast ultrasound is largely used, but there are a few valid indications for this imaging technique, primarily involving the differentiation between cystic and solid masses and the evaluation of palpable lesions not visible on MM (Jackson 1990; Kopans 2004).

Multiple areas of research have therefore been sought in order to select patients for biopsy and spare unnecessary surgical procedures. Among new imaging modalities, breast magnetic resonance imaging (MRI) and nuclear medicine breast imaging seem to be the most promising.

Breast scintigraphy, also called, is a supplemental breast exam that may be used in some patients to investigate a breast abnormality. This nuclear medicine test is not a primary investigative tool for BC, but can be helpful in selected cases after_mammography has been performed (Schillaci and Buscombe 2004; Schillaci 2005a).

6.1 Radiopharmaceuticals

SM is a diagnostic modality using radiopharmaceuticals to provide tumour-specific imaging of the breast: in fact, because the radiotracer accumulates differently in cancerous and non-cancerous tissues, breast scintigraphy can help physicians in determining whether cancer is present (Buscombe et al. 1997a; Schillaci and Scopinaro 1999).

Currently, the most widely used radiotracers for SM are Tc-99m sestamibi and Tc-99m tetrofosmin, which are small cationic complexes of technetium. Both these radiopharmaceuticals were introduced for myocardial perfusion imaging, and then they were proposed as a tumour-seeking agent (Spanu et al. 2005; Schomacker and Schicha 2000), because of their attractive advantages over traditional radionuclides employed for tumour imaging, such as Ga-67 and Tl-201: patients can be imaged earlier, they are available in a commercial kit form, and they are particularly suitable also for single photon emission computed tomography (SPECT) studies because of the favourable gamma emission characteristics of Tc-99m.

Tc-99m sestamibi uptake and retention in neoplastic cells depend on several factors such as regional blood flow, plasma and mithocondrial membrane potential, angiogenesis and tissue metabolism, with about 90% of tracer activity concentrated in the mitochondria (Carvalho et al. 1992; Delmon-Mongeon et al. 1990; Maublant et al. 1993; Scopinaro et al. 1994). Moreover, it was observed that Tc-99m sestamibi is a transport substrate for the P-glycoprotein (Pgp), a M_r 170,000 plasma membrane protein encoded by the multidrug resistance (MDR) gene that functions as an energy-dependent efflux pump for many drugs that are lipophilic and cationic at physiological pH (Piwnica-Worms et al. 1993). For Tc-99m tetrofosmin, similar mechanisms with respect to Tc-99m sestamibi have been suggested; however, in tumour cell lines tetrofosmin uptake depends on both cell membrane and mitochondria potentials with only a small fraction accumulating inside the mitochondria (Arbab et al. 1996). Tc-99m tetrofosmin shares with Tc-99m sestamibi also the property of being a substrate for the Pgp (Ballinger et al. 2001). Both radiopharmaceuticals proved to be suitable transport substrates also for functional MDR-related protein 1, suggesting their potential usefulness in the in vivo presence of multidrug resistance in neoplasms, which can help in predicting the response to chemotherapy and in the selection of proper management for patients (Van de Wiele et al. 2003).

6.2 Clinical Results

The best results in SM were achieved by imaging patients as proposed by Khalkhali et al. (1994) in the prone position instead of supine. Lateral breast prone images provide an excellent separation of deep breast structures from the myocardium or the abdominal organs (in particular the liver), which always show high uptake of the radiopharmaceuticals that may mask overlying breast activity. Moreover, prone imaging also allows evaluation of deep breast tissue adjacent to the chest wall that results in visualisation of more breast tissue and provides natural landmarks of breast contours, which are very important for lesions' localisation. The first series including a relatively large number of patients on the use of prone SM was evaluated in 59 patients in whom abnormal mammogram and physical examination warranted biopsy or fine-needle cytology of the breast (Khalkhali et al. 1994). In this group, the sensitivity of Tc-99m sestamibi breast imaging was 95.8%, specificity 86.8%, negative predictive value 97.1% and positive predictive value 82.1%, respectively. On the basis of these results, the authors concluded that SM is a highly sensitive test, able also to improve the specificity of mammography, and it is potentially useful to reduce the number of mammographically indicated biopsies.

Numerous studies have been published after this first report about the use of breast scintigraphy in the evaluation of patients with suspected BC. Recently, in order to establish an evidence base for its use clinically, a meta-analysis was performed on both single-site and multi-centre trials performed since January 1997 with both Tc-99m sestamibi and tetrofosmin (Hussain and Buscombe 2006). Using an on-line literature search all such trials containing 100 or more studies were identified; to prevent double counting of patients only the last published report from any centre was considered. A total of 2,424 patients were identified in the single-site trial group, the smallest study having 105 patients and the largest 353 patients. The overall sensitivity was 85% and the specificity was 84%. In the multi-centre trial studies, published data from 3,049 patients were included. The overall sensitivity in this group was also 85% and the specificity was 83%.

Another previous meta-analysis and review of the literature on the accuracy of SM in the diagnosis of BC included 64 unique studies published until December 1999 (Liberman et al. 2003). The articles considered in this review reported data on 5,340 patients with a total of 5,354 breast lesions identified as malignant (n=3,024) or benign (n=2,330) on the basis of fine-needle aspiration, excisional biopsy, core biopsy or mastectomy. The aggregated overall summary estimates were: sensitivity 85.2%, specificity 86.6%, negative predictive value 81.8%, positive predictive value 88.2% and accuracy 85.9%. The majority (80%) of the studies reported sensitivity and specificity values over 80%, with nearly half of them yielding values over 90%.

These results are confirmed by a recent multicenter prospective clinical trial evaluating the efficacy of Tc-99m sestamibi SM for diagnosing BC (Sampalis et al. 2003). A total of 1,734 women were submitted to breast scintigraphy, and, until the end of the study, 1,243 patients had complete data; histopathologic findings demonstrated malignancy in 201 of cases. Sensitivity and specificity of SM were estimated as 93% and 87%, respectively, with a diagnostic accuracy of 88%. Based on their results, both the cited review and the multicenter trial conclude that SM is highly accurate for detecting BC, and it may be used effectively as an adjunct to MM in the diagnosis of this disease.

In a study using receiver-operating-characteristics curve analysis on 374 suspicious breast lesions in 353 patients, the combination of mammography and SM produced more accurate results than either modality alone (Buscombe et al. 2001). Therefore, when there is a doubt about the accuracy of MM, scintigraphy is indicated as a second-line test in breast imaging.

6.3 Sensitivity

It is of the utmost importance to emphasise that the sensitivity of breast scintigraphy is strictly dependent on the size of the studied lesions. A three-centre study including 420 patients reported sensitivity of 26%, 56%, 95% and 97% for T1a, T1b, T1c and T2 BCs, respectively (Scopinaro et al. 1997). In particular, sensitivity was significantly different between malignant lesions >1 cm (46.5% for T1c and T2 cancers) and those inferior to this size (96% for T1c and T2 tumours). It has been reported (Waxman et al. 1995) that lesions greater than 12 mm are detected in more than 92% of cases, whereas smaller sized tumours are visualised only in 50% of cases. Similar results regarding sensitivity are obtained when breast lesions are grouped as palpable and nonpalpable, which always show a lower sensitivity (Scopinaro et al. 1997; Mekhmandarov et al 1998; Tolmos et al. 1998), as confirmed by the results of a multicentre clinical trial involving 673 patients in 42 North American institutions (Khalkhali et al. 2000). In this study, the institutional sensitivity for breast cancer detection was 87% and 61% for palpable and nonpalpable lesions, respectively. In the previously cited review sensitivity was 87.8% for patients with a palpable breast mass and 66.8% for patients without a palpable lesion (Liberman et al. 2003). These findings suggest that studies in which patient referral is biased to larger lesions will have more favourable sensitivities than studies in which the bias is toward smaller lesions, and clearly indicate that SM cannot be considered a screening procedure for BC detection. Moreover, a recent multivariate analysis of causes of false-negative scintimammographic results clearly indicates that the size of the tumour represents the most relevant independent parameter, and there are no reliable preoperative prognostic factors that are really useful for improving SM sensitivity in patients with small breast carcinomas (Lumachi et al. 2006). However, also biological factors, such as tumour type, determining the net radiotracer uptake in the cancer (Buscombe et al.

1997b) and the site of the lesions (i.e., near the chest wall) have to be taken into account for their visualisation by SM (Scopinaro et al. 1997).

Tumour size is crucial also for detecting ductal carcinoma in situ (DCIS). In the North American multicentre trial, the sensitivity of SM in patients with DCIS was 45.9%, in contrast to the 82% sensitivity for invasive cancers (Khalkhali et al. 2000). In particular, the sensitivity was 57.1% and 39.1% in patients with palpable and non-palpable DCIS, respectively. In another study, all the four DCISs evaluated were not visualised by breast scintigraphy (Obwegeser et al. 1999). However, in a systematic review of more than 350 patients with suspected BC that included 15 patients with proven DCIS (Cwikla et al. 2000a), the sensitivity of SM in the latter group of patients was, at 80%, almost double that of MM (43%).

6.4 SPECT

The acquisition of tomographic images, by means of SPECT, can play a role in increasing the sensitivity of planar scintimammography. However, different studies using SPECT for primary breast cancer imaging have reached discordant findings when compared to the results of planar scintigraphy. Although SPECT imaging provides better contrast resolution, it can be difficult to obtain accurate localisation of the lesion in some cases; on the contrary, prone images with planar lateral views provide natural landmarks of breast contours, which are very important for lesions' localisation (Schillaci et al. 1997a). The co-registration of SPECT with structural information obtained through radiological examinations allows the precise correlation of functional and anatomic data on the same image. The commercial availability of a hybrid gamma camera/CT scanner, which is able to provide, in addition to scintigraphic data, cross-sectional X-ray transmission images, has facilitated the fusion of anatomical maps and SPECT images (Schillaci 2005b). The first clinical applications of this new technology are very encouraging; in particular, when used for breast imaging, SPECT/CT correlative data have been demonstrated to be particularly useful in the more difficult cases, facilitating the interpretation of SPECT findings with a more accurate anatomical assessment of sites of abnormal activity (Schillaci et al. 2005a). Moreover, from a technical point of view, images should be reconstructed using iterative algorithms instead of back-projection methods (Garin et al. 2001).

It is interesting highlighting that the less satisfactory results were reported in studies employing SPECT prone dependent-breast imaging (Tiling et al. 1998; Buscombe et al. 1999). Good quality SPECT images can be obtained only with the patient in the supine position and the arms up, because SPECT with patients in prone position is clearly limited by geometric constraints of the patient, imaging table and gantry (Waxman 1997). The results of some studies using supine SPECT are more encouraging; in particular, in a study including 93 patients with breast lesions ≤1 cm, supine SPECT gave a significantly higher sensitivity than planar images both in T1b and nonpalpable BCs, without any decrease in specificity (Spanu et al. 2002).

The higher sensitivity of SPECT when compared to planar SM was reported in a recent paper aimed to evaluate the impact of SM on the management of patients with a doubtful or discordant triple diagnosis: mammography, ultrasound and fine-needle aspiration cytology (Mathieu et al. 2005). The study included 104 patients, either at initial presentation or after treatment. BC was proven in 69 cases: SM SPECT had a sensitivity of 88.4% and a specificity of 67%. Eleven cancers were detected by SPECT, although planar images were negative. SM SPECT correctly evaluated multicentricity or bilaterality in 8 of 11 patients and resulted in an increased tumour size in 8 patients. Overall, SM SPECT modified the patient management in 49% cases: SM made the diagnosis of cancer in 30 cases with doubtful or discordant triple diagnosis and ruled out malignancy in 28 cases.

6.5 Dedicated Breast Gamma Cameras

The problem of detecting small tumours is critical for the future development and clinical acceptance of SM, given that the other breast imaging modalities are increasingly used for the early identification of small suspicious lesions. Currently, SM is usually performed with a standard Anger camera, which is limited by its relatively poor intrinsic spatial resolution and by the sub-optimal detection geometry, because of the distance between the detector and the imaged breast.

The use of small field of view high-resolution cameras allows both greater flexibility in patient positioning (improving breast imaging by limiting the field of view and reducing image contamination from other organs, i.e., liver and heart) and breast compression, with an important increase in the target-to-background ratio (Schillaci et al. 2005b). In fact, the detector can be placed directly against the chest and a mild compression is possible, to reduce breast thickness and improve the camera's sensitivity. Moreover, by design, the dedicated cameras are also able to provide better intrinsic and extrinsic spatial resolution than standard ones, with an enhancement in contrast resolution of small lesions (Brem et al. 2002). These cameras can be easily attached to an adapter that fits on most upright mammography machines, replacing the radiographic Bucky.

The results obtained in a limited number of patients indicate a better sensitivity of high-resolution cameras when compared to conventional, large field of view cameras, especially in detecting small breast cancers (Brem et al. 2002; Scopinaro et al. 1999). In particular, the results of a study specifically designed to evaluate the usefulness of a dedicated breast-specific camera as a screening modality have been recently reported. In 37 women clinically and mammographically negative, with dense breasts and a family history of breast carcinoma (Coover et al. 2004), cancer that was otherwise undetectable by conventional methods was visualized in 3 out of 5 SM positive cases; only one of the three carcinomas identified with the specific gamma camera was detectable also with a standard camera. An important advantage is also the possibility of acquiring scintigraphic scans in the same mammographic views (craniocaudal and lateral oblique), making the comparison of the two kinds of images simpler.

Using the dedicated camera LumaGEM 3200S (Gamma Medica, Inc., Northridge, USA), 29 patients with lesions $\leq$1 cm were prospectively evaluated with a conventional gamma camera and the dedicated device (Schillaci et al. 2006). Four out of nine (44%) of the malignant lesions were detected with the standard gamma camera, whereas the high-resolution camera visualized all the BCs. The standard gamma camera and the dedicated one showed the same specificity: 19 out of 20 (95%) benign lesions were negative. The same dedicated device was used in a group of 40 women: Tc-99m sestamibi SM detected 33 out of 36 malignant lesions (sensitivity 92%) in 26 patients (Rhodes et al. 2005). In particular, the sensitivity was 86% in tumours sized less than 1 cm and 100% in larger ones, and 75% in T1a and 89% in T1b tumours. The specificity result was 64%, due to five false-positive findings (two fibroadenomas, one inflammatory fat necrosis, one radial scar and one normal breast parenvyma). Their data indicate that high-resolution imaging is able to visualise smaller and deeper breast cancers, overcoming the main limitations of conventional SM. To prospectively evaluate a high-resolution breast-specific gamma camera for depicting occult breast cancer in women at high risk for breast cancer, but with normal mammographic and physical examination findings, 94 women have been recently evaluated with Tc-99m sestamibi SM (Brem et al. 2005). Sixteen patients had abnormal scintigraphy: 14 of them had either benign findings at biopsy or no abnormality at US; in two patients, invasive carcinoma was diagnosed at US-guided biopsy. These results confirm that high-resolution breast-specific scintimammography can depict small ($\leq$1 cm), mammographically occult, nonpalpable lesions in women at increased risk for BC not otherwise identified.

6.6 Specificity

The specificity of SM is high both for palpable and nonpalpable lesions, due to the low number of false-positive results, which are mainly due to focal areas of radiopharmaceutical uptake in local inflammation, fibroadenomas and fibrocystic changes. The most common pathologic feature among false-positive findings is the hypercellularity of the lesions. Tc-99m sestamibi uptake in benign pathologies is strongly correlated with the presence of proliferative changes (Gupta et al. 1996). Because it has been shown that patients with hyperproliferative breast disease have a higher relative risk for development of cancer than those with nonproliferative benign breast, Waxman speculates that the false-positive scintimammographic results can reflect a premalignant potential. In particular, patients with atypical hyperplasia show higher incidence of positive scintigraphic findings (Waxman et al. 1997). Nevertheless, a negative SM in patients with palpable or >1-cm-sized lesions significantly reduces the probability of proliferative breast disease. In a recent paper aimed to assess tissue-specific effects on the uptake of Tc-99m sestamibi by breast lesions (Tiling et al. 2004), a targeted analysis of false scintigraphic diagnoses has been done. Surgical specimens from 75 patients (30 benign lesions, 8 of which had shown false-positive scintigraphic findings) were subjected to a distinct histopathologic/immunohistochemical reevaluation. Tissue-specific parameters, including cellular density, vascularity, signs of inflammation and proliferative activity, were visually scored and correlated with Tc-99m sestamibi uptake on scintimammograms. Only for a few specific histopathologic parameters, the authors found a statistically significant correlation with the uptake behaviour of a lesion; overall, the uptake pattern was determined by a combination of factors, with the extent of the inflammatory component of benign lesions playing a major role.

To improve the specificity of breast scintigraphy in differentiating malignant from benign lesions, a semiquantitative analysis with calculation of the count ratio of the target lesion to the controlateral normal area has been proposed. However, discordant results have been reported, because many benign abnormalities exhibit ratios similar to those of malignant ones (Khalkhali et al. 2001).

Moreover, also the phase of the menstrual cycle in which SM is performed has to be taken into account for improving specificity of the method in premenopausal women. In fact, we have noticed significant differences in tracer uptake pattern in the breast in the same patients evaluated in different phases of the cycle (personal observations), with less uptake in the mid-menstrual cycle period. However, this issue requires further evaluations to define the best time of imaging, also if a preliminary study indicated that SM is more specific if performed between 10 and 15 days following the last day of the menstrual cycle (Horne et al. 1999). The timing of acquiring SM in pre-menopausal women may also affect the performance of SM. In fact, when dichotomising patients as ≤ 50 or >50 years, despite a comparable sensitivity, higher specificity in the older population with palpable masses has been observed (Khalkhali et al. 2000). Other studies, however, have shown a much better sensitivity of SM in younger women when compared with MM, presumably due to the higher prevalence of high-grade ductal carcinomas in this age group, which displays the highest uptake of Tc-99m sestamibi, but often presents without calcification (Buscombe et al. 2002).

6.7 Clinical Indications

But, who is a candidate for SM? Breast scintigraphy is not a screening tool for BC; however, after a physical breast examination, MM and ultrasound are performed, SM may be appropriate for certain patients and helps in determining whether a patient has a suspicious breast lesion that would require a biopsy or not, thus decreasing the number of negative breast biopsies (Schillaci et al. 2005c). The appropriate clinical indications of SM are listed in Table 6.1, and the subgroups of patients that can really benefit from breast scintigraphy are now examined.

Table 6.1. Clinical indications of scintimammography. From Schillaci and Buscombe 2004

- Equivocal mammograms
- Dense breast
- Palpable abnormalities that cannot be imaged well with mammography
- Axillary lymph-node metastases of an adenocarcinoma of unknown primary origin
- Breast implants
- Parenchymal distortions of the breast.
- Doubtful microcalcifications
- Assessment of multicentric disease
- Breast iatrogenic architectural distortion
- Monitoring the response to neoadjuvant chemotherapy

6.7.1 Patients with Equivocal Mammograms

Breast scintigraphy was performed in 90 patients after classifying their mammograms as having a low, indeterminate or high probability of malignancy (Prats et al. 1999). SM was positive in all cancers with a low and indeterminate mammographic suspicion of malignancy and in 83.3% of highly suspicious cancers; specificity was 84.2%, 77.8% and 70% in the three groups, respectively. Based on these findings, the authors proposed a protocol with biopsy performed only on highly suspicious abnormalities and on those with low-indeterminate suspicion and positive breast scintigraphy or with negative SM and less than 1 cm in size. This approach would have resulted in a 34% reduction of the total number of biopsies performed and in a 65% reduction in the number of biopsies performed in the low-indeterminate groups.

The usefulness of SM in evaluating patients with low or indeterminate likelihood of cancer at MM is confirmed by a prospective study including 75 patients with minimal mammographic or physical examination findings (Polan et al. 2001). The overall sensitivity and specificity of breast scintigraphy in this series were 90% and 93.8%, respectively, suggesting that SM is useful both in early detection of breast cancer and in decreasing the number of unnecessary biopsies.

In the previously cited study (Sampalis et al. 2003), MMs were classified according to the American College of Radiology (ACR) Breast Imaging Reporting and Data System (BI-RADS), which provides a standardised reporting system for MM (Amercian College of Radiology 1995). On the basis of the level of suspicion, mammographically detected lesions are placed into one of five assessment categories (Table 6.2). Of the 696 BI-RADS 1 and 2 mammograms, SM accurately identified 77% of true-positive and 88% of true-negative lesions for malignancy, and falsely detected 2.3% of benign lesions as positive and 23% of malignant ones as negative. Among the 348 BI-RADS 3 and 4 mammograms, breast scintigraphy correctly diagnosed 88% of true-positive and 91% of true-negative lesions for malignancy, and falsely detected 8.8% of benign abnormalities as positive and 12.2% of malignant lesions as negative. In the 199 BI-RADS 5 lesions, SM accurately detected 98% of true positive and 67% of true negative abnormalities for malignancy, and falsely detected 33% of benign lesions as positive and 2% of malignant lesions as negative. The highest accuracy of SM (i.e., 90.5%) is reached in the group of BI-RADS 3 and 4 mammograms, including probably benign and suspected breast lesions. These results in a very large study population with a low prevalence of breast cancer (13%) indicate that a positive scintigraphy significantly increases the capacity to predict the presence of malignant disease. Moreover, the implementation of SM as an adjunct diagnostic tool could reduce both the number of unnecessary biopsies (a reduction of 62.1%) and the number of missed cancers (a reduction of 86%).

Table 6.2. BI-RADS final assessment categories. From Schillaci and Buscombe 2004

Category	Assessment	Description
1	Negative	Nothing to comment on
2	Benign findings	A benign finding described
3	Probably benign findings	Short-term follow-up recommended
4	Suspicious abnormality	Biopsy should be urged
5	Highly suggestive of malignancy	Appropriate action should be taken

6.7.2 Patients with Dense Breast

Radiographically dense breast tissue accounts for a large percentage of the cases of mammographically "missed" cancers (Birdwell et al. 2001). In particular, breast cancers presenting as masses without speculations or calcifications can be missed in dense breasts (Thurfjell 2002). Considering that about 25% of women have dense breasts, but that an elevated number of postmenopausal women receive hormone replacement therapy that causes an increase in breast density and younger women are included in screening protocols, this is an important problem. Moreover, women with dense breasts are also at increased risk for cancer because in a dense breast there is more glandular tissue and so more cells with the potential of a malignant transformation (Thurfjell 2002). SM can play a clinical role in this kind of patient because both Tc-99m sestamibi and Tc-99m tetrofosmin uptake is independent of the presence of dense breast tissue on MM (Schillaci and Scopinaro 1999; Schillaci et al. 1997b) (Fig. 6.1).

In a group of 67 patients with a suspicious palpable breast lesion but indeterminate MM due to extremely dense breast (grade IV according to the ACR classification), Tc-99m sestamibi imaging showed a sensitivity of 93.5%, a specificity of 91.7% and a diagnostic accuracy of 92.5% (Schillaci et al. 1999). Similar results were reported in patients with palpable breast masses that could not be adequately evaluated by MM due to radiographically dense tissue (Cutrone et al. 1999). MM yielded a sensitivity, specificity and accuracy of 73.9%, 53.3% and 63.2%, respectively, whereas SM resulted in a sensitivity of 95.6%, specificity of 91.1% and accuracy of 92.6%.

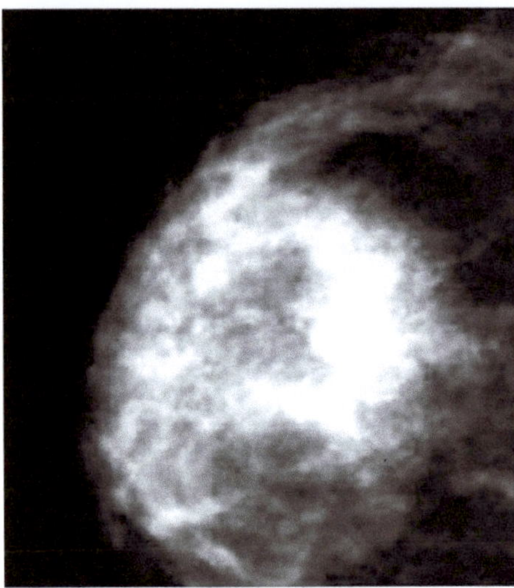
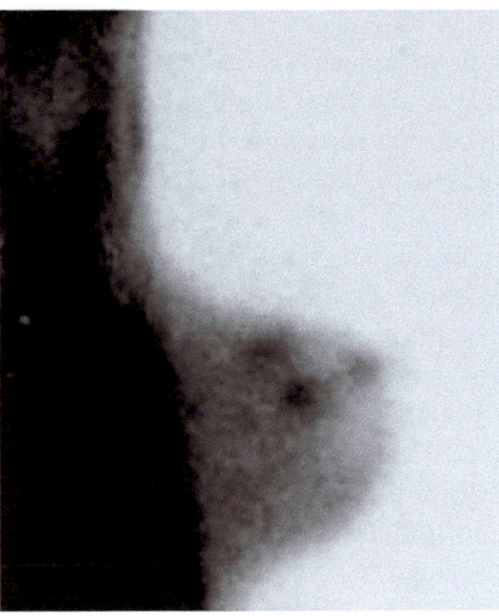

Fig. 6.1. A 44-year-old patient with very dense breast tissue in the right breast. Little can be seen on MM (*left-hand image*); however, SM (*right-hand image*) clearly reveals a 25-mm ductal carcinoma with two adjacent sites of DCIS. (Note that the transmission mammogram points in the opposite direction to the emission SM images). From Schillaci and Buscombe 2004

The accuracy of Tc-99m sestamibi breast imaging as an adjunct to MM and physical examination in detecting BC in patients with dense and fatty breast has been evaluated in a prospective multicenter study (Khalkhali et al. 2002). Of the 558 women enrolled, 47% had dense breasts according to the ACR criteria. The overall results showed that the accuracy of SM in visualizing breast cancer was similar for fatty and dense breasts. This finding confirms that the accuracy of breast scintigraphy is not affected by breast density and that the sensitivity of SM in dense breasts appears to be higher than that of mammography. Moreover, this study indicates that in women with dense breasts, a palpable mass and a negative mammography, a positive scintigraphy increases the probability of cancer from 15.6% before the nuclear medicine test to 37.5% after, whereas a negative SM decreases the probability of cancer from 15.6% to 6.9%. In patients with dense breasts, a palpable mass and a positive mammogram, a negative scintigraphy decreases the probability of cancer from 60.4% to 31.2%, whereas a positive SM increases the probability of cancer to 78%. In conclusion, in patients with a palpable mass that is not detected by mammography due to dense breast tissue, SM is appropriate because of its high sensitivity in palpable lesions.

6.7.3 Patients with Palpable Abnormalities that cannot be Imaged Well with MM

It is possible that a palpable mass is difficult to study with mammography, in particular in patients with lumpy breasts or fibrocystic changes. Glandular lumpy breasts with diffuse areas of increased and decreased density and fibrocystic breasts where it is difficult to determine the exact reason for highlighted abnormalities may often result in equivocal or not diagnostic MM. These patients are candidates for a breast biopsy or for a follow-up. Considering the very high accuracy of breast scintigraphy in evaluating palpable breast masses, this examination could be performed just after MM. The inclusion of SM in the work up of these patients would reduce their anxiety during the follow-up period (usually 6 months) and would be useful, especially in patients reluctant to undergo biopsy or when this procedure is relatively contraindicated (Waxman et al. 1997). Therefore, due to its higher specificity, SM rather than contrast-enhanced MRI may be suitable to further assess patients with indeterminate mammograms and to reduce the number of biopsies that give benign results (Tiling et al. 2005).

6.7.4 Patients with Axillary Lymph-Node Metastases of an Adenocarcinoma of Unknown Primary Origin

BC can manifest as isolated axillary node metastases, with negative MM and ultrasound and no clinical evidence of a primary tumour in the breast. In these patients, the frequency of finding an occult BC at MM is low. SM may be useful in this subset of the population for detecting the possible primary tumour within the breast. However, further study is needed to support this clinical indication of breast scintigraphy, in particular a comparison with MRI in the same group of patients would be of value, given that MRI results are satisfactory in this application (Orel and Schnall 2001).

6.7.5 Patients with Breast Implants

At MM, large portions of breast tissue can be obscured in patients with breast implants even when special compression techniques are employed. SM is not affected by the attenuation from the implant and can visualise any lesion within the breast tissue, and so can be useful when MM is not feasible or non-diagnostic (Fig. 6.2). A comparison with MRI in this group of patients would be very interesting, considering the diagnostic role of this technique in evaluating breast lesions overlying implants (McMahon et al. 2001).

6.7.6 Patients with Parenchymal Distortions of the Breast

In patients with focal architectural distortion, asymmetric breasts or ductal asymmetry, especially if at high risk for BC, SM may be advantageous compared to mammography because the diagnostic accuracy of scintigraphy is independent of structural characteristics and the anatomical appearances of breast tissue (Waxman et al. 1997).

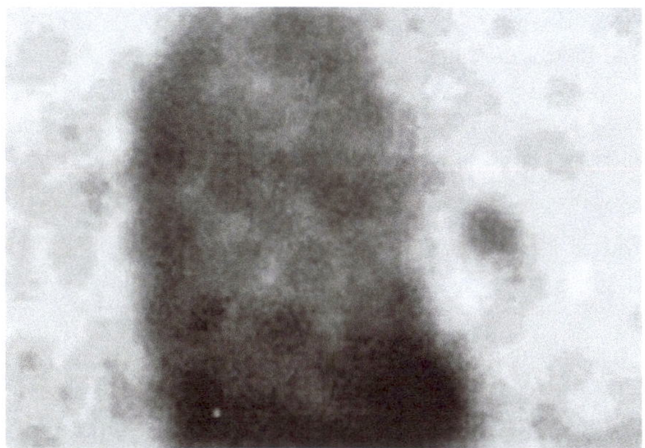

Fig. 6.2. Tomographic sagittal image showing a small focal area of Tc-99m sestamibi on the outside edge of a cosmetic breast prosthesis in a 32-year-old female. Excision confirmed a 15-mm ductal carcinoma. From Schillaci and Buscombe 2004

6.7.7 Patients with Doubtful Microcalcifications

BI-RADS classification of breast microcalcifications include clusters of tiny calcifications, all round or oval (category 3, probably benign lesions), granular microcalcifications (category 4, lesions with low-to-intermediate suspicion) and heterogeneous, allomorphic, branching, or casting calcifications (category 5, lesions highly suspect for malignancy). Despite the fact that microcalcifications are sometimes the only sign of the presence of cancer, the majority of them are benign; therefore, an examination able to accurately differentiate benign from malignant lesions, especially in category 4, would avoid many unnecessary biopsies.

The accuracy of breast scintigraphy in distinguishing between benign and malignant isolated clusters of microcalcifications has been evaluated in a series of 97 patients (Marini et al. 2001). Based on the level of suspicion of malignancy, the results of MM, SM and the combination MM-SM were divided in five groups. Seventy-four per cent of lesions with high scintigraphic suspicion of malignancy and only 9% with a low suspicion resulted in malignancy. These findings suggest that SM contributes to enhancing the diagnostic capability of MM and, in combination with mammography, may play a role in characterizing isolated clusters of microcalcifications in the breast (Fig. 6.3). If properly used, breast scintigraphy seems able, in selected cases, to help radiologists in choosing the follow-up rather than submitting patients to biopsy.

6.7.8 Assessment of Multicentric Disease

An accurate determination of the extent of BC is of the utmost importance in choosing the best surgical treatment. The ability in identifying the presence of multicentric disease preoperatively would assist in selecting the appropriate candidates for breast-conserving surgery, because mastectomy is indicated if there is multicentricity.

Like breast MRI, nuclear medicine may also be helpful to determine if multiple breast tumours are present. In fact, in those patients clinically and mammographically suspected of having unifocal carcinoma, up to 63% will have an additional malignant focus in the ipsilateral breast after detailed serial sectioning of the mastectomy specimen. It has

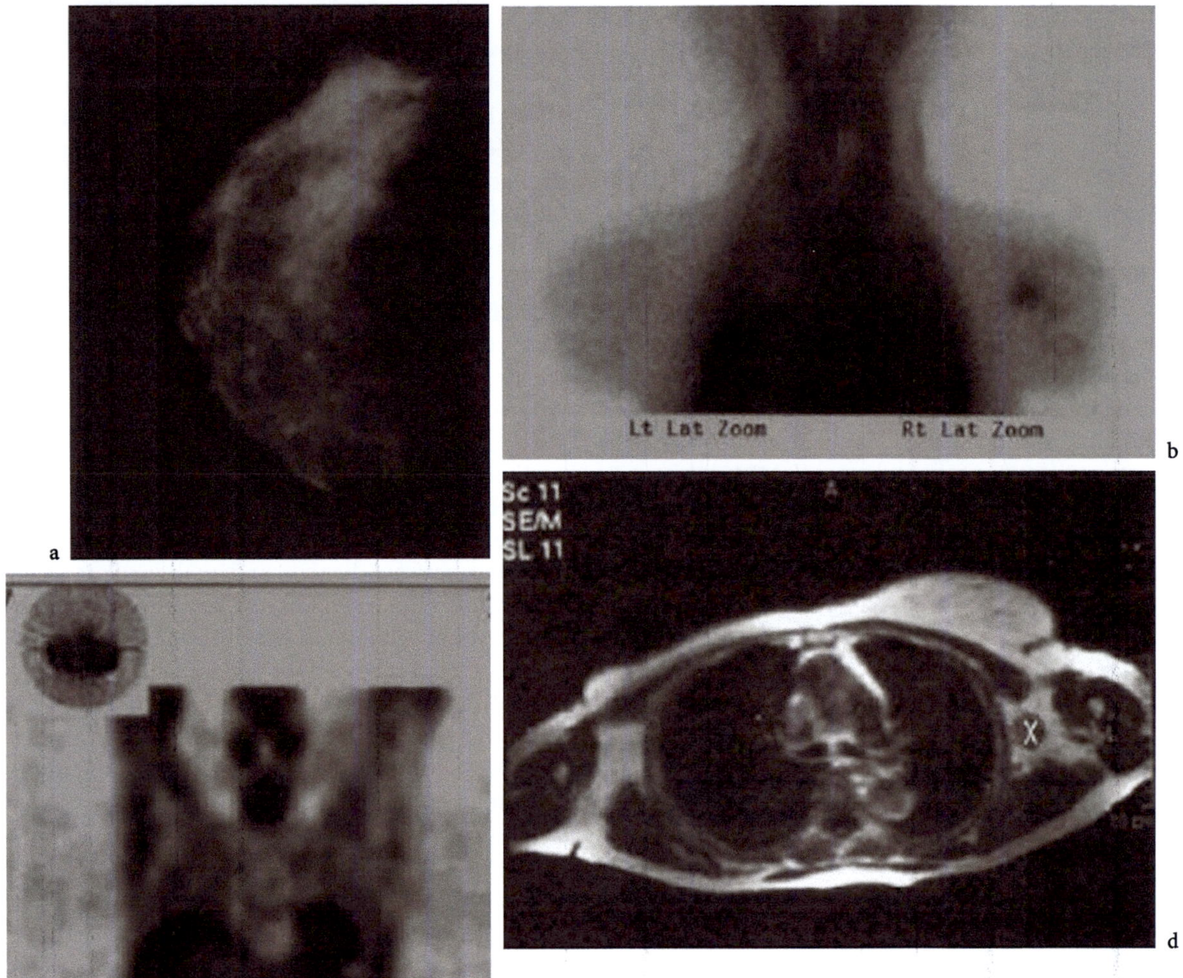

Fig. 6.3a–d. Craniocaudal view MM (**a**) of the right breast showing increased density and widespread microcalcifications, but no abnormality at the site of a palpable lesion. Planar prone lateral SM (**b**) shows a single area of focal uptake at the site of a 22-mm ductal carcinoma, confirmed by biopsy. The patient also underwent SPECT imaging (**c**), and focal uptake was seen in the left axilla; this was reported, but not biopsied. The patient had a right mastectomy and right axillary clearance. Follow-up MRI performed 6 months later (**d**) shows an abnormal left axillary lymph node (marked *X*). This was removed and found also to contain ductal breast cancer. From Schillaci and Buscombe 2004

been shown that SM will identify nearly three times the number of multi-focal tumours compared to MM and ultrasound alone (Cwikla et al. 2001). Although the overall sensitivity of breast scintigraphy in detecting BC is superior to that of physical examination and MM in identifying multicentric disease, it is not so high, especially in imaging small tumours (Vargas at al. 2001). Therefore, in this respect, nuclear medicine breast imaging is often of poor value; however, considering that MRI is sub-optimal (Tillman et al. 2002), SM may have limited applications in selected cases (Fig. 6.4).

6.7.9 Patients with Breast Iatrogenic Architectural Distortion

MM is less accurate in evaluating breasts that have been previously submitted to surgery, biopsy, radiation therapy or chemotherapy. Patients who have a scar within the breast due to these iatrogenic interventions are often difficult to study with MM, whereas a functional imaging technique such as breast scintigraphy is not affected by these morphologic changes. The only consistent series looking at

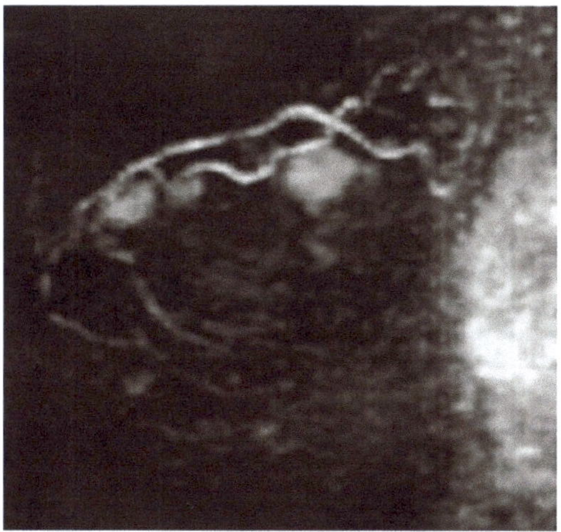
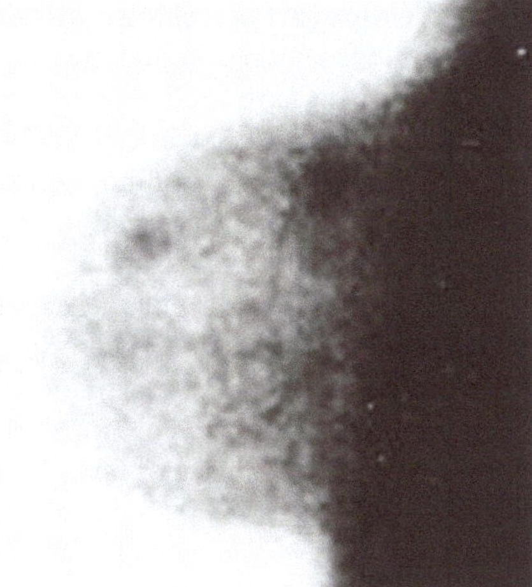

Fig. 6.4. Composite MRI image (*left image*) performed after gadolinium contrast showing the same multicentric tumour in the left breast as revealed on Tc-99m sestamibi SM (*right image*). From Schillaci and Buscombe 2004

recurrence within the breasts have shown that either alone or in combination with mammography, Tc-99m sestamibi SM is able to find almost double the number of intra-breast recurrences than relying on MM and ultrasound alone (Cwikla et al. 2000b; Yildiz et al. 2001). In addition other loco-regional disease outside of the breast such as lymph nodes may also be seen. Based on these results, the accuracy of SM in the assessment of patients with suspected recurrent BC is similar to that observed in patients with primary tumour. Recently, also Tc-99m tetrofosmin scintigraphy, in particular SPECT imaging, has been demonstrated to be useful in the follow-up of surgically treated BC patients for the detection of both loco-regional and distant recurrences (Spanu et al. 2003). Therefore, breast scintigraphy is an accurate non-invasive method to differentiate recurrent disease from fibrosis and scarring in patients previously submitted to surgery with or without radiotherapy; it can play a complementary role to conventional imaging procedures in this subset of patients.

6.7.10 Monitoring the Response to Neoadjuvant Chemotherapy

SM can be useful and effective in monitoring the response to neoadjuvant chemotherapy in patients with locally advanced breast cancer. In a series of patients in whom Tc-99m sestamibi scans were performed before and after neoadjuvant chemotherapy, using a simple region of interest method, it was possible to compare activity before and after the last cycle of cytotoxic chemotherapy. There was a reduction in activity in all patients after chemotherapy, but an additional drop was seen in those in whom there was a histological response (Cwikla et al. 1997, Takamura et al. 2001). Moreover, scintigraphic changes were a better predictor of the final histological response than MM or clinical examination. In particular, scintigraphy demonstrated clear superiority to MM in assessing patients with positive responses to neoadjuvant chemotherapy (Maini et al. 1997).

Tc-99m sestamibi imaging before the first chemotherapy and after the first or second cycle was used to predict the final result at the end of the treatment (Mankoff et al. 1999). This is important in breast cancer, as the response rate for neo-adjuvant chemotherapy in locally advanced disease is about 40%: therefore, 60% will not only risk potential side effects, but do so without any benefit. The patients would also have to wait for definitive and possibly curative surgery delayed until the end of the chemotherapy treatment. After 2 months the mean change in radiopharmaceutical uptake was -35% in patients with a final histological response compared to a mean increase of 17% in those ones who did not respond to therapy. When a complete pathologic response was obtained, the mean drop in Tc-99m sestamibi activity was 58%; moreover, a decrease of $\geq$40% in tracer activity after the second cycle allowed the identification of all patients with a complete response. It was more difficult to predict patients with a partial response, probably due to the small number of cases evaluated.

These findings are confirmed in a study in which patients with locally advanced and inflammatory BC were submitted to a scintigraphy protocol including two studies before and after neo-adjuvant chemotherapy. SM proved accurate in predicting tumour presence or absence after treatment, and useful for the in vivo detection of intrinsic and acquired chemo-resistant breast cancers, which is a very important factor for planning the best therapeutic options (Mezi et al. 2003). Moreover, it has been recently reported that high primary BC Tc-99m sestamibi uptake after neoadjuvant chemotherapy predicted poor survival, suggesting serial SM imaging may provide a useful quantitative surrogate end point for neoadjuvant chemotherapy trials in locally advanced BC (Dunnwald et al. 2005).

6.7 Cost Effectiveness

The cost effectiveness of SM has been extensively analysed in an article based on Medicare reimbursement values and quantitative methods of decision analysis (Allen et al. 2000). Decision-tree models were constructed to account for differences in competing strategies for BC diagnosis (MM alone or SM and MM). The use of the strategy including breast scintigraphy after MM demonstrated cost effectiveness over a large range; the cost saving comes at the expense of a small reduction in life expectancy. In particular, performing SM significantly lowered the number of breast biopsies in healthy patients. Therefore, these findings quantitatively verify the usefulness of SM in minimizing unnecessary biopsies.

6.8 Conclusions

MM remains the first imaging modality for the early detection of BC. SM can be a useful adjunct to non-diagnostic MM in some specific clinical applications, to improve patient selection for breast biopsy and reduce the number of negative biopsies, due to its capability to differentiate benign from malignant lesions. The main advantage of SM is its functional basis that makes radiopharmaceutical uptake not related with breast tissue density or with the presence of scar tissue or implants. The main limitation of SM is the low sensitivity for lesions sized less than 1 cm; the detection rate of small BCs will be improved by larger availability and diffusion of dedicated high-resolution breast-specific cameras.

References

Adler DD, Wahl RL (1991) New methods for imaging the breast: techniques, findings and potential. AJR Am J Roentgenol 164: 19–30

Allen MW, Hendi P, Schwimmer J et al (2000) Decision analysis for the cost-effectiveness of sestamibi scintimammography in minimizing unnecessary biopsies. Q J Nucl Med 44: 168–185

American College of Radiology (1995) Breast imaging reporting and data system (BI-RADS) 2nd edn. American College of Radiology, Reston

Arbab AS, Koizumi K, Toyama K et al (1996) Uptake of technetium-99m-tetrofosmin, technetium-99m-MIBI and thallium-201 in tumor cell lines. J Nucl Med 37: 1551–1556

Ballinger JR (2001) ^{99m}Tc-tetrofosmin for functional imaging of P-glycoprotein modulation in vivo. J Clin Pharmacol (Suppl): 39S–47S

Berlin L (2001) The missed breast cancer redux: time for educating the public about the limitations of mammography? AJR Am J Roentgenol 176: 1131–1134

Birdwell RL, Ikeda DM, O'Shaughnessy KF et al (2001) Mammographic characteristics of 115 missed cancers later detected with screening mammography and the potential utility of computer-aided detection. Radiology 219: 192–202

Brem RF, Schoonjans JM, Kieper DA et al (2002) High-resolution scintimammography: a pilot study. J Nucl Med 2002; 43: 909–915

Brem RF, Rapelyea JA, Zisman G et al (2005) Occult breast cancer: scintimammography with high-resolution breast-specific gamma camera in women at high risk for breast cancer. Radiology 237: 274–280

Buscombe JR, Cwikla JB, Thakrar DS et al (1997a) Scintigraphic imaging of breast cancer: a review. Nucl Med Commun 18: 698–709

Buscombe JR, Cwikla JB, Thakrar DS et al (1997b) Uptake of Tc-99m MIBI related to tumour size and type. Anticancer Res 17: 1693–1694

Buscombe JR, Cwikla JB, Thakrar DS et al (1999) Prone SPET scintimammography. Nucl Med Commun 20 :237–245

Buscombe JR, Cwikla JB, Holloway B et al (2001) Prediction of the usefulness of combined mammography and scintimammography in suspected primary breast cancer using ROC curves. J Nucl Med 42: 3–8

Buscombe JR, Kolasinska AD, Cwikla JB et al (2002) Does combining scintimammography and mammography in

the primary breast cancers than mammography alone in the under and over 50s? (abstract). J Nucl Med 43: 75P

Carvalho PA, Chiu ML, Kronauge JF et al (1992) Subcelluar distribution and analysis of Tc-99m MIBI in isolated perfused rat hearts. J Nucl Med 33: 1516–1521

Coover LR, Caravaglia G, Kuhn P (2004) Scintimammography with dedicated breast camera detects and localizes occult carcinoma. J Nucl Med 45: 553–558

Cutrone JA, Khalkhali I, Yospur LS et al (1999) Tc-99m sestamibi scintimammography for the evaluation of breast masses in patients with radiographically dense breasts. Breast J 5: 383–388

Cwikla JB,Buscombe JR, Barlow RV et al (1997) The effect of chemotherapy on the uptake of technetium-99m sestamibi in breast cancer. Eur J Nucl Med 24: 1175–1178

Cwikla JB, Buscombe JR, Hilson AJ (2000a) Detection of DCIS using ^{99m}Tc-MIBI scintimammography in patients with suspected primary breast cancer, comparison with conventional mammography. Nucl Med Rev Cent East Eur 3:41–45

Cwikla JB, Kolasinska A, Buscombe JR et al (2000b) Tc-99m MIBI in suspected recurrent breast cancer. Cancer Biother Radiopharm 15: 367–372

Cwikla JB, Buscombe JR, Holloway B et al (2001) Can scintimammography with ^{99m}Tc-MIBI identify multifocal and multicentric primary breast cancer? Nucl Med Commun 22: 1287–1293

Daniel B, Kopans DB (2004) Mammography screening is saving thousands of lives, but will it survive medical malpractice? Radiology 230: 20–24

Delmon-Mongeon LI, Piwinica-Worms D, Van der Abbeele AD et al (1990) Uptake of the cation hexakis (2-methoxyisobutilisonitrile)-technetium-99m by human carcinoma cell lines in vitro. Cancer Res 50: 2198–2202

Dunnwald LK, Gralow JR, Ellis GK et al (2005) Residual tumor uptake of [^{99m}Tc]-sestamibi after neoadjuvant chemotherapy for locally advanced breast carcinoma predicts survival. Cancer 103: 680–688

Garin E, Devillers A, Girault S et al (2001) Scintimammography: better detection of small-sized lesions with tomoscintigraphic than planar images, a phantom study. Nucl Med Commun 22: 1045–1054

Gupta P, Waxman A, Nguyen K et al (1996) Correlation of Tc-99m sestamibi uptake with histopathologic characteristics in patients with breast diseases (abstract). J Nucl Med 37: 250P

Holland R, Jan HC, Hendricks L et al (1983) Mammographically occult breast cancers: a pathological and radiologic study. Cancer 52:1810–1819

Horne T, Pappo I, Cohenpour M et al (1999) 99Tcm-MIBI scintimammography for the detection of breast malignancies: the contribution of the count ratio to specificity. Nucl Med Commun 20: 511–516

Hussain R, Buscombe JR (2006) A meta-analysis of scintimammography: an evidence-based approach to its clinical utility. Nucl Med Commun 27: 589–594

Jackson VP (1990) The role of US in breast imaging. Radiology 177: 305–311

Jemal A, Murray T, Ward E et al (2005) Cancer statistics, 2005. CA Cancer J Clin 55: 10–30

Khalkhali I, Vargas HI (2001) The role of nuclear medicine in breast cancer detection: functional breast imaging. Radiol Clin North Am 39:1053–1068

Khalkhali I, Mena I, Jouanne E et al (1994) Prone scintimammography in patients with suspicion of carcinoma of the breast. J Am Coll Surg 178: 491–497

Khalkhali I, Villanueva-Meyer J, Edell SL et al (2000) Diagnostic accuracy of ^{99m}Tc-sestamibi breast imaging: multicenter trial results. J Nucl Med 41: 1973–1979

Khalkhali I, Baum JK, Villanueva-Meyer J et al (2002) ^{99m}Tc sestamibi breast imaging for the examination of patients with dense and fatty breasts: multicenter study. Radiology 222: 149–155

Kopans DB (1992) The positive predictive value of mammography. AJR Am J Roentgenol 158: 521–526

Kopans DB (2004) Sonography should not be used for breast cancer screening until its efficacy has been proven scientifically. AJR Am J Roentgenol 182: 489–91

Liberman M, Sampalis F, Mulder DS et al (2003) Breast cancer diagnosis by scintimammography: a meta-analysis and review of the literature. Breast Cancer Res Treat 80: 115–126

Lumachi F, Ermani M, Marzola MC et al (2006) Relationship between prognostic factors of breast cancer and ^{99m}Tc-sestamibi uptake in patients who underwent scintimammography: Multivariate analysis of causes of false-negative results. Breast 15: 130–134

Maini CL, Tofani A, Sciuto R et al (1997) Technetium-99m-MIBI scintigraphy in the assessment of neoadjuvant chemotherapy in breast carcinoma. J Nucl Med 38: 1546–1551

Mankoff DA, Dunnwald LK, Gralow JR et al (1999) Monitoring the response of patients with locally advanced breast carcinoma to neoadjuvant chemotherapy using [technetium 99m]-sestamibi scintimammography. Cancer 85: 2410–2423

Marini C, Cilotti A, Traino AC et al (2001) Tc 99m-Sestamibi scintimammography in the differentiation of benign and malignant breast microcalcifications. Breast 10: 306–312

Mathieu I, Mazy S, Willemart B et al (2005) Inconclusive triple diagnosis in breast cancer imaging: is there a place for scintimammography? J Nucl Med 46:1574–1581

Maublant J, Zhang Z, Rapp M et al (1993) In vitro uptake of technetium-99m-teboroxime in carcinoma cell lines and normal cells: comparison with technetium-99m-sestamibi and thallium-201. J Nucl Med 34: 1949–1952

McMahon KE, Osborne DR, Davidson AL (2001) Role of breast magnetic resonance imaging in difficult diagnostic situations. Med J Aust 175: 494–497

Mekhmandarov S, Sandbank J, Coehn M et al (1998) Technetium-99m-MIBI scintimammography in palpable and nonpalpable breast lesions. J Nucl Med 39: 86–91

Mezi S, Primi F, Capoccetti F, Scopinaro F et al (2003) In vivo detection of resistance to anthracycline based neoadjuvant chemotherapy in locally advanced and inflammatory breast cancer with technetium-99m sestamibi scintimammography. Int J Oncol 22: 1233–1240

Monusturi Z, Herman PG, Carmody DP et al (1991) Limitations in distinguishing malignant from benign lesions of the breast by sistematic review of mammograms. Surgery 173: 438–442

Obwegeser R, Berghammer P, Rodrigues M et al (1999) A head-to-head comparison between technetium-99m-tetrofosmin and technetium-99m-MIBI scintigraphy to evaluate suspicious breast lesions. Eur J Nucl Med 26: 1553–1559

Orel SG, Schnall MD (2001) MR imaging of the breast for the detection, diagnosis, and staging of breast cancer. Radiology 220: 13–30

Polan RL, Klein BD, Richman RH (2001) Scintimammography in patients with minimal mammographic or clinical findings. Radiographics 21: 641–653

Prats E, Aisa F, Abos MD et al (1999) Mammography and ^{99m}Tc-MIBI scintimammography in suspected breast cancer. J Nucl Med 40: 296–301

Pwnica-Worms D, Chiu ML, Budding M et al (1993) Functional imaging of multidrug-resistant P-glycoprotein with an organotechnetium complex. Cancer Res 53: 977–984

Rhodes DJ, O'Connor MK, Phillips SW et al (2005) Molecular breast imaging: a new technique using technetiumTc scintimammography to detect small tumors of the breast. Mayo Clin Proc 80: 24–30

Sampalis FS, Denis R, Picard D et al (2003) International prospective evaluation of scintimammography with (99m)technetium sestamibi. Am J Surg 185: 544–549

Schillaci O (2005a) Is there a clinical role for scintimammography in breast cancer diagnosis? J Nucl Med 46: 1571–1573

Schillaci O (2005b) Hybrid SPECT/CT: a new era for SPECT imaging? Eur J Nucl Med Mol Imaging 32: 521–524

Schillaci O, Buscombe JR (2004) Breast scintigraphy today: indications and limitations. Eur J Nucl Med Mol Imaging 31 (Suppl) 1: S35–S45

Schillaci O, Scopinaro F (1999) Tc-99m sestamibi scintimammography: where is it now? Cancer Biother Radiopharm 14: 417–422

Schillaci O, Scopinaro F, Danieli R et al (1997a) 99Tcm-sestamibi scintimammography in patients with suspicious breast lesions: comparison of SPET and planar images in the detection of primary tumours and axillary lymph node involvement. Nucl Med Commun 18: 839–845

Schillaci O, Scopinaro F, Danieli R et al (1997b) Scintimammography with technetium-99m tetrofosmin in suspected breast cancer. Anticancer Res 17: 1623–1626

Schillaci O, Di Luzio E, Porfiri LM et al (1999) Role of Tc-99m sestamibi scintimammography in patients with indeterminate mammography due to dense breasts (abstract). Eur J Nucl Med 26: 986

Schillaci O, Manni C, Danieli R et al (2005a) Tc-99m sestamibi scintimammography with a hybrid SPECT/CT imaging system (abstract). Eur J Nucl Med Mol Imaging 32: S128

Schillaci O, Cossu E, Buonomo O et al (2005b) Dedicated breast camera: is it the best option for scintimammography? J Nucl Med 46: 550

Schillaci O, Danieli R, Romano P et al (2005c) Scintimammography for the detection of breast cancer. Expert Rev Med Devices 2: 191–196

Schillaci O, Cossu E, Romano P et al (2006) High-resolution gamma-camera for molecular breast imaging: first clinical results. Phys Med 21 (Suppl) 1: 113–116

Schomacker K, Schicha H (2000) Use of myocardial imaging agents for tumour diagnosis–a success story? Eur J Nucl Med 27: 1845–1863

Scopinaro F, Schillaci O, Scarpini M et al (1994) Technetium-99m sestamibi: an indicator of breast cancer invasiveness. Eur J Nucl Med 21: 984–987

Scopinaro F, Schillaci O, Ussof W et al (1997) A three center study on the diagnostic accuracy of ^{99m}Tc-MIBI scintimammography. Anticancer Res 17: 1631–1634

Scopinaro F, Pani R, De Vincentis G et al (1999) High-resolution scintimammography improves the accuracy of technetium-99m methoxyisobutylisonitrile scintimammography: use of a new dedicated gamma camera. Eur J Nucl Med 26: 1279–1288

Spanu A, Schillaci O, Meloni GB et al (2002) The usefulness of ^{99m}Tc-tetrofosmin SPECT scintimammography in the detection of small size primary breast carcinomas. Int J Oncol 21: 831–840

Spanu A, Farris A, Schillaci O et al (2003) The usefulness of ^{99m}Tc tetrofosmin scintigraphy in patients with breast cancer recurrences. Nucl Med Commun 24: 145–154

Spanu A, Schillaci O, Madeddu G (2005) ^{99m}Tc-cationic lipophilic complexes in malignant and benign tumors: the role of SPECT and pinhole-SPECT in breast cancer, differentiated thyroid carcinoma and hyperparathyroidism. Q J Nucl Med Mol Imaging 45: 145–169

Tabar LK, Vitak B, Chen HHT et al (2001) Beyond randomized controlled trials: organized mammographic screening substantially reduces breast cancer mortality. Cancer 91: 1724–1731

Takamura Y, Miyoshi Y, Taguchi T et al (2001) Prediction of chemotherapeutic response by technetium 99m-MIBI scintigraphy in breast carcinoma patients. Cancer 92: 232–239

Thurfjell E (2002) Breast density and the risk of breast cancer. N Engl J Med 347: 866

Tiling R, Tatsch K, Sommer H et al (1998) Technetium-99m-sestamibi scintimammography for the detection of breast carcinoma: comparison between planar and SPECT imaging. J Nucl Med 39: 849–856

Tiling R, Stephan K, Sommer H et al (2004) Tissue-specific effects on uptake of ^{99m}Tc-sestamibi by breast lesions: a targeted analysis of false scintigraphic diagnoses. J Nucl Med 45: 1822–1828

Tiling R, Kessler M, Untch M et al (2005) Initial evaluation of breast cancer using Tc-99m sestamibi scintimammography. Eur J Radiol 53: 206–212

Tillman GF, Orel SG, Schnall MD et al (2002) Effect of breast magnetic resonance imaging on the clinical management of women with early-stage breast carcinoma. J Clin Oncol 20: 3413–3423

Tolmos J, Cutrone JA, Wang B et al (1998) Scintimammographic analysis of nonpalpable breast lesions previously identified by conventional mammography. J Natl Cancer Inst 90: 846–849

Van de Wiele C, Rottey S, Goethals I et al (2003) ^{99m}Tc sestamibi and ^{99m}Tc tetrofosmin scintigraphy for predicting resistance to chemotherapy: a critical review of clinical data. Nucl Med Commun 24 :945–950

Vargas HI, Agbunag RV, Kalinowski A et al (2001) The clinical utility of Tc-99m sestamibi scintimammography in detecting multicentric breast cancer. Am Surg 67: 1204–1208

Waxman AD (1997) The role of ^{99m}Tc methoxyisobutylisonitrile in imaging breast cancer. Semin Nucl Med 27: 40–54

Waxman A, Nagaraj N, Kovalevsky M et al (1995) Detection of primary breast malignancy with Tc-99m methoxyisobutylisonitrile in patients with non-palpable primary malignancies: the importance of lesion size (abstract). J Nucl Med 36: 194P

Yildiz A, Garipagaoglu M, Gungor F et al (2001) The role of technetium-99m methoxyisobutyl isonitrile scintigraphy in suspected recurrent breast cancer. Cancer Biother Radiopharm 16: 163–169

^{99m}Tc-MIBI in the Evaluation of Breast Cancer Biology

7

Silvana Del Vecchio, Antonella Zannetti, Rosa Fonti,
Francesca Iommelli, and Marco Salvatore

CONTENTS

7.1 Introduction

Scintigraphic in vivo evaluation of complex cellular processes such as proliferation, apoptosis, receptor/ligand interactions, transport of substrates and metabolism of nutrients in human cancers is a wide and continuing evolving area of investigation in nuclear medicine (Denoyer et al. 2006; Been et al. 2004; Corsten et al. 2006; Weissleder 2006). A major purpose in this area is the non-invasive detection of well-known biochemical, molecular and histological markers of tumor aggressiveness, invasiveness and resistance to therapy, which may provide rational criteria for a fine tuning of therapeutic strategies in individual patients.

In the last decade, ^{99m}Tc-labeled lipophilic cations, originally developed as myocardial perfusion agents and subsequently used as tumor-seeking agents in a variety of human neoplasms, emerged as suitable tools to explore specific cellular processes and functions in malignant tumors. The class of ^{99m}Tc-labeled lipophilic cations includes several tracers such as ^{99m}Tc-MIBI, ^{99m}Tc-tetrofosmin and ^{99m}Tc-furifosmin, which share common biophysical, chemical and pharmacokinetic properties (Sharma 2004). In particular, ^{99m}Tc-MIBI and analogous ^{99m}Tc-labeled agents share similar mechanisms of uptake in both normal and malignant cells. A number of studies consistently show the passive influx of these lipophilic cations in response to large negative plasma membrane and mitochondrial membrane potentials as well as the reversible accumulation within mitochondria of both normal and malignant cells (Piwnica-Worms et al. 1990; Delmon-Moingeon et al. 1990; Carvalho et al. 1992).

Another common property of these tracers is the ability to interact with P-glycoprotein (Pgp), which is responsible for their active outward transport in the extracellular compartment (Piwnica-Worms et al. 1993). Human P-glycoprotein is a 170-kDa transmembrane protein that is encoded by the MDR1 gene and acts as an energy-dependent drug efflux pump of broad specificity (Szakacs et al. 2006). Overexpression of this protein confers resistance to a large number of chemotherapeutic agents including anthracyclines, Vinca alkaloids, epipodophyllotoxins, actinomycin D and taxol. A number of studies document that ^{99m}Tc-MIBI is a transport substrate of Pgp in a variety of tumor cells, and similar Pgp recognition properties have been reported for ^{99m}Tc-tetrofosmin and ^{99m}Tc-furifosmin (Sharma 2004) as well as positron-emitter labeled compounds (Bigott et al. 2005; Sharma et al. 2005; Elsinga et al. 2004). Several studies report that ^{99m}Tc-MIBI is a also a substrate for the multidrug resistance associated protein (MRP1), a multispecific organic anion transporter that differs from Pgp in that it has a substrate specificity for glutathione-, glucuronate- or sulfate-conjugates of drugs, and it is sensitive to glutathione depletion (Hendrikse 2000).

Because of the extensive literature on the use of ^{99m}Tc-MIBI for the biological characterization of breast lesions, the present chapter will primarily focus on the ability of this compound to trace specific cellular processes in breast cancer. However, the principles outlined for ^{99m}Tc-MIBI can be equally applicable to other agents of the same class of compounds. Clinical studies performed to correlate ^{99m}Tc-MIBI uptake or clearance with histological, molecular and biochemical markers of several cellular processes including apoptosis, proliferation, P-glycoprotein expression and neoangiogenesis will be reviewed and discussed. Since the existence of such correlations does not necessarily imply a direct dependence of the imaging findings from a specific cellular process or a cause-effect relationship, attempts will be made to define which cellular process directly affects ^{99m}Tc-MIBI uptake or clearance. Furthermore, efforts will be made to explain the apparent discrepancy in the results of different studies and to address specific issues such as the clinical relevance of correlations and the possibility to set criteria for daily clinical applications. Finally, the opportunity to translate the same principles to other human neoplasms will be taken into account by reporting parallel evidence of similar correlations in other types of cancer.

7.2 ^{99m}Tc-MIBI and Apoptosis: Biological Significance of False Negatives

Apoptosis is an energy-dependent, highly regulated process leading to selective cell death. Several stimuli including drugs, toxins, gamma irradiation, cytokines of the TNF family and growth factor withdrawal may trigger an apoptotic response. Three main apoptotic pathways originating from three different subcellular compartments have been identified as the death receptor-mediated pathway, the mitochondrial apoptotic pathway and the recently recognized endoplasmic reticulum pathway (Danial and Korsmeyer 2004). All pathways lead to the activation of the executioner caspases, which in turn cleave cellular substrates and cause the biochemical and morphological changes that are characteristic of apoptosis (Igney and Krammer 2002).

The mechanisms involved in the induction of apoptosis by most anticancer agents are believed to be largely mediated by the mitochondrial pathway (Johnstone et al. 2002). However, it has been increasingly recognized that the endoplasmic reticulum (ER) cooperates in drug-induced apoptosis and the interaction between mitochondria, and ER is an emerging topic of investigation (Bassik et al. 2004; Scorrano et al. 2000). When a death signal converges onto mitochondria, it causes an early increase in the permeability of the mitochondrial membrane and the release of cytochrome-c and other apoptogenic factors that trigger the downstream sequence of reactions (Kroemer and Reed 2000). Consistent evidence indicates that mitochondrial membrane permeabilization is regulated by the opposing actions of pro- and anti-apoptotic members of Bcl-2 family (Cory and Adams 2002). Although the complex interplay among these members remains controversial and several competing models have been proposed to explain how apoptogenic factors are released into the cytosol, it is generally accepted that this event results in mitochondrial dysfunction and dissipation of mitochondrial membrane potentials (Kroemer and Reed 2000; Cory and Adams 2002).

Due to the reversible accumulation of ^{99m}Tc-MIBI within mitochondria and the dependence of tracer uptake on mitochondrial membrane potentials, the relationship between ^{99m}Tc-MIBI uptake and apoptosis has been explored both in vivo and in vitro. In particular, we obtained consistent evidence that breast carcinomas that fail to accumulate ^{99m}Tc-MIBI, have high levels of the anti-apoptotic protein Bcl-2 (Del Vecchio et al. 2003). The expression of the anti-apoptotic protein was also inversely correlated with the early tumor-to-background ratio in malignant lesions capable of accumulating ^{99m}Tc-MIBI. A cause-effect relationship between Bcl-2 overexpression and reduction of ^{99m}Tc-MIBI uptake in breast carcinomas has also been confirmed by transfecting breast cancer cell lines with the human bcl-2 gene (Aloj et al. 2003). A dramatic reduction of ^{99m}Tc-MIBI uptake was observed in Bcl-2 overexpressing clones as compared to control cells. Interestingly, treatment with staurosporine, a potent inducer of apoptosis, caused an early, partial and transitory recover of tracer uptake in transfected cells.

Overexpression of the anti-apoptotic protein Bcl-2 has been reported in various types of cancer and correlates with relative resistance to chemotherapy and radiation therapy due to a defective apoptotic program (Reed 2006). In the breast, Bcl-2 is expressed in normal glandular epithelium and is upregulated by estrogen possibly by direct transcriptional induction (Teixeira et al. 1995). High levels of Bcl-2 have been found in a considerable percentage of breast carcinomas ranging between 32% and 86% (Arun et al. 2003). Recently, the expression of 13 biomarkers including Bcl-2 was evaluated in 930 breast cancers by immunohistochemistry on a tissue microarray, and positivity for Bcl-2 was reported to be a favorable prognostic marker in breast cancer independently of lymph node status, tumor size and grade combined in the Nottingham Prognostic Index (Callagy et al. 2006). Another recent study reported an inverse correlation between bcl-2 levels and rate of proliferation as determined by protein profiling using tissue microarray technology including Ki67 staining (Ruiz et al. 2006). Despite the recent reports on the positive prognostic role of Bcl-2, it remains controversial whether Bcl-2 overexpression is a significant independent predictor of response to treatment in breast cancer. There is evidence indicating that the ratio between Bcl-2 and the pro-apoptotic protein Bax, which is reported to be modulated in a p53-dependent manner, is a more reliable predictor of tumor response (Ziyaie et al. 2000). Also, pro-apoptotic members of Bcl-2 family were reported to be included in the clusters of genes associated with a pathological complete response to chemotherapy (Gianni et al. 2005). Finally, several studies reported that the absence of Bcl-2 in locally advanced breast cancer was significantly associated with a better pathological response to chemotherapy (Ogston et al. 2004; Pusztai et al. 2004; Prisack et al. 2005).

The exact mechanism by which Bcl-2 overexpression prevents ^{99m}Tc-MIBI uptake in breast carcinoma is presently unknown. However, a clue can emerge considering that Bcl-2 is an integral protein of the outer mitochondrial membrane and endoplasmic reticulum. At the mitochondrial level, it exerts a strong inhibitory effect on the permeabilization of mitochondrial membrane. Bcl-2 is reported indeed to inhibit cytochrome c release from mitochondria (Yang et al. 1997), the opening of mitochondrial permeability transition pore (Hirsch et al. 1997; Marzo et al. 1998), and the disruption of mitochondrial membrane potentials (Shimizu et al. 1998). However there is growing evidence that the Bcl-2 family controls apoptosis from the ER by regulating Ca2+ dynamics and crosstalk with mitochondria (Bassik et al. 2004; Scorrano et al. 2000; Oakes et al. 2005). At the endoplasmic reticulum level, the anti-apoptotic protein Bcl-2 can bind and sequester proapoptotic proteins, thus preventing the oligomerization and insertion of "multidomain" pro-apoptotic proteins such as Bax and Bak into the outer mitochondrial membrane and therefore pore formation and cytochrome-c release (Bassik et al. 2004; Scorrano et al. 2000; Oakes et al. 2005). Furthermore phosphorylated Bcl-2 predominantly localizes to the ER where it is reported to physically interact with inositol trisphosphate receptors I and III and directly or indirectly control the phosphorylation status and Ca2+ leak through these receptors (Oakes et al. 2005; Chen et al. 2004; Orrenius et al. 2003). Thus high levels of Bcl-2 in breast carcinomas may similarly affect the trafficking of ^{99m}Tc-MIBI cations across endoplasmic reticulum and prevent tracer uptake within mitochondria despite the stabilization of mitochondrial membrane potentials (Fig. 7.1).

There are several reports in the literature addressing the issue of ^{99m}Tc-MIBI uptake in cells or tumors undergoing apoptosis after exposure to drugs or gamma irradiation (Zhu et al. 2002; Vergote et al. 2001; Moretti et al. 2005). In particular, ^{99m}Tc-MIBI uptake has been reported to decrease in breast cancer cell lines after treatment with anti-cancer drugs (Vergote et al. 2001). The decrease of tracer uptake has been reported to be dose-dependent and time-dependent usually reaching a maximum at 72 h. Although cells may still appear viable, the downstream progression through the apoptotic cascade may lead to the disruption of mitochondrial membrane potential and dissipation of the driving force behind ^{99m}Tc-MIBI uptake.

Recently, we have obtained evidence that treatment of Bcl-2 transfected breast cancer cells and control parental cells with different anti-cancer agents results in opposite changes of ^{99m}Tc-MIBI uptake (unpublished data). After 24 h of drug exposure, Bcl-2 overexpressing clones show an increase of ^{99m}Tc-MIBI uptake as compared to untreated controls. Conversely, parental cells with no detectable levels of Bcl-2 show a reduction of tracer uptake after treatment.

The picture emerging from these findings is that, in the absence of biological barriers limiting the free diffusion of the tracer from blood to tumor, the uptake of ^{99m}Tc-MIBI reflects the status of mitochondrial membranes and endoplasmic reticulum. In particular it reflects the permeability of mitochondrial membrane, the preservation of mitochondrial membrane potentials and likely the integrity of interorganelle cross-talk. Alterations of these factors normally occur in cancer during drug-induced apoptosis and finally result in mitochondrial dysfunction with consequent reduction of ^{99m}Tc-MIBI

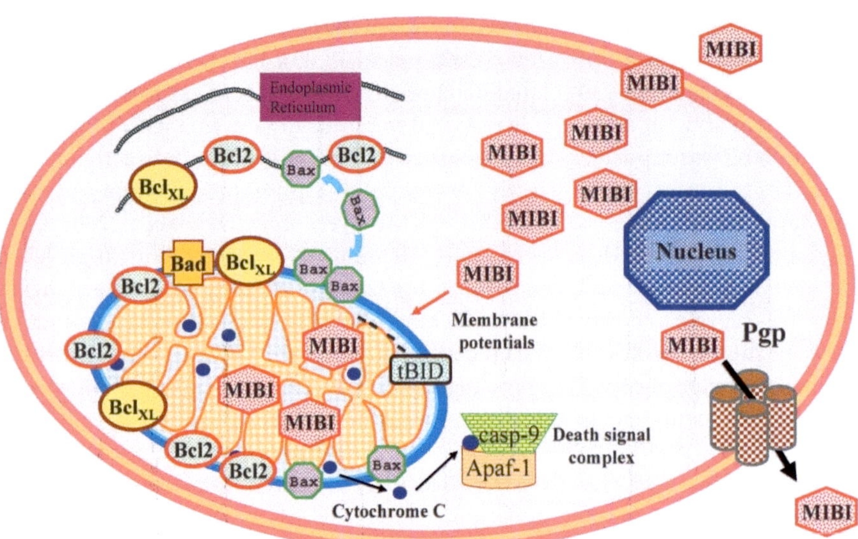

Fig. 7.1. Schematic representation of the uptake and efflux modalities of ^{99m}Tc-MIBI. Uptake: the passive movement of ^{99m}Tc-MIBI from the extracellular to the intracellular compartment and its reversible accumulation within mitochondria is driven by the electronegative plasma membrane and mitochondrial membrane potentials. Mitochondria are also main executioners of apoptosis, and mitochondrial membrane permeabilization is required for apoptosis. Permeability of mitochondrial membrane is regulated by the opposing actions of pro- and anti-apoptotic members of Bcl-2 family. The pro-apoptotic members such as Bax and Bad promote release of cytochrome c, whereas the anti-apoptotic members such as Bcl-2 and Bcl-X_L inhibit permeabilization of mitochondrial membrane and release of cytochrome c. Once in the cytosol, cytochrome c activates caspase-9 (casp-9) by binding to Apaf-1. High levels of Bcl-2 prevent ^{99m}Tc-MIBI to accumulate within mitochondria. Efflux: overexpression of P-glycoprotein in resistant tumor cells represents a powerful mechanism of ^{99m}Tc-MIBI extrusion from cells. The Pgp-dependent outward transport of the tracer can be visualized and estimated in ^{99m}Tc-MIBI positive malignant lesions

uptake. Overexpression of the antiapoptotic protein Bcl-2, with its dual inhibitory role on mitochondrial permeability and disruption of mitochondrial membrane potentials as well as its potential ability to control mitochondrial function from the endoplasmic reticulum, prevents ^{99m}Tc-MIBI accumulation in untreated breast carcinoma, and this effect may be counteracted during the early phases of drug-induced apoptosis allowing a transitory increase of tracer uptake.

Many well-known factors including tumor size, cellularity, blood supply and cell viability can cause false-negative results at scintimammography. How and when false-negative results at ^{99m}Tc-MIBI scan may provide a piece of information on breast cancer biology? A possible way to address this issue is to perform a stress test. In other words, a ^{99m}Tc-MIBI scan performed before and immediately after treatment with anti-cancer agents may reveal changes in tracer accumulation, which depends on Bcl-2 levels in mitochondrial and ER membranes. For instance, ^{99m}Tc-MIBI negative lesions, which become positive early after treatment with anti-cancer agents, would presumably express high levels of Bcl-2. A decrease of tumor-to-background ratio in ^{99m}Tc-MIBI positive lesions after treatment would indicate the absence of significant levels of Bcl-2. Further studies are needed to validate this hypothesis and to translate this approach into clinical applications. However, many clinical studies have highlighted the prognostic value of absent or reduced early ^{99m}Tc-MIBI uptake in different types of tumors. In particular, the absent or reduced early ^{99m}Tc-MIBI uptake in lung cancer predicts poor response to chemotherapy and radiation therapy independently of tracer clearance (Bom et al. 1998; Yamamoto et al. et al. 1998; Yuksel et al. 2002; Nishiyama et al. 2000). Also, lymphoma lesions not visualized at ^{99m}Tc-MIBI scan are refractory to subsequent chemotherapy (Kapucu et al. 1997; Kao et al. 2001).

7.3 ^{99m}Tc-MIBI and Proliferation: Biological Significance of True Positives

Several studies have been undertaken to elucidate the relationship between ^{99m}Tc MIBI uptake and proliferation in breast cancer. Cutrone et al. (1998) evaluated several histological variables, including tumor cell proliferation, in 42 surgical excised breast lesions. They found a moderate, but significant correlation between degree of ^{99m}Tc-MIBI uptake and cellular proliferation in such lesions. In malignant lesions with a diameter lower than 1.5 cm, Bonazzi et al. (2001) found that breast carcinomas with detectable ^{99m}Tc-MIBI uptake showed an increased proliferative activity as compared to ^{99m}Tc-MIBI negative malignant lesions. In 42 breast carcinomas with a diameter higher than 1.8 cm, we could not find any significant difference in mitotic index between MIBI-positive and MIBI-negative lesions, but the apoptotic index was dramatically reduced in MIBI-negative malignant lesions (Del Vecchio et al. 2003). Furthermore, a strong, significant and direct correlation between the rate of proliferation and the apoptotic index was found in MIBI-positive lesions, and the apoptotic index was significantly and directly correlated with the early tumor-to-background ratio, whereas proliferation showed a borderline correlation. Evidence of a strong and direct correlation between the proliferation rate and ^{99m}Tc-MIBI uptake has been reported also for brain tumors (Nagamachi et al. 2001; Ak et al. 2003).

These observations, taken together, raised the question whether proliferation is more important than apoptosis in determining the degree of ^{99m}Tc-MIBI uptake in malignant breast tumors. Although cell proliferation and cell death appear to be opposing and mutually contradictory processes, substantial evidence indicates that their pathways are generally coupled in human malignancies (Lowe et al. 2004). Many dominant oncogenes, which are well known promoters of cell proliferation, actually also possess proapoptotic activity, and their mitogenic and pro-apoptotic properties are often genetically inseparable (Pelengaris et al. 2002; Nahle et al. 2002). Similar findings have been reported for certain functionally inactive tumor suppressors (Lowe et al. 2004; Hickman et al. 2002). Therefore in cells with deregulated oncogenes or inactive suppressors, the activation of the proliferative machinery by appropriate growth signals primes also the cellular apoptotic program or alternatively sensitizes growing cells to apoptotic signals. In the absence of further alterations impairing the apoptotic response such as, for instance, Bcl-2 overexpression, the enhanced proliferative activity in response to growth signals is accompanied by an enhanced apoptotic response to death signals in malignant tumors. In this respect, a direct and significant correlation between the proliferative and apoptotic index has been reported in breast cancer (de Jong et al. 2000; Archer et al. 2003). Therefore it is not surprising that both the proliferative and apoptotic indexes have been found to correlate directly with ^{99m}Tc-MIBI uptake. Furthermore, detection of apoptosis in tumor tissues is usually performed by staining of DNA fragments or by counting cells with peculiar morphological changes and identifies the fraction of cells that had already completed the apoptotic program. Although directly correlated to the rate of proliferation, this fraction is usually limited in breast cancer, accounting for less than 5–10% of total tumor cells. At present, we do not have any marker to recognize cells that have been primed for apoptosis or sensitized to death signals by deregulated oncogenes or inactive suppressors. It remains to be elucidated whether early ^{99m}Tc-MIBI uptake can be a surrogate marker to identify such cells.

7.4 ^{99m}Tc MIBI and P-Glycoprotein Expression: Biological Significance of Tracer Clearance

Despite the large number of anticancer drugs that have been developed and tested, multidrug resistance remains the primary cause of treatment failure in cancer patients. Multiple cellular mechanisms may contribute to the development of the multidrug-resistant phenotype using different modes of action. Reduced uptake of water-soluble drugs, altered metabolism of drugs, increased repair of DNA damage, reduced apoptosis and enhanced efflux of hydrofobic drugs through energy-dependent transporters may potentially cause resistance of cancer cells (Szakacs et al. 2006). One of the most extensively studied mechanisms of multidrug resistance in human tumors involves the overexpression of P-glycoprotein (Pgp), a member of the ATP-binding cassette (ABC) family of transporters. A number of physiological, biochemical and genetic studies indicates that high levels of Pgp enable cancer cells to extrude many chemotherapeutic agents, circumventing their lethal effects (Gottesman et al. 2002). The human genoma contains 48 genes that encode ABC transporters, which have been divided into seven subfamilies named from ABCA through ABCG, and at least 12 ABC transporters have a role in drug resistance in cultured tumor cells. Whether each of these transporters has a role in clinical anticancer drug resistance in patients remains to be established (Leonard et al. 2003). The association of high levels of Pgp (ABCB1) with poor clinical outcome appears to be consolidated in many human cancers including breast carcinoma, sarcoma and certain types of leukemia. In particular, a meta-analysis of 31 breast cancer trials showed a three-fold reduction in response to chemotherapy among tumors expressing Pgp after treatment (Trock et al. 1997).

The clinical relevance of Pgp in determining breast cancer response to treatment and the availability of ^{99m}Tc-labeled compounds such as ^{99m}Tc-MIBI, ^{99m}Tc-tetrofosmin and 9mTc- furifosmin prompted investigating whether these tracers could detect and monitor Pgp expression and function in vivo (Fig. 7.1).

The first issue addressed by clinical studies in breast cancer was whether ^{99m}Tc-MIBI uptake is reduced in Pgp-overexpressing tumors (Moretti et al. 1996; Kostakoglu et al. 1997; Sun et al. 2000; Kao et al. 2001). Although the results of these studies indicated an inverse relationship between net tracer uptake and Pgp levels, the time-dependence of such relationships was not proven since delayed images were not obtained in these studies.

A tracer kinetic analysis was performed over a 4-h period in a series of 30 untreated patients with ^{99m}Tc-MIBI-positive breast carcinomas and revealed a direct statistically significant correlation between tracer efflux and Pgp levels (Del Vecchio et al. 1997). A threshold value could also be established to discriminate Pgp-overexpressing tumors from breast carcinomas with basal levels of Pgp, and this threshold corresponded to a time to half clearance of 204 min. Tracer clearance was also tested for its ability to predict response to subsequent treatment in patients with locally advanced breast cancer candidates for neoadjuvant chemotherapy (Ciarmiello et al. 1998). A rapid clearance of ^{99m}Tc-MIBI from tumors was significantly associated with a highly cellular macroscopic residual tumor at pathological examination of surgical specimens indicating a lack of tumor response to neoadjuvant chemotherapy. On the contrary, the prolonged retention of the tracer was associated with an effective pathological tumor response to treatment in two-thirds of the patients. Similar findings have been obtained by Sciuto et al. (2002) in 30 patients with locally advanced breast cancer undergoing neoadjuvant chemotherapy. They used early (10 min) and delayed (4 h) ^{99m}Tc-MIBI uptake ratio to derive the washout rate and found that a cut-off of 45% provides a satisfactory discrimination between responders and non-responders.

Takamura et al. (2001) evaluated 46 patients with locally advanced or recurrent breast carcinoma and determined both early and delayed tumor-to-background ratios on SPECT images. After chemotherapy, tumor response was determined by clinical examination. Both early and delayed tumor-to-background ratios were significantly higher in responders than in non-responders. Conversely, Pgp levels determined by immunoperoxidase on biopsy specimens prior to treatment were significantly lower in responders than in non-responders.

Mubashar et al. (2002) evaluated early and delayed uptake ratios in 20 patients with breast carcinoma before and after treatment with toremifene, an antiestrogen with Pgp-modulating property. An inverse correlation between the delayed uptake ratio and Pgp expression in tumors was confirmed before treatment. Although a clear cut-off value of tumor-to-background ratio between Pgp-overexpressing and Pgp-negative tumors could not be established, analysis of the change between early and delayed scan appeared to be a better predictor of Pgp status. After toremifene treatment, the authors found that the delayed uptake ratio significantly increased only in Pgp-overexpressing tumors, whereas it decreased in tumors with low Pgp levels. Interestingly, three of the four patients whose tumors were not visualized before toremifene failed to accumulate ^{99m}Tc-MIBI also after treatment with the Pgp-modulator.

There are several reports in the literature correlating a single early uptake ratio of ^{99m}Tc-MIBI with response to treatment (Cayre et al. 2002). Although the absent or reduced uptake of ^{99m}Tc-MIBI in breast carcinoma is indeed correlated with a poor response to therapy, it is not clear, in the absence of a direct evidence of Pgp expression in individual tumors, whether resistance is due to the overexpression of Pgp or to other Pgp-independent mechanism of resistance such as Bcl-2 overexpression altering MIBI uptake. In order to distinguish in vivo Pgp-dependent from Pgp-independent mechanisms of multidrug resistance, the faster decline of tracer uptake over time should be demonstrated and estimated in individual patients. This should be taken into account when setting the criteria for a standardized procedure allowing the functional imaging of Pgp in clinical practice and the selection of patients that may benefit from treatment with Pgp inhibitors.

Once patients with high efflux of Pgp substrates have been identified, two alternative approaches can be adopted, namely inhibition of Pgp function or use of drugs that are able to evade efflux. Despite the considerable efforts to develop drugs that inhibit the function of efflux transporters that lead to the identification of first, second and third generation of Pgp inhibitors, clinical trials with these drugs did not show significant clinical benefit in term of overall survival and response rate (Szakacs et al. 2006). However, phase III trials with the last generation of inhibitors showing greater substrate specificity, lower toxicity and improved pharmacokinetic profiles are currently ongoing. ^{99m}Tc-MIBI has been used to test the effect of Pgp inhibitors in patients. An enhanced liver uptake of ^{99m}Tc-MIBI was reported following administration of several Pgp inhibitors (Chen et al. 1997; Peck et al. 2001; Agrawal et al. 2003). This finding has been ascribed to Pgp inhibition at physiological sites of protein expression and considered as a surrogate marker of effective Pgp inhibition (Wong et al. 2005; Hendrikse et al. 2004). An increased accumulation of ^{99m}Tc-MIBI in drug resistant tumors has also been reported after the administration of third generation inhibitor XR9576 (Agrawal et al. 2003; Pusztai et al. 2005).

On the other end, the number of drugs that are able to evade efflux is currently limited, and most anticancer agents of the MDR spectrum are practically irreplaceable in chemotherapy regimens (Szakacs et al. 2006). Therefore the clinical impact of functional imaging of multidrug resistance still remains unexploited and appears to mainly rely upon the development of novel anticancer agents designed to escape efflux mechanisms.

7.5 ^{99m}Tc-MIBI and Tumor Blood Supply

Since a prerequisite of ^{99m}Tc-MIBI uptake is an effective delivery of the tracer to the tumor mass, several studies have been undertaken to evaluate the relationship between ^{99m}Tc-MIBI uptake and tumor blood supply. Mankoff et al. (2002) evaluated ^{99m}Tc-MIBI kinetics and blood flow in locally advanced breast carcinoma. They studied 37 patients with ^{99m}Tc-MIBI and ^{15}O-water PET imaging and found a direct correlation between early ^{99m}Tc-MIBI uptake and blood flow in agreement with the findings reported for myocardial perfusion studies. Conflicting results have been reported on neoangiogenesis as a factor affecting ^{99m}Tc-MIBI uptake. The formation of new blood vessels is invariably required for growth of breast cancer, and it has a recognized role as an indicator of node metastases and survival (Weidner et al. 1991; Neri and Bicknell 2005; Jain et al. 2006). Cutrone et al. (1998) found no significant difference in microvessel density in ^{99m}Tc-MIBI-positive and ^{99m}Tc-MIBI-negative malignant lesions. When neoangiogenesis was compared with tumor-to-background ratio, a direct correlation has been found in 31 untreated breast cancer patients (Yoon et al. 1999). Scopinaro et al. evaluated microvessel density in 19 untreated breast carcinomas and correlated this histological variable with nodal metastases and ^{99m}Tc-MIBI findings (Scopinaro et al. 1994). The enhanced density of newly formed blood vessels was associated with both nodal metastases and detectable ^{99m}Tc-MIBI uptake in the primary tumors. No correlation between intratumoral microvessel density and ^{99m}Tc-MIBI uptake ratio could be found in patients with breast carcinomas in two independent studies (Kim et al. 2002; Bekis et al. 2005). These findings, taken together, indicate that, although a preserved blood supply is required for tracer delivery to breast carcinoma, it is still controversial whether ^{99m}Tc-MIBI uptake can be used as an indicator of tumor angiogenesis.

7.6 Clinical Implications

All the cellular processes that have been examined in relation to scintigraphic findings with ^{99m}Tc-MIBI are indeed relevant for tumor response to treatment. Most anticancer drugs exert their lethal effect by inducing apoptosis mainly through the mitochondrial pathway that is governed by members of the Bcl-2 family. The lack of ^{99m}Tc-MIBI uptake in palpable malignant lesions of the breast may indicate the presence of high levels of the anti-apoptotic protein Bcl-2 in the mitochondrial membrane or endoplasmic reticulum. Whether this observation is relevant to predict poor tumor response in breast carcinomas remains to be established in perspective clinical studies.

Conversely, a high early uptake in untreated breast carcinoma is correlated with the rate of proliferation. A high growth fraction usually indicates a more aggressive tumor behavior, but also a better and more rapid tumor response to treatment. An orthodox concept in oncology suggests indeed that cytotoxic agents are more effective against rapidly proliferating cells. Therefore a high early ^{99m}Tc-MIBI uptake ratio in breast cancer, when associated with high tracer retention, would indicate an effective tumor response to subsequent chemotherapy.

In addition, an enhanced tracer clearance in ^{99m}Tc-MIBI-positive malignant lesions of the breast is indicative of a Pgp-mediated outward transport of the tracer. Therefore tumors with a fast tracer clearance are likely to become refractory to subsequent chemotherapy due to the drug transport activity of Pgp. Since the clearance of ^{99m}Tc-MIBI cannot be obviously evaluated in negative ^{99m}Tc-MIBI malignant lesions, the expression of Pgp in those tumors will remain indeterminate. An important step toward the clinical application of functional imaging of Pgp in breast cancer is the standardization of the procedure. On the basis of the reported observations, the most reliable and direct index of Pgp function appears to be the tracer washout or clearance. Furthermore, some cut-off values of clearance and washout have been reported to correctly discriminate between responders and non-responders in patients with locally advanced breast cancer, and these values may be used in larger clinical studies with the aim to confirm this evidence.

Although the influence of neoangiogenesis on ^{99m}Tc-MIBI uptake is still controversial, it is worth to noting that a preserved tumor blood supply is relevant not only for tracer delivery, but also to limit tumor hypoxia, which can contribute to treatment failure.

7.7 Conclusions

Both the uptake and efflux mechanisms of ^{99m}Tc-MIBI and analogous ^{99m}Tc-labeled agents in breast carcinomas involve cellular processes that are important for tumor response to treatment. The tracer uptake reflects the status of mitochondria and endoplasmic reticulum, in terms of permeability of mitochondrial membrane, preservation of mitochondrial membrane potentials and integrity of cross-talk between the two cellular organelles. Mutations or altered expression of key molecules participating in the apoptotic process may profoundly affect the function of mitochondria and endoplasmic reticulum and hence tracer uptake both in basal conditions and during drug-induced apoptosis. In the absence of such alterations, apoptosis and proliferation are coordinately modulated in breast cancer, and this may explain the additional relationship between the tracer uptake and rate of proliferation. Although apparently contradictory, both processes are considered important to sensitize cells to the lethal effects of drugs. Accordingly, malignant breast lesions, which are able to accumulate and retain the tracer, will likely respond to therapy. The role of ^{99m}Tc-MIBI and analogous agents in predicting tumor response is reinforced by a number of studies evaluating its ability to trace the activity of Pgp. In this case the tracer efflux reflects the Pgp-mediated outward transport of the tracer, and this clearance mimics the kinetic behavior of anti-cancer drugs of the MDR spectrum.

In conclusion, on the basis of the imaging parameter chosen for the analysis of the ^{99m}Tc-MIBI scan in breast cancer patients, the biological information provided may be related to different cellular processes, but all of them appear ultimately related to the susceptibility of breast carcinoma to treatment. Nevertheless it remains important to discriminate on the images alterations of the uptake mechanism from enhancement of tracer clearance because these observations may orient clinicians towards a very different adjustment of therapy. A number of efforts have been focused on the development of Pgp-inhibitors and Bcl-2 antagonists. The appropriate selection of patients based on the mechanism primarily involved in the development of a multi-drug resistant phenotype would hopefully improve the efficacy of individually tailored therapeutic strategies.

Acknowledgments

This work was partly supported by FIRB-MIUR, Ministero della Salute and the European Molecular Imaging Laboratories (EMIL, LSH-2004-503569) network.

References

Agrawal M, Abraham J, Balis FM et al (2003) Increased 99mTc-sestamibi accumulation in normal liver and drug-resistant tumors after the administration of the glycoprotein inhibitor, XR9576. Clin Cancer Res 9:650-656

Ak I, Gulbas Z, Altinel F et al (2003) Tc-99m MIBI uptake and its relation to the proliferative potential of brain tumors. Clin Nucl Med 28:29-33

Aloj L, Zannetti A, Caraco C et al (2004) Bcl-2 overexpression prevents (99m)Tc-MIBI uptake in breast cancer cell lines. Eur J Nucl Med Mol Imaging 31:521-527

Archer CD, Parton M, Smith I et al (2003) Early changes in apoptosis and proliferation following primary chemotherapy for breast cancer. Br J Cancer 89:1035-1041

Arun B, Kilic G, Yen C et al (2003) Correlation of Bcl-2 and p53 expression in primary breast tumors and corresponding metastatic lymph nodes. Cancer 98:2554-2559

Bassik MC, Scorrano L, Oakes SA et al (2004) Phosphorylation of BCL-2 regulates ER Ca2+ homeostasis and apoptosis. Embo J 23:1207-1216

Been LB, Suurmeijer AJ, Cobben DC et al (2004) [^{18}F]FLT-PET in oncology: current status and opportunities. Eur J Nucl Med Mol Imaging 31:1659-1672

Bekis R, Degirmenci B, Aydin A et al (2005) Correlation between ^{99m}Tc-MIBI uptake and angiogenesis in MIBI-positive breast lesions. Nucl Med Biol 32:465-72

Bigott HM, Prior JL, Piwnica-Worms DR et al (2005) Imaging multidrug resistance P-glycoprotein transport function using microPET with technetium-94m-sestamibi. Mol Imaging 4:30-39

Bom HS, Kim YC, Song HC et al (1998) Technetium-99m-MIBI uptake in small cell lung cancer. J Nucl Med 39:91-94

Bonazzi G, Cistaro A, Bello M et al (2001) Breast cancer cellular proliferation indexes and 99mTc-sesta Mibi capture: what correlation? J Exp Clin Cancer Res 20:91-94

Callagy GM, Pharoah PD, Pinder SE et al (2006) Bcl-2 is a prognostic marker in breast cancer independently of the Nottingham Prognostic Index. Clin Cancer Res 12:2468-2475

Cayre A, Cachin F, Maublant J et al (2002) Single static view 99mTc-sestamibi scintimammography predicts response to neoadjuvant chemotherapy and is related to MDR expression. Int J Oncol 20:1049-1055

Chen CC, Meadows B, Regis J et al (1997) Detection of in vivo P-glycoprotein inhibition by PSC 833 using Tc-99m sestamibi. Clin Cancer Res 3:545-552

Chen R, Valencia I, Zhong F et al (2004) Bcl-2 functionally interacts with inositol 1,4,5-trisphosphate receptors to regulate calcium release from the ER in response to inositol 1,4,5-trisphosphate. J Cell Biol 166:193-203

Ciarmiello A, Del Vecchio S, Silvestro P et al (1998) Tumor clearance of technetium 99m-sestamibi as a predictor of response to neoadjuvant chemotherapy for locally advanced breast cancer. J Clin Oncol 16:1677-1683

Corsten MF, Hofstra L, Narula J et al (2006) Counting heads in the war against cancer: defining the role of annexin A5 imaging in cancer treatment and surveillance. Cancer Res 66:1255-1260

Cory S, Adams JM (2002). The bcl2 family: regulators of the cellular life-or-death switch. Nat Rev Cancer 2:647-656

Cutrone JA, Yospur LS, Khalkhali I et al (1998) Immunohistologic assessment of technetium-99m-MIBI uptake in benign and malignant breast lesions. J Nucl Med 39: 449-453

Carvalho PA, Chiu ML, Kronauge JF et al (1992) Subcellular distribution and analysis of technetium-99m-MIBI in isolated perfused rat hearts. J Nucl Med 33:1516-1522

Danial NN, Korsmeyer SJ (2004) Cell death: critical control points. Cell 116:205-219

de Jong JS, van Diest PJ, Baak JP (2000) Number of apoptotic cells as a prognostic marker in invasive breast cancer. Br J Cancer 82:368-373

Del Vecchio S, Ciarmiello A, Potena MI et al (1997) In vivo detection of multidrug-resistant (MDR1) phenotype by technetium- 99m sestamibi scan in untreated breast cancer patients. Eur J Nucl Med 24:150-159

Del Vecchio S, Zannetti A, Aloj L et al (2003) Inhibition of early 99mTc-MIBI uptake by Bcl-2 anti-apoptotic protein overexpression in untreated breast carcinoma. Eur J Nucl Med Mol Imaging 30:879-887

Delmon-Moingeon LI, Piwnica-Worms D, Van den Abbeele AD et al (1990) Uptake of the cation hexakis(2-methoxyisobutylisonitrile)-technetium- 99m by human carcinoma cell lines in vitro. Cancer Res 50:2198-2202

Denoyer D, Perek N, Le Jeune N et al (2006) Spectrum of radiopharmaceuticals in nuclear oncology. Curr Cancer Drug Targets 6:181-196

Elsinga PH, Hendrikse NH, Bart J et al (2004) PET studies on P-glycoprotein function in the blood-brain barrier: how it affects uptake and binding of drugs within the CNS. Curr Pharm Des 10:1493-1503

Fuster D, Munoz M, Pavia J et al (2002) Quantified 99mTc-MIBI scintigraphy for predicting chemotherapy response in breast cancer patients: factors that influence the level of 99m Tc-MIBI uptake. Nucl Med Commun 23:31-38

Gianni L, Zambetti M, Clark K et al (2005) Gene expression profiles in paraffin-embedded core biopsy tissue predict response to chemotherapy in women with locally advanced breast cancer. J Clin Oncol 23:7265-7277

Gottesman MM, Fojo T, Bates SE (2002) Multidrug resistance in cancer: role of ATP-dependent transporters. Nat Rev Cancer 2:48-58

Hendrikse NH (2000) Monitoring interactions at ATP-dependent drug efflux pumps. Curr Pharm Des 6:1653-1668

Hendrikse NH, Kuipers F, Meijer C et al (2004) In vivo imaging of hepatobiliary transport function mediated by multidrug resistance associated protein and P-glycoprotein. Cancer Chemother Pharmacol 54:131-138

Hickman ES, Moroni MC, Helin K (2002) The role of p53 and pRB in apoptosis and cancer. Curr Opin Genet Dev 12:60-66

Hirsch T, Marchetti P, Susin SA et al (1997) The apoptosis-necrosis paradox. Apoptogenic proteases activated after mitochondrial permeability transition determine the mode of cell death. Oncogene 15:1573–1581

Igney FH, Krammer PH (2002) Death and anti-death: tumour resistance to apoptosis. Nat Rev Cancer 2:277–288

Johnstone RW, Ruefli AA, Lowe SW (2002) Apoptosis: a link between cancer genetics and chemotherapy. Cell 108:153–164

Jain RK, Duda DG, Clark JW et al (2006) Lessons from phase III clinical trials on anti-VEGF therapy for cancer. Nat Clin Pract Oncol 3:24–40

Kao CH, Tsai SC, Liu TJ et al (2001) P-Glycoprotein and multidrug resistance-related protein expressions in relation to technetium-99m methoxyisobutylisonitrile scintimammography findings. Cancer Res 61:1412–1414

Kao CH, Tsai SC, Wang JJ et al (2001) Evaluation of chemotherapy response using technetium-99M-sestamibi scintigraphy in untreated adult malignant lymphomas and comparison with other prognosis factors: a preliminary report. Int J Cancer 95:228–231

Kapucu LO, Akyuz C, Vural G et al (1997) Evaluation of therapy response in children with untreated malignant lymphomas using technetium-99m-sestamibi. J Nucl Med 38:243–247

Kim SW, Park SS, Ahn SJ et al (2002) Identification of angiogenesis in primary breast carcinoma according to the image analysis. Breast Cancer Res Treat 74:121–129

Kostakoglu L, Elahi N, Kiratli P et al (1997) Clinical validation of the influence of P-glycoprotein on technetium-99m-sestamibi uptake in malignant tumors. J Nucl Med 38:1003–1008

Kroemer G, Reed JC (2000) Mitochondrial control of cell death. Nat Med 6:513–519

Leonard GD, Fojo T, Bates SE (2003) The role of ABC transporters in clinical practice. Oncologist 8:411–424

Lowe SW, Cepero E, Evan G (2004) Intrinsic tumour suppression. Nature 432:307–315

Mankoff DA, Dunnwald LK, Gralow JR et al (2002) [Tc-99m]-sestamibi uptake and washout in locally advanced breast cancer are correlated with tumor blood flow. Nucl Med Biol 29:719–727

Marzo I, Brenner C, Zamzami N et al (1998) Bax and adenine nucleotide translocator cooperate in the mitochondrial control of apoptosis. Science 281:2027–2031

Moretti JL, Azaloux H, Boisseron D et al (1996) Primary breast cancer imaging with technetium-99m sestamibi and its relation with P-glycoprotein overexpression. Eur J Nucl Med 23:980–986

Moretti JL, Hauet N, Caglar M et al (2005) To use MIBI or not to use MIBI? That is the question when assessing tumour cells. Eur J Nucl Med Mol Imaging 32:836–842

Mubashar M, Harrington KJ, Chaudhary KS et al (2002) 99mTc-sestamibi imaging in the assessment of toremifene as a modulator of multidrug resistance in patients with breast cancer. J Nucl Med 43:519–525

Nagamachi S, Jinnouchi S, Nabeshima K et al (2001) The correlation between ^{99m}Tc-MIBI uptake and MIB-1 as a nuclear proliferation marker in glioma – a comparative study with 201Tl. Neuroradiology 43:1023–1030

Nahle Z, Polakoff J, Davuluri RV et al (2002) Direct coupling of the cell cycle and cell death machinery by E2F. Nat Cell Biol 4:859–864

Neri D, Bicknell R (2005) Tumour vascular targeting. Nat Rev Cancer 5: 436–446

Nishiyama Y, Yamamoto Y, Satoh K et al (2000) Comparative study of Tc-99m MIBI and TI-201 SPECT in predicting chemotherapeutic response in non-small-cell lung cancer. Clin Nucl Med 25:364–369

Oakes SA, Scorrano L, Opferman JT et al (2005) Proapoptotic BAX and BAK regulate the type 1 inositol trisphosphate receptor and calcium leak from the endoplasmic reticulum. Proc Natl Acad Sci USA 102:105–110

Ogston KN, Miller ID, Schofield AC et al (2004) Can patients' likelihood of benefiting from primary chemotherapy for breast cancer be predicted before commencement of treatment? Breast Cancer Res Treat 86:181–189

Orrenius S, Zhivotovsky B, Nicotera P (2003) Regulation of cell death: the calcium-apoptosis link. Nat Rev Mol Cell Biol 4:552–565

Peck RA, Hewett J, Harding MW et al (2001) Phase I and pharmacokinetic study of the novel MDR1 and MRP1 inhibitor biricodar administered alone and in combination with doxorubicin. J Clin Oncol 19:3130–3141

Pelengaris S, Khan M, Evan G (2002) c-MYC: more than just a matter of life and death. Nat Rev Cancer 2:764–776

Piwnica-Worms D, Chiu ML, Budding M et al (1993) Functional imaging of multidrug-resistant P-glycoprotein with an organotechnetium complex. Cancer Res 53:977–984

Piwnica-Worms D, Kronauge JF, Chiu ML (1990) Uptake and retention of hexakis (2-methoxyisobutyl isonitrile) technetium(I) in cultured chick myocardial cells. Mitochondrial and plasma membrane potential dependence. Circulation 82:1826–1838

Prisack HB, Karreman C, Modlich O et al (2005) Predictive biological markers for response of invasive breast cancer to anthracycline/cyclophosphamide-based primary (radio-)chemotherapy. Anticancer Res 25:4615–4621

Pusztai L, Krishnamurti S, Perez Cardona J et al (2004) Expression of BAG-1 and BcL-2 proteins before and after neoadjuvant chemotherapy of locally advanced breast cancer. Cancer Invest 22:248–256

Pusztai L, Wagner P, Ibrahim N et al (2005) Phase II study of tariquidar, a selective P-glycoprotein inhibitor, in patients with chemotherapy-resistant, advanced breast carcinoma. Cancer 104:682–691

Reed JC (2006) Drug Insight: cancer therapy strategies based on restoration of endogenous cell death mechanisms. Nat Clin Pract Oncol 3:388–398

Ruiz C, Seibt S, Al Kuraya K et al (2006) Tissue microarrays for comparing molecular features with proliferation activity in breast cancer. Int J Cancer 118:2190–2194

Sciuto R, Pasqualoni R, Bergomi S et al (2002) Prognostic value of (99m)Tc-sestamibi washout in predicting response of locally advanced breast cancer to neoadjuvant chemotherapy. J Nucl Med 43:745–751

Scopinaro F, Schillaci O, Scarpini M et al (1994) Technetium-99m sestamibi: an indicator of breast cancer invasiveness. Eur J Nucl Med 21:984–987

Scorrano L, Oakes SA, Opferman JT et al (2003) BAX and BAK regulation of endoplasmic reticulum Ca2+: a control point for apoptosis. Science 300:135–139

Sharma V (2004) Radiopharmaceuticals for assessment of multidrug resistance P-glycoprotein-mediated drug transport activity. Bioconjug Chem 15:1464–1474

Sharma V, Prior JL, Belinsky MG et al (2005) Characterization of a ^{67}Ga/^{68}Ga radiopharmaceutical for SPECT and PET of MDR1 P-glycoprotein transport activity in vivo: validation in multidrug-resistant tumors and at the blood-brain barrier. J Nucl Med 46:354–364

Shimizu S, Eguchi Y, Kamiike W et al (1998) Bcl-2 prevents apoptotic mitochondrial dysfunction by regulating proton flux. Proc Natl Acad Sci USA 95:1455–1459

Sun SS, Hsieh JF, Tsai SC et al (2000) Expression of mediated P-glycoprotein multidrug resistance related to Tc-99m MIBI scintimammography results. Cancer Lett 153:95–100

Szakacs G, Paterson JK, Ludwig JA et al (2006) Targeting multidrug resistance in cancer. Nat Rev Drug Discov 5:219–234

Takamura Y, Miyoshi Y, Taguchi T et al (2001) Prediction of chemotherapeutic response by Technetium 99m-MIBI scintigraphy in breast carcinoma patients. Cancer 92:232–239

Teixeira C, Reed JC, Pratt MA (1995) Estrogen promotes chemotherapeutic drug resistance by a mechanism involving Bcl-2 proto-oncogene expression in human breast cancer cells. Cancer Res 55:3902–3907

Trock BJ, Leonessa F, Clarke R (1997) Multidrug resistance in breast cancer: a meta-analysis of MDR1/gp170 expression and its possible functional significance. J Natl Cancer Inst 89:917–931

Vergote J, Di Benedetto M, Moretti JL et al (2001) Could ^{99m}Tc-MIBI be used to visualize the apoptotic MCF7 human breast cancer cells? Cell Mol Biol (Noisy-le-grand) 47:467–471

Weidner N, Semple JP, Welch WR et al (1991) Tumor angiogenesis and metastasis-correlation in invasive breast carcinoma. N Engl J Med 324:1–8

Weissleder R (2006) Molecular imaging in cancer. Science 312:1168–1171

Wong M, Evans S, Rivory LP et al (2005) Hepatic technetium Tc 99m-labeled sestamibi elimination rate and ABCB1 (MDR1) genotype as indicators of ABCB1 (P-glycoprotein) activity in patients with cancer. Clin Pharmacol Ther 77:33–42

Yamamoto Y, Nishiyama Y, Satoh K et al (1998) Comparative study of technetium-99m-sestamibi and thallium-201 SPECT in predicting chemotherapeutic response in small cell lung cancer. J Nucl Med 39:1626–1629

Yang J, Liu X, Bhalla K et al (1997) Prevention of apoptosis by Bcl-2: release of cytochrome c from mitochondria blocked. Science 275:1129–1132

Yoon JH, Bom HS, Song HC et al (1999) Double-phase Tc-99m sestamibi scintimammography to assess angiogenesis and P-glycoprotein expression in patients with untreated breast cancer. Clin Nucl Med 24:314–318

Yuksel M, Cermik F, Doganay L et al (2002) ^{99m}Tc-MIBI SPET in non-small cell lung cancer in relationship with Pgp and prognosis. Eur J Nucl Med Mol Imaging 29:876–881

Zhu X, Wu H, Xia J et al (2002) The relationship between (99m)Tc-MIBI uptakes and tumor cell death/proliferation state under irradiation. Cancer Lett 182:217–222

Ziyaie D, Hupp TR, Thompson AM (2000) P53 and breast cancer. Breast 9:239–246

Sentinel Node Detection in Pre-Operative Axillary Staging

8

Giovanni Paganelli, Giuseppe Trifirò, Oreste Gentilini, Mattia Intra, Giuseppe Viale, and Umberto Veronesi

CONTENTS

8.1 Introduction

Sentinel lymph node (SLN) localisation and biopsy represent one of the most important developments in surgery and have already produced important changes in the management of patients affected by early infiltrating breast carcinoma. Sentinel lymph node biopsy (SLNB) was first applied in melanoma patients by Morton and colleagues (Morton et al. 1992); they intra-operatively injected the patent with vital blue dye close to the primary lesion, and the blue-stained SLN was later found by dissection, following tracer diffusion.

Subsequently this technique was proposed as a method of disease staging in breast cancer patients (Giuliano et al. 1997) in order to permit the use of less aggressive surgical treatment that would not compromise quality of life. In fact, removal of axillary nodes in the presence of breast cancer is performed for staging and not with curative intent (Fisher et al. 2002), and axillary dissection is burdened by a significant rate of immediate and delayed possible complications such as lymphoedema, paraesthesia, pain and restriction of arm motion. Nevertheless, information on axillary nodes is important in determining the appropriate type of adjuvant treatment, and SLNB has been proposed as an alternative to routine axillary clearance for the determination of nodal status. Today, more than 10 years after the pioneering reports of Krag (Krag 1993; Giuliano 1994), SLNB has become a new standard of care for axillary node staging in breast cancer. A widely accepted consensus exists in the literature that SLNB is "feasible and accurate, works well in a wide range of practice settings, is sufficiently robust to withstand variations in technique, increases staging accuracy by allowing enhanced pathologic analysis, has less morbidity than complete axillary lymph node dissection (CAD), and gives local control comparable of that of CAD" (Cody 2003).

Despite the fact that for several years SLNB has been routinely performed in clinical practice, the correct indications for SLNB still represent an unsolved question. In fact, to ensure a high SLN accuracy and a low false-negative rate, in the early experience of the 1990s (the developmental phase of validation) SLNB was strictly limited to patients with small unique invasive tumours and clinically negative axillary lymph nodes. Nevertheless, with the increased experience gained and the widespread use of the technique, the indications for SLNB have since been extended to encompass most patients with non-metastatic disease previously excluded for technical or theoretical reasons. So, most of the "historical" relative contraindications for SLNB are now being questioned, and the initial restrictive selection of patients is now progressively enlarging. Several new clinical situations are presenting in the clinical practice as possible, previously unexpected, indications so that someone is actually asking "does anybody not need a SLNB?" (Cody 2003).

The concept of the "sentinel lymph node" implies that lymphatic metastasis is not a random event, but rather is based on an orderly and predictable pattern of lymph flow from the primary site to the regional lymph node basin. Sequential progression of tumour cells is assumed to occur, with the first lymph node (the SLN) filtering the afferent lymph and thereby entrapping the tumour cells. Both experimental evidence and clinical data support the hypothesis that there is an orderly and predictable pattern of lymphatic drainage from the breast to the regional lymph nodes and progressive involvement of the axillary lymph nodes. In fact, lymphatic spread within the axilla generally proceeds from the first Berg level to the third, and skip metastases are infrequent (Veronesi et al. 1990; Zurrida et al. 1999).

Several studies have demonstrated that lymphoscintigraphy in combination with gamma probe-guided surgery is the best procedure to identify and remove the SLN in breast cancer patients (Veronesi et al. 1997), being more suitable and sensitive than blue dye mapping. The method of lymphoscintigraphy to be used for SLN localisation is still controversial. We have already described a reliable lymphoscintigraphic technique in previous works (Paganelli et al. 1998; De Cicco et al. 1998).

8.2 Lymphoscintigraphy

In recent years, hundreds of studies have been published on lymphoscintigraphy in breast cancer, and the reported experience and data have often been discordant. The main areas of controversy concern radiopharmaceuticals, the site of injection and mode of administration, the optimal activity and the appropriate radiotracer volume.

Three types of radiopharmaceutical preparations are commonly employed for lymphoscintigraphy: ^{99m}Tc-sulphur colloid is the most commonly used in the United States, either unfiltered (size about 15–5,000 nm) or filtered. Some authors (Hill et al. 1999; Cody and Borgen 1999) still claim the superiority of the unfiltered over the filtered preparation (Krag et al. 1993). In Europe, ^{99m}Tc-nanocolloid is more frequently used, with particles between 4 and about 100 nm (95% of the particles are <80 nm). Finally, ^{99m}Tc-antimony trisulphide (3–30 nm) is widely employed for SLN procedures (Wilhelm et al. 1999) in Australia and Canada. It is generally considered that radiocolloid with most of the particles ranging between 100 and 200 nm in size represents the best compromise between fast and efficient lymphatic drainage and satisfactory retention in the SLN (Mariani et al. 2001).

The site of injection is the most crucial parameter, and heavily affects the final choice of the other two main parameters, volume and activity. Intratumoural injection (Tanis et al. 2003) represents a natural extension of the technique developed earlier with vital blue dye: it is generally characterised by a relatively large volume of radiotracer (at least 4 ml) and a relatively high injected activity of radiocolloid (37–370 MBq). Interstitial administration can be performed using peritumoral/intraparenchymal injection and subdermal/intradermal injection (Roumen et al. 1999) (Fig. 8.1). The principle of intraparenchymal administration is to inject the tracer in a site immediately adjacent to the tumour, that is, in the space with a supposedly normal lymphatic system, which is the only possible drainage pathway for fluids, particles and cells leaving the tumour via the extravascular route. Finally, peri-areolar/subareolar tracer injection (Klimberg et al. 1999) is based on the existence of a lymphatic plexus around each lobule of the mammary gland that follows the path of the galactophore ducts, converging to the areola to form the Sappey subareolar plexus, which is part of the general subcutaneous plexus (Spratt et al. 1965). It is in fact reasonable to assume that these various techniques are complementary (Alazraki et al. 2000).

Several technical aspects of lymphoscintigraphy have been optimised by our group, based on detailed investigations (De Cicco et al. 1998; Paganelli et al. 2002; De Cicco et al. 2004; Luini et al. 2002). In a large series of patients we performed a comparative study using antimony sulphide colloids with a particle size of <50 nm, colloidal particles of HSA sized <80 nm and colloidal particles of HSA sized 0.2–1 µm, administered either subdermally or peritumourally in a volume ranging from 0.2 to 3 ml and with very low activity (De Cicco et al. 1998). The results suggested the use of larger colloidal particles (0.2–1 µm) to be most appropriate because while only one or two SLNs were identified, smaller colloids were often trapped in several nodes and retained in the lymphatic channels, which would cause the surgeon problems in distinguishing between the true SLN and other radioactive sources (Paganelli et al. 1998).

The likelihood of visualising a lymphatic duct and a draining lymph node increases when the radiocolloid is injected in the skin overlying the mammary gland, because lymphatic drainage from the skin is richer and faster than drainage from the remaining breast parenchyma (Borgstein et al. 1998). Axillary SLNs can therefore be efficiently visualised as early as 20–30 min after intradermal injection of radiocolloid, thus making the entire lymphoscintigraphic procedure highly practicable. Nevertheless, convenient timing is not the only factor that makes the intradermal administration route such an attractive option for SLNB in early breast cancer. Reliability of this approach for SLN identification has a sound anatomical and physiological basis. With this administration approach, a small volume of tracer (between 0.2–0.3 ml), containing 10–15 MBq of ^{99m}Tc-colloid, is injected as a single aliquot in the skin directly overlying the tumour. Based on how deeply the injection is performed, tracer administration is defined as intradermal when the needle is almost tangential to the skin surface and a classical urticarial wheal ensues, and as subdermal when injection is a little deeper (this is signalled by reduced resistance to penetration of the needle) and the wheal is less obvious. Clearly, there is some overlap between these two modalities and the two terms are often used interchangeably, also because of the wide variation in the thickness of the skin overlying the breast as a function of individual characteristics, breast size and age of the patient.

Some investigators perform peri-areolar tracer injection (usually with the injection of four aliquots) as a modification of the subdermal route. However sound its pathophysiological basis may be (due to the rich connections of the subareolar plexus with the general subcutaneous plexus), we do not favour this technique, in part because it causes some discomfort to patients. This approach may also demonstrate sites of drainage of the breast per se as opposed to specific drainage of the tumour.

Advantages of the intradermal-subdermal injection technique are its practicability (it requires a minimum of training), the administration of a small volume using a single injection, the fast visualisation of lymphatic drainage pathways and the low administered activity, which results in fewer technical problems during lymphoscintigraphic imaging and intraoperative gamma probe counting. Some studies have compared the lymphoscintigraphic pattern and the performance in respect of SLN identification when using both the intradermal and the peritumoral approach in the same patients (Klimberg et al. 1999; Borgstein et al. 1997; Borgstein et al. 2000; Roumen et al. 1999). Although the two techniques are reported to yield virtually equivalent results in the vast majority of patients (Klimberg et al. 1999; Borgstein and Meijier 1998; Keshtgar and Ell 1999), some authors have reported a sizeable proportion of discordant results concerning SLNs in the axilla and/or in the internal mammary chain (IMC) (Roumen et al. 1999; Morton and Chan 2000). Whatever method is used, we believe that, with rare exceptions, lymphoscintigraphy must be able to localise axillary SLNs.

a b

Fig. 8.1a,b. Right anterior oblique view early (**a**) and delayed (**b**). Injection site at the inferior internal quadrant. Note that the lymphatic route drains around the areola to the axillary SLN. Nipple is marked with +

8.3 Internal Mammary Chain

The internal mammary lymphatic trunks originate from the anterior pre-pericardial lymph nodes lying upon the upper surface of the diaphragm. These nodes receive the lymph from the anterior and superior portion of the liver via the falciform ligament, from the anterior portion of the diaphragm, and from the upper portion of the rectus abdominis muscle, as well as from the lower inner sector of the adjacent mammary gland (Handley and Trackray 1954). The main efferent lymphatic vessels from the breast to the internal mammary route emerge from the deep portion and from the medial edge of the mammary gland.

When lymphoscintigraphy is performed after subdermal/intradermal radiocolloid injection, the detection of SLNs outside the axilla is an unlikely event, occurring in 1–2% of cases (Noguchi et al. 2000; Cox et al. 1999). We performed a pilot study in order to establish whether a deep injection can visualise the IMC nodes in a high percentage of cases, according to our standard lymphoscintigraphic protocol. Three points emerged from this study as regards to IMC lymphoscintigraphy and localisation:

A deep injection (under the tumour) is a suitable way of administering ^{99m}Tc-colloids to visualise IMC nodes;

Uptake by the IMC nodes occurred in 65% of lesions located in the inner quadrant;

An involved SLN in the IMC was found in 8.5% of the evaluated cases. According to the UICC staging classification, these cases "migrated" from N0 (two cases) and N1 (three cases) to N3. Without internal mammary sampling, these patients would have been understaged (Paganelli et al. 2002).

8.4 Randomised Trials

Six prospective randomised trials have been designed to validate SLNB. Actually, most centres and surgeons adopted SLNB as standard practice in the treatment of early breast cancer before the publication of these trials. This approach has been accepted because it has been clearly demonstrated that axillary clearance is performed for information purposes rather than with curative intent (Fisher et al. 2002).

The results of the first prospective randomised study have been published by Veronesi and co-workers (2003). Five hundred and sixteen women with primary breast cancer <2 cm in size were randomly assigned to undergo either SLNB and simultaneous axillary dissection (AD) or SLNB followed by AD only in the event of a positive SLNB. The primary endpoint of the study was the predictive power of the status of the SLN, measured in terms of the percentage of cases of axillary involvement detected by SLNB in relation to the percentage found by routine AD. A SLN was positive in 32.3% in the AD group and in 35.5% in the SLN group. In the AD group, the overall accuracy, the sensitivity and the specificity of the SLN was 96.9%, 91.2% and 100%, respectively. The false negative rate of 8.8% and the negative predictive value of 95.4% were consistent with previous studies (Veronesi et al. 1997; Giuliano et al. 1994; Krag et al. 1998). There was less pain and better arm mobility in patients who underwent SLNB only than in those who also underwent AD. After a median follow-up of 46 months, disease-free and overall survival rates were not significantly different between the two groups. In particular, overt axillary metastases were not detected in patients who had undergone SLNB only.

In the U.S. two studies have been launched (Wilke and Giuliano 2003; Ross 2001). The National Surgical Adjuvant Breast and Bowel Project (NSABP) trial B-32 (Krag and Julian 2002) has been designed in order to evaluate whether SLNB alone is equivalent to AD in terms of long-term control of regional disease, disease-free survival and overall survival, as primary end-points, with accrual of 5,500 patients with clinically negative axillae and a pathologically negative SLN. The American College of Surgeons-Oncology Group (ASOCOG) study (protocol Z0011) has now stopped accrual for a trial evaluating survival in women with pathologically positive SLNs who are randomly assigned to either AD or observation alone (Grube and Giuliano 2001; Brady Breast Study 2003).

In Europe three additional trials are ongoing. The European Organisation on Research and Treatment of Cancer (EORTC) is enrolling women in the AMAROS (After Mapping of the Axilla: Radiotherapy or Surgery?) trial comparing complete AD with axillary radiotherapy in women with positive SLNs; the target is accrual of 3,485 patients within 3 years (Hurkmans et al. 2003).

The Medical Research Council in the United Kingdom has funded the Axillary Lymphatic Mapping Against Nodal Axillary Clearance (ALMANAC) trial, where around 1,300 women with clinically negative axillary nodes are expected to be randomised either to conventional surgery or to SLNB. The primary endpoints are axillary morbidity, health economics and quality of life following SLNB as compared to conventional axillary procedures (Clarke et al. 2001).

Finally, the clinical and prognostic value of SLN micrometastases is being evaluated in the International Breast Cancer Study Group (IBCSG) trial 23.01, in which about 1,960 women with a diagnosis of micrometastases or isolated tumour cells only in the SLN are being randomly assigned to either complete AD or no further axillary treatment.

8.5 Sentinel Lymph Node Biopsy: When and Where?

The rapid spread of SLNB has led to its use in clinical settings previously considered contraindications to SLNB. All these clinical scenarios are now listed and discussed separately.

8.6 SLNB after Primary Chemotherapy

Former papers on SLNB after primary chemotherapy (PC) reported that the false negative rate of SLNB was higher in patients who had received PC than in those who had not (Bedrosian et al. 2000; Cohen et al. 2000; Nason et al. 2000; Brady 2002). More recent and larger studies have demonstrated that, with increasing experience, the identification and false-negative rates of SLNB are similar to those reported in the absence of PC (Breslin et al. 2000; Stearns et al. 2002; Mamounas 2003; Schwartz and Meltzer 2003). The paper with the largest cohort published on this topic reports the experience collected within the National Surgical Adjuvant Breast and Bowel Project multicentric trial (Krag and Julian 2002), in which 428 patients underwent lymphatic mapping after neoadjuvant chemotherapy. Success rate for the identification and removal of a sentinel node was 84.8%. Success rate increased significantly with the use of radioisotope (87.6% to 88.9%) versus with the use of lymphazurin alone (78.1%, P=0.03). Of the 343 patients who had SLNB and axillary dissection, the SLNs were positive in 125 patients and were the only positive nodes in 70 patients (56.0%). Of the 218 patients with negative SLNs, nonsentinel nodes were positive in 15 (false negative rate, 10.7%, 15 of 140 patients). There were non significant differences in false-negative rate according to clinical patient and tumor characteristics, method of lymphatic mapping or tumor response to chemotherapy. The authors concluded that the results were comparable to those obtained in multicentric studies evaluating SLNB before systemic therapy and that the sentinel node concept is also applicable after neoadjuvant chemotherapy.

Therefore, in women with a clinically negative axilla before the start of PC, SLNB might be considered after the completion of medical treatment if no progression has occurred. In patients with suspicious axillary nodes at presentation which have been "downstaged" to N0 by medical treatment, SLNB might also be considered an option in the hands of surgeons with extensive experience in this procedure. SLNB is obviously not recommended for patients whose axillary nodes remain clinically suspicious after PC. PET scan might be an useful tool to properly select those patients in which SLNB can be performed, even though this still represents a matter of research.

Some considerations might be added regarding the opportunity to gain pathological information on the nodal status before starting preoperative treatment. Axillary status before PC provides prognostic information that could be missed following PC, therefore it would be wise to perform axillary staging before PC in the event of a clinically negative axilla. Afterwards, if the node(s) were negative, axillary dissection following PC could be avoided, whereas in the case of a positive SLN, AD would be part of the surgical plan after medical treatment. This approach might also overcome the concern regarding the debated lower identification rate and sensitivity of SLNB after PC (Sabel et al. 2003).

On the other hand, it is conceivable that the prognostic value of axillary staging following PC is even higher, since it already mirrors response to treatment. Moreover, performing SLNB before PC would lead to AD in patients with positive SLNs, thus increasing the frequency of AD since PC may "sterilise" axillary node metastases in about 20% of patients (Fisher et al. 1997).

8.7 Multicentric/Multifocal Breast Cancer

Multifocal disease seems to be associated with a higher rate of nodal involvement than unifocal lesions of similar size (Andea et al. 2002). Multiple foci of carcinoma, particularly when located in different quadrants of the breast, have been considered a relative contraindication to SLNB because of concerns that these tumours might involve more than one dominant lymphatic trunk draining to axillary nodes, and thus lead to an increased false-negative rate (Anderson 2003; Reintgen et al. 2002). In our initial experience with 163 women, 2 of the 4 patients with false-negative SLNB had multifocal disease (Veronesi et al. 1997). Ozmen et al. (2002), in a study conducted on 111 patients, 21 of whom had multifocal tumours, reported an accuracy of 93.7% with a false negative rate of 11.3% in the whole cohort of patients. Multifocality and tumour size (>2 cm) were significantly associated with decreased accuracy and increased false negative rates. Klimberg et al. (1999), however, reported that the rate of identification of the SLN was equal following either subareolar or peritumoural injection, and therefore multicentric cancers might drain first to the subareolar area and then to the SLN in the axilla, through a network of lymphatic vessels connecting different quadrants with the subareolar area (Grant et al. 1959). Schrenk and Wayand (Schrenk and Wayand 2001) performed SLNB with either blue dye alone or blue dye and radiolabelled colloid injected in the subareolar area in 21 women with multicentric breast carcinoma who were prospectively evaluated and candidates for standard AD. The authors found a 100% identification rate of SLNs and no false-negative SLNBs.

Two papers from the Memorial Sloan-Kettering Cancer Center have addressed the issue of SLNB in multicentric breast cancer. In the first (Kim et al. 2002), five patients with two tumours in distinct quadrants were injected at one site with technetium-labelled sulphur colloid and at the second site with isosulphan blue dye. Having identified at least one node that was both hot and blue within the axilla in all cases, the authors suggested that the lymphatic drainage of the entire breast coincides with the drainage of the tumour bed, regardless of its location. In the second paper, Tousimis et al. (2003) considered 70 patients with multicentric/multifocal breast carcinoma who were submitted to mastectomy and SLNB with planned AD. The accuracy of SLNB was 96%, and the sensitivity, 92% (false negative rate 8%); these results are comparable to those of published studies carried out in women presenting with unifocal disease. All three patients with inaccurate SLNB had dominant invasive tumour larger than 5 cm, and in one case axillary disease was palpable at surgery.

In the study by Kumar et al. (2003) on 48 patients with multicentric/multifocal breast carcinoma, success rate, sensitivity, negative predictive value and accuracy were 93%, 100%, 100% and 100% using the radiocolloid probe, 87%,100%, 100% and 100% using blue dye, and 93.5%, 100%, 100% and 100% using combined methods. The authors concluded that SLN localisation maintained a high negative predictive value in multicentric/multifocal breast cancer, as opposed to the common belief that a higher rate of false negative results occurs in this subset of patients, and they proposed its routine use instead of AD in these patients, too.

Recently a multi-institutional validation study has been published by the Austrian Sentinel Node Study Group (Knauer et al. 2006), comparing 142 patients with multicentric cancer to 3,216 patients with unicentric breast cancer. The authors reported sensitivity, negative predictive value and overall accuracy of 96.0%, 93.3% and 97.3%, respectively, concluding that multicentric breast cancer is a new indication for SLNB without routine ALND in controlled trials.

The initial experience of our institute has been also recently reported (Gentilini et al. 2006). Between 2001 and 2004, 42 patients with multicentric breast cancer and a clinically negative axilla underwent lymphatic mapping either by a single subareolar or a double peritumoral/subdermal injection of 99 Tc-HAS nanocolloids. Mean number of SLNs identified by lymphoscintigraphy was 1.36 (range 1–5) and mean number of SLNs removed at surgery was 1.55 (range 1–5), with an identification rate of 100%. The mean number of hot spots identified by lymphoscintigraphy was similar in patients who underwent single or double injections (1.36 and 1.35, respectively). In 21 of 42 patients the SLN was positive, and in 7 of these 21 patients the SLN was the only positive node. After a median follow-up of 24 months no overt axillary metastases occurred in patients with negative SLN. We concluded that the number of SLNs is not dependent on the number and site of injections. In our institute SLNB is our standard procedure for nodal staging in patients with multicentric breast cancer and a clinically negative axilla.

8.8 Previous Breast Biopsy

Some authors have suggested that altered lymphatic drainage decreases the likelihood of successful lymphatic mapping and, indeed, that SLNB for breast cancer may be less accurate after excisional biopsy of the primary tumour (Borgstein et al. 1998; McMaster et al. 1998; Ollila and Giuliano 1998). Other authors (Wong et al. 2002; Miner et al. 1999) claim that neither biopsy type nor type of definitive surgical procedure significantly affects the accuracy of SLN biopsy for breast cancer, and that SLNB can be performed accurately after excisional biopsy and is equally effective in patients undergoing partial mastectomy or total mastectomy. At EIO (Luini et al. 2005) we examined the accuracy of SLNB by following the axillary relapses after the procedure in 543 patients who had undergone a breast biopsy before SLNB. All the patients received SLNB by lymphoscintigraphy performed on the biopsy area. We followed these patients with a clinical assessment every 6 months and instrumental examinations every year, particularly focusing on the research of axillary relapse of disease. In 70.4% of cases, the sentinel node was negative, and only three patients underwent further axillary dissection. The sentinel node was identified in 99% of cases and this was the only positive node in 61.5% of cases with positive axillary nodes. The median follow-up was 2 years; four nodal recurrences were observed: three axillary lymph node relapses and one loco-regional. In conclusion, SLNB accuracy after a previous breast biopsy is comparable with the results obtained in validation studies. SLNB after a previous breast biopsy can be considered a standard procedure. Lymphoscintigraphy identifies the sentinel node in 99% of patients.

8.9 Previous Axillary Surgery

Since SLNB is routinely performed in the clinical practice as standard procedure for axillary staging of patients with primary operable breast cancer and clinically uninvolved axillary lymph nodes, the occurrence of an ipsilateral breast tumour reappearance (IBTR) in patients with previous histologic negative SLN represents a quite new clinical situation, destined to dramatically increase. In case of limited IBTR, the risk of metastases in the residual axillary nodes is very low and a complete axillary dissection could be an unnecessary over-treatment in the majority of these patients. Most authors consider a previous axillary surgery, and in particular SLNB, a definitive contraindication to a new SLNB, but no data are currently available to support or refute this concept. Therefore, several inappropriate axillary dissections are commonly offered to IBTR patients.

In the Memorial Sloan-Kettering Cancer Center experience (Port et al. 2002), a previous axillary surgery, either a partial level I-II axillary dissection or a previous successful or failed lymph node biopsy, did not hamper the identification of a SLN, especially when fewer than ten nodes were removed during the earlier procedure. In their series the sec-SLNB was guided by using a combined dye-isotope mapping technique, the overall identification rate was 75% and the number of sec-SLNs removed was 2.3/patient. The rate of SLN identification is significantly lower than in our series (100% of SLN identification), probably due to the larger extent of previous surgical treatment on the axilla. In fact, when the sec-SLNB was performed after a level I-II axillary dissection or an inadequate axillary dissection, the identification rate was only 66.6% while, if the sec-SLNB was performed after a previous SLNB, the identification rate was higher (87.5%).

At the European Institute of Oncology in Milan, between January 2000 and June 2004, 79 patients, previously treated with BCS and a negative SLNB for early breast cancer, developed, during the follow-up, a local recurrence amenable to re-operation (re-operative BCS or salvage total mastectomy). Eighteen of these patients, nine with invasive carcinoma and nine with DCIS, were offered a sec-SLNB due to a clinically negative axillary status, after an average of 26.1 months from the primary event. We defined as true local recurrence (TLR) the tumours re-appearing close to the skin scar or in the index breast quadrant, and as new ipsilateral primary tumours (NIPT) those occurring in the other breast quadrants. Accordingly, 12 tumours of our series were considered TLR and 6 NIPT. A sec-SLNB was not offered to the majority (61/79) of the patients with local recurrences due to the clinical presentation of the disease (multicentric disease, inflammatory disease, metastatic disease, suspicious axillary lymph nodes at clinical examination) or simply because a sec-SLNB was not considered, at that time, technically feasible or clinically acceptable. All the patients offered a sec-SLNB accepted the surgical procedure and signed an informed consent.

Lymphoscintigraphy was performed using the standard technique in our institution. In case of NIPT the technique did not differ from that already described. The 10–12 MBq of ^{99m}Tc-labeled colloidal particles of human albumin were injected in correspondence of the skin projection of the tumour, subdermally, the day before surgery or the same day. In case of TLR, the injection technique was the same used in presence of a skin scar for a previous surgical biopsy: one single subdermal injection close to the skin scar towards the axilla. In both cases, TLR and NIPT, lymphoscintigraphy was then carried out acquiring planar images in anterior and oblique anterior views, collecting 150 K counts, at 15 and 30 after the injection. More delayed acquisition at 120 min were carried out only if SLNs were not previously evident.

Four of the nine patients with DCIS developed an invasive recurrence and two of the nine patients with invasive carcinoma developed a DCIS recurrence. In total, 7 DCIS and 11 invasive recurrences underwent sec-SLNB. At the preoperative lymphoscintigraphy, at least one new axillary SLN (total 20; average 1.1/patient) was visualized in all 18 cases. No other sites of drainage outside the axilla (e.g., lymph nodes of the internal mammary chain) were observed. In all patients one or more SLNs were surgically removed (average 1.3/patient). Metastases were identified in the SLNs of two patients with invasive recurrence and a complete axillary dissection followed. In 1 patient the sec-SLN was the only metastatic lymph node, while in the other patient, 12 additional metastatic axillary lymph nodes were identified. Comparing the characteristics of the SLNs in the 12 TLRs and 6 NIPTs, in terms of number of SLNs visualized at lymphoscintigraphy or identified at surgery, and interval time between radioisotope injection and scintigraphic visualization, no differences were observed. In particular, the SLNs were visualised at lymphoscintigraphy within 120 min from the radioisotope injection in all 18 cases and no further administrations were necessary. At a median follow up of 12.7 months, no axillary recurrences occurred in the 16 patients who had not undergone completion axillary dissection.

The SLN is, by definition, the first node or nodes directly draining the lymph from the breast carcinoma area. Although usually an axillary node, and most commonly in the central group of level I, the SLN may be at level II (behind the pectoralis minor muscle) or level III (infraclavicular), or may even be an intramammary node, an interpectoral (Rotter's) node, or an internal mammary node. To be anatomically and oncologically effective and to correctly predict the histological status of the axilla, SLNB requires, at minimum, the presence of an intact lymphatic flow from the site of the primary tumour (or recurrence). A previous axillary surgery could partially and/or temporarily interrupt and modify the lymphatic flow, thus making it more difficult to correct identify the SLN. In case of partial interruption of the lymph flow, an axillary SLN may still be identified. In fact, several studies (Goyal and Mansel 2004) support the hypothesis that breast tumours drain through a few common afferent lymphatic channels to a common axillary SLN, regardless of tumour location and number of tumour foci. The breast drains to the axilla as a single unit through few major lymphatic trunks coming from a subareolar plexus. If one or more trunks are interrupted, an alternative path to the SLN may be utilized successfully for the radioisotope migration. In case of complete lymphatic interruption, the physiological restoring of the anatomy of the lymphatic drainage makes the obstacle only temporary. In fact, when an adequate period of time elapses between the first axillary surgery and the breast recurrence, the lymphatic net has time to be re-built and a new lymphatic "bridge" can connect the breast and the operated axilla. Such a post-operatively "collateralization" of lymphatics occurs as a physiological compensatory mechanism. The new lymphatic pathway allows identifying a novel SLN, true "sentinel" *hic et nunc* of the new tumour as the first SLN was of the first carcinoma. These considerations could introduce a new dynamic concept of SLN: not "*one SLN for ever*", but "*always a new SLN*". In our series, a new SLN was detected at lymphoscintigraphy in 99% of the patients after a median interval of 26.1 months (range 4–61 months) from the primary axillary operation.

What is the adequate period of time that must elapse from the first SLNB to consider a sec-SLNB effective? Of course it is impossible to quantify the minimal interval of time between the two events, the time of the restoring of the anatomy of the lymphatic drainage being unkown. Nevertheless, a very early IBTR after BCS must probably be considered a residual tumour more than a true recurrence. In these cases, the first SLN maintains the same predictive value for both the first tumour and the recurrence, and a sec-SLNB could not be useful.

In case of NIPT the technique did not differ from the one already described, implying a single subdermal injection in correspondence of the projection of the tumour. In case of TLR, the radioisotope injection technique was the same used in case of a skin scar from a previous surgical biopsy, i.e., one single subdermal injection close to the scar towards the axilla. In our experience on 534 patients previously submitted to surgical biopsy, this method allows identifying the SLN in 98.5% of cases. Comparing the two groups of patients, no differences were observed in terms of number of SLNs visualized at lymphoscintigraphy and interval time between radioisotope injection and scintigraphic visualisation. In the NIPT group, the number of SLNs identified at surgery was slightly higher than in the TLR group, but the small number of patients does not allow drawing any significant conclusions.

In conclusion, we recommend performing a lymphoscintigraphy in case of local recurrence after BCS, even if a SLNB has been previously performed. Whenever a SLN is identified at lymphoscintigraphy, the axillary dissection, and its morbidity and sequelae, could be avoided also in these patients, without losing the important prognostic information of the axillary status. Furthermore, it should be emphasized that the lymphoscintigraphic technique, adopted at EIO, allows to distinguish prior to surgery the patients candidate to SLNB or AD. In case of lack of preoperative visualization of SLN, the axillary dissection must be considered only after a careful evaluation of all the patient and tumoral characteristics, increasing the axillary metastatic risk. Moreover, axillary ultrasonography with fine-needle aspiration cytology and PET can be very useful tools to predict the axillary lymphnodal status.

8.10 Ductal Carcinoma in Situ and SLNB

In the presence of ductal carcinoma in situ (DCIS), AD is not indicated since this is an intra-epithelial neoplasm that typically does not have the potential for metastasis. The prevalence of axillary metastases, which is lower than 2% (Schnitt et al. 1988), does not justify the significant morbidity associated with lymph node removal. The techniques of lymphatic mapping and SLNB, however, have also been applied to patients with DCIS, resulting in some series in an unexpectedly high rate of detection of metastases. Pendas et al. (2000) reported a 5.7% rate in 87 patients, though after exclusion of micro-invasion this rate decreased to 4.6%. Of the 76 patients with high-risk DCIS described by Klauber-DeMore et al. (2000), 12% had metastases in the SLN, but further evaluation allowed exclusion of patients with invasion and the actual rate was lowered to 6.6%. In the paper by Cox et al. (2001), a 13% rate of positive SLNs was found in 195 patients with pure DCIS, but lack of data on the extent of sampling makes comparison difficult.

At European Institute of Oncology in Milan, between March 1996 and December 2003, 508 consecutive patients affected by pure DCIS (DCIS with microinvasion were excluded) were submitted to lymphoscintigraphy, SLN biopsy and histologic examination. SLN metastases were detected in 9 of the 508 patients (1.8%). The SLNs were the only affected nodes in the eight patients who underwent subsequent complete axillary dissections. Five of the nine patients with SLN positive had only micrometastases (<2 mm). The low number of positive SLN patients and the subsequent imbalance in the two groups make impossible any kind of comparison between the two groups of patients, with the sole exception of histological pattern and tumour size. In particular, the risk of lymph node metastases does not seem to be correlated with clinical presentation, grade, sex steroid hormone receptor status, proliferative index (Ki67) or type of surgery. Only tumour size and subhistotype comedocarcinoma seem to be relevant in predicting the risk of SLN metastases: the median tumour size in the SLN-positive group was 22.3 mm, while in SLN-negative 12.1 mm. Furthermore, 22.2% in the SLN-positive group were comedocarcinomas, while 10.2% in the SLN-negative DCIS patient group. Another interesting observation is that seven (77.8%) out of the nine patients with a metastatic SLN had undergone a previous breast biopsy: two patients had undergone an open surgical biopsy elsewhere, and five patients were subjected to vacuum-assisted biopsy in our institution. In two of these five latter patients, an artefactual dislocation of tumour cells within the stroma along the needle tract was identified. On the other hand, only 58.9% of patients with negative SN were previously submitted to an invasive diagnostic procedure. The chance of a passive transport of dislocated epithelial cells to the SLN following an invasive pre-operative manoeuvre has been reported, but still represents a hotly debated issue, with unresolved clinical implications (Carter et al. 2000). However, a pre-operative invasive manoeuvre could remove or hide micro-invasive foci in the sampled DCIS. After 46 months of follow-up, no loco-regional or systemic event was observed in the nine SLN-positive patients. In conclusion, due to the low prevalence of metastatic involvement (1.8%), SLNB should not be considered a standard procedure in the treatment of all patients with DCIS. In pure non-comedo DCIS completely excised by radical surgery with free margins of resection, SLNB should be avoided since not only is it unnecessary, but it could also jeopardize a successive re-SLNB in case of invasive recurrence. A very extensive and accurate histological examination of the tumour in DCIS is compulsory to exclude micro-invasive foci and, finally, to decrease the prevalence of unexpected SLN metastases. Less thorough sampling and examination of large tumours may miss (micro) invasive foci. SLNB could be considered in case of DCIS where there exists a strong doubt of invasion at the definitive histology, such as large solid tumours or diffuse or pluricentric microcalcifications undergoing mastectomy. In this case a successive SLNB could not be proposed. Moreover, if the trend is statistically confirmed with a wider population, large comedo-DCIS, presenting superior risk of SLNs metastasis, could be scheduled for SLNB. If the SLN is micrometastatic complete axillary dissection is not unavoidable.

8.11 SLNB in Men's Breast Cancer

Male breast cancer is a rare disease, accounting for fewer than 1% of all breast cancers and fewer than 1% of all annual cancer deaths in males (Greenlee et al. 2000). Because of the low number of patients with this disease, treatment for breast cancer in males has been extrapolated from treatment protocols for breast cancer in females. Men are more likely than women to have a delay between the onset of symptoms and a diagnosis of breast cancer, possibly because of the limited public awareness of breast cancer in men. This delay in diagnosis may contribute to men presenting at later stages than do women and nodal involvement is present in up to 60% of male breast cancer patients (Joshi et al. 1996). Despite recent advances in the application of SLN biopsy for axillary staging in female breast cancer patients, modified radical mastectomy remains the standard of care for male breast cancer patients in most institutions. Men are at no less risk for the development of the morbidities associated with axillary dissection. The potential impact for the male, though no more or less than the female, may be somewhat different. For males, since they frequently have vocations in which the physical activity may be more pronounced the impact may be more devastating. So far six papers have been published about SLNB in males (De Cicco et al. 2004; Cimmino et al. 2004; Albo et al. 2003; Port et al. 2001; Gennari et al. 2001; Mullan and Kissin 2001) with only a few patients reported. The detection rate was 100% in all the studies. We reported the largest experience with 18 male patients who underwent SLNB with ALND performed only in case of positive SLN (De Cicco et al. 2004). Other groups performed a backup ALND in some patients with no false negative in a very limited and not significant sample of patients so that it is impossible to draw conclusions about the false negative rate of SLNB in male patients with breast cancer. Although a large clinical trial on the use of SLNB in male breast cancer patients would be interesting, we do not believe it is necessary to design a specific study to validate SLNB in males. Tumour biology, prognostic factors, and outcomes have been reported to be equivalent in male and female breast cancer patients, providing a scientific basis for the extrapolation of treatment for males with breast cancer from treatment algorithms for females with this disease (Gradishar 2000). Since there are no biological or anatomical issues that would alter the lymphatic drainage in men with respect to women, SLNB should be applied also to male patients with breast cancer and a clinically negative axilla, unless there is an overwhelming evidence to prove the opposite.

8.12 Pregnancy

In a recent review on BCdP, it was stated that axillary dissection is preferred because nodal metastases are commonly found, nodal status affects the choice of adjuvant chemotherapy and SNB poses an unknown risk to the foetus from the radioisotope (Woo et al. 2003).

Indeed, when breast cancer is diagnosed during pregnancy axillary lymph nodes are frequently positive, but when the tumour is diagnosed at an early stage a considerable proportion of patients have a node-negative disease. Therefore they might benefit from the sentinel node biopsy procedure.

Furthermore, the decision-making process regarding adjuvant treatment in pregnancy is limited. In fact, tamoxifen and other endocrine agents are generally not recommended (Halakivi-Clarke et al. 2000), and some drugs such as metotrexate are strongly contraindicated during pregnancy, whereas anthracyclines can be administered during the second and the third trimester (Berry et al. 1999). From this standpoint, axillary staging gives important prognostic information and allows better local control, but should not influence the type of adjuvant treatment during pregnancy.

In order to evaluate the safety of lymphoscintigraphy and SLNB in pregnant patients, we carried out a study (Gentilini et al. 2004) by conducting a simulation in 26 premenopausal non-pregnant patients, who underwent peritumoral injection of approximately 12 MBq of ^{99m}Tc-HSA nanocolloids. Static (15 min and 16 h post injection (p.i.) and whole body (16 h p.i.) scintigraphic images were acquired. Activity concentration in the urine (0–2, 2–4, 4–8, 8–16 h p.i.) was evaluated by a gamma-counter. Activity in the blood stream was measured at 4 and 16 h p.i. Thermoluminescent dosimeters (TLD) were placed on the injection site before tracer injection, the epigastrium, and at the umbilicus and hypogastrum, and were removed before surgery.

Scintigraphic imaging showed no diffusion of radiotracer except in the injection site and in the sentinel node. The biological pharmacokinetic data showed that a very small amount of the injected activity circulates in the blood pool and is excreted by the urinary system (less than 2%). Considering the physical decay of the radiotracer, we can confirm that the level of radioactivity in the body is absolutely negligible at each time after the administration, proving no significant risk to the foetus. In 23/26 patients, all absorbed dose measurements resulted lower than TLD sensitivity (<10 Gy); in the remaining 3 patients, the absorbed doses to the epigastrium, umbilicus and hypogastrium resulted to be 100–1,000 fold lower than the threshold for a deterministic effect. We concluded that, according to our protocol, lymphoscintigraphy and sentinel node biopsy can be safely performed also during pregnancy, since specific evaluations of radiation protection do not indicate significant risks to the foetus at any phase of a potential pregnancy.

Moreover, some practical recommendations might be given in order to further minimise the exposure of the foetus, such as avoiding contact with other patients being potential sources of radioactivity (e.g., by scheduling pregnant patients as the first procedure of the day, and keeping the patient in a single-bed room), and reducing the time interval between lymphoscintigraphy and surgery, with a subsequent possible reduction of the administered activity. Thus, in pregnant patients SLNB can be performed within 2–3 h post injection of 3–5 MBq of ^{99m}Tc radiocolloids.

Consistent results were reported also by the M.D. Anderson group (Keleher et al. 2004). The maximum absorbed dose to the embryo/foetus in pregnant women undergoing breast lymphoscintigraphy with 92.5 MBq (2.5 mCi) of technetium Tc-99m sulphur colloid was found to be 0.0043 Gy under the most adverse conditions in the theoretical model (all the injected radiopharmaceutical travels immediately to the bladder and is eliminated through the process of physical decay). The potentially largest absorbed dose with lymphoscintigraphy remained approximately 12 to 23 times less than the threshold associated with reported risk of foetal adverse effects associated with radiation exposure. The authors concluded that the use of technetium Tc-99m sulphur colloid for pregnant patients with a clinically negative axilla is theoretically safe for the developing embryo/foetus.

8.13 Pathology

The histopathological examination of each SLN must be particularly accurate to avoid a false-negative or a false-positive diagnosis. We have devised a very accurate protocol for the examination of axillary SLNs, which can be applied either to frozen sections for an intraoperative diagnosis or to fixed and embedded SLNs (Viale et al. 1999). Upon receipt of the SLN, the pathologist must remove the perinodal fibrous-fatty tissue and bisect the lymph node along the major axis. Small lymph nodes (up to 5-mm thick) may be processed uncut, while larger lymph nodes are sliced in 3- to 4-mm-thick slices.

From each moiety or slice of the SLN, 15 pairs of sections are cut at 50-mm intervals; whenever lymph node tissue is left, additional pairs of sections, cut at 100-mm intervals, are obtained until the node has been completely sectioned. One section from each pair is stained with haematoxylin and eosin (H&E) and examined. The mirror section is kept for possible immunohistochemical staining to ascertain the nature of any atypical cells, suspicious for malignancy, that are detected in the H&E preparations. We perform a rapid assay (Chilosi et al. 1994), based on a single incubation step with a monoclonal antibody to cytokeratins (MNF116) directly coupled to peroxidase via a polymer (EPOS Dako, Glostrup, Denmark). We normally avoid performing a traditional intraoperative examination of the SLNs, whereby only one to three frozen sections are examined and the rest of the node is left for the subsequent examination of permanent sections. In this event, a high ratc of false-negative intraoperative diagnoses is to be expected, with the need for a second operation to achieve complete AD in almost 17% of patients.

The above-described extensive histopathological examination of the SLN has been designed to identify in the SLNs even micrometastatic disease (i.e., tumour foci up to 2 mm in size) or isolated tumour cells (ITCs), which can escape detection by less accurate evaluation. ITCs are defined as single neoplastic cells or small clusters of cells not larger than 0.2 mm that do not typically show evidence of metastatic activity (e.g., proliferation or stromal reaction) or penetration of vascular or lymphatic sinus walls (Hermanek et al. 1999). These cells are more commonly identified with the use of immunohistochemical reactions, but may also be recognised in routinely stained sections. The actual prognostic value of axillary lymph node micrometastases is still the subject of debate, though most recent findings indicate that they correlate with a worse overall survival (International Breast Cancer Study Group 1990; Dowlatshahi et al. 1997; Cote et al. 1999). From a practical point of view, however, the first question to be addressed is whether the detection of micrometastases in the SLN should dictate completion of AD, or whether the risk of additional metastases to non-sentinel lymph nodes is low enough to allow axillary clearance to be spared, as has been suggested (Chu et al. 1999; Reynolds et al. 1999). We (Viale et al. 2001) and others (Turner et al. 2000) have demonstrated that the risk of additional metastases to non-sentinel axillary lymph nodes in the presence of micrometastatic disease in the SLN actually ranges from 22% to 25%, and that when ITCs are present in the SLN, patients have no less than a 15% risk of additional metastases. Accordingly, outside of randomised clinical trials designed to test the value of AD in these patients, the current practice in our institute is to complete AD in all patients with SLN micrometastases or ITCs. A randomised clinical trial has recently been launched by the International Breast Cancer Study Group (IBCSG) to assess whether patients with micrometastatic SLNs should necessarily undergo complete AD for a more extensive evaluation of the lymph node status, or whether the information obtained by examination of the SLN only, coupled with the morphological and biological characteristics of the primary tumour, is sufficient to plan proper adjuvant treatment.

More recently, molecular biology assays have also been adopted for the identification of so-called occult metastases, i.e., metastases not detected by morphological methods, including immunohistochemistry (Masuda et al. 2000; Bostick et al. 1998; Bostick et al. 1998; Kataoka et al. 2000). Micrometastases in axillary lymph nodes detected by RT-PCR have been reported to be clinically significant, being an independent predictor of survival in a retrospective series of patients (Viale et al. 2001). Some researchers have indicated that detection of tumour mRNA markers in the SLNs of breast carcinoma patients may be more accurate than histological examination in predicting axillary lymph node status, or have recommended reverse transcription-polymerase chain reaction (RT-PCR) as a more feasible and practical assay than extensive histological examination for an accurate diagnosis of SLN metastases, with a similar detection sensitivity (Turner et al. 2000; Masuda et al. 2000; Bostick et al. 1998).

We have compared the results of RT-PCR assays with those obtained by our extensive histopathological examination of the SLN from 123 patients (Manzotti et al. 2001). A multiple-marker RT-PCR assay of five different tumour mRNA markers (cytokeratin 19, CEA, maspin, mammaglobin and MUC-1) showed a good sensitivity (95.6%), but a poor specificity (66.3%) when compared with histology, and a lower predictive value with respect to the status of the remaining non-sentinel axillary lymph nodes. In particular, we observed a high prevalence of positive RT-PCR assays in histologically uninvolved SLNs, possibly due to the occurrence of low-level expression of genes by illegitimate transcription in normal resident cells of the SLN. To overcome this limitation, we are currently exploiting the use of quantitative real-time RT-PCR assays for differentiating the low-level "illegitimate" transcription of some mRNA markers by non-neoplastic tissues from the expected higher expression in neoplastic cells.

8.14 Conclusion

In the near future, new and more precise evaluations of the gene expression profiling of breast cancer probably will allow all the complete prognostic information we need to understand the biological behaviour of the tumour, and will make pointless whatever diagnostic surgical invasive procedure on the axilla (microarray). Waiting for this moment, when clinically and oncologically it appears indicated or useful to know the histologic status of the axilla, SLNB is a reasonable option for most breast cancer patients with nonmetastatic disease. The suitability of SLNB has been studied and established in the settings of DCIS, in multifocal and multicentric disease, following neo-adjuvant chemotherapy, after excisional or core-needle biopsy or after small or large volumes of resection and finally after a previous SLNB when a local recurrence occurs. SLNB has been recently demonstrated to be safe and sure in pregnancy and can be also considered in patients with clinically suspicious axillary nodes if preoperative palpation or US-guided FNA is nondiagnostic (Specht et al. 2005). Only for a small subset of patients at both ends of the tumoral spectrum, those with pure low grade DCIS radically resected and those with inflammatory cancer, the jury is still out. Moreover, due to the high sensitivity that PET showed to predict the axillary SLN status when it was applied preoperatively before performing SLNB, an axillary positive PET should directly suggest a CAD.

Of course, in order to guarantee the best results, more and more a large amount of SLNB experience and a correct standardisation and validation of all the phases of the technique (surgery, pathology, radiology and nuclear medicine) are required. In fact, it should be considered that introduction of the SLNB procedure in any given institution requires a combined effort that involves at least three different specialties, nuclear medicine, surgical oncology and pathology, with the addition of health physics. However experienced a specialist is, there will be a definite, significant learning curve that depends on how rapidly the different operators develop the attitude that they are working as a single team. Thus, the learning curve should be related to the team rather than to the individual specialists, who will have to gain confidence in all the various steps of the procedure and at the same time rely on each other's contribution to the entire process.

Paradoxically, in the most breast cancer patients the new fundamental question seems to be not "is SLNB correct in this patient?" but "am I able to correctly perform SLNB in this patient?" Probably, the inability to correctly perform SLNB actually remains the only contraindication to SLNB.

References

Alazraki NP, Styblo T, Grant SF et al (2000) Sentinel node staging of early breast cancer using lymphoscintigraphy and the intraoperative gamma-detecting probe. Semin Nucl Med 30:56–64

Albo D, Ames FC, Hunt KK et al (2003) Evaluation of lymph node status in male breast cancer patients: a role for sentinel lymph node biopsy. Breast Cancer Res Treat 77: 9–14

Andea AA, Wallis T, Newman LA et al (2002) Pathologic analysis of tumor size and lymph node status in multifocal/multicentric breast carcinoma. Cancer 94:1383–1390

Anderson BO (2003) Sentinel lymphadenectomy in breast cancer: an update on the NCCN Clinical Practice Guidelines. J Natl Compr Cancer Network 1:S64–S70

Bedrosian I, Reynolds C, Mick R et al (2000) Accuracy of sentinel lymph node biopsy in patients with large primary breast tumors. Cancer 88:2540–2545

Berry D, Theriault R, Holmes F et al (1999) Management of breast cancer during pregnancy using a standardized protocol. J Clin Oncol 17:855–861

Borgstein PJ, Meijr S, Pijpers R (1997) Intradermal blue dye to identify sentinel lymph node in breast cancer. Lancet 349:1668–1669

Borgstein P, Meijier S (1998) Historical perspective of lymphatic tumour spread and the emergence of the sentinel node concept. Eur J Surg Oncol 24:85–89

Borgstein PJ, Pijpers R, Comans EF et al (1998) Sentinel lymph node biopsy in breast cancer: guidelines and pitfalls of lymphoscintigraphy and gamma probe detection. J Am Coll Surg 186:275–283

Borgstein PJ, Meijer S, Pijpers RJ et al (2000) Functional lymphatic anatomy in breast cancer: echoes from the past and the periareolar blue method. Ann Surg 232:81–89

Bostick PJ, Huynh KT, Sarantou T et al (1998) Detection of metastases in sentinel lymph nodes of breast cancer patients by multiple-marker RT-PCR. Int J Cancer 79:645–651

Bostick PJ, Chatteriee S, Chi DD et al (1998) Limitations of specific reverse-transcriptase polymerase chain reaction markers in the detection of metastases in the lymph

nodes and blood of breast cancer patients. J Clin Oncol 16:2632–2640
Brady EW (2002) Sentinel lymph node mapping following neoadjuvant chemotherapy for breast cancer. Breast J 8:97–100
Brady Breast Study announcements. Durham, N.C.: American College of Surgeons Oncology Group, 2003. (Accessed July 18, 2003 at www.asocog.org/studies/organ_site/breast/.)
Breslin TM, Cohen L, Sahin A et al (2000) Sentinel lymph node biopsy is accurate after neoadjuvant chemotherapy for breast cancer. J Clin Oncol 18:3480–3486
Carter BA, Jensesn RA, Simpson JF et al (2000) Benign transport of breast epithelium into axillary lymph nodes after biopsy. Am J Pathol 113:259–265
Chilosi M, Lestani M, Pedron S et al (1994) A rapid immunostaining method for frozen sections. Biotech Histochem 69:235–239
Chu KU, Turner RR, Hansen NM et al (1999) Do all patients with sentinel node metastasis from breast carcinoma need complete axillary node dissection? Ann Surg 229:536–541
Cimmino VM, Degnim YC, Sabel HS et al (2004) Efficacy of sentinel lymph node biopsy in male breast cancer. J Surg Oncol 86:74–77
Clarke D, Khonji NI, Mansel ER (2001) Sentinel node biopsy in breast cancer: ALMANAC trial. World J Surg 25:819–822
Cody HS 3rd, Borgen PI (1999) State-of-the-art approaches to sentinel node biopsy for breast cancer: study design, patient selection, technique, and quality control at Memorial Sloan-Kettering Cancer Center. Surg Oncol 8:85–91
Cody HS 3rd (2003) Sentinel lymph node biopsy for breast cancer: does anybody not need one? Ann Surg Oncol 10(10):1131–1132
Cohen LF, Breslin TM, Kuerer HM et al (2000) Identification and evaluation of axillary sentinel lymph nodes in patients with breast carcinoma treated with neoadjuvant chemotherapy. Am J Surg Pathol 24:1266–1272
Cote RJ, Peterson HF, Chaiwun B et al (1999) Role of immunohistochemical detection of lymph-node metastases in management of breast cancer. Lancet 354:896–900
Cox CE, Bass SS, Reintgen DS (1999) Techniques for lymphatic mapping in breast carcinoma. Surg Oncol Clin North Am 8:447–468
Cox CE, Nguyen K, Gray RJ et al (2001) Importance of lymphatic mapping in ductal carcinoma in situ (DCIS): why map DCIS? Am J Surg 67:513–519
De Cicco C, Cremonesi M, Luini A et al (1998) Lymphoscintigraphy and radioguided biopsy of the sentinel axillary node in breast cancer. J Nucl Med 39:2080–2084
De Cicco C, Baio SM, Veronesi P et al (2004) Sentinel node biopsy in male breast cancer. Nucl Med Commun 25:139–143
Dowlatshahi K, Fan M, Snider HC et al (1997) Lymph node micrometastases from breast carcinoma. Reviewing the dilemma. Cancer 80:1188–1197
Fenaroli P, Tondini C, Motta T et al (2000) Axillary sentinel node biopsy under local anesthesia in early breast cancer. Ann Oncol 11:1617–1618
Fisher B, Brown A, Mamounas E et al (1997) Effect of preoperative chemotherapy on local-regional disease in women with operable breast cancer: findings from National Surgical Adjuvant Breast and Bowel Project B-18. J Clin Oncol 15:2483–2493
Fisher B, Jeong JH, Anderson S et al (2002) Twenty-five-year follow up of a randomized trial comparing radical mastectomy, total mastectomy, and total mastectomy followed by irradiation. N Engl J Med 22:567–575
Gennari R, Renne G, Travaini L et al (2001) Sentinel node biopsy in male breast cancer: future standard treatment? Eur J Surg 167:461–462
Gentilini O, Cremonesi M, Trifirò G et al (2004) Safety of sentinel node biopsy in pregnant patients with breast cancer. Ann Oncol 15:1348–1351
Gentilini O, Trifirò G, Soteldo J et al (2006) Sentinel lymph node biopsy in multicentric breast cancer. The experience of the European Institute of Oncology. Eur J Surg Oncol 32(5):507–510
Giuliano AE, Kirgan DM, Guenther JM et al (1994) Lymphatic mapping and sentinel lymphadenectomy for breast cancer. Ann Surg 220:391–401
Giuliano AE, Jones RC, Brennan M et al (1997) Sentinel lymphadenectomy and breast cancer. J Clin Oncol 15:2345–2350
Goyal A, Mansel RE (2004) Multifocality and sentinel node biopsy in breast cancer. Eur J Surg Oncol 30:3–4
Gradishar WJ (2000) Male breast cancer. In: Harris JR, Lippman ME, Morrow M, Osborne CK (eds) Diseases of the breast. Lippincott Williams & Wilkins, Philadelphia, pp 661–667
Grant RN, Tabah EJ, Adair FE (1959) The surgical significance of the subareolar plexus in cancer of the breast. Surgery 33:71–78
Greenlee RT, Murray T, Bolden S et al (2000) Cancer statistics 2000. CA Cancer J Clin 50:7–33
Grube BJ, Giuliano AE (2001) Observation of the breast cancer patient with a tumor-positive sentinel node: implications of the ASOCOG Z0011 trial. Semin Surg Oncol 20:230–237
Halakivi-Clarke L, Cho E, Onojafe I et al (2000) Maternal exposure to tamoxifen during pregnancy increases carcinogen-induced mammary tumorigenesis among female rat offspring. Clin Cancer Res 6:305–308
Handley RS, Trackray AC (1954) Invasion of internal mammary lymph nodes in carcinoma of the breast. Br Med J 1:61–63
Hermanek P, Hutter RVP, Sobin LH et al (1999) International Union Against Cancer. Classification of isolated tumour cells and micrometastasis. Cancer 86:2668–2673
Hill AD, Tran KN, Yeung H et al (1999) Sentinel lymph node biopsy in breast cancer: unfiltered radioisotope is superior to filtered. J Am Coll Surg 188:377–381
Hurkmans CW, Borger JH, Rutgers EJ et al (2003) Quality assurance of axillary radiotherapy in the EORTC AMAROS trial 10981/22023. Radiother Oncol 68:233–240
International (Ludwig) Breast Cancer Study Group (1990) Prognostic importance of occult axillary lymph node micrometastases from breast cancer. Lancet 335:1565–1568
Joshi MG, Lee AK, Loda M et al (1996) Male breast carcinoma: an evaluation of prognostic factors contributing to a poorer outcome. Cancer 77: 490
Kataoka A, Mori M, Sadanaga N et al (2000) RT-PCR detection of breast cancer cells in sentinel lymph nodes. Int J Oncol 16:1147–1152

Keleher A, Wendt III R, Delpassand E et al (2004) The safety of lymphatic mapping in pregnant breast cancer patients using Tc-99m sulphur colloid. Breast J 10:492–495
Keshtgar MRS, Ell PJ (1999) Sentinel lymph node detection and imaging. Eur J Nucl Med 1999 26:57–67
Kim HJ, Heerdt AS et al (2002) Sentinel node drainage in multicentric breast cancers. Breast J 8:356–361
Klauber-DeMore N, Tan LK, Liberman L et al (2000) Sentinel lymph node biopsy: is it indicated in patients with high-risk ductal carcinoma-in-situ and ductal carcinoma-in-situ with microinvasion? Ann Surg Oncol 7:636–642
Klimberg VS, Rubio IT, Henry R et al (1999) Subareolar versus peritumoural injection for location of the sentinel lymph node. Ann Surg 229:860–864
Knauer M, Konstantiniuk P, Haid A et al (2006) Multicentric breast cancer: a new indication for sentinel node biopsy – a multi-institutional validation study. J Clin Oncol 24:3374–3380
Krag DN, Weaver DL, Alex JC et al (1993) Surgical resection and radiolocalization of the sentinel lymph node in breast cancer using a gamma-probe. Surg Oncol 2:335–340
Krag DN, Weaver D, Ashikaga T et al (1998) The sentinel node in breast cancer – a multicenter validation study. N Engl J Med 339:941–946
Krag DN, Julian T (2002) Expert perspectives: update on NSABP B-32, a randomized phase III clinical trial to compare sentinel node resection to conventional axillary dissection for clinically node-negative breast cancer. Breast Dis Year Book Q 13:113–114
Kumar R, Jana S, Heiba SI et al (2003) Retrospective analysis of sentinel node localization in multifocal, multicentric, palpable, or nonpalpable breast cancer. J Nucl Med 44:7–10
Luini A, Gatti G, Frasson A et al (2002) Sentinel lymph node biopsy performed with local anesthesia in patients with early-stage breast carcinoma. Arch Surg 137:1157–1160
Luini A, Galimberti V, Gatti G et al (2005) The sentinel node biopsy after previous breast surgery: preliminary results on 543 patients treated at the European Institute of Oncology. Breast Cancer Res Treat 89(2):159–163
Mamounas EP (2003) Sentinel lymph node biopsy after neoadjuvant systemic therapy [review]. Surg Clin North Am 83:931–942
Manzotti M, Dell`Orto P, Maisonneuve P et al (2001) Reverse transcription-polymerase chain reaction assay for multiple mRNA markers in the detection of breast cancer metastases in sentinel lymph nodes. Int J Cancer 95:307–312
Mariani G, Moresco L, Viale G et al (2001) Radioguided sentinel lymph node biopsy in breast cancer surgery. J Nucl Med 42:1198–1215
Masuda N, Tamaki Y, Sakita I et al (2000) Clinical significance of micrometastases in axillary lymph nodes assessed by reverse transcription-polymerase chain reaction in breast cancer patients. Clin Cancer Res 6:4176–4185
McMaster KM, Giuliano AE, Ross MI et al (1998) Sentinel-lymph-node biopsy for breast cancer – not yet the standard of care. N Engl J Med 339:990–995
Miner TJ, Shriver CD, Jaques DP et al (1999) Sentinel lymph node biopsy for breast cancer: the role of previous biopsy on patients eligibility. Am Surg 65:493–499
Morton DL, Wen DR, Wong JH et al (1992) Technical details of intraoperative lymphatic mapping for early stage melanoma. Arch Surg 127:392–399
Morton DL, Chan AD (2000) The concept of sentinel node localization: how it started. Semin Nucl Med 30:4–10
Mullan MH, Kissin MW (2001) Positive sentinel node biopsy in male breast carcinoma. ANZ J Surg 71:438–440
Nason KS, Anderson BO, Byrd DR et al (2000) Increased false negative sentinel node biopsy rates after preoperative chemotherapy for invasive breast carcinoma. Cancer 89:2187–2194
Noguchi M, Tsugawa K, Miwa K (2000) Internal mammary chain sentinel lymph node identification in breast cancer patient. J Surg Oncol 73:75–80
Ollila DW, Giuliano AE (1998) Intraoperative lymphatic mapping and sentinel lymphadenectomy using isosulfan blue dye. Breast Dis 8:297–300
Ozmen V, Muslumanoglu M, Cabioglu N et al (2002) Increased false negative rates in sentinel lymph node biopsies in patients with multifocal breast cancer. Breast Cancer Res Treat 76:237–244
Paganelli G, De Cicco C, Cremonesi M et al (1998) Optimized sentinel node scintigraphy in breast cancer. Q J Nucl Med 42:49–53
Paganelli G, Galimberti V, Trifirò G et al (2002) Internal mammary node lymphoscintigraphy and biopsy in breast cancer. Q J Nucl Med 46:138–144
Pendas S, Dauway E, Giuliano R et al (2000) Sentinel node biopsy in DCIS patients. Ann Surg Oncol 7:15–20
Port ER, Fey JV, Cody III HS et al (2001) Sentinel lymph node biopsy in patients with male breast carcinoma. Cancer 91:319–323
Port ER, Fey J, Gemignani ML et al (2002) Reoperative sentinel lymph node biopsy: a new option for patients with primary or locally recurrent breast carcinoma. J Am Coll Surg 195:167–172
Reintgen D, Giuliano R, Cox G (2002) Lymphatic mapping and sentinel lymph node biopsy for breast cancer. Cancer J 8:S15–S21
Reynolds C, Mick R, Donohue JH et al (1999) Sentinel lymph node biopsy with metastasis: can AD be avoided in some patients with breast cancer? J Clin Oncol 17:1720–1726
Ross MI (2001) Sentinel lymph node dissection in early-stage breast cancer: ongoing prospective randomized trials in the USA. Ann Surg Oncol 8:778–818
Roumen RM, Geuskens LM, Valkenburg JG (1999) In search of the true sentinel node by different injection techniques in breast cancer patients. Eur J Surg Oncol 25:347–351
Roumen RM, Geuskens LM, Valkenburg JG (1999) In search of the true sentinel node by different injection techniques in breast cancer patients. Eur J Surg Oncol 25:347–351
Sabel MS, Schott AF, Kleer CG et al (2003) Sentinel node biopsy prior to neoadjuvant chemotherapy. Am J Surg 186:102–105
Schnitt SJ, Silen W, Sadowsky NL et al (1988) Ductal carcinoma in situ. N Engl J Med 318:898–902
Schrenk P, Wayand W (2001) Sentinel-node biopsy in axillary lymph-node staging for patients with multicentric breast cancer. Lancet 357:122
Schwartz GF, Giuliano AE, Veronesi U (2002) Consensus Conference Committee. Proceedings of the consensus conference on the role of sentinel lymph node biopsy in carcinoma of the breast, April 19–22, 2001, Philadelphia, Pennsylvania. Cancer 94:2542–2551
Schwartz GF, Meltzer AJ (2003) Accuracy of axillary sentinel lymph node biopsy following neoadjuvant (induc-

tion) chemotherapy for carcinoma of the breast. Breast J 9:374–379

Specht MC, Fey JV, Borgen PI et al (2005) Is the clinically positive axilla in breast cancer really a contraindication to sentinel lymph node biopsy? J Am Coll Surg.200(1):10–14

Spratt JS, Schieber W, Dillard B (1965) Anatomy and surgical technique of groin dissection. St. Louis: CV Mosby

Stearns V, Ewing CA, Slack R et al (2002) Sentinel lymphadenectomy after neoadjuvant chemotherapy for breast cancer may reliably represent the axilla except for inflammatory breast cancer. Ann Surg Oncol 9:235–242

Tanis PJ, Valdes Olmos RA, Muller SH et al (2003) Lymphatic mapping in patients with breast carcinoma: reproducibility and lymphoscintigraphic results. Radiology 228:313–315

Tousimis E, Van Zee KJ, Fey JV et al (2003) The accuracy of sentinel lymph node biopsy in multicentric and multifocal invasive breast cancers. J Am Coll Surg 197:529–535

Turner RR, Chu KU, Qi K et al (2000) Pathologic features associated with nonsentinel lymph node metastases in patients with metastatic breast carcinoma in a sentinel lymph node. Cancer 89:574–581

Veronesi P, Intra M, Vento AR et al (2005) Sentinel lymph node for localized ductal carcinoma in situ. Breast 14:520–522

Veronesi U, Luini A, Galimberti V et al (1990) Extent of axillary involvement in 1446 cases of breast cancer. Eur J Surg Oncol 16:127–133

Veronesi U, Paganelli G, Galimberti V et al (1997) Sentinel-node biopsy to avoid AD in breast cancer with clinically negative lymph-nodes. Lancet 349:1864–1867

Veronesi U, Paganelli G, Viale G et al (2003) A randomized comparison of sentinel-node biopsy with routine axillary dissection in breast cancer. N Engl J Med 349:546–553

Viale G, Bosari S, Mazzarol G et al (1999) Intraoperative examination of axillary sentinel lymph nodes in breast carcinoma patients. Cancer 85:2433–2438

Viale G, Maiorano E, Mazzarol G et al (2001) Histologic detection and clinical implications of micrometastases in axillary sentinel lymph nodes for patients with breast carcinoma. Cancer 92:1378–1384

Wilhelm AJ, Mijnhout GS, Franssen EJF (1999) Radiopharmaceuticals in sentinel lymph-node detection – an overview. Eur J Nucl Med 26:S36–S42

Wilke LG, Giuliano AE (2003) Sentinel lymph node biopsy in patients with early-stage breast cancer: status of the National Clinical Trials. Surg Clin North Am 83:901–910

Wong SL, Edwards MJ, Chao C et al (2002) The effect of prior breast biopsy method and concurrent definitive breast procedure on success and accuracy of sentinel lymph node biopsy. Ann Surg Oncol 9:272–277

Woo JC, Yu T, Hurd TC (2003) Breast cancer in pregnancy: a literature review. Arch Surg 138:91–99

Zurrida S, Morabito A, Galimberti V et al (1999) Importance of the level of axillary involvement in relation to traditional variables in the prognosis of breast cancer. Int J Oncol 15:475–480

State of the Art of Current Modalities for the Diagnosis of Breast Lesions

9

Cosimo Di Maggio

CONTENTS

9.1 Introduction: a Critical Analysis of the Diagnostic Methods in Breast Diseases

The risks of unjustified use of such techniques and the lack of rational clinical application have increased with the availability of many diagnostic techniques. Errors of this nature would affect the diagnostic accuracy and therefore reduce the possibilities for treatment. It is not uncommon for women and also for general practitioners to be misinformed about which is the most suitable technique, or rather what is the best combination of the various techniques; for this reason, inappropriate tests are often requested or tests which would in fact make a useful contribution to safeguarding the women's health.
This work has the following aims: to state precisely the real diagnostic contribution of each method, both radiological and otherwise, and suggest methods of application and indications consistent with the state of the art and to suggest the most effective and rational blends of the various techniques and organisation of diagnostic activities.

9.1.1 Breast Self-Examination

Women are still being advised to carry out periodic breast self-examination (BSE) although it has been well documented that this test does not provide early diagnosis (though it may anticipate the diagnosis) and that there is no evidence of a reduction in the mortality of women who practice BSE compared to those who do not (Hartmann 2005; Weiss 2003). In informing women how to carry out BSE, general practitioners and specialists should ensure that both its advantages and its limitations are explained (Table 9.1), so as to avoid both false reassurance and false alarms. Women should not be blamed for not

Table 9.1. Breast self examination (bse)

Limitations
does not provide early diagnosis
no proof of efficacy
creates anxiety if carried out or feeling of guilt if not
Advantages
awareness of own breasts
getting to know the problems of breast cancer
women performing self examination give a diagnostic contribution to clinicians
early diagnosis in the absence of other more sensitive and effective techniques
Conclusions
encourage women particularly those younger than 40 to carry out periodic self-examination
not blame women for not wishing to carry out BSE

wishing to carry out BSE. Since BSE may provide useful information in certain cases (when the lesion appeared, its volumetric development over time, etc.), the clinician would do well not to overlook findings reported by women who practice BSE.

From the methodological viewpoint, it is time to set aside commonplaces and teach women that BSE consists of two parts: an inspection to be carried out in front of the mirror and palpation to be carried out in the supine position and not in the shower, as often happens. Because of the length of time it takes for the tumour to grow, it would be better to explain to women that almost monthly self-palpation not only creates anxiety, but may actually delay the perception of nodes because the hand becomes accustomed to their slow growth. For this reason, it would be more logical to suggest that checks should be performed every 3 months during the fertile period, at the end of the menstrual stage.

9.1.2 Clinical Examination

The clinical examination should only be performed by trained medical personnel in a suitable environment (Lamarque et al. 1997) and should be preceded by careful examination of the patient's case history, including the assessment of possible risk factors (Cuzick 2003).

9.1.2.1 Signs and Medical Report

The most typical signs of cancer are the presence of a hard swelling with irregular or indistinct edges, skin involvement, fixation to the pectoral muscle or the chest wall, bloody discharge, axillary adenopathy (which is, however, non-specific if N2 cases are excluded) and the eczematous appearance of the nipple in Paget's disease. The relevant signs of the benign or malignant lesions (Figs. 9.1, 9.2) should be described in the concluding report. As regards nodular lesions, the report should always state the dimensions in centimetres, measured with callipers, and the site, with reference to the four quadrants and the areolar region. The conclusive diagnostic judgement (negative, benign or suspicious) should always be precisely indicated. In the case of suspicious signs, it is necessary to supply the data for the staging system or the TNM category directly.

9.1.2.2 Results

Sensitivity is relatively low for T1 forms (approximately 70%, but considerably lower for lesions of less than 1 cm) and therefore the clinical examination is of little use for the early diagnosis of tumours (Kolb et al. 2002). Its contribution is often limited to the perception of the existence of pathology, but it greatly facilitates the search for and recognition of lesions, preventing them from being overlooked. The specificity of this test is also somewhat limited; there would be a high bioptic cost if the decision on whether to perform a biopsy were to be based solely on the clinical examination.

It is obvious, therefore, that the clinical examination alone is not sufficient to exclude the presence of tumours and that any clinical signs, even if they are in the slightest way suspicious, should lead to the performance of other tests. Even today, a strong clinical suspicion of neoplasia constitutes good grounds for a biopsy, except in cases where mammography or other diagnostic techniques afford a sure diagnosis of benignity, as may occur in the presence of lipoma, calcific fibroadenoma, fat necrosis, etc.

It should be borne in mind that although the diagnostic contribution of the clinical examination is limited, its contribution in terms of giving accurate information to women, stimulating active involvement and renewing the relationship between

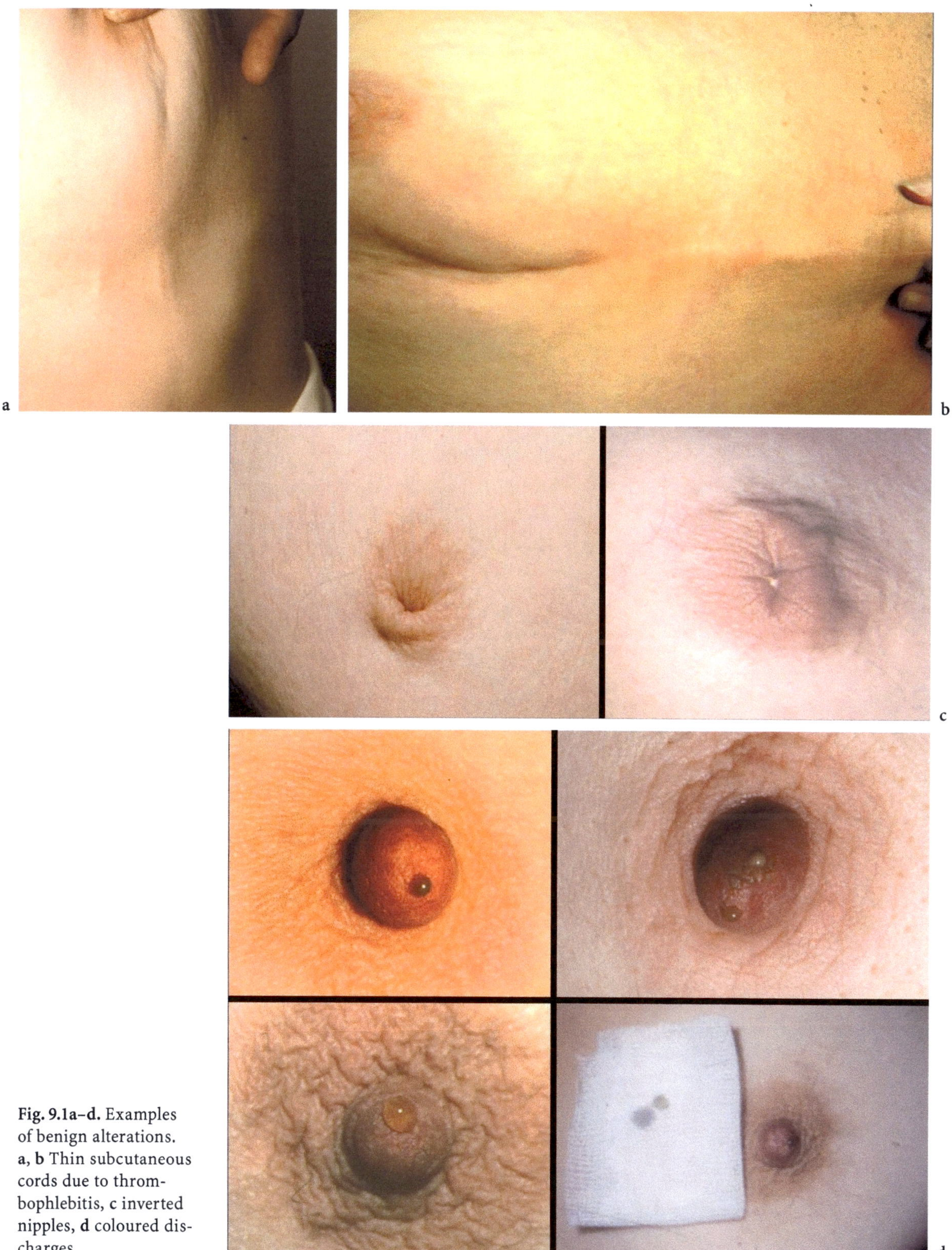

Fig. 9.1a–d. Examples of benign alterations. **a, b** Thin subcutaneous cords due to thrombophlebitis, **c** inverted nipples, **d** coloured discharges

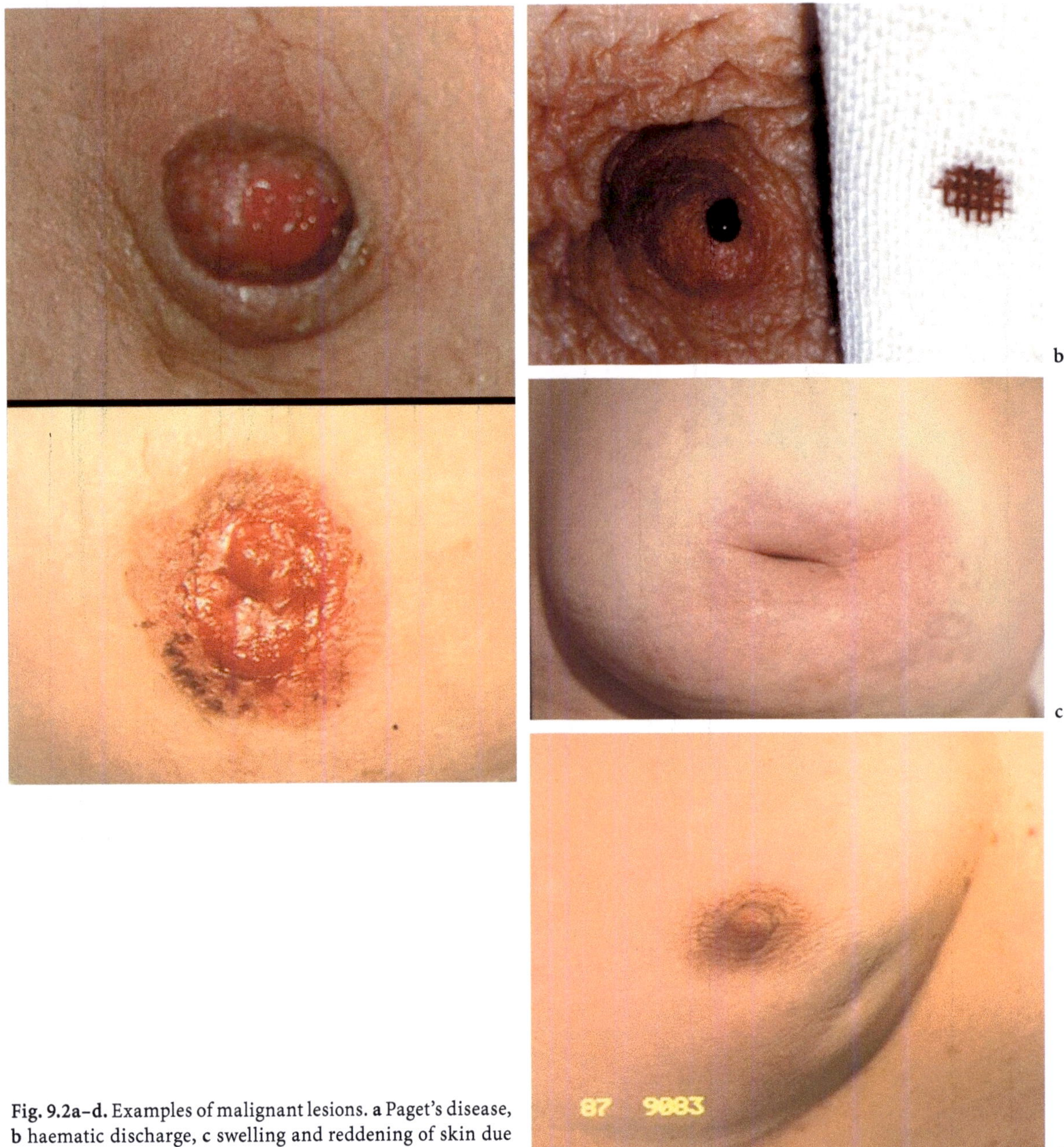

Fig. 9.2a–d. Examples of malignant lesions. **a** Paget's disease, **b** haematic discharge, **c** swelling and reddening of skin due to inflammatory carcinoma, **d** spontaneous skin retraction

doctor and patient, is irreplaceable (Berlin 2001). Under the pressure of economic problems, the human contribution which stems from the clinical examination is often overlooked. The effort to achieve lower mortality rates at an acceptable cost has made us forget that perhaps the greatest benefit of diagnostic activity lies not so much in the detection of disease as in the peace of mind that is derived from a negative diagnosis (Di Maggio 1993).

9.1.2.3 Indications

As well as offering an opportunity to talk to the patient about the problem of breast cancer, the clinical examination provides a guide to the performance of instrumental diagnostic investigations and helps in their interpretation. It is still a fundamental and irreplaceable examination when a symptom is present. In such cases, the clinical examination should always precede instrumental investigations and should receive equal attention in the interpretative summary. For this reason, it is essential that the clinical examination is carried out by the physician who is to perform the instrumental investigation even if the patient has already been examined by other physicians.

9.1.3 Mammography

Mammography should be performed using the right equipment and methodology in order to acquire images which contain a wealth of information while delivering a limited radiation dose (ISTISAN 1995; EUREF 1999; Hendrick et al. 1999; Perry 2001; Cole et al. 2003; Gambaccini and Baldelli 2003; Gennaro et al. 2003; Gennaro and di Maggio 2006). In many diagnostic centres, digital technology is now widely used. The advantages of digital mammography include the possibility of obtaining high-quality images at lower doses than are required for analogue mammography, the capacity to compensate for errors in exposure (Fig. 9.3a,b) and the broader dynamic range. However, while digital mammography provides images of a medium to high standard and

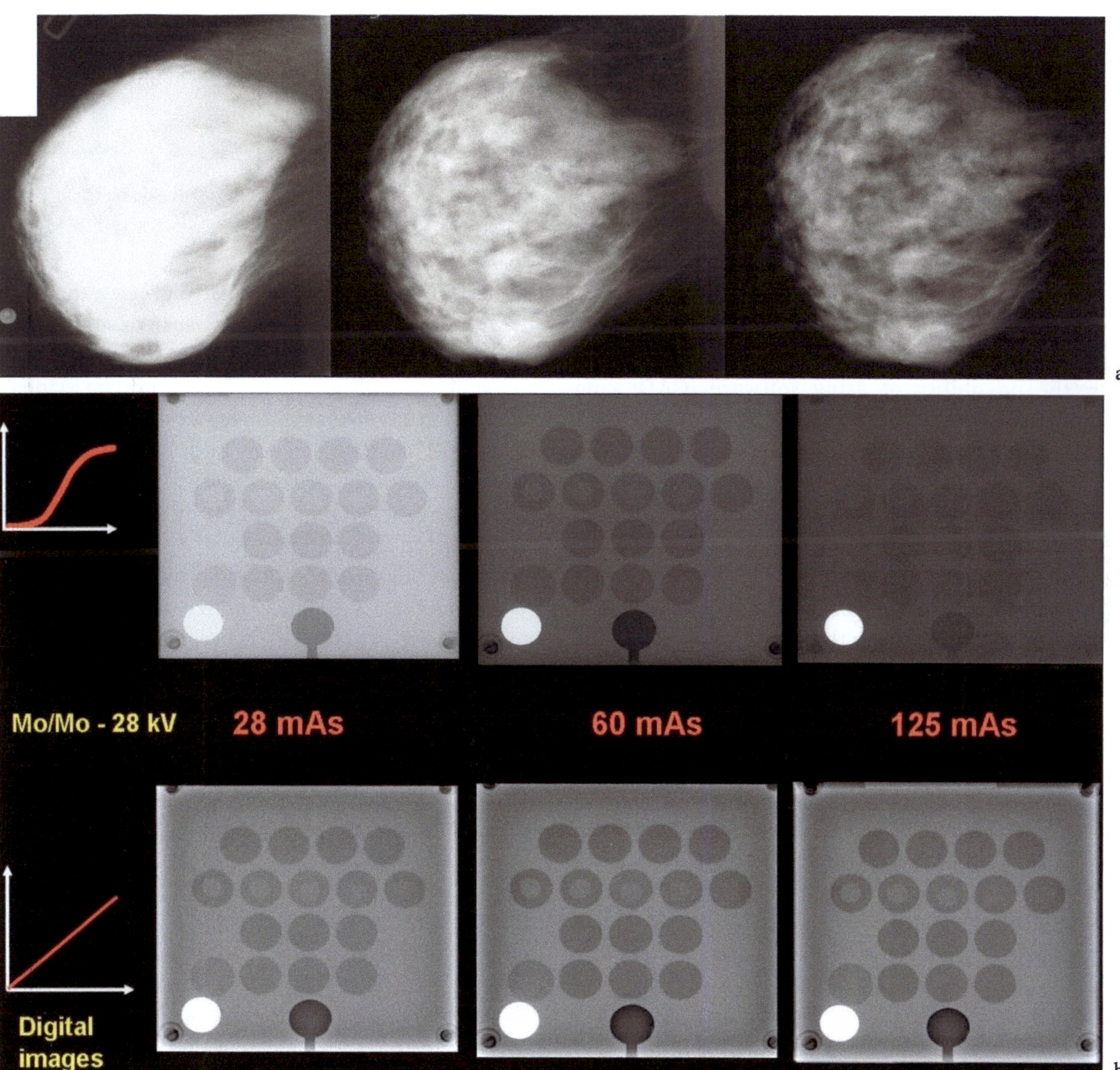

Fig. 9.3. **a** Film-screen mammography: different parameters of exposure generate images with different optical density (underexposure leads to false radio density and subsequently the masking of possible small lesions), **b** screening/film versus digital mammography: in digital mammography the optical density of the images is always the same despite the different exposure values

facilitates perception of possible alterations above all in dense breasts (James 2004; Pisano 2000; Di Maggio et al. 2004; Pisano et al. 2005), the spatial resolution of digital images is currently lower than that of analogue ones; this sometimes makes it more difficult to categorise a lesion. The availability of numerous second-level diagnostic tests minimises this drawback, since the chief requirement for a first-level test is its ability to detect the presence of a possible lesion. Indeed, the task of basic mammography, whether performed in the course of a screening programme or in a clinical context, is mainly that of selection. Attempting a diagnosis almost always comes later, on the basis of supplementary radiographs or further investigations.

The advantage of the easier perception of the signal afforded by digital mammography is increased by:

- the use of a review workstation that, thanks to the elaboration of the images on the monitor, makes it possible to optimise the brightness and contrast of the interested area, rotate images, electronically magnify small areas, on the spot use of software capable of visualising the images with different algorithms and thus emphasize small differences in density (contrast enhancement);
- the possibility of using software (CAD: computer-aided detection) (Baker et al. 2003; Brem et al. 2003; Ciatto et al. 2003; Freer and Ulissey 2001; Lechener et al. 2002; Stines et al. 2002) capable of circumscribing with greater sensitivity small changes in density with morphological features suggestive of tumours. Such systems do not have a diagnostic task; their job is only to show items which might escape the radiologist's attention, but which the radiologist must later interpret without being influenced by the results obtained using CAD.

The most promising development in digital mammography is the "TOMOSYNTHESIS". This method is based on the successive automatic acquisition of multiple radiograms with different obliquities; the digital reconstruction of images seems to be able to highlight those lesions that are masked by overlapping structures (Fig. 9.4).

The carcinogenic risk from mammography is similar to that which can be hypothesised for all other radiological investigations and should always be assessed on a cost/benefit basis (Feig 1997; Gregg 1977). In the case of mammography, the danger of not recognising small carcinomas, in the highest risk age group, is vastly greater than the hypothetical risk posed by exposure to small doses of radiation. At our current state of knowledge, we can state that, while every effort should be made to keep radiation doses as low as possible or to reduce them still further (Dendy and Brugmans 2003; Law and Faulkner 2002), the decision on whether or not to resort to mammography should be based above all on quantification of the expected benefit rather than on the possible hypothetical risk. A special case is that of women with deleterious mutation BRCA1 since their breasts may be subject to greater sensitivity to ionising radiation (Sharan et al. 1997). The decision to use mammography on these patients, especially if they are young, should be made with care, and numerous trials are taking place to clarify whether magnetic resonance imaging may be used as a routine technique instead of mammography.

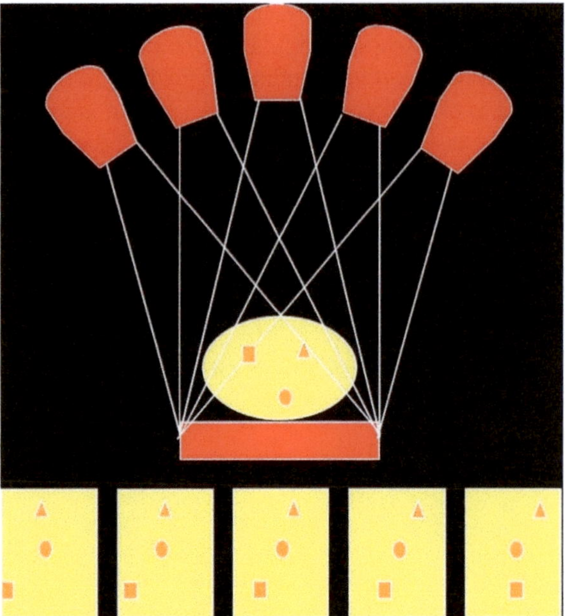

Fig. 9.4. Summary of how the tomosynthesis works

9.1.3.1 Signs and Medical Report

The most common signs of neoplasia are nodular opacities (64%), microcalcifications (19%) and structural distortions (17%) (Tavassoli and Devilee 2003) (Fig. 9.5a,b). Other indirect signs of neoplasia, such as cutaneous inspissation and retraction, nipple retraction or an increase in vascularisation, are of little

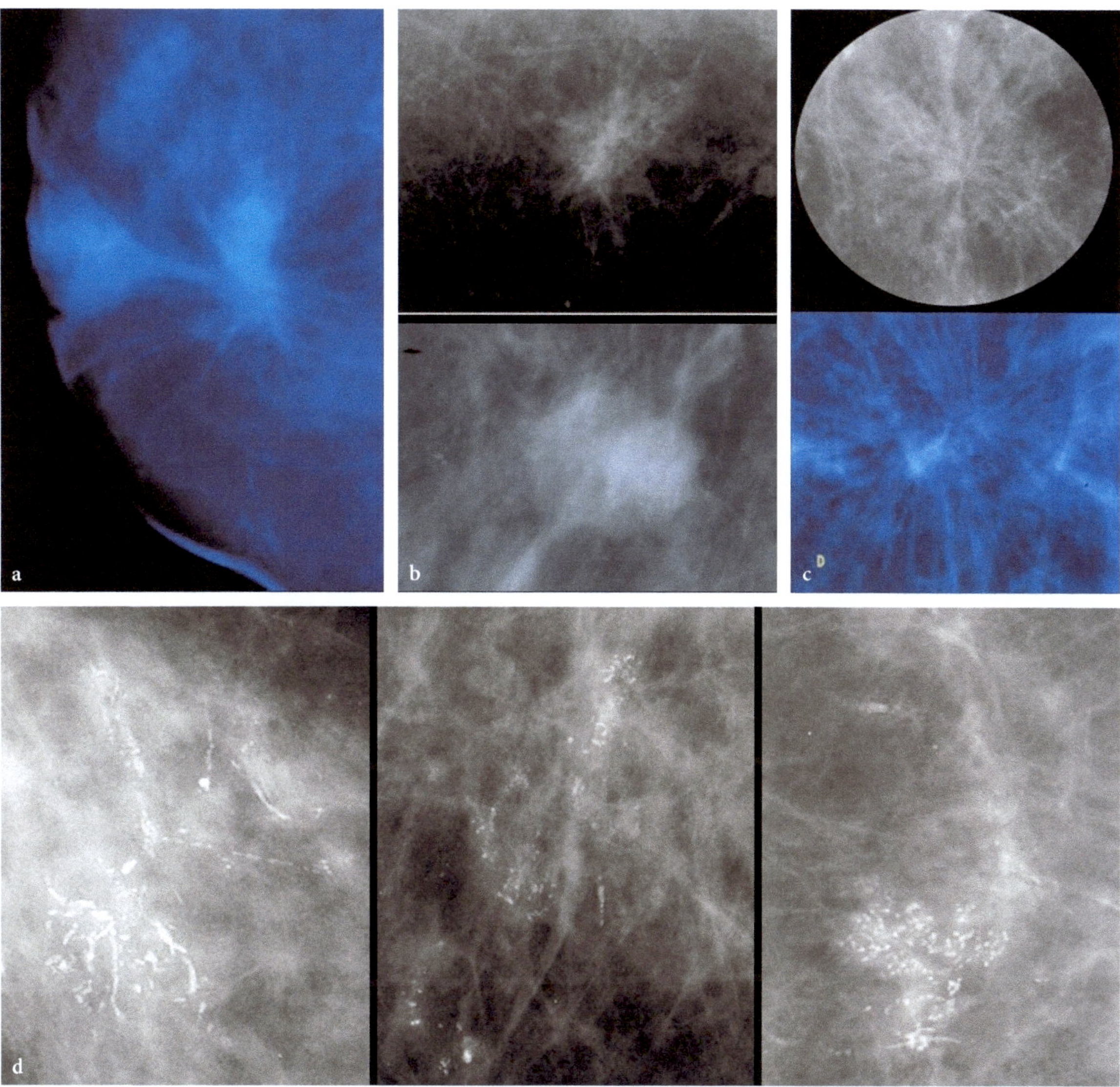

Fig. 9.5a–d. Examples of breast carcinomas. **a** Mass with irregular edges, **b** nodular opacities, **c** structural distortions, **d** microcalcifications

diagnostic importance since they are often associated with voluminous and clinically evident neoplasia.

Special cases are lobular carcinomas and inflammatory carcinomas. Owing to the preservation of the glandular architecture and the limited stromal reaction, lobular carcinomas frequently do not show particular features on mammography (Amici et al. 2000). Inflammatory carcinomas almost always begin acutely with clinical signs, and it is often impossible to find even minor signs of them on previous radiographs. The mammography report should be drawn up according to the requirements for rationalisation and clarity of the informational content:

- Less significant findings (benign calcifications, microcysts, intramammary lymph nodes, etc.) may be omitted since they are often a source of needless anxiety. It is better to indicate the presence and extension of the anatomical radiopaque structures that can mask the mass (Fig. 9.6).
- Noteworthy findings should be clearly reported, with precise indication of the site of the lesion, its dimensions, the possible presence of several lesions and lesion location(s). No indelible marks

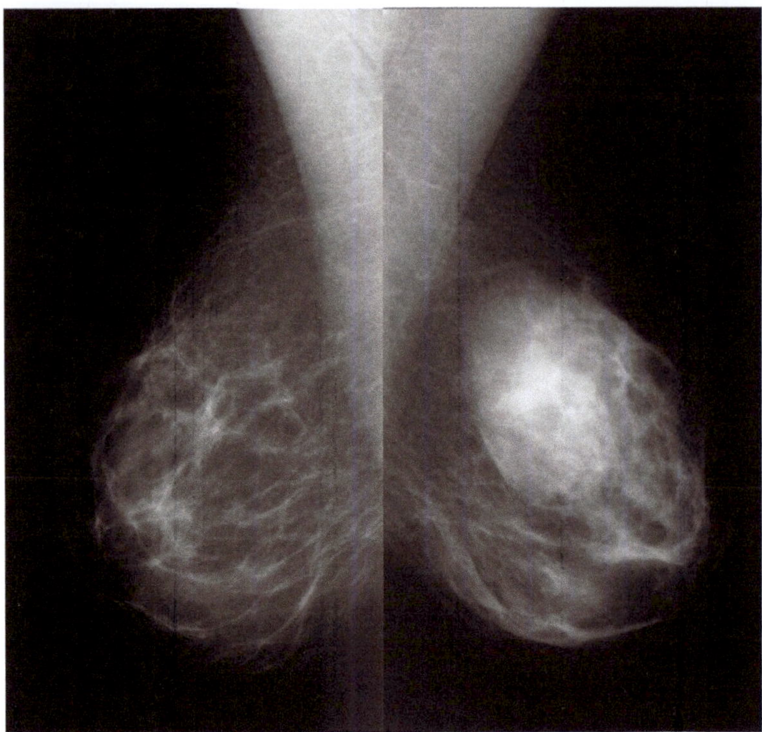

Fig. 9.6. Example of different distributions of radio-opaque structures (morphologic variant): radio density may mask some lesions

should be made on the original radiograph. In the presence of clinical signs, it should be specified whether or not there are corresponding changes on the mammogram.

- The radiologist must clearly indicate both the diagnostic orientation and, especially in the case of small subclinical lesions, whether the finding requires further investigation or a biopsy. In such situations it is always best to specify which type of guide (ultrasound or stereotactic) is preferable for taking the cyto-/histological specimen.

Table 9.2. Assessment Of Breast Lesions Based On ACR-BIRADS Categories

Negative/ benign finding	(cat. 1-2)	Stop
Probably benign finding	(cat. 3)	Additional Tests/Initial short-term (6 months) follow-up
Suspicious abnormality	(cat. 4)	Percutaneous Needle Sampling
Suggestive of malignancy	(cat. 5)	Surgical Treatment

In order to avoid distorted interpretations as regards both the diagnostic hypothesis and the possible continuation with tests for diagnosis, the radiologist must sum up the conclusions in a five-category classification ranging from negative (class 1) or certainly benign (the diagnostic strategy stops) to an ever-increasing possibility of pathology (BI-RADS classes) (American College of Radiology 2003; ANAES 1998; Lattanzio and Simonetti 2002) (Table 9.2):

- In the presence of a lesion classified as benign (BI-RADS 2), no further tests are required and, if carried out, would only give rise to anxiety and false positives.
- In the presence of a probably benign picture (BI-RADS 3) (less than a 2% risk of malignancy), the radiologist should clearly indicate whether s/he feels it necessary to order other diagnostic tests or whether a short-interval follow-up is sufficient. In view of the consequences of a possible error of interpretation, the radiologist should keep track not only of the symptoms, but also of the dimensions of the alterations found. In these cases the radiologist, wherever s/he may be operating (clinical diagnostics or screening), must never forget that s/he is the only person responsible for the successive choices since they are based on the radiological semeiotics. These choices should be clearly communicated to and shared with the patient and other specialists.

- In the presence of a lesion classified as BI-RADS 4 (risk of malignancy between 2% and 70%), further diagnostic tests should be carried out (ultrasound, fine-needle aspiration cytology). If these tests prove negative, the radiologist should re-examine the radiographs and write a new report leading to an "integrated conclusive summary".
- In the presence of a lesion classified as BI-RADS 5, it is imperative to indicate surgical removal and therefore the histological diagnosis of the entire lesion. Other diagnostic tests may be useful only to assist in planning the surgical operation or to confirm the diagnosis in the case of non-surgical treatment.

In conclusion, in many cases the refined semeiotics of mammography permit diagnosis of the histological type, but the particular tasks of mammography are above all (1) the detection of possible lesions, (2) the search for "objective signs" of deviation from assumed normality (pathological semeiotics), and (3) the classification of the findings into one of the five categories mentioned above so that both the diagnostic hypothesis and the appropriate course of diagnostic and therapeutic action are clearly identified.

9.1.3.2 Results

Mammography has a sensitivity of more than 85%. However, the results are affected by the technical execution and the methodology used in the test. The accuracy is reduced if the adipose component is not well represented. In such cases it is very useful and sometimes indispensable to combine the test with a clinical examination or ultrasound (Burrel et al. 1996). Carrying out a clinical examination at the same time may also reveal the presence of possible neoplasia in peripheral sites which might not be included in the standard routine projections.

9.1.3.3 Indications

Mammography enables exploration of the entire breast and offers the greatest sensitivity, in particular for tumours in the initial stage of development. For this reason it is the only test which can be used as the basic technique in a screening programme.

If the clinical examination produces evident findings, it is always appropriate to carry out mammography in patients older than 35–40 years. It enhances the diagnostic accuracy of the clinical signs, better defines the extension of possible suspicious lesions and enables the discovery of non-palpable contiguous or contralateral lesions.

9.1.4 Ultrasound

Ultrasound involves the use of high-frequency probes (greater than or equal to 10 MHz), linear or annular, and surface focussed. The recent introduction of machines with a digital platform has greatly improved the definition and detail of the ultrasound image, thanks in particular to the use of new multi-frequency broad-band transducers, the possibility of recording the harmonic tissue frequencies, and the use of a wide field of view and compound scanning (Giuseppetti 2002; Merritt 2001; Rizzatto 2001).

The examination should be performed carefully, exploring both breasts, in every quadrant, using different angles and exercising different pressure. Nowadays, the ultrasound scan may be enhanced by echo signal amplifiers, substances injected intravenously which increase the acoustic signal (Fig. 9.7a). Using special impulses, these substances generate harmonic frequencies which reveal both the macro-circulation and the micro-circulation and therefore give a more precise evaluation of vascularisation, if employed with the latest equipment with the appropriate software. The ability of this technique to detect the more homogeneous and regular vascularity of benign lesions as compared with carcinomas, where it is possible to reveal the presence of arteriovenous shunts, improves the accuracy of diagnostic differentiation between benign and malignant lesions on the basis of the signal/time intensity curve (Fig. 9.7b) (Jakobsen 2001; Martinez et al. 2003; Moon et al. 2000; Wittingam 1999). The use of echo signal amplifiers is, however, still at the stage of clinical validation. The current literature shows that the use of these substances improves sensitivity, but leads to a considerable reduction in specificity and an increase in costs.

The elastosonography is a recently introduced ultrasound technique. Dedicated instruments allow assessing variations in tissue elasticity during manual compression (Fig. 9.8a). By means of the chromatic scale utilised, the stiff tissue, typical of carcinomas, is highlighted in blue and the benign tissue in green. Instead, different to the other lesions, the colours of cysts appear in different layers (Figs. 9.8b, 9.9) (Itoh et al. 2006; Giuseppetti et al. 2005).

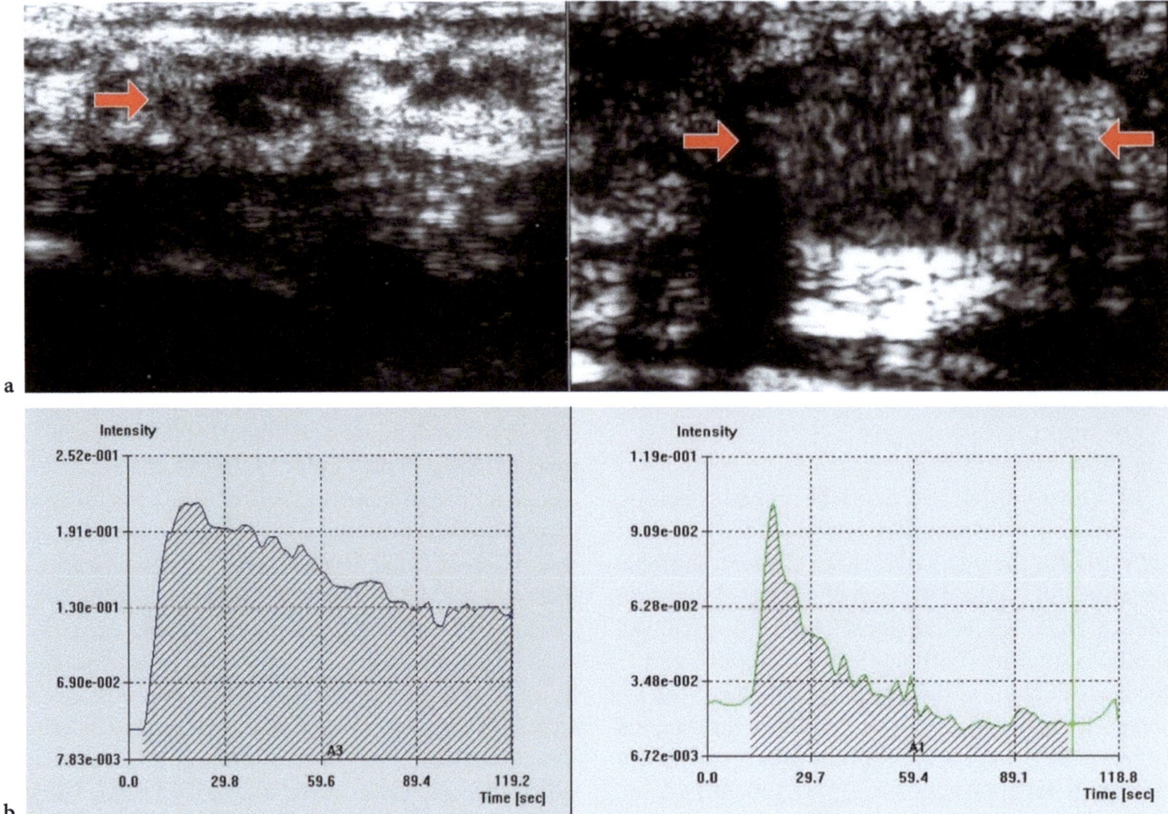

Fig. 9.7. a Ultrasound scan before and after echo-amplifiers (marked increase of the acoustic signal in the lesion). **b** Wash-in/wash-out curve in the benign lesion (slow initial increase in enhancement and slow wash-out) and in the malignant lesion (fast initial increase in enhancement and fast wash-out)

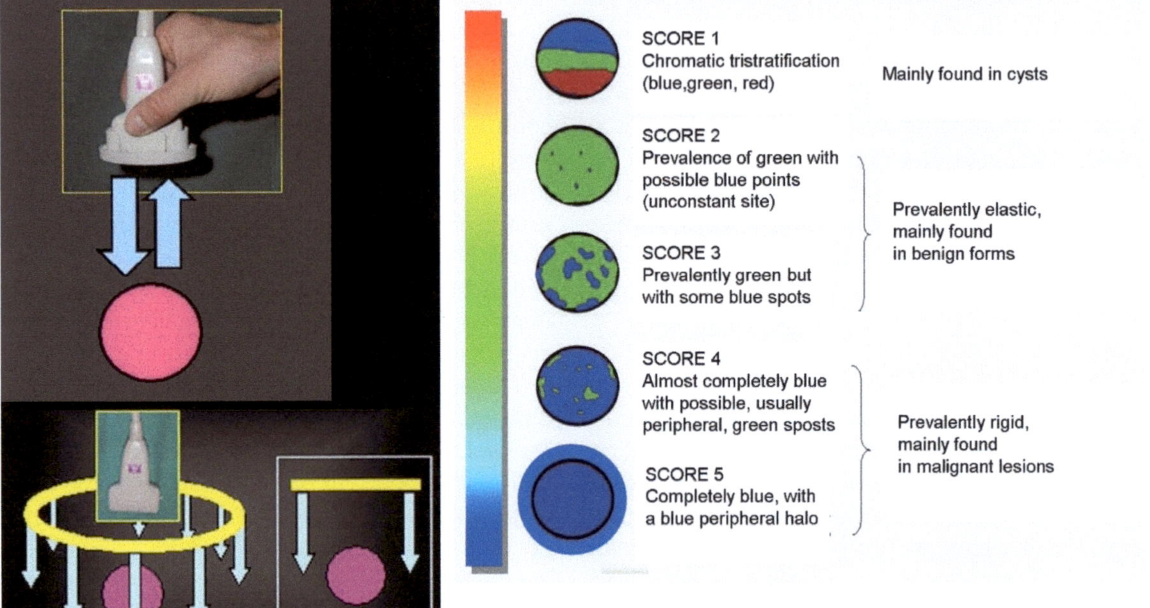

Fig. 9.8. a Method of elastosonography. **b** Elastosonography. The Italian score based on the chromatic-morphology of the breast lesions

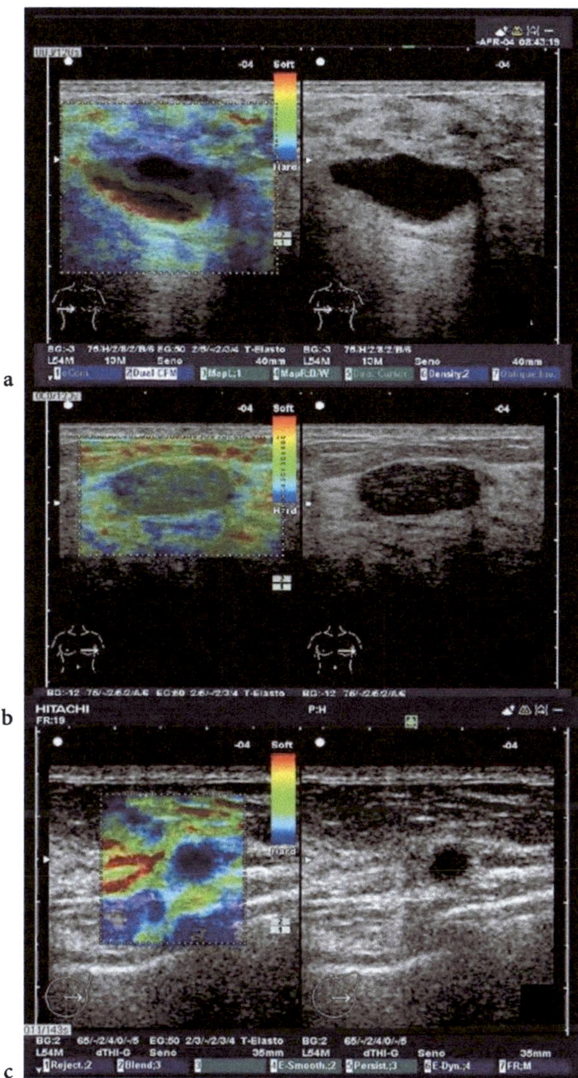

Fig. 9.9a–c. Paradigmatic findings of elastosonography: **a** cyst, **b** benign node, **c** carcinoma

9.1.4.1
Signs and Medical Report

Differential diagnosis is based on the morphology, structure, vascularisation and perilesional reaction. The American College of Radiology, in the fourth edition (2003) of BI-RADS, subdivided the ultrasound diagnostic hypotheses into five categories with an increasing probability of risk of carcinoma, similar to what already occurs for mammography. More specifically, the findings relevant to classification of nodules as suspicious or benign may be summarised as follows:

- Nodules of a very suspicious nature: irregular morphology, poorly defined edges, inhomogeneous echo structure, posterior acoustic attenuation, hyperechogenicity of the surrounding fat, anarchic and plentiful vascularisation with more than one pole (Fig. 9.10)
- Benign type nodules: regular or oval morphology, well-defined edges, internal echoes absent (cysts) or weak and uniform, underlying echoes enhanced (cysts) or normal, surrounding echo structure preserved, vascularisation absent or peripheral and limited with only one pole (Fig. 9.11).

Problems in the diagnosis derive, as usually happens, from ultrasound images that are difficult for the radiologist to classify as either malignant or definitely benign (Fig. 9.12a). The colour-power Doppler may prove to be useful, even if not decisive in these cases. In the presence of vascular peduncles needle aspiration is recommended (Fig. 9.12b), whereas, in the absence of vascular peduncles, a careful short-term follow-up would be more advisable especially if the lesion is less than 6–7 mm in diameter, has morphological ultrasound structure type cysts and the patient is on hormonal therapy (Fig. 9.12c).

The operator should describe the site of the lesions found, their nature (whether solid, liquid or mixed), their dimensions, their depth and possible involvement of the skin and the pectoral muscle. The description of the lesions as regards their physical acoustic features (anechoic, hyperechoic, hypoechoic, etc.) is optional and of no great utility, whereas it is essential to include diagnostic conclusions. The conclusions drawn from the ultrasound scan are essential since they are the result of direct evaluation of the images on the monitor by the operator and cannot be deduced from photographic reproductions.

Where there are also clinical or mammographic lesions, the report should also state whether they correspond to the lesion identified by ultrasound.

9.1.4.2
Results

When used together with mammography, ultrasound improves diagnostic accuracy, increasing both the sensitivity (to as high as 90%) (Fig. 9.13 a,b) and the specificity (to as high as 98%) (Fig. 9.13c,d) (Cilotti et al. 1997; Kaplan 2001; Moy et al. 2002; Zonderland et al. 1999). Despite the continuing technological development, ultrasound remains a complementary

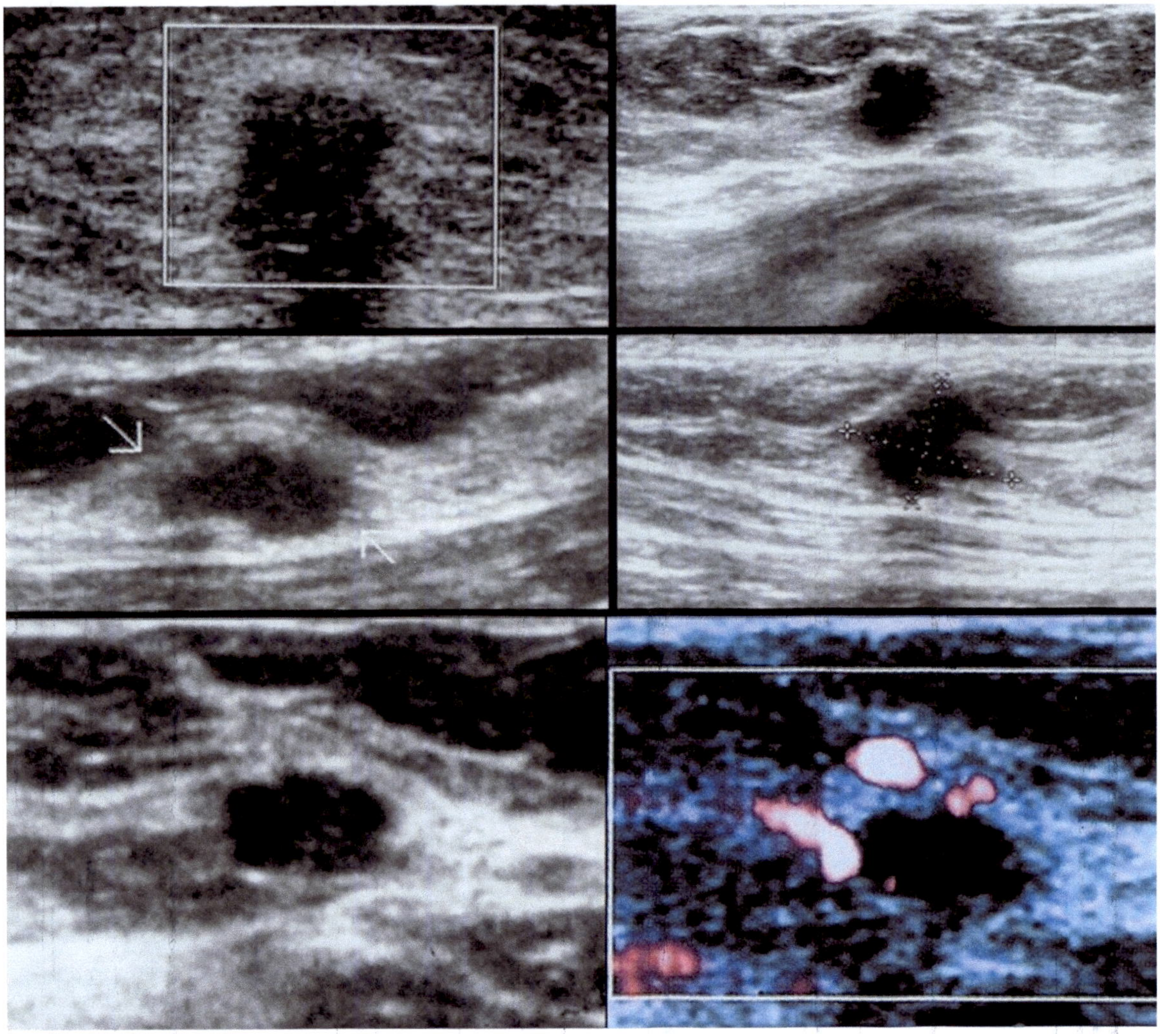

Fig. 9.10. Conventional B-mode ultrasound: findings of lesions highly suggestive of malignancy

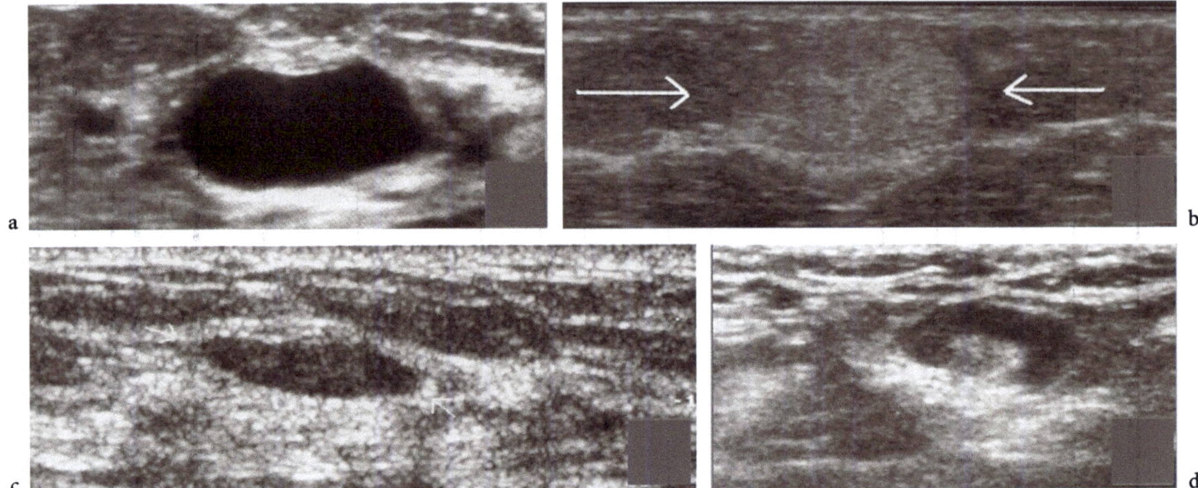

Fig. 9.11a–d. Conventional B-mode ultrasound: findings of benign lesions: **a** cyst, **b** lypoma, **c** fibroadenoma, **d** intramammary lymph node

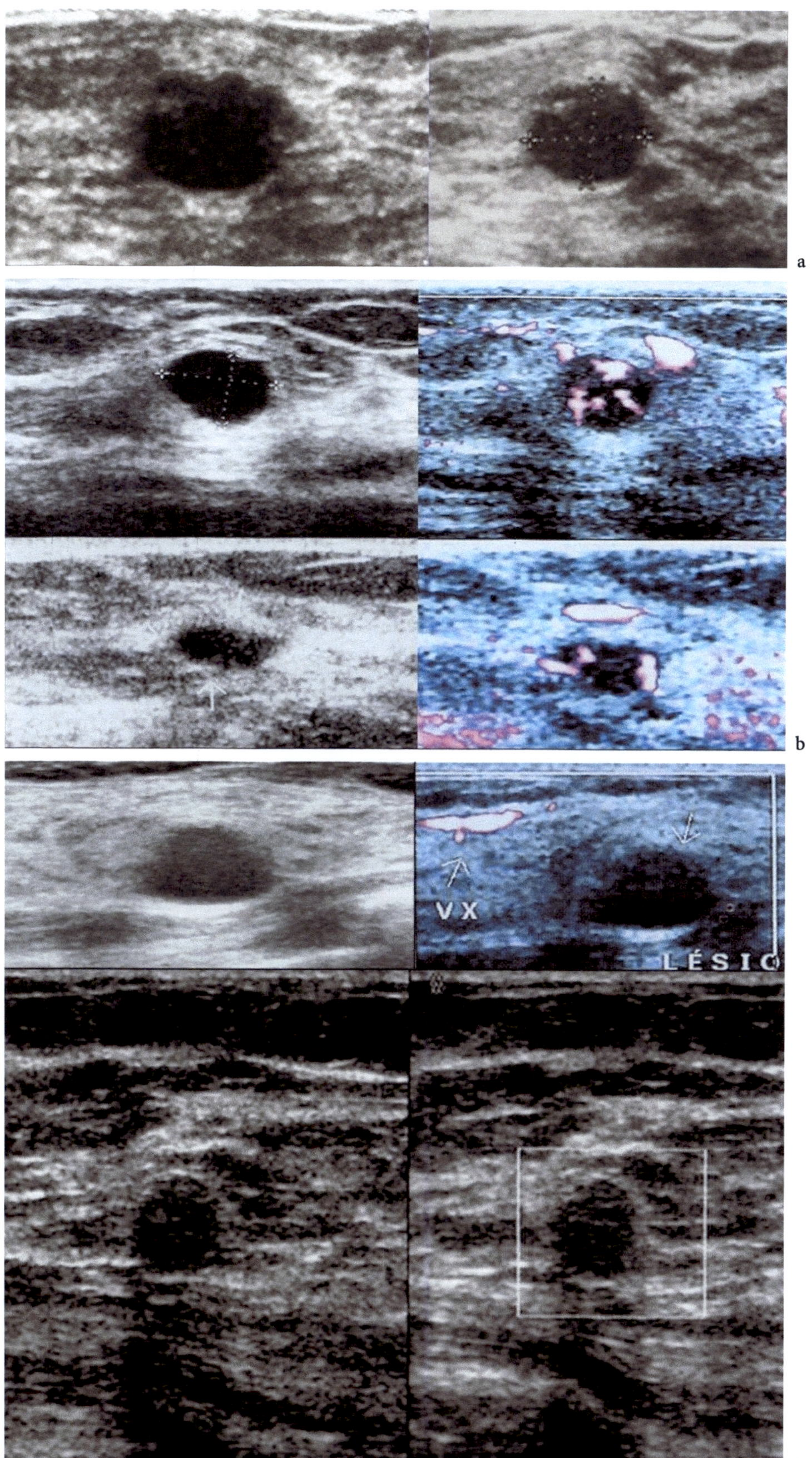

Fig. 9.12. **a** Undetermined ultrasound benign-like lesions: unhomogeneously hypoechogeneity, microlobulated or quite well-defined edges, also with posterior enhancement. **b** Undetermined lesions at standard ultrasound, but with numerous vascular peduncles (histological diagnosis: carcinomas). **c** Undetermined lesions at standard ultrasound, but not vascularised (benign lesions at needle sampling)

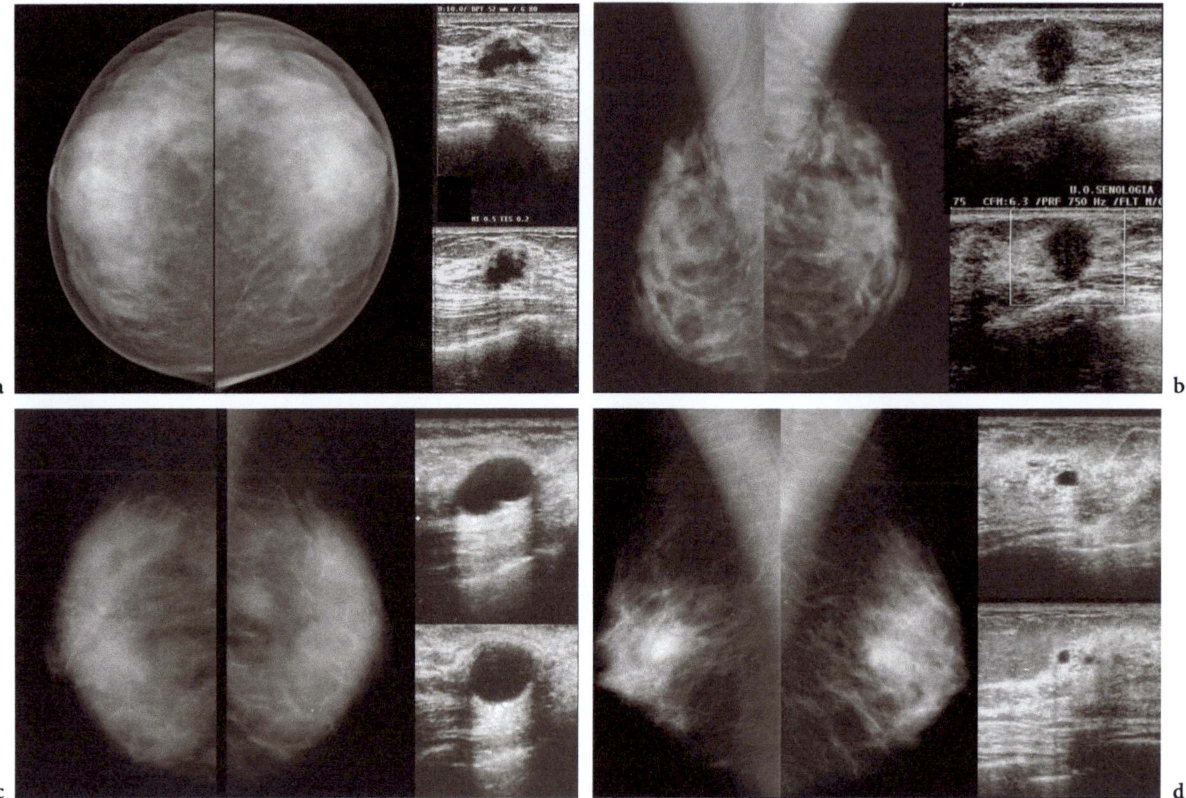

Fig. 9.13. a,b Examples of mammographic dense breasts; the carcinoma is identifiable only with ultrasound. **c,d** Examples of suspect lesions at mammography. Ultrasound instead characterises the lesion as cysts and provides an accurate diagnosis. No need for the patient to undergo needle sampling.

examination to mammography and cannot be used as a sole diagnostic test, except in certain specific situations (Feig 1992).

The most obvious limitations of ultrasound lie in the identification and characterisation of preclinical tumour lesions. On the other hand, it possesses extremely high specificity in the diagnosis of cysts and may be considered a first-line technique for non-oncological situations as well, such as inflammation and trauma. In screening programmes, there is no scientific justification for the use of ultrasound as the exclusive or preliminary diagnostic test (Balu-Maestro et al. 2003).

The use of colour power Doppler provides additional, but still debatable information, in the differential diagnosis between benign and malignant pathologies. It is, however, of use in the diagnostic differentiation between fibrosis and relapse.

The main contribution of the elastosonography consists in the characterisation of the small lesions almost certainly benign identified at ultrasound (e.g., small dense cysts, benign solid nodes) avoiding needle sampling (Fig. 9.14).

9.1.4.3 Indications

The indications for breast ultrasound suggested by the American College of Radiology in 1995, and updated in 1999 and 2001 (American College of Radiology (2000\2001) may be summed up as follows:

- Identification and characterisation of the lesions (whether palpable or not) and the further investigation of dubious clinical and/or mammographic findings.
- Guidance for interventional procedures (preoperative marking of lesions, cytological or histological sampling). One of the most recent indications is ultrasound-guided needle aspiration of axillary lymph nodes found to be suspicious on ultrasound, in order to prevent the excision of the sentinel lymph node if positive

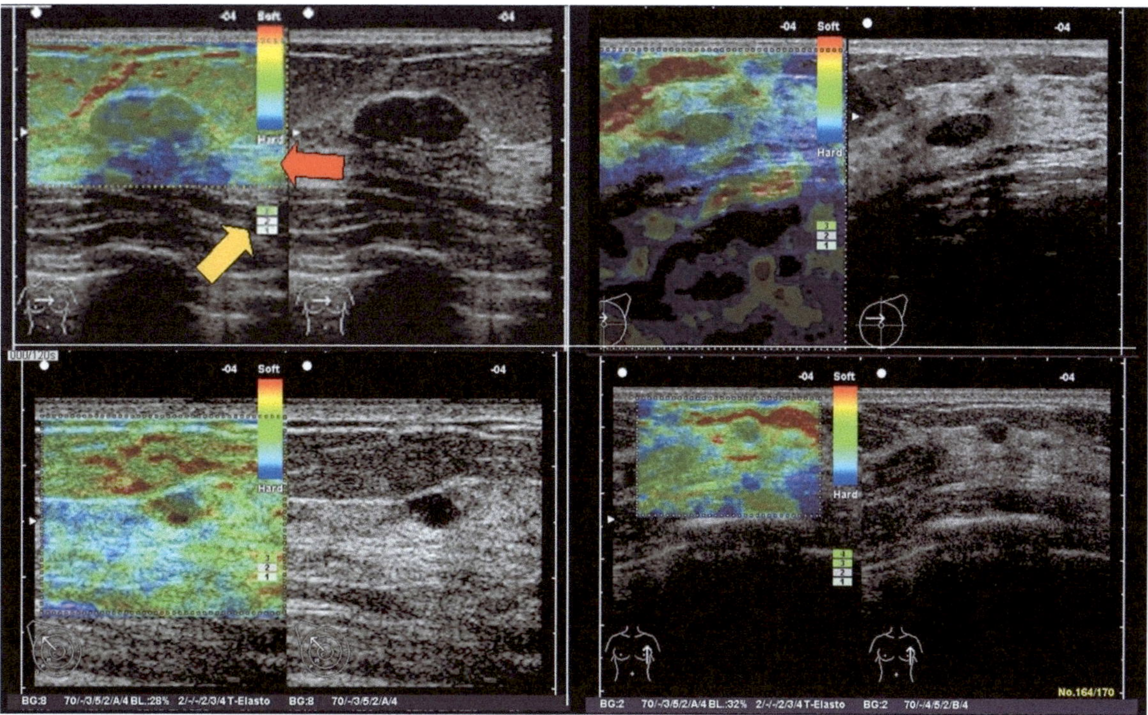

Fig. 9.14. Small nodes presenting as benign at elastosonography (cytological confirmation)

- Evaluation of breast implants.
- First-level investigation for evaluation of lesions in young women (under circa 30 years of age) and women who are breastfeeding or pregnant.

The use of ultrasound as a method of screening should at present be regarded as the exclusive province of clinical research.

9.1.5 Pneumocystography

Pneumocystography consists in obtaining radiographs after the emptying of a cyst and injection of air into it; the walls of the cyst can thus be studied and possible vegetation revealed. At present, pneumocystography should be performed only to resolve doubts which persist after the ultrasound scan.

9.1.6 Ductogalactography

Ductogalactography consists in the injection of a radiopaque hydrosoluble contrast medium into the secretion duct followed by radiography. It reveals defects in the filling of the duct due to vegetation within the duct (Fig. 9.15), but cannot provide certain differential diagnosis between benign and malignant lesions. This test is indicated in cases of bloody, mixed serous and bloody, or transparent secretions, especially if unilateral and from a single duct and when occurring in the presence of suspicious cytology. It is not indicated when there are other types of secretion since the probability of otherwise hidden neoplasia in such cases is negligible.

9.1.7 Magnetic Resonance Imaging

Magnetic resonance imaging (MRI) of the breast may only be performed with the appropriate equipment, including suitable hardware and software. The examination should be simple, fast and panoramic (a simultaneous bilateral study). It should guarantee high-quality images and provide a dynamic investigation with the possibility of subsequent processing of the images (subtraction, MIP, MPR, etc.) as well as measurement of the signal intensity-time (SI/T) curves.

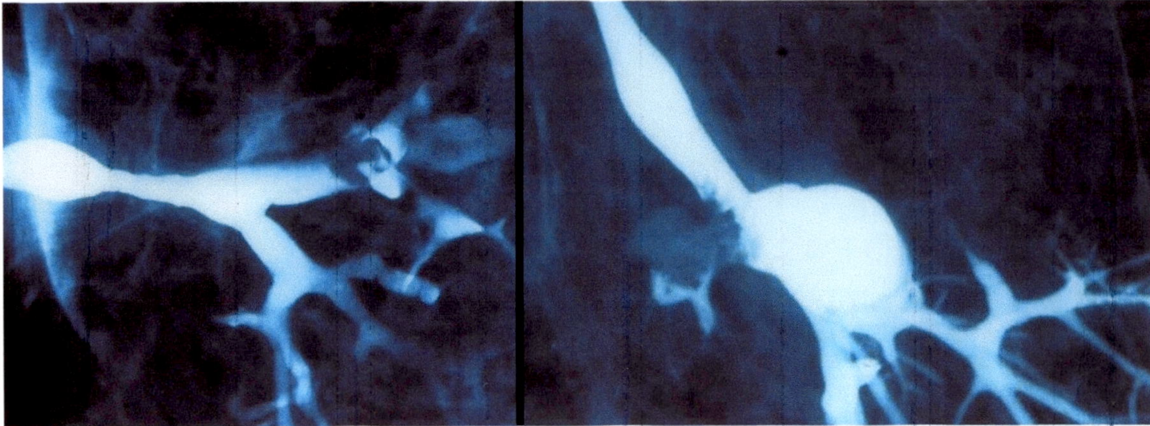

Fig. 9.15. Galactography: presence of defects in the filling of the duct due to intraductal proliferation.

The diagnostic accuracy of MRI depends on the technical and acquisitional features, but also to a very great extent on the image processing. Processing should therefore be considered one of the main stages of the technique (Del Maschio et al. 2002; Morris 2002).

Reparative processes lead to focal or diffuse inflammatory reactions, with hypervascular areas and a consequent enhancement effect which is sometimes difficult to distinguish from that due to malignant lesions. MRI should therefore generally be performed at least 6 months after surgery and 12 months after radiotherapy. If necessary, however, the examination may be carried out in the few days immediately following the operation (since, during the first 30–70 h, none of the reparative processes have taken place), and it is useful when there is some doubt as to whether the lesion has been removed.

Hormone, physiological and pharmaceutical stimulation greatly affects the MR image. For this reason the examination should preferably be performed in the second or third week of the menstrual cycle, and, in menopausal patients, 1 or 2 months after possible replacement hormone treatment has been suspended. If this methodology is not observed, there is an increased risk of false positives. When MRI reveals lesions which did not appear on the conventional investigations, the matter can often be resolved by a second targeted ultrasound scan, guided by the MR images. When diagnostic doubt persists and cannot be resolved by second-look ultrasound (or mammography), it is advisable to repeat MRI 1 or 2 months later, in the suitable period for fertile women, before undertaking surgery (Teifke et al. 2003).

It is also generally advisable for MRI to precede needle aspiration or needle biopsy since these manoeuvres may alter the behaviour of the precontrast signal and contrast enhancement. However, the methodological timing is still a matter of debate. It is believed to be best to take the specimen using the needle prior to MRI where there are unifocal lesions: if the specimen proves negative and the integrated negative diagnosis is deemed sufficiently accurate, normal follow-up with ordinary first-level tests may be considered sufficient. In contrast, where suspicious or clearly multifocal lesions exist, MRI should, if possible, precede needle aspiration.

9.1.7.1
Signs and Medical Report

Identification of lesions is based on visualisation of the areas of greatest vascularisation on images produced by subtraction. Once the possible lesions have been identified, the images are evaluated from the morphological viewpoint and the functional characteristics are assessed by means of SI/T curves.

Characterisation of breast lesions using MRI is based above all on contrast enhancement dynamics after the administration of paramagnetic contrast medium. The presence of enhancement is closely correlated with the dynamics of the contrast medium in the lesion, which appear to be determined by the volume and permeability of the vessels, as well as by the width of the interstitial space. Since these characteristics are intrinsic to the process of angiogenesis of malignant lesions, MRI of the breast may be assumed to be a suitable method for the discovery and quantification of the angiogenic process itself.

The parameters to consider are: morphology, edges, enhancement characteristics (homogeneous, inhomogeneous, centripetal, centrifugal), the intensity of the initial signal, and the course of the SI/T curve (Fig. 9.16). As regards morphology, the criteria for malignancy are the same as for conventional techniques: irregular lesions with ill-defined edges. The functional aspect of malignant lesions is characterised by the enhancement features: inhomogeneous, with a centripetal, rapid and intense, but brief course. A typical feature of malignant lesions is intense enhancement at the first measurement after injection of the contrast medium, with an increase in signal intensity of more than 70%–100% compared to the initial value; there is therefore an initially steep SI/T curve which decreases rapidly, giving an early wash-out, i.e. a fading out of the contrast medium. Benign lesions have a regular morphology and regular edges and show homogeneous enhancement with a slow and progressive course.

The report should state the presence of areas of enhancement, the lesion site, the lesion dimensions, the hypothesis as to its nature and the relation of the lesion to the surrounding tissue. Since MRI is often performed to resolve diagnostic doubts emerging from conventional methods, such tests should be referred to, a diagnostic conclusion should be expressed and specific suggestions should be made for further possible investigations.

It should be stressed that MRI cannot be proposed as the first diagnostic examination for breast pathologies and that the specific indications for this modality should be followed in order to prevent an excess of doubtful cases and false positives.

9.1.7.2
Results

MRI of the breast is characterised by very high sensitivity, of between 95% and 100% for infiltrating carcinomas and approximately 80% for in situ ductal carcinomas. The negative predictive value for infiltrating carcinomas approaches 100%. All authors agree on these values, but there is incomplete agreement on the specificity, which is approximately 80% using state of the art equipment.

9.1.7.3
Indications

Currently, breast MRI should be regarded as a technique to be used only in combination with mammography and ultrasound. There are a number of principal indications:

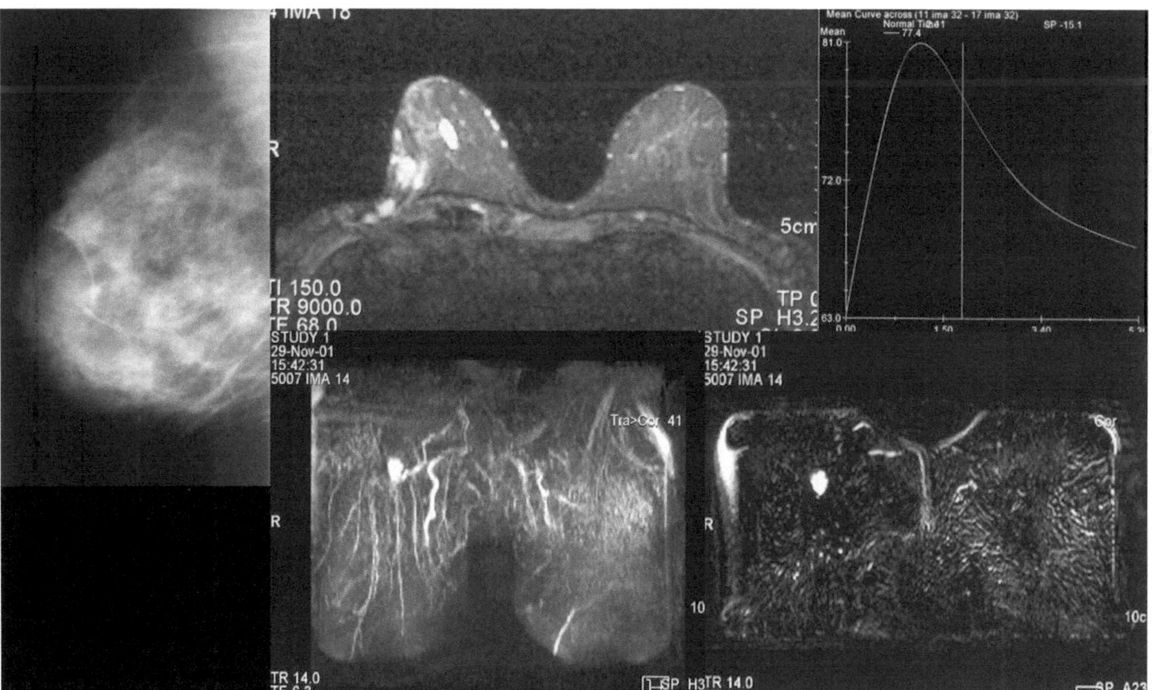

Fig. 9.16. Example of carcinoma highlighted at MRI in mammographic dense breast

- The study of women with a genetic or high family risk of breast carcinoma. Owing to the ability of MRI to detect characteristics associated with the process of angiogenesis, use of MRI in conjunction with conventional techniques allows the identification of some tumours which would not otherwise be recognised (the contribution in this respect is particularly valuable in women with radiologically dense breasts) (Kuhl et al. 2000; Podo et al. 2002; Tilanus-Linthorst et al. 2000).
- The search for unknown primitive carcinomas when conventional methods are negative (Schorn et al. 1999).
- Preoperative assessment or local staging in the case of breast carcinomas diagnosed using traditional techniques. MRI is the most accurate technique for correctly defining the relationship between surrounding tissue and the size and number of lesions, thus affording the identification of multifocality/multicentricity and contralateral lesions. The literature reports that multifocal/multicentric lesions not detected by conventional imaging techniques were identified using MRI in 16–37% of cases and that synchronous occult contralateral lesions were identified in 5–10% of the patients studied. In brief, MRI changed the therapeutic approach to the patient in between 11% and 51% of cases (Oellinger et al. 1993; Slanetz et al. 1998).
- Monitoring of breast lesions treated with neoadjuvant presurgical chemotherapy (MRI permits more precise definition of the dimensions of the residual tumour and its differentiation from necrotic and fibrotic components) (Panizza et al. 1997; Rieber et al. 1997; Wasser al. 2003).
- Follow-up after breast-conserving surgery and/or radiotherapy, wherever conventional methods raise doubts regarding the differential diagnosis of fibrosis and relapses. The sensitivity of MRI in distinguishing between relapse and fibrosis ranges from 93% to 100%, and the specificity from 88% to 100% (Dao et al. 1993; Solomon et al. 1998).
- Evaluation of women with breast implants. MRI is the most effective technique for studying the state of the implant (integrity, fibrous capsule, dislocation, silicon migration); according to the literature, MRI has a 75% sensitivity and specificity in the recognition of ruptured implants. In addition, MRI allows assessment of the native breast and especially the regions hidden by the implant that are difficult to explore using mammography or ultrasound (Ahn et al. 1993; Gorzica et al. 1994; Reynolds et al. 1994).
- Evaluation of breasts that are difficult to interpret using conventional techniques or for which different diagnostic approaches have yielded discrepant findings.
- As a guide for the taking of cyto-/histological specimens of lesions that can only be revealed by MRI. Combined use of new stereotactic equipment and surface bobbins and non-magnetic needles now makes it possible to perform cytological and microhistological sampling pre-operative marking of lesions (Liberman et al. 2003; Panizza et al. 2003; Wald et al. 1993).

Contra-indications to MRI include inflammation, which is indistinguishable from malignant alterations, and all the other usual contra-indications (pacemakers, metallic plates, etc.).

At our present state of knowledge, the most debated issue as regards the indications for MRI is whether or not it should be routinely used when a breast carcinoma has been diagnosed by conventional techniques and breast-conserving treatment proposed. The literature would appear to suggest that MRI should routinely be performed prior to conservative surgical interventions. However, it is clearly too early to impose such a protocol, both because it would be difficult to offer the test to every woman with a carcinoma in its initial phase and above all because we still do not have clear scientific evidence of the advantages in terms of survival. Until such evidence becomes available, each case should be carefully assessed and, before a decision is made on whether to use MRI, the patient should be made fully aware that if further foci are discovered, it will no longer be possible to avoid mastectomy, even though quadrantectomy and radiotherapy might offer the same results.

9.1.8 Needle Sampling

9.1.8.1 Fine-Needle Aspiration for Cytological Analysis

Cytology is performed on: secretions from the nipple, the contents of cysts, material obtained from scarification of erosive lesions of the nipple, and aspiration samples of palpable or non-palpable solid tumefaction when it is not definitely benign. The slide should bear the data essential for identifying the patient, placed there prior to the test.

Fine-needle aspiration cytology (FNAC) may involve the use of a needle alone or a needle attached to a syringe, with the syringe mounted on a handle. Complications are typically negligible (infection, haemorrhage) and more serious complications (pneumothorax) are extremely rare if the methodology is appropriate. In theory, it is possible that dissemination of neoplastic cells might occur as a result of FNAC, but no such cases have been described in the literature on breast carcinoma.

Signs and Medical Report

A descriptive diagnosis is optional and, in this case, the cytopathological report should be clear and succinct. By contrast, the diagnostic conclusion is obligatory and should be codified into five classes:

- C1: findings insufficient for a diagnostic judgement
- C2: findings negative for tumour cells
- C3: findings dubious; lesions probably benign, but presence of atypia
- C4: suspicious findings, peremptory indications for surgical biopsy
- C5: positive findings for malignant tumour cells (an area of tumour cells unequivocally malignant, already recognisable when only slightly enlarged) with almost absolute positive prediction (>99%).

Results

The sensitivity of FNAC for breast cancer (suspicious + positive cases, excluding insufficient findings from consideration) is 90–95%, and it has a positive predictive value of more than 99%. The rate of insufficient findings in cases of cancer is less than 10%. When FNAC yields a positive finding, intraoperative histological confirmation may be omitted. When a suspicious finding is obtained (in the literature the predictive value of suspicious findings ranges between 40% and 80%), surgical biopsy is required, regardless of the clinical evidence. Given the possibility of false-negative cytology, a negative cytological analysis is not sufficient to avoid a surgical biopsy if other diagnostic tests are either dubious or suspicious (Di Maggio et al. 2003; Helbich et al. 2003; Pisano et al. 2001; Sauer et al. 2003).

If the sensitivity, specificity and predictive values achieved at a treatment centre are not comparable with the foregoing rates, it is necessary to critically review sampling, smear staining and interpretation and possibly to compare one's own practice with that at a more experienced centre.

9.1.8.2
Needle Biopsy for Histological Analysis (Percutaneous Biopsy)

The specimen is taken using a wide-calibre needle and therefore special methodological precautions are required (informed consent, accurate anamnesis regarding coagulation disorders or allergy to anaesthetics, local anaesthesia and possible general sedation, cutaneous incision, subsequent manual compression for 10_15 min and radiography of specimens). In fact, not all of these precautions should always be carried out, but the methodology is undoubtedly more invasive than in FNAC. The average time for the procedure ranges from 15 to 60 min; a report is only available several days later.

Nowadays, various techniques are available for percutaneous biopsy, including multiple sampling with automatic or semi-automatic guillotine cutting needles with a 14- to 20-G calibre, the advanced breast biopsy instrumentation (ABBI) system, which allows removal of a core of breast tissue up to 2 cm in size, and the Mammotome breast biopsy system, allowing removal of samples with gentle suction.

Percutaneous biopsy allows histological analysis of the lesion, providing information on tumour invasiveness and certain parameters related to its aggressiveness; it yields a low number of insufficient findings. The expected results are influenced by the type of lesion (node or calcification), by the calibre of the needle and by the number of pieces taken. It should always be borne in mind, in the interests of correct programming of surgery and treatment, that in 10–30% of cases with a microhistological diagnosis of carcinoma in situ, subsequent surgical removal will reveal the presence of invasive carcinoma (Jackman et al. 2001).

9.1.8.3
Indications for Needle Aspiration/Biopsy and Choice of Method

Palpable lesions: Although FNAC almost always enables the diagnostic problem of palpable lesions to be resolved, it is preferable, except in certain specific cases, to use aspiration not as a sole clinical test, but after evaluation of the mammogram (or at least the ultrasound scan). This ensures that FNAC is carried out only when necessary, at the right time and in the right place.

Non-Palpable Lesions

Needle aspiration should be performed with an ultrasound or a radiostereotactic guide. In some centres, it is possible to use an MRI guide. In all cases where the lesion, though discovered through mammography, can be recognised with a targeted ultrasound scan and where there is certainty that the lesion on the ultrasound image corresponds to that on mammography, ultrasound-guided aspiration is to be preferred because it is simpler, faster, more agreeable for the patient and less expensive.

The increasingly frequent findings of non-palpable lesions and their small size require that diagnostic procedures should be very strictly applied, that the recommendation for aspiration must be justified, and that the choice of method (FNAC versus percutaneous biopsy) must be rational (Deurloo et al. 2003; Di Maggio et al. 2003; Nori 2003; Parker et al. 2001). In the presence of lesions of a dubious nature, therefore, the radiologist should use second- and third-level examinations (targeted radiography, mammographic enlargement, possible ultrasound scan studies with a contrast medium, digital processing, MRI, etc.) to try to characterise the lesions as well as possible.

The following considerations may justify aspiration and help in selection of the method:

- Needle sampling should be deemed necessary if the expected findings might change the subsequent diagnostic approach or treatment (follow-up control or excision, interval between check-ups). In the presence of nodes with a diameter of less than 1 cm, classified 3 or 4A at mammography or ultrasound according to BI-RADS and classified negative or benign at needle aspiration, it is advisable to avoid surgical excision and perform only a short-term follow-up: this choice reduces anxiety in the majority of patients, reduces costs and avoids possible alterations in structural scarring that may cause diagnostic difficulties in future check-ups (Fig. 9.17). Similar considerations should be adopted in the case of hyperplasia without atypia (Jacobs 2002).
  - Instead, in the case of atypical ductal hyperplasia, surgical excision is always recommended since the differential diagnosis between ADH and low-grade DCIS is difficult and in many cases foci of ADH can be found at DCIS margins. When ADH is diagnosed at needle aspiration subsequently a diagnosis of DCIS in a reasonable number of cases is made (from 19% to 44%) (Hartmann 2005).
  - Needle sampling may also be recommended even when the mammogram is clearly suspicious or positive, in order to obtain a definitive preoperative diagnosis so that the patient can be better informed as to the type of surgical operation that will be performed or to avoid a two-stage operation (first, a diagnostic biopsy and then a radical intervention).
- The choice among the various methods should be based both on the scientific evidence avail-

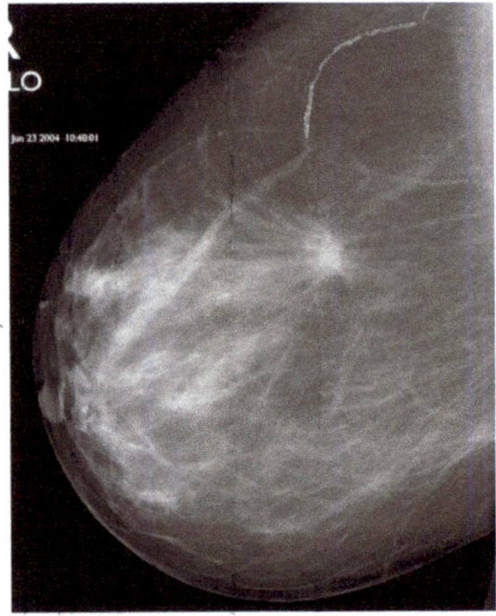

a

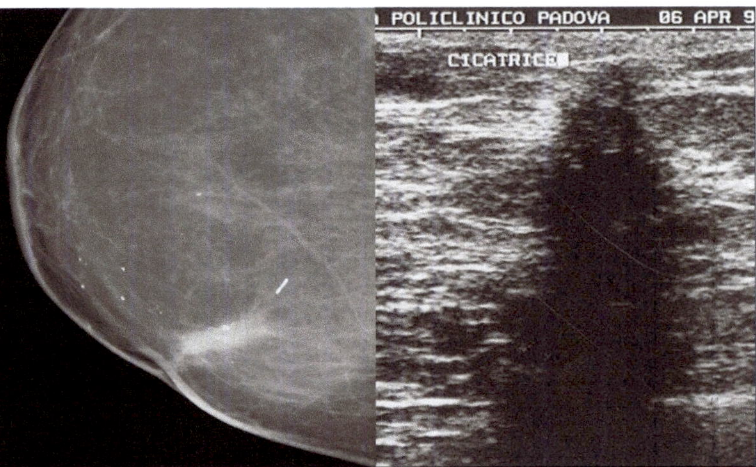

b

Fig. 9.17a,b. Images simulating a carcinoma, but caused by scar alterations after surgery

able (evaluation of the contributions they offer for diagnosis, knowledge of the prognostic factors and knowledge of the invasiveness of the carcinoma) and on personal experience.

It is always worth bearing in mind that, if a choice can or has to be made, it is best to employ the less invasive method in cases in which the results will tend to coincide or in which the particular information that may be obtained using the more invasive technique (e.g., tumour invasiveness or aggressiveness, histological type) is not indispensable or can be obtained during the surgical intervention without prejudicing it and the prognosis.

To sum up, the following guidelines may be suggested: given the grounds for needle aspiration, the method of choice to obtain further diagnostic information will in most cases be FNAC (less invasive, less costly), with percutaneous biopsy reserved for cases without a definitive diagnostic evaluation (cases that are classified as C1/C3, or which are the subject of disagreement between the radiologist and the pathologist) and cases in which information is required that cytology cannot provide (invasiveness, aggressiveness).

It should be stressed that the choice of method lies with the operators (the radiologist, pathologist and surgeon), who may prefer FNAC or percutaneous biopsy, according to their own experience. In many cases, moreover, the choice should be discussed and agreed upon on a case-by-case basis in the multidisciplinary unit.

9.2 Suggested Diagnostic Procedure for Self-Referrals

9.2.1 Women Who are Symptom-Free

9.2.1.1 Under 40 Years of Age

There are no particular recommendations regarding the preventive control except to note that the women involved are at high risk (genetic/familial high risk) and are part of a specific programme of diagnostic surveillance. Rigorous check-up is also recommended in women submitted to previous treatment for Hodgkin's disease (Hill 2005; Travis 2003, 2005). Routine ultrasound scans are unjustified in the absence of objective signs.

9.2.1.2 Over 40 Years of Age

It is recommended that mammography should be performed at intervals of between 1 and 2 years. Mammography at 1-year intervals, in combination with routine breast and ultrasound examination, is justifiable for women with radiologically dense breasts owing to the greater difficulty in discovering a possible tumour and because the radiological density appears to be associated with a greater risk of tumour development (Boyd et al. 1995, 2002; Harvey and Bovbierg 2004; Mandelson et al. 2000).

As regards the clinical and instrumental surveillance of the group of women with a genetic risk of breast carcinoma, there are as yet no recommendations grounded in hard scientific evidence. It is advisable for such women to attend centres where there are working groups devoted to the problem.

Given that mammography has limitations, especially in younger women, the usefulness of routinely combining MRI with ultrasound and mammography is currently being assessed. At present it is widespread practice to advise that check-up visits should begin at 30 or at the same age as the youngest family member affected. Currently, diversified diagnostic procedures and intervals according to the level of risk (e.g., genetic risk for breast cancer) are being evaluated. Periodic tests may also be advisable in males over the age of 50 when there is a family history of breast cancer.

9.2.2 Women with Symptoms

9.2.2.1 Under 35 Years of Age

Due to the low incidence of breast carcinoma in patients aged less than 35 years, the clinical examination performed by the general practitioner may be sufficient to clear up any doubts and allay needless anxiety. In the presence of real focal pathology, which is not suspicious clinically, ultrasound and possible needle aspiration may be deemed sufficient. If the suspicion persists, the diagnostic evaluation should continue with mammography and other techniques if necessary.

9.2.2.2 Over 35 Years of Age

In patients aged over 35 years who have relevant symptoms, mammography in combination with clinical examination and, preferably, ultrasound will afford a correct diagnosis in most cases. The use of ultrasound has the advantage that it will avoid failure to diagnose carcinomas that cannot be revealed radiographically. Ultrasound is indispensable both when there is difficulty in exploring the breast radiographically (dense breasts) and when mammography or the clinical examination reveals nodules whose nature is unclear.

If the difficulty in classifying the images persists or if suspicious elements emerge, needle aspiration should be performed (percutaneous cytology or biopsy). It will be necessary to decide on a case-by-case basis whether or not needle aspiration should be preceded by MRI or breast scintigraphy.

9.3 Operational Models (Organisation of Diagnostic Procedures)

The organisation of the procedures used in diagnosing breast pathologies should take account of three objectives:

- To diagnose most small tumours at an early stage so as to ensure a reduction in the mortality and a better quality of life
- To achieve correct diagnosis of benign growths in order to avoid additional anxiety and unnecessary biopsies
- To reassure healthy women and give them peace of mind

From the methodological point of view, two ways of proceeding can be considered:

- Creation of breast diagnostic units (BDUs)
- Implementation of mammographic screening programmes

9.3.1 Breast Diagnostic Units (BDUs)

Only the centralisation of diagnostic activity in a single site (a BDU), catering for both women who present spontaneously, with or without symptoms, and women selected through screening, enables administrators to optimise resources and to provide personalised procedures so that a definitive diagnosis can be obtained at low cost and with minimum inconvenience for the patient (Di Maggio 1991). It is convenient to arrange for two sets of procedures: one set for women with symptoms and another for those without (Di Maggio 1996, 2004).

Patients with evident clinical symptoms are inducted into a set of procedures that includes a preliminary clinical examination, then mammography and, in rapid succession, any other tests (ultrasound, needle sampling) needed to reach a conclusive diagnosis. Communicating rooms need to be available.

Naturally, the sequence of the diagnostic procedures may require modification in accordance with the presumed pathology and the patient's age. The result is given to the patient at the end of the tests, except in cases in which it is necessary to take a sample with a needle (the analysis of which should also be carried out in the same centre).

In the event of a positive result, it is the radiologist who provides the first explanations and prepares the patient for the subsequent therapeutic procedures (Figs. 9.18, 9.19). The referring doctor is, of course, informed immediately (with the patient's consent) and is directly involved.

Women without clinical symptoms who spontaneously present with a view to prevention undergo the same set of diagnostic procedures on the first occasion as patients with symptoms. In most cases, clinical examination and mammography are sufficient to conclude the diagnostic process in these women. The date of the next check-up and follow-up procedures are established when the results are given.

Women without symptoms who are found to be in a healthy state are offered one of two differing sets of subsequent procedures:

- Women with breasts that are more difficult to examine are invited to return for annual check-ups with mammography and ultrasound.
- Women with breasts that are mainly adipose can be monitored by mammography alone at 2-yearly intervals. In this case, interpretation of the radiographs is deferred and double reading is essential.

The diagnostic activity must be carefully monitored. The patient should come away from the BDU with a definitive diagnosis and not with a request for further diagnostic testing.

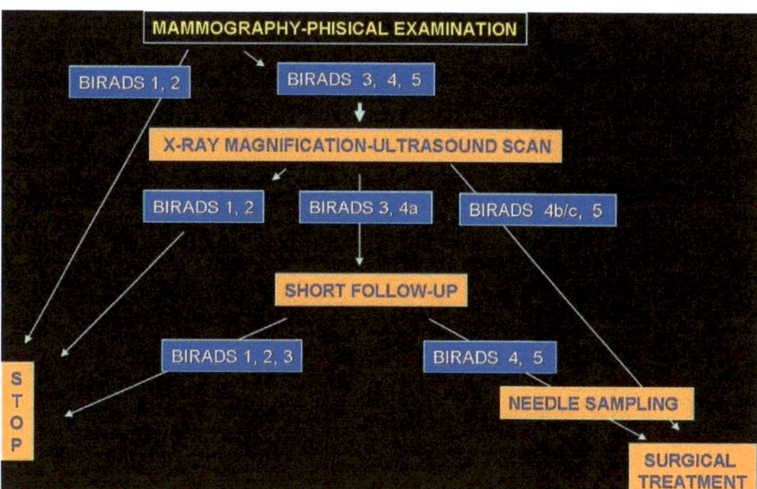

Fig. 9.18. Practice guidelines in breast disease assessment

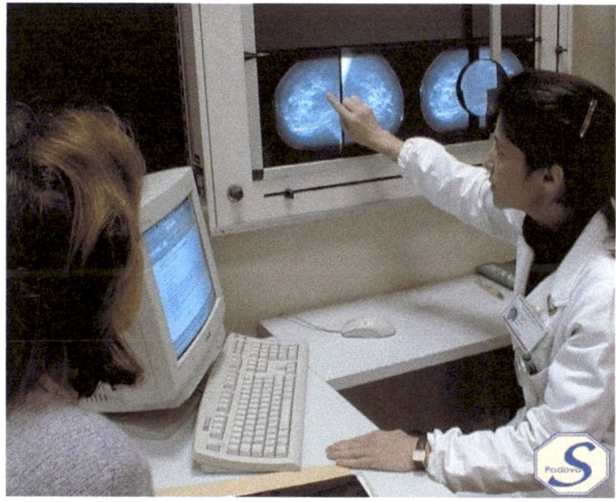

Fig. 9.19. Consultation with the patient at the end of the exam reduces anxiety that may occur from the moment of the diagnosis until the start of therapy

9.3.2 Mammographic Screening

The purpose of mammographic screening is not diagnosis as such, but the selection of women "probably affected by a tumour". The sole objective of the screening programme is to obtain a reduction in mortality at an acceptable cost; it is therefore to be undertaken only if its effectiveness has been demonstrated, if funds are available, if the cost is acceptable and if it is competitive in relation to other public health initiatives. For the same reasons, the programme is not directed at all women, but only at those in the age band at greatest risk.

As far as breast cancer is concerned, screening programmes have now been operative for very many years and their effectiveness is proven; the cost per life saved would also appear to be acceptable (Duffy 2002; Nystrom et al. 2002; Peto et al. 2000; Shapiro 1977; Vanara et al. 1995). Screening programmes can be credited with having demonstrated that prompt diagnosis results in a reduction in mortality and that good results can be obtained only if all steps of the programme are optimised and all results are periodically checked. Although the efficacy of mammographic screening has been proven over many years, it cannot be said that the population is adequately covered. However, it has to be borne in mind that is not possible, within a limited time, to fully implement a programme that requires broad participation among the population, growth of awareness, sufficient economic resources and an adequate number of well-trained professional figures (radiologists and radiographers) (EUREF 2001/2006; Sickles et al. 2002).

The negative aspects of a programme of mammographic screening are well known (di Maggio et al. 1994; Fletcher and Elmore 2003; Wald et al. 1993): prolonged awareness of illness when therapy is not able to yield the desired results, over-diagnosis and over-treatment, false reassurance in the event of false-negative results, anxiety inducement in the event of false-positive results and the possible risk associated with radiation, over-diagnosis and over-treatment (De Koning et al. 2006; Warren and Eleti 2006; Zackrisson et al. 2006).

Overdiagnosis is: the diagnosis of a tumour through screening that would never have been diagnosed if screening had not been carried out since progression is very slow. Overdiagnosis leads to: surgical interventions, useless drug therapy, intensive follow-up and negative psycho-physical consequences.

Overdiagnosis should not be confused with early diagnosis (excess of observed incidence with screening), which means anticipating the diagnosis of tumours that would have become clinically evident in the future.

The operating methodology for a screening programme is today rigorously codified (Advisory Committee on Cancer Prevention 2000; American Cancer Society 1999–2003; Piscioli and Cristofolini 1996; Bancej et al. 2003) exclusive mammography bi-annually, deferred reading, recall with further diagnostic testing of women with a doubtful diagnosis expressed even by only one of the two readers, and limitation to women aged between 50 and 69.

Some considerations with respect to current screening methodology include: Mammography is offered as the sole test, at 2-yearly intervals and with deferred reading. This allows a reasonable number of examinations per hour to be completed and reduces the number of working hours required of radiologists, but it leads to less thorough and sensitive diagnostics, as well as to the need for follow-up in uncertain cases. The limited sensitivity of mammographic screening used as the sole test on a bi-annual basis is clearly attested to by the rather high rate of so-called interval cancers (Maijd et al. 2003; Marra et al. 1999; Raja et al. 2001; Sylvester et al. 1977). It has been sufficiently documented that a good proportion of these cancers would be picked up if shorter intervals were used (Bauce et al. 1998; Feig 1997; Michaelson et al. 1999; Rosen et al. 2002; Zappa et al. 2002) if the screening were combined with other tests (Cilotti et al. 1997; Kaplan 2001; Kolb et al. 1998; Moy et al. 2002; Zonderland et al. 1999). It therefore seems reasonable to consider the possibility that, for women with breasts that are not amenable to X-ray scanning, the screening protocol should be modified to include routine ultrasound scans.

Very useful, but perhaps less feasible for reasons of cost and lack of personnel, would be the inclusion of the medical radiologist at the time of the first examination. The implementation of a concurrent clinical examination and ultrasound scan, when necessary, would lead to a 7–10% reduction in diagnostic errors (Bancej et al. 2003; D'Angelo et al. 1996) and thus also in the incidence of interval cancers (Kopans 2004; Guthrie 1999). Furthermore, it would obviate the need to recall patients for second-level tests, which causes anxiety, and would offer the woman receiving the information the kind of human contribution that can only be ensured by the presence of the doctor.

As stated above, women aged 50–69 are prioritised as subjects for screening, but in view of the longer life expectancy of women in good health and past the age of 70, it may be advisable to continue actively screening women who attended previous tests up to the age of 74.

The decision as to whether the age at which the first "invitation to screening" is offered should be lowered to 45 can be left to the health authorities, taking into account available resources and working in collaboration with the scientific society. There is a general consensus that women should be given the opportunity to undergo periodic tests at this age since the results of recent studies, although not conclusive, have indicated the possible effectiveness of early diagnosis in this age range as well. Naturally, the women concerned must be adequately informed of the possible benefits, but also of the possible negative effects (diagnostic overestimation of risk, anxiety) (Bjurstam et al. 1997; Smart et al. 1995).

9.4 Concluding Considerations on Procedures for Timely Diagnosis of Breast Cancer

Procedures for early diagnosis must be implemented in such a way that the entire geographic area in question is adequately covered, and women who undergo checkups, whether spontaneously or as directed by their own doctors, must be assured of good quality diagnosis. In order to obtain the greatest advantage from the diagnostic activities while containing the negative effects, every procedure aimed at achieving a timely diagnosis must take place within the context of a well-organised and supervised programme and must be supported by thorough training programmes for the operators. All the diagnostic programmes must therefore be backed up by adequate planning, and all the necessary resources, in terms of both professional support and institutional structures, must be guaranteed, including the health care functions subsequent to the diagnosis, namely therapy and follow-up to an appropriate standard.

Whenever the prerequisites for implementation of a high-quality screening programme within a limited period are lacking, it is essential that priority is given to measures aimed at reorganising and rationalising the diagnostic activities already available within that geographical area, reconstituting them into dedicated structures in the form of BDUs. It is necessary to create a network of BDUs evenly distributed across the territory since a network of this kind represents an indispensable preliminary phase in a programme that will extend to the population as a whole. The institution of a BDU network and the initiation of a screening programme may be perceived as a single project to be implemented at the regional level.

In view of the fact that the diagnosis of breast lesions is currently based on tests that rely largely or exclusively on the expertise of the radiologist, and given that the apparatus is costly and that its use must be supervised and carried out in an integrated fashion, it is appropriate for clinical and organisational responsibility for the diagnostic procedures to be entrusted to the radiologist, assisted by a physician or general practitioner and a pathologist. It is also necessary, when disease is found, for interdisciplinary expertise to be available so that the most suitable form of treatment can be identified more easily.

Possible non-standard modes of organisation should also be carefully evaluated (Dilhuydy et al. 2003; Di Maggio et al. 2001); this lies within the remit of the respective technical committees. Similarly, the diagnostic protocol to be used can be modified with a view to increasing the sensitivity of screening (Consiglio dell'Unione Europea 2003).

Finally, it would be desirable for each region to set up an ***interdisciplinary body of reference for quality assurance***. The function of such a body would be to ensure that work on breast pathology reaches a high level of quality and that this level is maintained throughout the region in question. Naturally, in order to guarantee the desired quality, it is necessary to allocate adequate resources and to ensure the availability of suitably qualified personnel.

One of the most urgent problems is to guarantee the quality of the procedures employed in breast pathology diagnostics, both in the clinical context and in screening. Attention needs to be paid specifically to the need to extend quality control to diagnostic centres that do not operate under the auspices of a screening programme, since today most women still undergo tests autonomously outside the organised programmes. Some quality assurance activities can be undertaken as part of the activities of the health service, but others will require specific, targeted funding and will need to cover training activities, data collection and the compilation of proper annual reports to be presented at the regional level.

References

Advisory Committee on Cancer Prevention (2000) Recommendations on cancer screening in the European Union. Eur J Cancer 36:1473–1478

Ahn CY, Shaw WW, Narayanan K et al (1993) Definitive diagnosis of breast implant rupture using magnetic resonance imaging. Plast Reconstr Surg 94:681–691

American Cancer Society 1999–2003. Guidelines for clinical cancer prevention

American College of Radiology (2000\2001) ACR standard for performance of the breast ultrasound examination. In: Standards of the American College of Radiology. Reston, Va, 389–392

American College of Radiology (2003) Illustrated breast imaging reporting and data system (BI-RADS), 4th edn. Reston, VA, ACR

Amici F, Baldassarre S, Giuseppetti GM (2000) Imaging in senologia – Testo Atlante. Milano, Paletto

ANAES (Agence National d'Accreditation e d'Evaluation de la Santè) (1998) Recommandations pour la pratique clinique. Synthèse des recommandations cancer du sein. Paris, ANAES

Baker JA, Rosen EL, Lo JY et al (2003) Computer-aided detection (CAD) in screening mammography. AJR 181:1083–1088

Balu-Maestro C, Chapellier C, Bleuse A (2003) Place de l'échographie dans le dépistage du cancer du sein. J Le Sein 13:127–134

Bancej C, Decker K, Chiarelli A, et al (2003) Contribution of clinical breast examination to mammography screening in the early detection of breast cancer. J Med Screen 10:16–21

Bauce A, Benesso S, Galiano A (1998) Relazione tra densità mammografica, età delle pazienti e sensibilità. Radiol Med 5 (suppl 1):271

Berlin L (2001) The missed breast cancer redux: time for educating the public about the limitation of mammography? AJR 176:1131–1134

Bjurstam N, Bjorneld L, Duffy SW et al (1997) The Gothenburg Breast Screening Trial. Cancer 80:2091–2099

Boyd NF, Byng JW, Jong RA (1995) Quantitative classification of mammographic densities and breast cancer risk: results from the Canadian National Breast Screening Study. J Natl Cancer Inst 87:670–675

Boyd NF, Dite GS, Stone J et al (2002) Heritability of mammographic density, a risk factor for breast cancer. N Engl J Med 347:886–894

Brem RF, Baun J, Lechner M et al (2003) Improvement in sensitivity of screening mammography with computer-aided detection: a multiinstitutional trial. AJR 181:687–693

Burrel HC, Pinder SE et al (1996) The positive predictive value of mammographic signs. Clin Radiol 51:277–281

Ciatto S, Rosselli del Turco M, Burke P et al (2003) Comparison of standard and double reading and computer-aided detection (CAD) of interval cancers at prior negative screening mammograms: blind review. Br J Cancer 89:1645–9

Cilotti A, Bagnolesi P et al (1997): Comparison of the diagnostic performance of high-frequency ultrasound in non-palpable lesions of the breast. Eur Radiol 7:1240–1244

Cole EB, Pisano ED, Kistner EO et al (2003) Diagnostic accuracy of digital mammography in patients with dense breast. Radiology 226:153–160

Consiglio dell'Unione Europea (2003) Raccomandazioni del 2-12-2003 sullo screening dei tumori. 2003/878/CE G.U. Unione Europea 16.12.2003 L 327/34–37

ISTISAN (1995) Controllo di qualità in mammografia: aspetti tecnici e clinici. Istituto superiore di sanità. ISTISAN 95/12 (ISSN 1123-3117), Roma

Cuzick J (2003) Epidemiology of breast cancer-selected highlights. Breast 12:405–411

D'Angelo I, Pindaro L, Glorioso V et al (1996) Progetto primavera. Risultati del primo passaggio. In: Piscioli F,Cristofolini M (eds) Modelli operativi di prevenzione secondaria del carcinoma mammario. Trento, Temi, pp 209–221

Dao TH, Rahmouni A, Campana F et al (1993) Tumor recurrences versus fibrosis in the irradiated breast: differentiation with dynamic gadolinium enhancement MR imaging. Radiology 187:751–755

De Koning HJ, Draisma G, Fracheboud J et al (2006) Overdiagnosis and overtreatment of breast cancer. Microsimulation modelling estimates based on observed screen and clinical data. Breast Cancer Res 8:202

Del Maschio A, De Gaspari A, Panizza P (2002) Risonanza magnetica in senologia. Radiol Med 104:253–261

Dendy PP, Brugmans MJP (2003). Low dose radiation risks. Br J Radiol; 76:674–677

Deurloo EE, Tanis PJ, Gilhuijs KG et al (2003) Reduction in the number of sentinel lymph node procedures by preoperative ultrasonography of the axilla in breast cancer. European Journal of Cancer 39:1068–1073

Dilhuydy MH, Monnereau A, Barreau B (2003) Le dépistage «à la française». Action programmée ou aménagement du diagnostic précoce individuel? J Le Sein 2: 83–90

Di Maggio C (1991) Il servizio di senologia diagnostica. Radiol Med 81:585–591

Di Maggio C (1993) Lo screening mammografico, questo sconosciuto. Atti LXIX Cong. Soc. It. di Ginecologia (SIGO) Padova La Garangola 122–126

Di Maggio C (1996) La diagnosi del tumore della mammella: linee guida ed aspetti organizzativi (UFSD). In: Piscioli F,Cristofolini M (eds) Modelli operativi di prevenzione secondaria del carcinoma mammario. Trento, Temi, pp 361–379

Di Maggio C, Giuseppetti G, Gozzi G et al (1994) La mammografia nelle quarantenni: verso un chiarimento definitivo. Radiol Med 87:731–735

Di Maggio C, Fioretti P, La Grassa M et al (2001) Screening mammografico o diagnostica clinica? Proposta di un modello unificato. Radiol Med 101:326–333

Di Maggio C, La Grassa M, Pescarini L et al (2003) Interventistica radio-stereoguidata tradizionale e digitale. In: Nori J, Mazzocchi M (eds) Senologia. Stato dell'arte in interventistica. Napoli, Idelson-Gnocchi, pp 9–18

Di Maggio C, La Grassa M, Pescarini L et al (2003) Indicazioni al prelievo con ago ed alla scelta metodologica. In: Nori J, Mazzocchi M (eds) Senologia. Stato dell'arte in interventistica. Napoli, Idelson-Gnocchi, pp 33–41

Di Maggio C, Gennaro G, La Grassa M et al (2004). Mammografia digitale. Radiol Med 107 (suppl 2):15–20

Di Maggio C et al (2004) CHARTA SENOLOGICA. Radiol Med 108:569–587

Duffy SW, Tabar L, Chen HH et al (2002) The impact of organized mammography service screening on breast carcinoma mortality in seven Swedish counties. Cancer 95:458–469

EURWF (2001) European Guidelines for Quality Assurance in Mammography Screening. Terza Quarta edizione, 4th edn. EUREF, Gennaio

Feig SA (1977) Can breast cancer be radiation induced? In: Logan WW (ed) Breast carcinoma. NewYork, Wiley Medical, pp 5–14

Feig SA (1992) Breast masses: mammographic and sonographic evaluation. Radiol Clin North Am 30:67–94

Feig SA (1997) Increased benefit from shorter screening mammography intervals for women ages 40–49 years. Cancer 80:2035–2039

Fletcher SW, Elmore JG (2003) Mammographic screening for breast cancer. N Engl J Med 348:1672–80

Freer TW, Ulissey MJ (2001) Screening mammography with computer-aided detection: prospective study of 12,860 patients in a community breast center. Radiology 220:781–786

Gambaccini M, Baldelli P (2003) Mammografia digitale. Principi fisici e sviluppi futuri. Radiol Med 106:454–466

Gennaro G, Baldelli P, Taibi A, Di Maggio C, Gambaccini M (2003) Patient dose in full-field digital mammography: an Italian survey. Eur Radiol; published online 12 August 2003

Gennaro G, di Maggio C (2006) Dose comparison between screen/film and full-field digital mammography. Eur Radiol DOI 10.1007/S00330-006-0314-2

Giuseppetti GM (2002) L'ecografia senologica. Radiol Med 104:1–12

Giuseppetti GM, Martegani A, Di Cioccio B, Baldassarre S (2005) Elastosonografia nella caratterizzazione delle lesioni nodulari della mammella: esperienza preliminare. Radiol Med 1-2:69–76

Gorzica DC, De Bruhl ND, Mund DF, Basset LW (1994) Linguine sign at MR imaging: it represents collapsed silicone implant shell? Radiology 191:576–577

Gregg EC (1977) Radiation risks with diagnostic X-rays. Radiology 123:447–453

Guthrie TH (1999) Breast cancer litigation: an update with practice guidelines. Breast J 5:335–339

Hackshaw AK, Paul EA (2003) Breast self-examination and death from breast cancer: a meta-analysis. Br J Cancer 88: 1047–53

Hartmann LC (2005) Benign breast disease and the risk of breast cancer. N Engl J Med 353:229–237

Harvey JA, Bovbierg VE (2004) Quantitative assessment of mammographic breast density: relationship with breast cancer risk. Radiology 230:29–41

Helbich TH, Matzek W, Fuchsjager MH (2003) Stereotactic and ultrasound-guided breast biopsy. Eur Radiol; published online 13 November 2003

Hendrick RE, Basset L, Bosco MA et al (1999) Mammography quality control manual. Reston, Va, American College of Radiology

Hill DA (2005) Breast cancer risk following radioterapy for Hodgkin's lymphoma. Blood 106:3358–3365

Itoh A, Ueno Ei, Tohno E et al (2006) Breast disease: clinical application of US elastography for diagnosis. Radiology 239:341–350

Jackman RJ, Burbank F, Parker SH et al (2001) Stereotactic breast biopsy of nonpalpable lesions: determinants of ductal carcinoma in situ underestimation rates. Radiology 218:497–502

Jacobs T (2002) Nonmalignant lesions in breast core needle biopsies. To excise or not to excise? Am J Surg Pathol 26:1095–1110

Jakobsen JA (2001) Ultrasound contrast agents: clinical application. Eur Radiol 11:1329–1337

James JJ (2004) The current status of digital mammography. Clin Radiol 59:1–10

Kaplan SS (2001) Clinical utility of bilateral whole-breast US in the evaluation of women with dense breast tissue. Radiology 221:641–649

Kolb T, Lichy J, Newhouse JH (1998) Occult cancer in women with dense breast: normal mammographic and physical examination findings: detection with screening US. Radiology 207:191–199

Kolb TM, Lichy J, Newhouse JH (2002) Comparison of the performance of screening mammography, physical examination, and breast US and evaluation of factor that influence them: an analysis of 27,825 patient evaluations. Radiology 225:165–175

Kopans DB (2004) Mammography screening is saving thousands of lives, but will it survive medical malpractice? Radiology 230:20–24

Kuhl CK, Schmutzer RK, Leutner C et al (2000) Breast MR imaging screening in 192 women proved or suspected to be carriers of a breast cancer susceptibility gene: preliminary results. Radiology 215:267–279

Lamarque JL, Cherifcheikh J, Laurent JC et al (1997) La qualité en mastologie: criterès, contrôle. Montpelier, Manosmed, Tome I, Sauramps médical

Lattanzio V, Simonetti G (2002) Mammografia: guida alla refertazione ed alla codifica dei risultati Re.Co.R.M. Napoli, Idelson-Gnocchi srl

Law J, Faulkner K (2002) Concerning the relationship between benefit and radiation risk, and cancers detected and induced, in a breast screening programme. Br J Radiol 75:678–684

Lechener M, Nelson M, Elvecrog E (2002) Comparison of two commercially available computer-aided detection (CAD) systems. Appl Radiol 31:31–35

Liberman L, Morris EA, Dershaw DD et al (2003) Fast MRI-guided vacuum-assisted breast biopsy: initial experience. AJR 181:1283–1293

Maijd AS, Shaw de Paredes E, Doherty RD et al (2003) Missed breast carcinoma: pitfalls and pearl. Radiographics 23:881–895

Mandelson MT, Oestreicher N, Porter PL et al (2000) Breast density as a predictor of mammographic detection: comparison of interval- and screen-detected cancers J Natl Cancer Inst 92:1081–1087

Marra V, Frigerio A, Di Virgilio MR, Coll E (1999) Il carcinoma mammario diagnosticato nello screening mammografico nei passaggi di incidenza. Radiol Med 98:342–346

Martinez AM, Medina CJ, Bustos C et al (2003) Assessment of breast lesions using Doppler with contrast agents. Eur J Gynaecol Oncol 24:527–30

Merritt CRB (2001) Technology update. Radiol Clin North Am 39:385–397

Michaelson JS, Halpern E, Kopans DB (1999) Breast cancer computer simulation method for estimation of optimal intervals for screening. Radiology 212:551–560

Moon WK, Im JG, Noh DY, Han MC (2000) Non-palpable breast lesion: evaluation with power Doppler US and microbubble contrast agent-initial experience. Radiology 217:240–6

Morris EA (2002) Breast cancer imaging with MR. Radiol Clin North Am 40:349–355

Moy L, Slanertz P, Moore MA et al (2002) Specificity of mammography and ultrasound in the evaluation of a palpable abnormality: retrospective review. Radiology 225:176–181

Nori J, Mazzocchi M (2003) Senologia. Stato dell'arte in interventistica. Napoli, Idelson-Gnocchi

Nystrom L, Andersson I, Bjurstam N et al (2002) Long-term effects of mammography screening: updated overview of the Swedish randomised trials. Lancet 359:909–19

Oellinger H, Heins S, Sander B et al (1993) Gd-DTPA-enhanced MRI of breast: the most sensitive method for detecting multicentric carcinomas in female breast? Eur Radiol 3:223–226

Panizza P, De Corbelli F, De Gaspari A et al (2003) MR-guided stereotactic breast biopsy: technical aspects and preliminary results. Radiol Med 106:232–44

Panizza P, De Gaspari A, Vanzulli A et al (1997) Role of MR mammography (MRM) in planning preoperative chemotherapy treatment and analyzing results. Eur Radiol 7:242

Parker SH, Klaus AJ, Schilling KJ et al (2001) Sonographically guided directional vacuum-assisted breast biopsy using a handled device. AJR 177:405–408

Perry NM (EUSOMA Working Party) (2001) Quality assurance in the diagnosis of breast disease. Eur J Cancer 37:159–172

Peto R et al (2000) UK and USA breast cancer deaths down 25% in year 2000 AD ages 20–69 years (letter). Lancet 20:1822

Pisano ED (2000) Current status of full field digital mammography. Radiology 214:26–28

Pisano ED, Fajardio LL, Caudry DJ et al (2001) Fine-needle aspiration biopsy of nonpalpable lesion in a multicenter clinical trial. Radiology 219:785–792

Pisano ED, Gatsonis C, Hendrick E et al (2005) For the Digital Mammographic Imaging Screening Trial (DMIST) Investigators Group. N Engl J Med 353:1773–1783

Piscioli F, Cristofolini M (1996) Modelli operativi di prevenzione secondaria del carcinoma della mammella. Trento, Tipolitografia Temi

Podo F, Sardanelli F, Canese R et al (2002) The Italian Multi-Centre Project on Evaluation of MRI and Other Imaging Modalities in Early Detection of Mammary Tumors in Subjects at High Genetic Risk. J Exp Clin Cancer Res 21/3:115–124

Raja MA, Hubbard A et al (2001) Interval breast cancer: is it a different type of breast cancer? Breast 10:100–108

Reynolds HE, Buckwalter KA, Jackson VP et al (1994) Comparison of mammography, sonography, and magnetic resonance imaging in the detection of silicone-gel breast implant rupture. Ann Plast Surg 33:247–257

Rieber A, Zeitler H, Rosenthal H et al (1997) MRI of breast cancer: influence of chemotherapy on sensitivity. Br J Radiol 70:452–458

Rizzatto G (2001) Towards a more sophisticated use of breast ultrasound. Eur Radiol 11:2425–2435

Rosen EL, Baker JA, Soo MS (2002) Malignant lesions initially subjected to short-term mammographic follow-up. Radiology 223:221–228

Rosselli del Turco M (1999) Programmi di screening per il carcinoma mammario. In: Veronesi U e Coll (eds) Senologia oncologica. Milano, Masson, pp 165–176

Sauer T, Myrvold K, Lomo J et al (2003) Fine-needle aspiration cytology in nonpalpable mammographic abnormalities in breast cancer screening. Breast 12:314–319

Schorn C, Fischer U, Luftner-Nagel S et al (1999) MRI of the breast in patients with metastatic disease of unknown primary. Eur Radiol 9:470–473

Shapiro S (1977) Evidence on screening for breast cancer from a randomized trial. Cancer 39:2772–2782

Sharan SK, Morimatsu M, Albrecht U et al (1997) Embryonic lethality and radiation hypersensitivity mediated by Rad51 in mice lacking Brca2. Nature 386: 804–810

Sickles EA, Wolverton DE, Dee KE (2002) Performance parameters for screening and diagnostic mammography: specialist and general radiologists. Radiology 224:861–869

Slanetz PJ, Edmister WB, Weisskoff RM et al (1998) Occult contralateral breast cancer detected by breast MR. Radiology 209:416

Smart CR, Hendrick RE, Rutledge JH et al (1995) Benefit of mammography screening in women ages 40 to 49 years. Cancer 75/7:1619–1626

Solomon B, Orel SG, Reynolds C et al (1998) Delayed development of enhancement in fat necrosis after breast conservation therapy: a potential pitfall of MR imaging of the breast. AJR 170:966–968

Stines J, Noel A, Levy L, et al (2002) Digital mammography and computer-assisted diagnosis. J Radiol 83:581–590

Sylvester PA, Vipond MN, Kutt E (1977) Rate and classification of interval cancers in the breast screening programme. Ann R Coll Surg Engl 79:276–277

Tavassoli FA, Devilee P (2003) Pathology and genetics of tumours of the breast and female genital organs. IARC (International Agency for Research on Cancer)–WHO–OMS. Lyon, IARC Press

Teifke A, Lehr HA, Vomweg TW et al (2003) Outcome analysis and rational management of enhancing lesions incidentally detected on contrast-enhanced MRI of the breast. AJR 181:655–662

Tilanus-Linthorst MM, Obdeijn IM, Bartels KC et al (2000) First experience in screening women at high risk for breast cancer with MR imaging. Breast Cancer Res Treat 63:53–60

Travis LB, Hill D, Dores GM et al (2003) Breast cancer following radiotherapy and chemotherapy among young women with Hodgkin's disease. JAMA 290:465–475

Travis LB, Hill D, Dores GM et al (2005) Cumulative absolute breast cancer risk for young women treated for Hodgkin's lymphoma. J Natl Cancer Inst 97:1428–1437

Vanara F, Ponti A, Frigerio A et al (1995) Analisi dei costi di un programma di screening mammografico. Epidemiologia e prevenzione 19:318–329

Viehweg P, Heinig A, Amaya B et al (2002) MR-guided interventional breast procedures considering vacuum biopsy in particular. Eur Radiol 42/1:32–39

Wald NJ, Chamberlain J, Hackshav A (1993) Report of the European Society for Mastology on Breast Cancer Screening. Breast 2:209–216

Warren R, Eleti A (2006) Overdiagnosis and overtreatment of breast cancer. Is overdiagnosis an issue for radiologists? Breast Cancer Research 8:205

Wasser K, Sinn HP, Fink C et al (2003) Accuracy of tumor size measurement in breast cancer using MRI is influenced by histological regression induced by neoadjuvant chemotherapy. Eur Radiol 6:1213–1223

Weiss NS (2003) Breast cancer mortality in relation to clinical breast examination and breast self-examination. Breast J 9:86–89

Wittingam TA (1999) Tissue harmonic imaging. Eur Radiol 9:323–326

Zackrisson S, Andersson I, Janzon L et al (2006) Rate of overdiagnosis of breast cancer 15 years after end of Malmo mammographic screening trial: follow-up study. BMJ 332:689–692

Zappa M, Falini P, Bonardi D et al (2002) Monitoring interval cancers in mammographic screening: the Florence district programme experience. Breast 11:301–305

Zonderland HM, Coerkamp EG, Hermans J et al (1999) Diagnosis of breast cancer: contribution of US as an adjunct to mammography. Radiology 213:413–422

New Trends of MRI in Breast Cancer Diagnosis

10

Daniele Vergnaghi, Giovanna Trecate, and Siranoush Manoukian

CONTENTS

10.1 Introduction

Magnetic resonance imaging (MRI) was first applied to the evaluation of breast parenchyma in the late 1980s, mainly in women with proven carcinomas. Heywang and coworkers (1986) discovered that breast cancer is associated with significant enhancement following the intravenous injection of contrast medium (gadolinium dimeglumine, e.g., Gd-DTPA). The pathophysiological basis of this enhancement has been extensively investigated. Folkman first described the biological rule of capillary vessels for the nutrition of normal tissues and arrived at the discovery that malignant tissues need a supplementary inflow of nutritional factors. For this reason, they are able to release some specific proteins that induce new vessel growth (vascular endothelial growth factor, VEGF) (Folkman 1985, Folkman et al. 1987; Folkman 2002; Weidner et al. 1991; Hanahan et al. 1996; Gimbrone et al. 1972).

The new, malignant vascular dragnet has an anarchic distribution, and the single capillary structure shows pathological wall architecture. The results of angiogenetic activity in MRI are then summarized in an increased vascularity leading to a grown inflow of contrast material and in a major permeability leading to a precocious wash out of gadolinium.

In radiological practice, the angiogenetic consequence is then represented by the early and stronger uptake of contrast medium within cancer foci. This fundamental concept led to establishing a new manner of diagnostic approach that introduces the dynamic analysis of breast parenchyma beside its morphologic evaluation. Dynamic analysis consists of the acquisition of one pre-contrast and a series of post-contrast sequences, covering both breasts, at the highest possible temporal resolution.

The earliest studies were performed with T1-weighted spin echo sequences with an imaging time of approximately 5 min and slice thickness of 5 mm. Limited numbers of slices were available for the dynamic evaluation, and slices were interleaved by a small gap. The result was a reduction in spatial resolution.

With the development of fast T1-weighted gradient echo pulse sequences, dynamic imaging of the entire breast with thinner and contiguous sections has become possible. The analysis of the same voxel over several minutes generates a signal intensity curve that quantifies the rate and velocity of any enhancing region. Starting from this double possibility of morphologic and dynamic analysis, two different schools evolved, both of them with good results in terms of diagnosis. The European school focused attention on dynamic evaluation and the distinction of benign from malignant lesions on the basis of their enhancement characteristics at high temporal resolution. The US school based the diagnosis on the analysis of morphological characteristics exhibited by malignant disease at high spatial resolution.

At the dawn of MR imaging, optimization of both spatial and temporal resolution was impossible: high temporal resolution implied a sensible loss in number and thickness of slices, thus compromising the sensitivity for small and multifocal breast carcinomas. On the other hand, the cost of high spatial resolution was represented by a sensible elongation of time acquisition for each sequence. Moreover, high anatomical resolution analysis needs in general to be performed only on one breast and in the sagittal plane. Beside to improve the detectability of smaller enhancing lesions, the US school prefers fat suppression sequences, adding further scan time. Thanks to progressive technology advances, the two strategies today can converge rather than compromise each other.

New emerging techniques such as parallel imaging that uses multiple MRI received coil elements to encode spatial information, and new macromolecular contrasts that diffuse less rapidly than gadolinium may in fact improve very high spatial and temporal resolution. Nowadays, a satisfactory compromise is attempted between time acquisition sequences that do not exceed 1 min and are provided with slice thickness of 1 or 2 mm and a 512 matrix. Both breasts are represented in axial or coronal plane. The main advantage of coronal acquisition is the reduction of acquisition time as it allows a rectangular FOV. This plane allows also a better view of the axilla, and it is thus preferable after breast conservative therapies. On the other hand, it is more sensible than the breathing motion.

The axial plane follows vascular structures of the breast parenchyma better, which is helpful in distinguishing blood vessels from ductal disease. Further, it better describes the region of the nipple. On the other hand, it is more sensible than cardiac pulsation artifacts.

Maximum intensity projection (MIP) is a dedicated software that can be very helpful in distinguishing blood vessels from suspicious lesions. Moreover, new diagnostic strategies always continue to be improved by imaging technology.

For non-palpable breast lesions that are only detectable on MRI, it may be difficult to obtain adequate material for pathological examination. Thus, MRI-guided wire localization and needle biopsy have been developed to obtain interesting results (Landheer et al. 2006). Recently, also spectroscopy has been applied to breast evaluation searching for molecular peak differences between malignant lesions and benign or normal tissues (Hsiang et al. 2005; Manton et al. 2006).

Last introduced was diffusion-perfusion imaging (Charles-Edwards et al. 2006; Marini et al. 2007). Based on thermal movement of the molecules, diffusion of water in tissues is measured to obtain diffusion imaging in MR. Diffusion contrast on MRI represents the strength of water molecular microscopic motion. To create diffusion contrast, there are some dedicated sequences that switch to different gradients giving a specific coefficient. The diffusion coefficient is a measure of the velocity of diffusion within different tissues. Diffusion imaging calculates the average of diffusion coefficient for each voxel, deriving the so-called apparent diffusion coefficient map. The ADC map is exploitable today to differentiate benign from malignant lesions, where the augmented cellularity of cancer restricts water motion into reduced extracellular spaces.

As introduced before, both morphological and dynamic parameters have to be integrated to better assess the characterization of enhancing lesions. The first distinction should be between mass and non-mass enhancement. In the first case morphologic patterns to consider are the characteristics of margins (smooth or spiculated) and edges (well or ill defined) and enhancement uptake (homogeneous or inhomogeneous rim enhancement). Also the distribution of the enhancement mass is important (single, multiple, scattered or clumped). If non-mass enhancement is recognized, this can be regional, diffuse, linear or branching. Dynamic patterns are represented on the time/intensity curve, where we can read the precocity and rate of enhancement, signal intensity behavior and eventual wash out.

Kuhl distinguishes three types of time/intensity curve according to the most common behavior of signal intensity within breast lesions. In synthesis, she points out how these curves reflect angiogenetic processes. Within this group, the most suggestive for malignancy is in fact the curve with rapid, strong and early wash in that raises up to significant rates and is followed by a typical washout. The current trend is to follow the recently published MRI Lexicon (MRI BIRADS) (Ikeda 2001).

High soft tissue contrast and high spatial resolution are the most important factors at the basis of high sensitivity of MRI, even in dense breast tissue. Faced with high sensitivity, MRI specificity achieves less encouraging results. In fact, both morphologic and dynamic overlaps exist between benign and malignant lesions.

Benign diseases in fact are often well vascularized. MRI semiology aims at the detection of foci with quantitative major inflow of gadolinium, but MRI software cannot make a qualitative distinction between high benign vascularization and neoangiogenetic vessels.

According to these considerations, it should be underlined that MRI cannot be proposed as the first diagnostic approach to breast analysis. To reduce false-positive results sometimes related to hormonal influences, it must be remembered that breast MRI examination should be performed within the 2nd or the 3rd week of the ovarian cycle and eventually 1 or 2 months after suspension of replacement hormone treatment.

Current indications where MRI is believed to integrate with conventional imaging for ruling out more information include:

- evaluation of patients with axillary metastatic lymph nodes and undetectable primitive cancer by means of mammography or sonography
- staging of the extent of cancer when a single focus has been diagnosed and breast conservative therapy is considered
- follow-up after breast conserving surgery and radiotherapy
- surveillance of women at a high risk of genetically induced breast cancer
- assessing tumor response to neoadjuvant chemotherapy
- evaluation of breast implants
- evaluation of breast with questionable findings at conventional imaging

Among these indications, staging of DCIS and invasive cancer, detection of cancer recurrence and surveillance of high-risk women are more often applied in clinical diagnostics.

10.2 Staging

Accurate staging of breast carcinoma is of primary relevance to plan the best treatment options. Knowledge of the tumor extent can decide which patients can be addressed to mastectomy and which others to breast conservation. The main factors that influence the choice of surgical therapy include first of all tumor size and tumor volume related to breast volume. Tumor location and its relationship with the surrounding anatomical structures are also relevant features. Psychological factors cannot be underestimated, and they may also influence therapeutic strategies. Contraindications for breast conservation include multicentric disease (cancer involving multiple quadrants) and a previous surgical conservative action (Winchester and Cox 1992). Multifocal disease (multiple cancer foci within the same quadrant) can theoretically be addressed to quadrantectomy. Breast conservative surgery combined with radiation therapy has been shown not to change mortality in patients with stage 1 and 2 (following the tumor node metastasis system), but the recurrence frequency is higher (1%–2% per year) than recurrence rate in patients who undergo mastectomy (Veronesi et al. 1981).

Incomplete excision of eventual smaller cancer foci not detected at conventional imaging may be the reason for these relapses. The incidence of multicentric focal breast cancer is reported to range from 9% to 75% (Baker 1982; Holland et al. 1985). In patients with clinically occult, non-palpable breast cancer detected by mammography, Schwartz et al. (1980) reported a multicentricity incidence rate of 44%. Moreover, accurate assessment of the disease decreases the rate of positive margins after lumpectomy.

It has been demonstrated that incomplete tumor excision can be another reason for higher recurrence rates (Scmidt-Ullrich et al. 1989; Blamey 1989). Hence, the more detailed the information about the true extension of the disease is, the lower the possibility of cancer recurrence. Possible pitfalls for conventional imaging are related to parenchyma density, nodular structure, presence of scar related to previous surgery or biopsy and prosthesis. Moreover, some histology may easily remain undetected. This happens for lobular infiltrative cancer, which infiltrates without significant stoma reaction and for extensive intraductal non-calcified component associated with the more evident infiltrative component.

MRI imaging gives more diagnostic opportunities because of its high spatial resolution, which allows the depiction of smaller lesions and high soft tissue contrast that removes the problem of breast density.

At the basis of MRI global major sensitivity is the fact that this technique recognizes cancer by detecting its pathologic vascularization, known as neoangiogenesis, while conventional imaging demonstrates only morphologic changes within the parenchyma. Moreover, MRI is a multiplanar diagnostic tool, and this is very helpful to recognize the involvement of other anatomical structures surrounding the parenchyma, such as skin, musculature or chest wall.

Many studies have documented the high sensitivity of MRI in the detection of invasive breast cancer. The reported rates rise up to 94–99% (Oellinger et al. 1993; Harms et al. 1989; Heywang et al. 1989; Boetes et al. 1995; Mumtaz et al. 1997). This sensitivity allows a better measurement of the primary tumor, which determines the chemotherapy choice, and a better evaluation of the margins of cancer.

Concerning multifocal-multicentric disease, some authors confirmed the superiority of MRI in detecting unsuspected smaller cancer foci not detectable at conventional imaging (Oellinger et al. 1993; Harms et al. 1989; Heywang et al. 1989; Boetes et al. 1995; Mumtaz et al. 1997).

Nowadays, in clinical practice, when conventional imaging has demonstrated a probably malignant lesion and breast-conserving therapy is considered, preoperative breast MRI should be recommended to localize additional breast cancer foci.

Moreover, MRI is indicated in case of lobular cancers, knowing the difficulties of diagnosing this pathological histotype at mammography and sonography. Recently, some authors (Fischer et al. 1999; Lee et al. 2003; Liberman et al. 2003) indicated that MRI preoperative analysis introduces some relevant information about the true extent of the disease (Fig. 10.1).

Concerning axillary lymph nodes, there is still little information that we can receive by MRI analysis both because of the site of the axilla that is exposed to cardiac pulsation artifact and because actual contrast medium cannot differentiate between benign or malignant nodes.

It has to be remembered that the sensitivity for detection DCIS is reported to be lower than that for invasive carcinoma (Gilles et al. 1995; Orel et al. 1997; Soderstrom et al. 1996; Ikeda et al. 2000). This can be related both to the kind of sequences applied at the study of the breast and to the too many tiny angiogenetic factors associated with the smaller lesion. For this reason, a suspicious mammographic finding should be biopsied despite a negative MRI examination (Westerhof et al. 1998). In contrast with high sensitivity, false-positive findings have to be accounted for. Specificity rates range in fact from 37% to 97% (Harms et al. 1989; Heywang et al.1989; Fischer et al. 1999; Orel et al. 1995; Kaiser and Zeitler 1989; Orel et al. 1994).

At the basis of this problem, there is the fact that if MRI can demonstrate focal areas of major vascularization, it still gives only a quantitative evaluation without discrimination between high benign vascularization (inflammatory disease, dysplasia) and neoplastic neoangiogenesis.

The false-positive findings may become a serious problem when it is necessary to decide whether to apply conservative or radical surgery or when there is a suspected lesion in the contralateral breast. For this reason, histological proof of all suspected lesions seen on MRI must be taken by percutaneous or surgical biopsy before deciding on conservative or demolitive surgery.

For smaller lesions, seen only at MRI, there are two possibilities. The first is a careful ultrasound second look on the basis of the MRI report (Panizza et al. 1997). Sometimes this procedure leads to recognizing the foci of cancer. The second choice is the MRI-guided wire localization and needle biopsy.

In conclusion, MRI can be very helpful in staging breast cancer and thus in planning the therapeutic approach. Due to the high sensitivity of MRI in detecting invasive carcinoma, a negative MRI evaluation can reliably exclude the presence of cancer (Morris et al. 1997). Because of its lower specificity, MRI cannot replace conventional imaging, but it remains a complementary analysis.

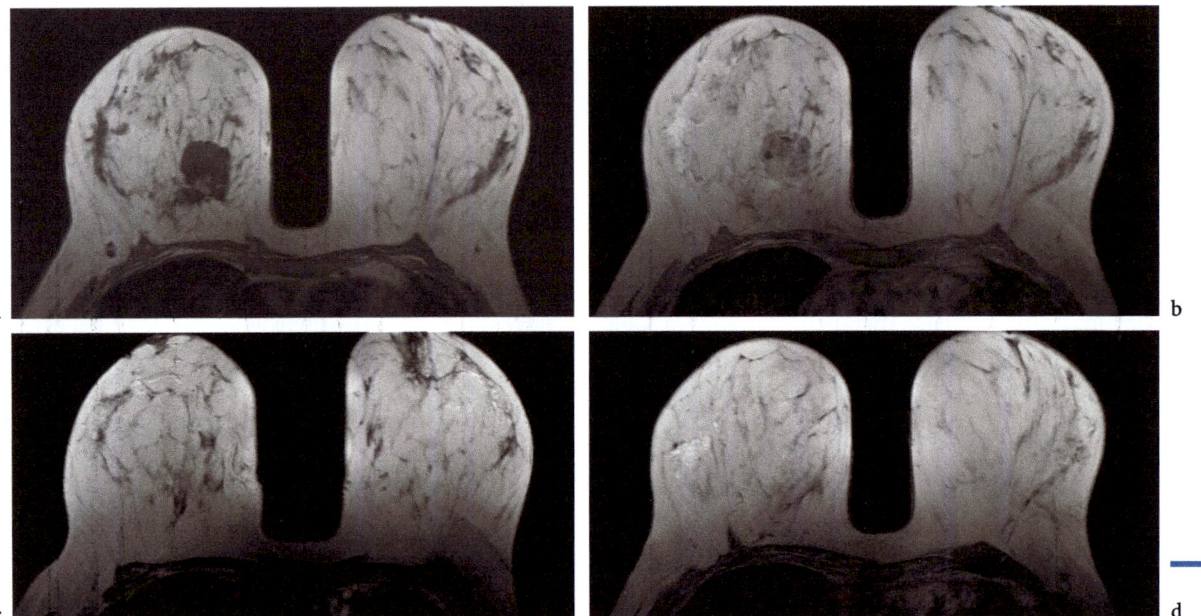

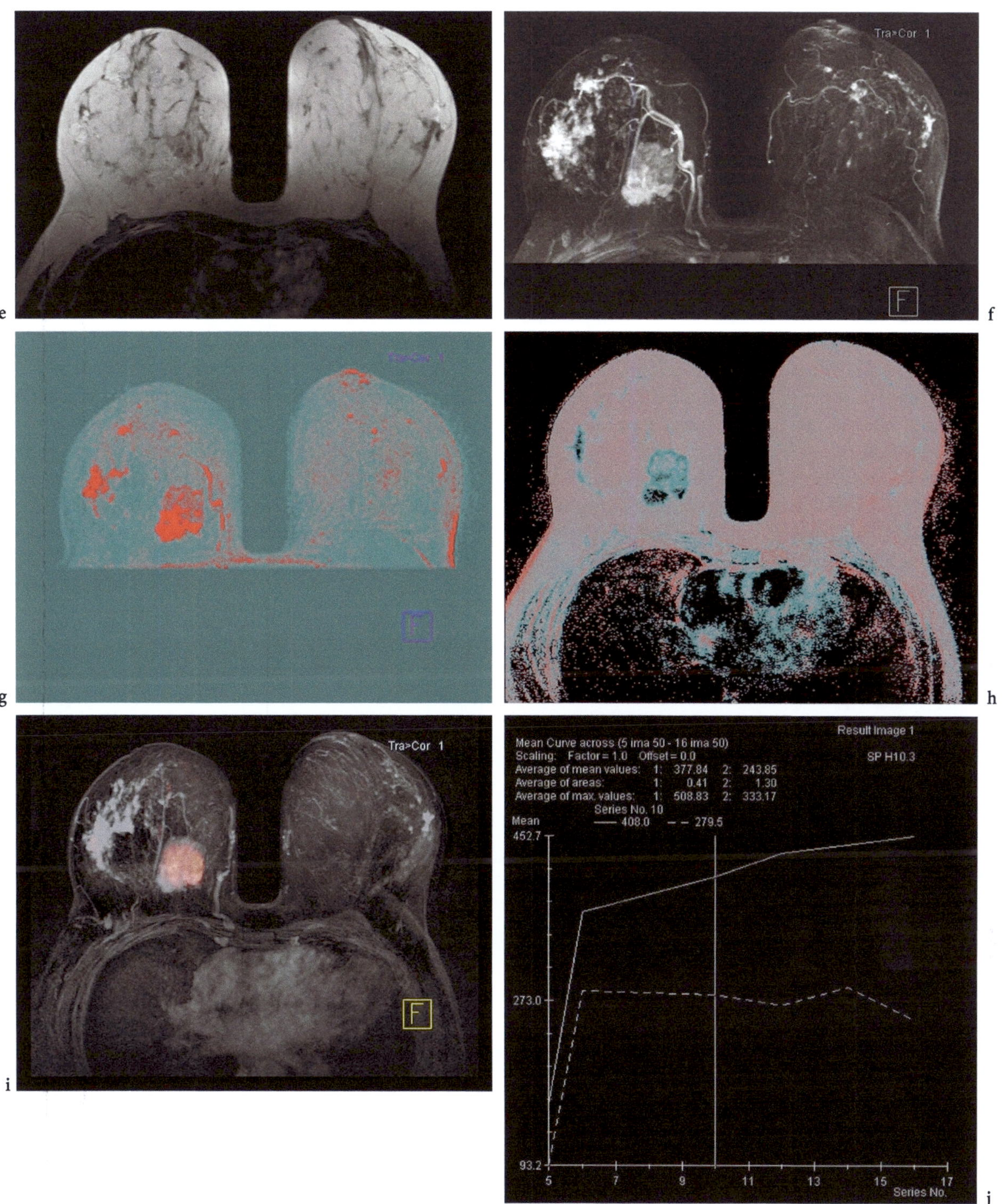

Fig. 10.1a–j. Mass enhancement due to a ductal invasive carcinoma in the upper medial quadrant of the right breast. T1 (**a**) and T1 intermediate postcontrast sequence (**b**) with slice thickness of 1.8 mm. **c–e** T1 intermediate postcontrast sequence. Both breasts show also a highly suspicious multiple clumped foci of enhancement in the outer quadrants of both breasts that histology confirmed to be intraductal extension of the disease. Notice the high anatomical detail provided with very small slice thickness. **f** Note on MIP reconstruction the higher vascularity of the invasive histotype. **g,h** Wash-in and wash-out maps point out the high vascularity of larger tumor lesions. **i** This image represents an assemblage of MIP reconstruction and diffusion map. It highlights the different vascularization between normal parenchyma and neoplastic tissue. **j** Time intensity curve on the larger lesion confirms its suspected nature

10.3 DCIS

Microcalcifications can be the only sign of clinically occult breast carcinoma, and in most cases such findings are supported by ductal carcinoma in situ (DCIS). DCIS is a neoplastic, but not infiltrative lesion, and it consists of an atypical proliferation of epithelial calls without invasion through the basement membrane into the periductal connective tissue (Page and Rogers 1992).

DCIS is not a single entity, but a heterogeneous group of lesions that may differ in biological behavior, growth pattern and histopathological features. Several schemes of classifications have been proposed for DCIS.

Traditionally, it was classified on the basis of the architectural growth pattern and cell type within two main subgroups: comedo type if associated with the presence of comedonecrosis within ducts and non-comedo type. More recently, Holland et al. (1994) introduced a new pathologic classification based on the cytonuclear and architectural growth pattern, which distinguishes among well, intermediate or poorly differentiated DCIS. Silverstein proposed the Van Nuys classification, which considers the presence or the absence both of high nuclear grade and comedo-type necrosis.

These histopathological classifications are directed at recognizing the degree of aggressiveness of DCIS for better therapeutic management. Due to the peculiarity of its calcium deposits, mammography is the most sensitive technique to depict DCIS. With the advent of mammographic screening, the percentage of diagnosed DCIS breast cancer has risen from about 1% to 15–25% (Ernster et al. 1996; Silverstein et al. 1996). The mammographic classification follows the LeGal scheme, which distinguishes microcalcifications in five subtypes on the basis of their morphology and with growing malignant predictive value (LeGal et al. 1984).

Although it has high sensitivity, mammography may "lose" both multifocal non-calcified lesions and wider intraductal extent (Stomper and Connolly 1992; Holland et al. 1990). Moreover, radiological patterns can be non-specific in distinguishing those benign entities that can also produce calcium deposits. With the advent of MRI, huge hope was addressed to the resolution of these diagnostic problems. If sensitivity of MRI in depicting invasive carcinomas rose to satisfactory results (Heywang et al.1989; Kaiser and Zeitler 1989; Drew et al. 1999), sensitivity rates were less encouraging (Gilles et al. 1995; Viehweg et al. 2000; Heywang 1994).

The analysis of these data (Orel et al. 1997; Zuiani et al. 2002) led us to find that the reason for these differences were the tumor size, the tumor grade, some tumoral histological features or different MRI parameters applied in MR imaging. Concerning tumor size, if the DCIS is smaller than the voxel of MR imaging, breast normal parenchyma may hide the lesion. However, some DCIS greater than 1 cm have been described as not enhancing at MRI (Boetes et al. 1995; Stomper et al. 1995).

This directed attention to possible biological differences, mainly on the differences between comedo and non-comedo types. Boetes first underlined that non-comedo enhanced less than the comedo type (Boetes et al. 1995), but later other authors found the same behavior (Gilles et al. 1995; Orel et al. 1995; Heywang 1994; Stomper et al. 1995) in both of these subtypes. Last, angiogenesis has once again been demonstrated to be the most important factor for MR imaging.

It has been established that malignant lesions release angiogenetic factors (vascular endothelial growth factor, VEGF) that induce sprouting and growth of pre-existing capillaries and the formation of new vessels. However, angiogenesis starts for tumor lesions exceeding 2 mm in diameter. Thus, very small lesions with a few angiogenic changes may not enhance at MRI evaluation (Gilles et al. 1995). Thanks to the development of MRI machines, breast coils and sequences, it has become easier to detect and better diagnose even smaller foci of DCIS (Fig. 10.2).

Nowadays, with the most modern MRI devices that allow applying a slice thickness of 1 or 2 mm, it is possible to reveal the smaller intraductal extension (Figs. 10.2, 10.3).

When associated with enhancement, DCIS may reveal slight differences both in morphologic and dynamic behavior if compared with invasive carcinomas. Considering morphology, DCIS may appear as a linear enhancement, simple or branched according to the anatomy of the ducts (Figs. 10.3, 10.4).

It may show a nodular enhancement, single or multiple. Nodular enhancement representing DCIS mainly has well-defined margins, while spiculated edges and rim enhancement are more frequently associated with invasive cancer. In our experience, when the morphological pattern is represented by multiple nodular enhancement, these are usually unilateral, very small (3D sequences mandatory), more frequently clumped (Trecate et al. 2002), and very close each other, representing an organized pathological entity, growing along the architecture of ducts. The last morphological pattern of DCIS is represented by a regional enhancement (Fig. 10.5).

Multiple nodular and regional enhancements are unfortunately also often associated with benign disease, especially with the group of dysplasia (Fig. 10.6).

There are some factors that can help the differential diagnosis. Multiple, stippled or regional enhancement represented in both breasts and with a scattered, anarchic distribution is in fact more frequently related to dysplasia. Despite these parameters, it is often quite impossible to distinguish between the benign and malignant nature of enhancement.

Also considering dynamic curves, DCIS may exhibit two orders of differences if compared to infiltrative carcinoma. These differences may even stress the difficulty in the differential diagnosis between DCIS and dysplasia.

The first is represented by dynamic curves that may mimic benign lesions: lack of early contrast enhancement and absence of a peak within the first 2 min (Kuhl et al. 1999; Trecate et al. 2002). The explanation of this phenomenon is given once more by angiogenesis. Lesions that are too small with few angiogenic changes seem unable to provide the MRI device's software with enough valuable pixels to allow elaboration of a typically malignant curve shape. The quantitative analysis of these curves, however, reveals in general a significant increase in signal intensity (in our experience =/˜70%) (Trecate et al. 2002).

The second problem is represented by those well-vascularized benign diseases whose dynamic curves reproduce the malignant shape: speed of uptake, peak of enhancement and significant percentage of uptake. A possible explication for such behavior is still debated.

Some authors underline that some benign lesions have been demonstrated to be able to induce angiogenesis (Heywang 1994). It must be remembered that many benign lesions are simply associated with high vascularization. This behavior is at the basis of the decrease in specificity registered for MRI. MRI signal intensity and dynamic curves correspond in fact to quantitative parameters, but they are not able to distinguish between the benign or malignant nature of the enhancement.

In conclusion, MRI cannot be considered as a reliable technique to state the nature of microcalcifications because there are too many morphologic and dynamic overlaps between benign and malignant lesions. The practical consequence is that MRI is not recommended for evaluating mammographic indeterminate microcalcifications. On the other hand, when mammographic microcalcifications are suspected, the high sensitivity of MRI may be very helpful in determining the true extent of the disease and its eventual multifocality.

10.4 Breast Cancer Recurrence

Several studies have demonstrated no differences in disease-free survival for tumorectomy and radial therapy versus mastectomy (Veronesi et al. 1981; Sarrazin et al. 1984; Fisher et al. 1985) with better cosmetic and psychological outcomes. Breast conservative surgery combined with radiation therapy has therefore become the treatment of choice for early stage T1 and T2. The remaining breast parenchyma is however at risk of recurrence. Follow-up for these patients includes a periodical physical examination and mammography every 6 months during the first 2 years and every year thereafter. The rate of local tumor recurrence is 1–2% year (Dershaw 1995; Neff et al. 1996). Some patients are at higher risk for inadequate treatment mostly in the presence of invasive cancer with an extensive intraductal component or for large pure intraductal carcinomas. Moreover, previous cancer is known as a risk factor for cancer in the contralateral breast (Gajalakshmi et al.1999; Belli et al. 2002) (Fig. 10.7).

Because the survival rate is directly related to the size of tumor recurrence, its early detection should be mandatory to improve the prognosis. Several studies have demonstrated a lack of specificity of mammography in detecting local recurrence (Stomper et al. 1987; Dershaw et al. 1990; Solin et al. 1990). Breast parenchyma encounters in fact some changes after surgery and irradiation. Post-irradiation mammographic findings are related firstly to vascular dilatation and capillary damage that promote increased blood flow with edema and later to parenchyma retraction due to fibrosis. Also calcifications may occur.

Postoperative mammographic changes are represented by hematoma, fat tissue necrosis, scar tissue development and parenchyma distortion. All of these findings may hide or mimic true cancer relapse (Fig. 10.8).

Heywang-Köbrunner (1993) first investigated MRI enhancement of breast tissue during variable time intervals after therapy. She described that up to 9 months after therapy differentiation between post-therapeutic changes and recurrence is frequently impossible because of the strong enhancement of the all-glandular tissue. Ten to 18 months after therapy, this enhancement subsides slowly, while after 18 months, no significant enhancement was encountered in normal breast in her study.

Nowadays, conventional ranges of 6 months after surgery and 12 months after radiotherapy are commonly considered as acceptable to avoid problematic enhancement post-therapy. Morphologic and dynamic patterns of cancer recurrence are the same as cancer at its first presentation: nodular, linear or regional enhancement, with early and intense uptake.

However, because of a possible previous scar or fibrosis, fader enhancement within morphologic suspected patterns should be considered with caution. In case of suspected recurrence, the MRI rule is to establish a differential diagnosis between cancer tissue supported by angiogenesis and fibrotic scar known to have a very poor vascularization.

For this reason, beside the high sensitivity of the technique, also specificity raises up to interesting levels within this chapter of breast disease.

In conclusion, contrast-enhanced MRI has been demonstrated to improve the diagnostic accuracy in cancer relapse detection, especially in those cases where mammographic or clinical diagnosis is uncertain due to dense or irregularly shaped tissue. In case of mammographic, sonographic or clinical suspicion of local tumor recurrence, MRI should be performed before biopsy is planned. If non-contrast enhancement occurs, biopsy may not be necessary because of the high negative predictive value of the technique.

10.5 MRI in Women with High Genetic Risk of Breast Cancer

Although the majority of breast cancer is considered sporadic, arising in women without a significant family history, nearly 5% to 10% of all breast cancers are actually attributable to an inherited predisposition. Today some highly penetrant genes have been discovered, and although *BRCA*1 and *BRCA*2 are actually the main genes identified, they explain less than one third of all the hereditary breast cancer cases; the remaining genes are still to be identified (Narod and Foulkes 2004).

*BRCA*1 and *BRCA*2 germline mutations confer a lifetimerisk of breast cancer ranging from 60 to 80% in different studies. *BRCA* carriers usually develop breast cancer at a younger age, with much of this risk occurring between 30 and 50 years (Antoniou et al. 2003). Moreover, carriers face an almost 30% risk of contralateral breast cancer at 10 years following a first diagnosis (Pierce et al. 2006). *BRCA* mutations also confer a lifetime risk for ovarian cancer, about 40% for *BRCA*1 mutations and 20% for *BRCA*2 mutations, respectively (Antoniou et al. 2003). Breast cancer associated with *BRCA*1 mutations often shows adverse histopathological features such as a high proliferation rate, high nuclear grading and hormone receptor negativity, and may display a more aggressive biological behavior than sporadic breast cancer (Foulkes et al. 2006) (Fig. 10.9).

Given the substantial risk faced by women with a hereditary predisposition to breast cancer, adapted strategies are crucial for their management. Primary prevention, based on prophylactic bilateral mastectomy, appears to be the most effective way to avoid breast cancer, with a risk reduction of at least 90%. Although marked differences exist between different countries, prophylactic mastectomy is not usually considered the first choice for the majority of carrier women,

Fig. 10.2. a–c Suspicious microcalcifications of the left breast. Microcalcifications are located in the deepest portion of the parenchyma, almost close to pectoral fascia. Note their low visibility on middle oblique projection because of their position. **d–g** Subtraction images with slice thickness of 2.5 mm. MRI revealed tiny pathological multiple foci even anteriorly to the site of microcalcifications, both between upper and between lower quadrants of the left breast. Note the lower anatomical detail with thicker slices. **h** Time-intensity curves of small enhancing foci. Histology confirmed intraductal extended DCIS

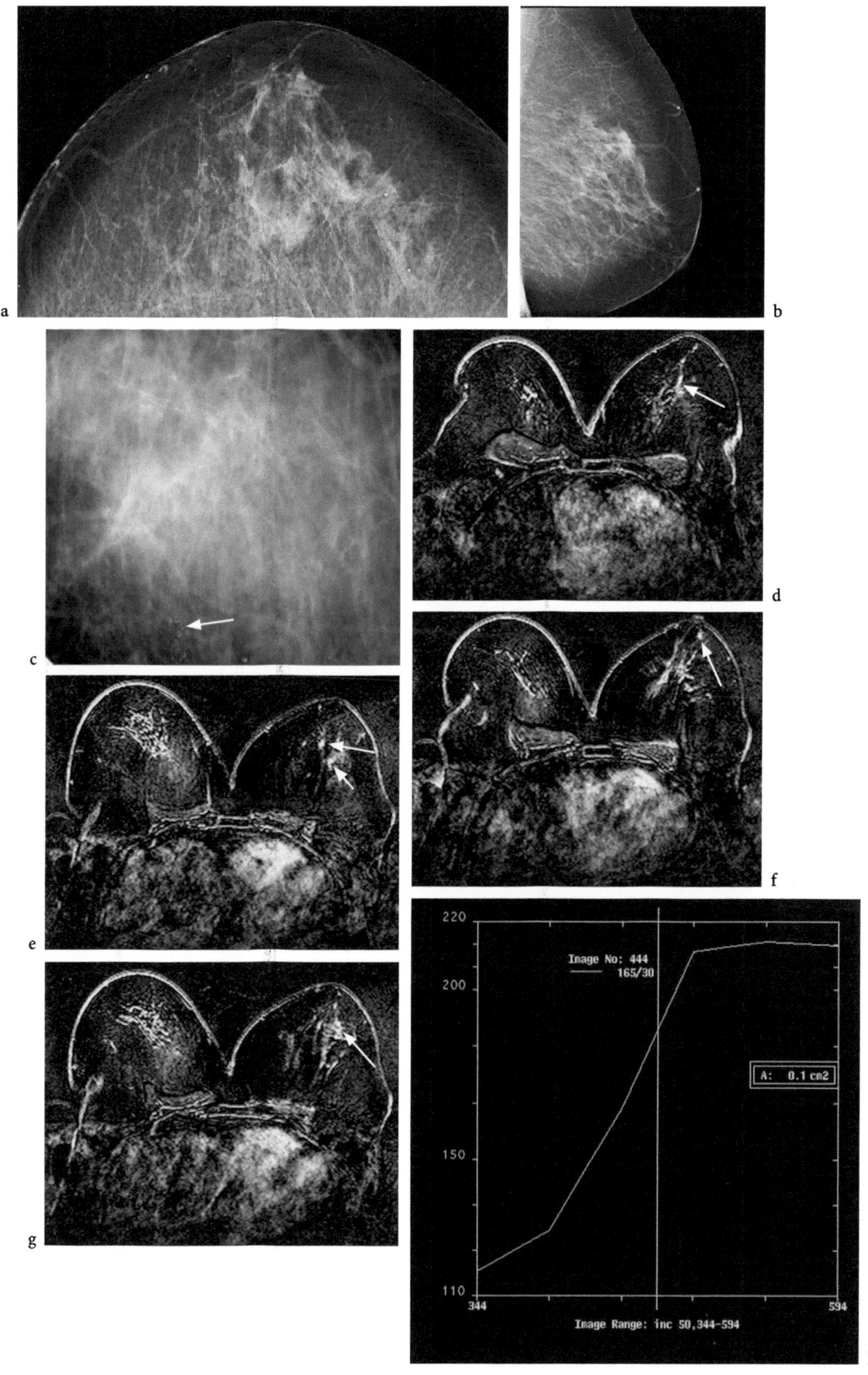
a
b
c
d
e
f
g
h
220
200
150
110
344
594
Image No: 444
165/30
A: 0.1 cm2
Image Range: inc 50,344-594

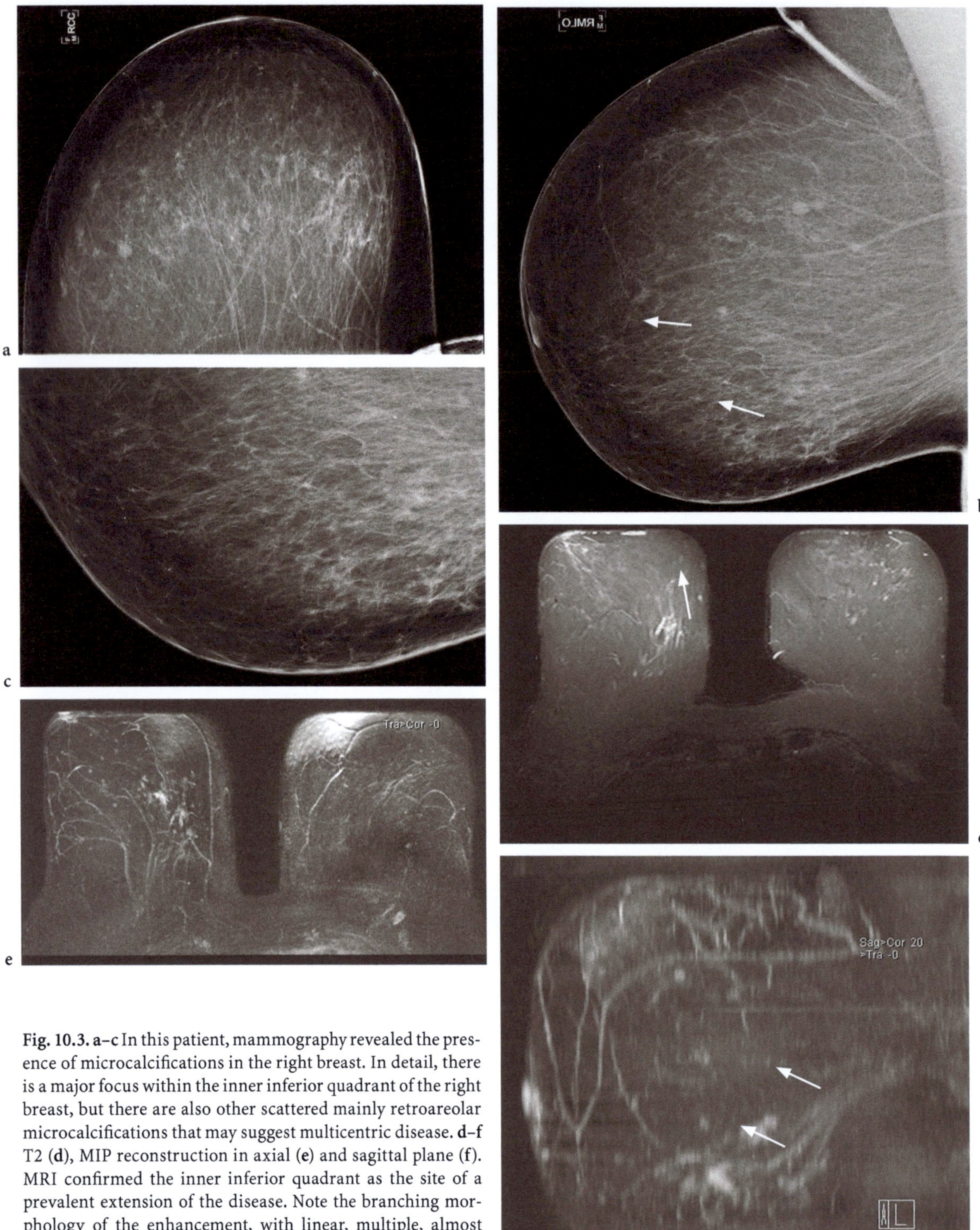

Fig. 10.3. a–c In this patient, mammography revealed the presence of microcalcifications in the right breast. In detail, there is a major focus within the inner inferior quadrant of the right breast, but there are also other scattered mainly retroareolar microcalcifications that may suggest multicentric disease. **d–f** T2 (**d**), MIP reconstruction in axial (**e**) and sagittal plane (**f**). MRI confirmed the inner inferior quadrant as the site of a prevalent extension of the disease. Note the branching morphology of the enhancement, with linear, multiple, almost contiguous irregular ducts. They are shown within the parenchyma as ductal structures stuffed with pathological cells. Moreover, there are other multiple nodular small enhancements in the external lower quadrant and in the middle of the parenchyma. These are less organized, very small, and more difficult to correctly identify as benign or as extension of the disease

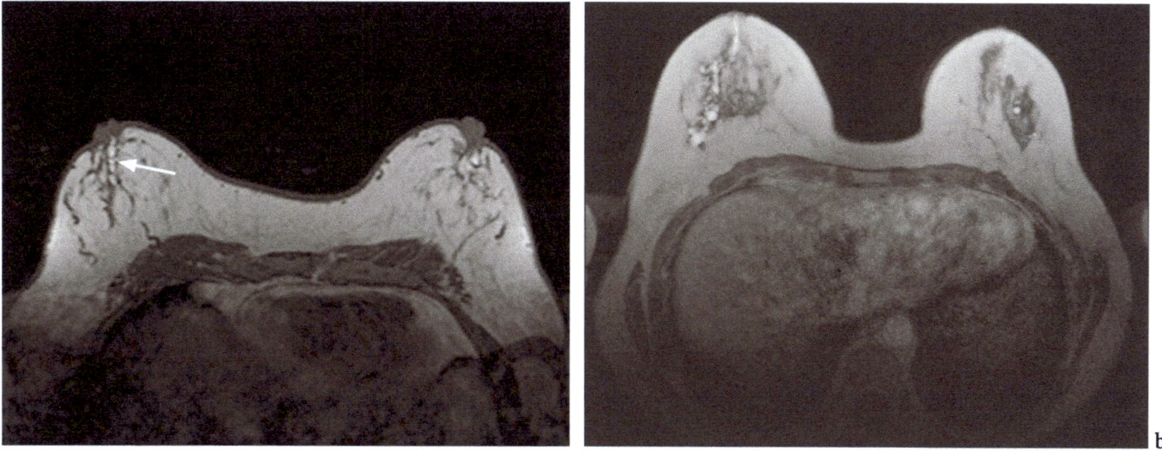

Fig. 10.4a,b. Ductal retroareolar images. Some examples of ductal hyperintensity on T1 sequences within some main ducts in patients with hematic nipple discharge

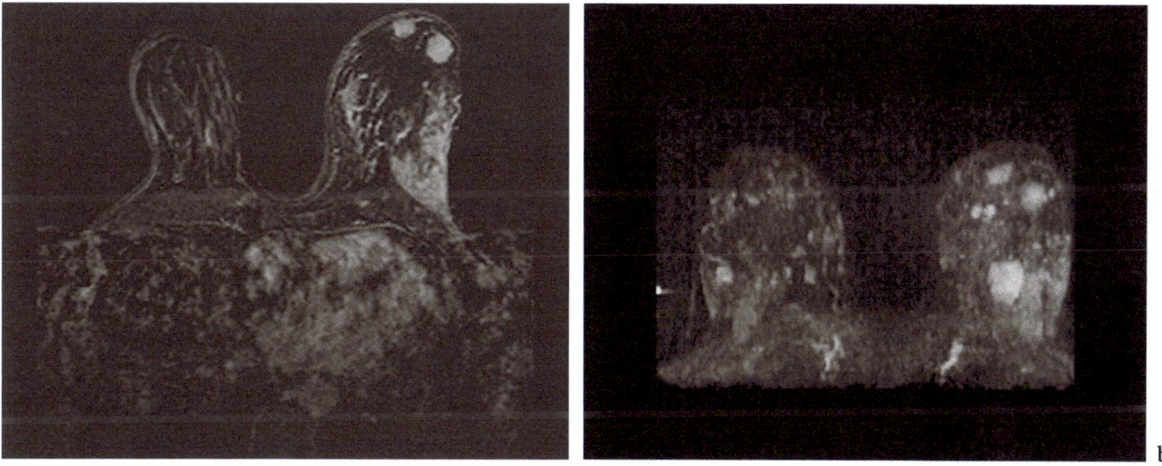

Fig. 10.5. a Regional non-mass enhancement on a subtracted image in the upper external quadrant of the left breast close to some benign fibroadenomas. b The same finding after MIP reconstruction

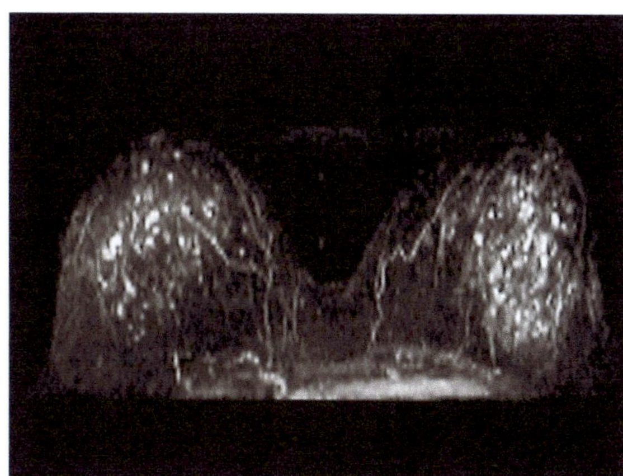

Fig. 10.6. Typical multinodular diffuse bilateral enhancement. This presentation is often associated with highly vascularized benign dysplasia. It is also true that among all of these enhancing lesions, it is quite impossible to rule out eventual small intraductal foci

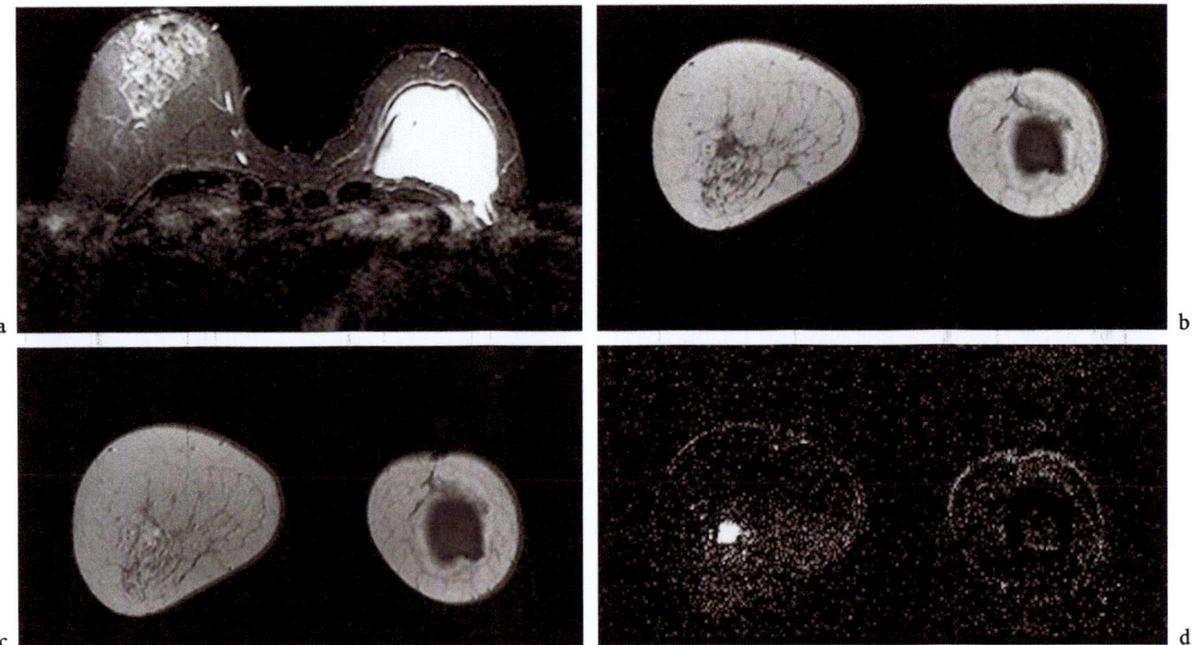

Fig. 10.7. a T2 in axial plane, T1 (**b**) and T1 postcontrast (**c**) in coronal plane and subtracted (**d**) coronal images. Patient with previous left mastectomy for invasive ductal carcinoma and contemporary right breast reduction. MRI executed to analyze left breast implant integrity revealed cancer recurrence in the right breast

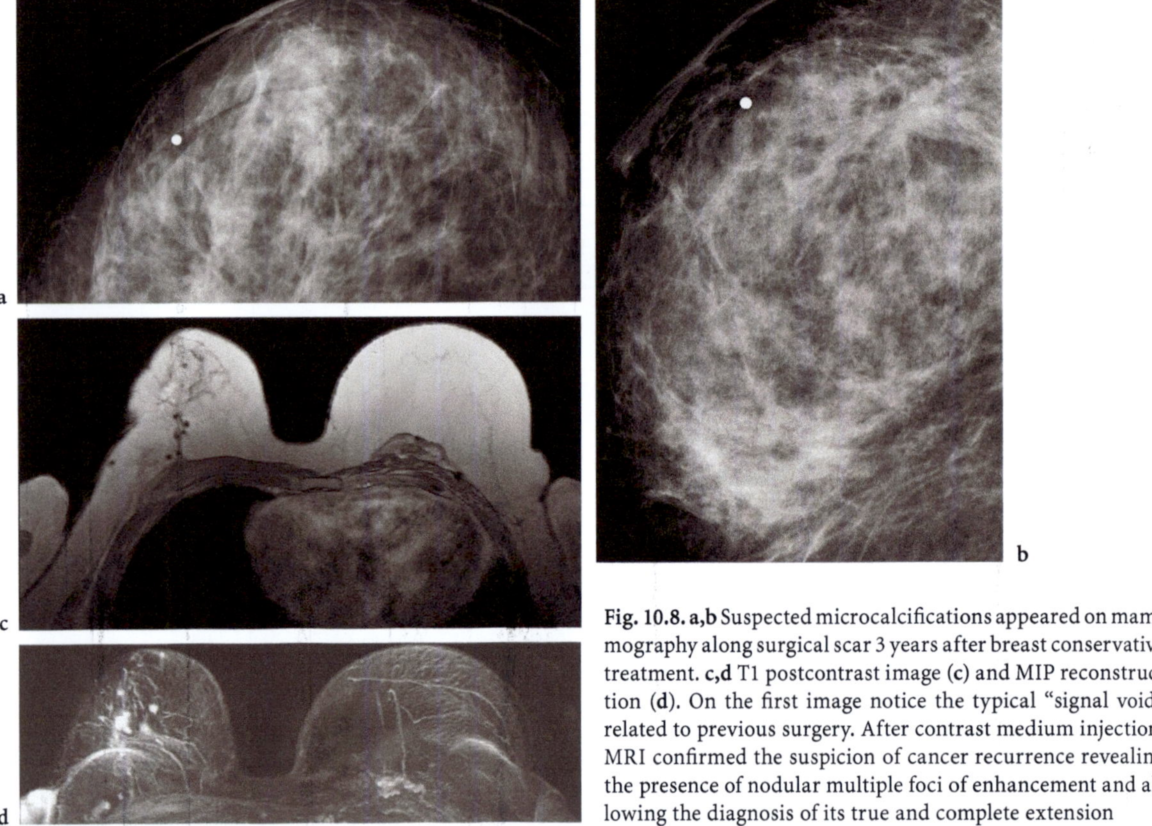

Fig. 10.8. a,b Suspected microcalcifications appeared on mammography along surgical scar 3 years after breast conservative treatment. **c,d** T1 postcontrast image (**c**) and MIP reconstruction (**d**). On the first image notice the typical "signal void" related to previous surgery. After contrast medium injection, MRI confirmed the suspicion of cancer recurrence revealing the presence of nodular multiple foci of enhancement and allowing the diagnosis of its true and complete extension

because of its irreversibility and its strong psychological and emotional impact. Considering other preventive measures, beside an unquestionable impact on ovarian and tubal cancer, prophylactic annexiectomy also appears to reduce the risk of breast cancer in premenopausal women. On the side of chemoprevention, the effectiveness of tamoxifen is still under investigation (Smith and Robson 2006).

For all these reasons, secondary prevention is still a fundamental strategy in high risk women. Routine mammography is currently the most effective screening method within the general population, and especially for postmenopausal women in whom involution of the parenchymal tissue has started. However, due to the early onset of hereditary breast disease, these women need to begin screening at a much younger age, when the breast parenchyma is dense and mammography is less sensitive in disease detection. Consequently, mammographic screening in young women, even if associated with US, might not be sufficient to guarantee an early diagnosis of genetically related breast cancers (Smith and Robson 2006; Saslow et al. 2007). Furthermore, *BRCA*-related gene products are implicated in the repair mechanism of DNA damage and, although the possible biological effect of frequent mammograms is still unknown, there is concern about a possible increase in radiosensitivity in this group of women. The need for these women to start diagnostic surveillance at a young age and continue for their whole

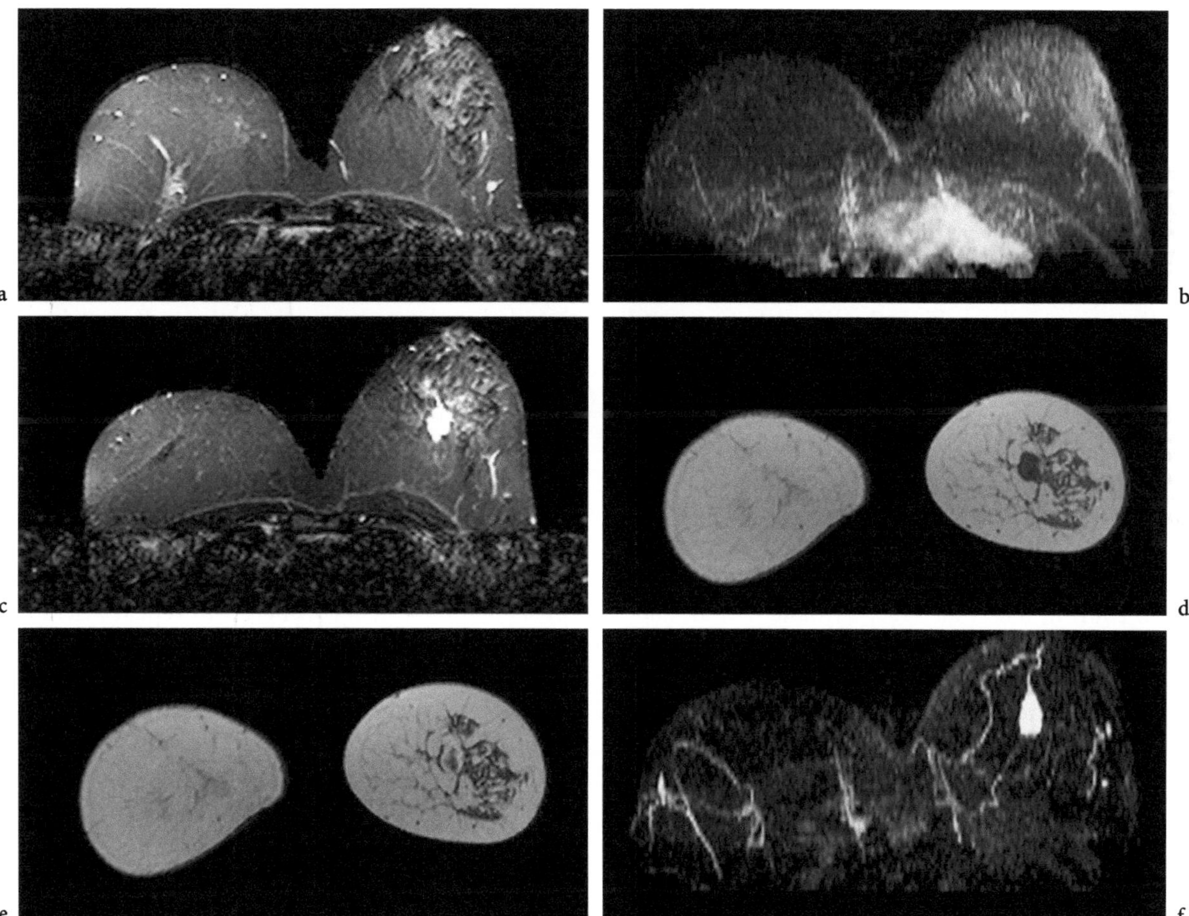

Fig. 10.9a–f. Aggressive biological behavior of breast cancer associated with *BRCA* mutation. In this *BRCA1* mutated 54-year-old patient, 2 cm ductal invasive cancer sprouted within 1 year. **a,b** T2 image (**a**) and MIP reconstruction (**b**). Negative MRI evaluation at the enrollment of the patient. **c–f** T2 in axial plane (**c**), T1 (**d**), T1 postcontrast (**e**) in coronal plane and MIP reconstruction (**f**). One year later a 2-cm ductal invasive cancer had sprouted in the left breast. Notice very high T2 hyperintensity as usually seen in benign disease and rim enhancement that is typical for malignancy

lifetime should be taken into account, considering the possible biological damage from X-ray over a more sensitive background (Narod and Foulkes 2004). For these reasons the attention has moved to other investigative techniques, and recent studies show that US and MRI, compared with mammography, improve early breast cancer detection in women at a high genetic risk (Kuhl et al. 2000; Sim et al. 2004; Warner et al. 2001; Leach et al. 2005; Sardanelli et al. 2007).

The major advantages of the technique are related to a better evaluation of dense breast in comparison with mammography, to the avoidance of X-ray-based methods, to the possibility of vascular characterization of very small lesions and to the availability of easier biopsy tools under US guidance. In our experience (Trecate et al. 2006), *BRCA* cancer-related patterns showed no significant differences in regards to sporadic breast cancer, both for mammography and ultrasound.

Considering MRI, an interesting finding in these hereditary cancers is that the lesions often show a very high T2 signal intensity, which in the general population is mostly indicative of benign lesions. Kuhl (2000) also underlined this possible behavior in breast cancer in a high-risk population. The biological explanation is unknown, but it represents another features of the natural history of this disease, which significantly differs from sporadic breast cancer. In our experience genetically predisposed population, it was present in 7 of 11 detected cancers (63%) among genetically predisposed women. The first published results on the inclusion of MRI in secondary prevention confirmed that the sensitivity of MRI in detecting genetically related breast cancers is very high, certainly higher than that of mammography (Sim et al. 2004; Warner et al. 2001; Leach et al. 2005; Sardanelli et al. 2007). The high spatial and contrast resolution of MRI allow detection of very small lesions without any influence of breast parenchymal density (Fig. 10.10).

For these reasons it may happen that some cancers are depicted only by MRI. It frequently happens when the lesions are smaller than 1 cm, the glandular parenchyma is irregularly nodular at mammography or scar tissue due to previous surgery and radiotherapy is present. Lobular carcinoma or reconstructive prosthesis may also hide cancer foci at conventional imaging. Such favorable sensitivity values, which reflect MRI's capacity to depict very tiny breast abnormalities, imply on the other hand a reduction of specificity.

False-positive results are often related to hormonal influences within normal parenchyma. For this reason current diagnostic protocols prescribe second-look ultrasound in case of suspicious MRI results when conventional imaging and clinical examination are negative. A positive result on second look justifies ultrasound-guided biopsy, while a negative result prompts to repeat MRI after an interval shorter than 6 months (Sardanelli et al. 2007).

At the beginning of our experience, we accounted for one 43-year-old patient who was *BRCA2* mutated. All conventional images and clinical examination were negative, while MRI showed two areas of intense and irregular enhancement within the left parenchyma. The right breast was completely negative, while dysplasia or benign disease related to hormonal influences is generally observed in the parenchyma of both breasts. The left breast lesions were suspect for malignancy. At a careful second look with ultrasound, both parenchyma were still judged negative for neoplastic disease. It was decided to keep the patient under surveillance with an additional MRI examination after 3 months. At this time, the result was impressive as both breasts were completely negative.

These observations, together with similar findings in other young women seen at our institution, led us to some considerations. It may happen that breast parenchyma, although evaluated by MRI in the correct period of the ovarian cycle (Kuhl 2000), shows suspicious enhancing areas that are related to hormonal influences. This phenomenon may be observed uni- or bilaterally. Therefore, when MRI shows any focal or diffuse uncertain enhancing area that is confirmed as negative by conventional images even at a careful second look, it seems better to repeat MRI after 3 to 6 months to avoid unnecessary biopsies. As the specificity of MRI can never be as high as its sensitivity, the introduction of MRI screening for individuals at high genetic risk should not encourage women at average risk to undergo regular MRI as a screening tool. On the other hand, for individuals at high genetic risk for whom intensive screening starting at a young age is recommended, the integration of MRI in surveillance protocols has become of primary importance as it seems to achieve the largest number of early diagnoses (Kuhl et al. 2000; Lee et al. 2003; Warner et al. 2001; Stoutjesdijk et al. 2001; Podo et al. 2002; Tilanus-Linthorst et al. 2000).

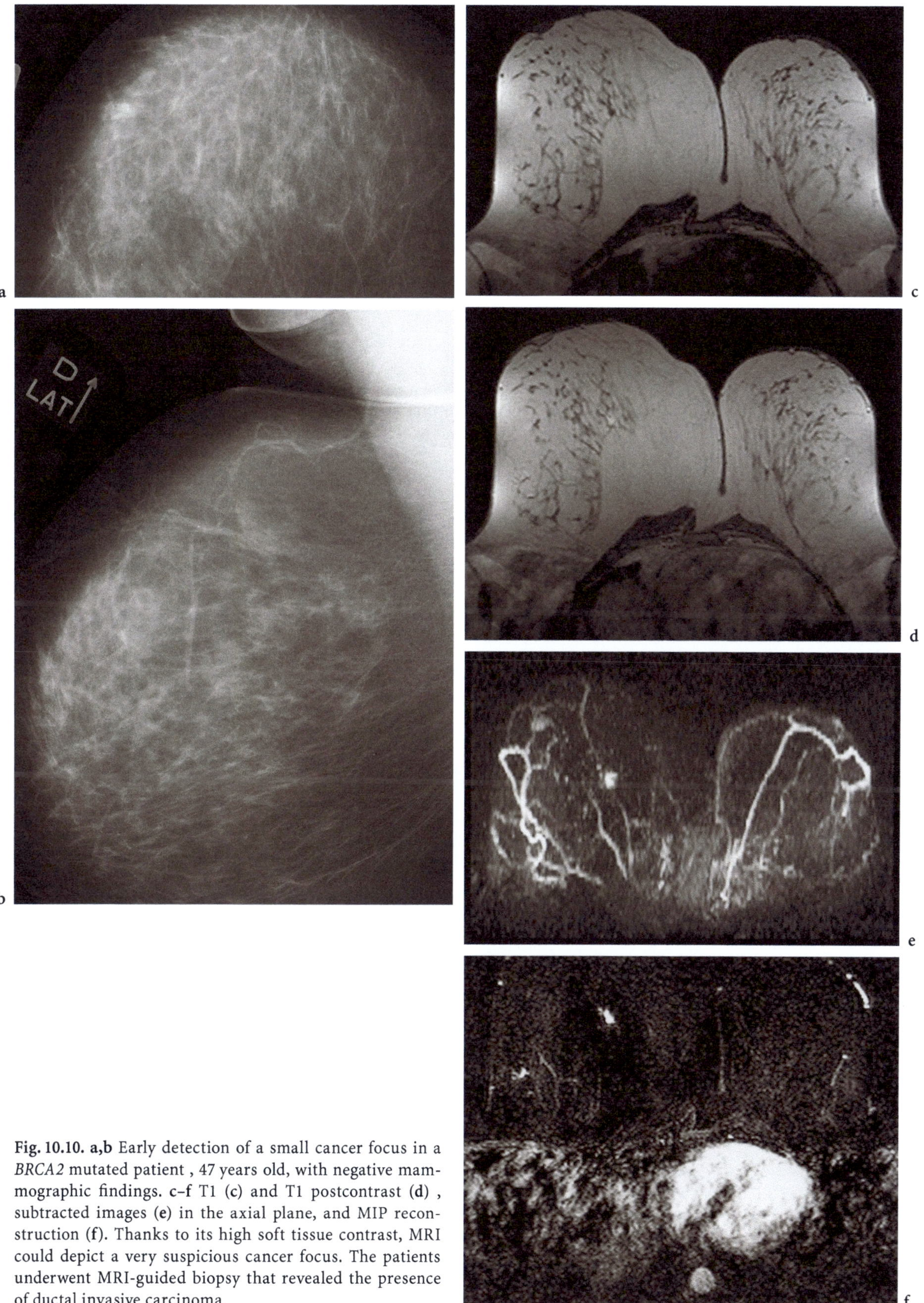

Fig. 10.10. a,b Early detection of a small cancer focus in a *BRCA2* mutated patient , 47 years old, with negative mammographic findings. **c–f** T1 (**c**) and T1 postcontrast (**d**) , subtracted images (**e**) in the axial plane, and MIP reconstruction (**f**). Thanks to its high soft tissue contrast, MRI could depict a very suspicious cancer focus. The patients underwent MRI-guided biopsy that revealed the presence of ductal invasive carcinoma

Reference

Antoniou A, Pharoah PD, Narod S et al (2003) Average risks of breast and ovarian cancer associated with BRCA1 or BRCA2 mutations detected in case series unselected for family history: a combined analysis of 22 studies. Am J Hum Genet 72:1117–1130

Baker LH (1982) Breast cancer detection demonstration project: 5 year summary report. Cancer J Clin 32:194–225

Belli P, Costantini M, Romani M et al (2002) Magnetic resonance imaging in breast cancer recurrence. Breast Cancer Res Treat 73:223–235

Blamey RW (1989) Factors influencing local recurrence after excision and radiotherapy for primary breast cancer. Br J Surg 76:890–894

Boetes C, Mus RDM, Holland R et al (1995) Breast tumours: comparative accuracy of MR imaging relative to mammography and US for demonstrating extent. Radiology 197:743–737

Charles-Edwards EM, deSouza NM (2006) Diffusion-weighted magnetic resonance imaging and its application to cancer. Cancer Imaging 6:135–143

Dershaw DD (1995) Mammography in patients with breast cancer treated by breast conservation (lumpectomy with or without radiation). Am J Roentgenol 164:309–316. Review

Dershaw DD, McCormick B, Cox L et al (1990) Differentiation of benign and malignant local tumor recurrence after lumpectomy Am J Roentgenol 155:35–38

Drew PJ, Chatterje S, Turnbull LW et al (1999) Dynamic contrast enhanced magnetic resonance imaging of the breast is superior to triple assessment for the preoperative detection of multifocal breast cancer. Ann Surg Oncol 6:599–603

Ernster VL, Barclay J, Kerlikowske K et al (1996) Incidence of and treatment for ductal carcinoma in situ of the breast. JAMA 275:913–918

Fischer U, Kopka L, Grabbe E (1999) Breast carcinoma: effect of pre-operative contrast-enhanced MR imaging on the therapeutic approach. Radiology 213:881–888

Fisher B, Bauer M, Margolese R et al (1985) Five-year results of a randomized clinical trial comparing total mastectomy and segmental mastectomy with or without radiation in the treatment of breast cancer. N Engl J Med 312:665–673

Folkman J (1985) Tumor angiogenesis. Adv Cancer Res 43:175–199

Folkman J (2002) Role of angiogenesis in tumor growth and metastasis. Semin Oncol 29 (6 Suppl 16):15–18

Folkman J, Klagsbrun M (1987) Angiogenic factors. Science 235:422–447

Foulkes WD, Stefansson IM, Chappuis PO et al (2003) Germline BRCA1 mutations and a basal epithelial phenotype in breast cancer. J Natl Cancer Inst 95:1482–1485

Gajalakshmi CK, Shanta V, Hakama M (1999) Survival from contralateral breast cancer. Breast Cancer Res Treat 58:115–122

Gilles R, Zafrani B, Guinebretiere JM et al (1995) Ductal carcinoma in situ: MR imaging-histopathologic correlation. Radiology 196(2):415–419

Gimbrone MA, Leapman SB, Cotran RS, Folkman J (1972) Tumor dormancy in vivo by prevention of neovascularization. J Exp Med 73:461–473

Hanahan D, Folkman J (1996) Patterns and emerging mechanism of the angiogenic switch during tumorigenesis. Cell 86:353–364

Harms SE, Flamig DP, Hesley KL et al (1993) MR imaging of the breast with rotating delivery of excitation off resonance: clinical experience with patologic correlation. Radiology 187:493–501

Heywang SH (1994) Contrast-enhanced magnetic resonance imaging of the breast. Invest Radiol 29:94–104

Heywang SH, Hahn D, Schmidt H et al (1986) MR imaging of the breast using Gd-DTPA. J Comput Assist Tomogr 10:199–204

Heywang SH, Wolf A, Pruss E et al (1989) MR imaging of the breast with Gd-DTPA: use and limitations. Radiology 171:95–103

Heywang-Köbrunner SH, Schlegel A, Beck R et al (1993) Contrast-enhanced MRI of the breast after limited surgery and radiation therapy. Am J Roentgenol 17:891–900

Holland R, Veling SHJ, Mravunac M et al (1985) Histologic multifocality of Tis, T1-2 breast carcinomas (implications for clinical trials of breast conserving therapy). Cancer 56:979–990

Holland R. Hendriks JH, Verbeek A et al (1990) Extent, distribution, and mammographic/histological distribution of breast ductal carcinoma in situ. Lancet 335:519–522

Holland H, Peterse JL, Millis RR et al (1994) Ductal carcinoma in situ: a proposal for a new classification. Semin Diagn Pathol 11:167–180

Hsiang D, Shah N, Yu H et al (2005) Coregistration of dynamic contrast enhanced MRI and broadband diffuse optical spectroscopy for characterizing breast cancer. Technol Cancer Res Treat 4:549–558

Ikeda DM (2001) Progress report from the American College of Radiology Breast MR Imaging Lexicon Committee. Magn Reson Imaging Clin N AM 9:295–302

Ikeda DM, Birdwell RL, Daniel BL (2000) Potential role of magnetic resonance imaging and other modalities in ductal carcinoma in situ detection. Semin Breast Dis 3:50–60

Kaiser WA, Zeitler E (1989) MR imaging of the breast: fast imaging sequences with and without Gd-DTPA. Radiology 170:681–686

Kuhl CK (2000) MRI of breast tumors. Eur Radiol 10:46–58

Kuhl CK, Mielcareck P, Klaschik S et al (1999) Dynamic breast MR imaging: are signal intensity time course data useful for differential diagnosis of enhancing lesions? Radiology 211:101–110

Kuhl CK, Schmutzler RK, Leutner CC, Kempe A, Wardelmann E, Hocke A, Maringa M, Pfeifer U, Krebs D, Schild HH (2000) Breast MR imaging screening in 192 women proved or suspected to be carriers of a breast cancer susceptibility gene: preliminary results. Radiology 215:267–279

Landheer ML, Veltman J, van Eekeren R et al (2006) MRI-guided preoperative wire localization of nonpalpable breast lesions. Clin Imaging 30:229–233

Leach MO, Boggis CR, Dixon AK, Easton DF, Eeles RA, Evans DG, Gilbert FJ, Griebsch I, Hoff RJ, Kessar P, Lakhani SR, Moss SM, Nerurkar A, Padhani AR, Pointon LJ, Thompson D, Warren RM; MARIBS study group (2005) Screening with magnetic resonance imaging and mammography of a UK population at high familial risk of breast cancer: a prospective multicentre cohort study. Lancet 365:1769–1778

Lee SG, Orel SG, Woo IJ et al (2003) MR imaging screening of the contralateral breast in patients with newly diagnosed breast cancer: preliminary results. Radiology 226:773–778

LeGal M, Chavanne G, Pellier D (1984) Valeur diagnostique des microcalcifications groupées découvertes par mammographie. Bull cancer 71:57–64

Liberman L, Morris EA, Kim CM et al (2003) MR imaging findings in the contralateral breast of women with recently diagnosed breast cancer. Am J Roentgenol 180(2):333–341

Manton DJ, Chaturvedi A, Hubbard A et al (2006) Neoadjuvant chemotherapy in breast cancer: early response prediction with quantitative MR imaging and spectroscopy. Br J Cancer 94:427–435

Marini C, Iacconi C, Giannelli M et al (2007) Quantitative diffusion-weighted MR imaging in the differential diagnosis of breast lesion. Eur Radiol 17:2646–2655

Morris EA, Schwartz LH, Dershaw DD et al (1997) MR imaging of the breast in patients with occult primary breast carcinoma. Radiology 205(2):437–440

Mumtaz H, Hall-Craggs MA, Davidson T et al (1997) Staging of symptomatic primary breast cancer with MR imaging. Am J Roentgenol 169:417–424

Narod SA, Foulkes WD (2004) BRCA1 and BRCA2: 1994 and beyond. Nat Rev Cancer 4:665–676. Review

Neff PT, Bear HD, Pierce CV et al (1996) Long-term results of breast conservation therapy for breast cancer. Ann Surg 223:709–716; discussion 716–717

Oellinger H, Heins S, Sander B (1993) The most sensitive method for detecting multicentric carcinomas in female breast? Eur Radiol 3:223–226

Orel SG, Schnall MD, Powell CM (1995) Staging of suspected breast cancer: effect of MR imaging and MR-guided biopsy. Radiology 196:115–122

Orel SG, Mendonca MH, Reynolds C et al (1997) MR imaging of ductal carcinoma in situ. Radiology 202(2):413–420

Orel SG, Schnall MD, LiVolsi VA et al (1994) Suspicious breast lesions: MR imaging with radiologic-pathologic correlation. Radiology 190:485–493

Page DL, Rogers L (1992) Combined histologic and cytologic criteria for the diagnosis of mammary atypical ductal hyperplasia. Hum Pathol 23:1095–1099

Panizza P, DeGaspari G, Vanzulli A et al (1997) Accuracy of post-MR imaging second-look sonography in previously undetected breast lesions. Radiology 205(P):489

Pierce LJ, Levin AM, Rebbeck TR et al (2006) Ten-year multi-institutional results of breast-conserving surgery and radiotherapy in BRCA1/2-associated stage I/II breast cancer. J Clin Oncol 24:2437–2443

Podo F, Sardanelli F, Canese R et al (2002) The Italian multi-centre project on evaluation of MRI and other imaging modalities in early detection of breast cancer in subjects at high genetic risk. J Exp Clin Cancer Res 21(3 Suppl):115–124

Sardanelli F, Podo F, D'Agnolo G et al (2007) Multicenter comparative multimodality surveillance of women at genetic-familial high risk for breast cancer (HIBCRIT study): interim results. Radiology 242:698–715

Sarrazin D, Le M, Rouesse J et al (1984) Conservative treatment versus mastectomy in breast cancer tumors with macroscopic diameter of 20 millimeters or less. The experience of the Institut Gustave-Roussy. Cancer 53:1209–1213

Saslow D, Boetes C, Burke W, Harms S, Leach MO, Lehman CD, Morris E, Pisano E, Schnall M, Sener S, Smith RA, Warner E, Yaffe M, Andrews KS, Russell CA; American Cancer Society Breast Cancer Advisory Group (2007) American Cancer Society guidelines for breast screening with MRI as an adjunct to mammography. CA Cancer J Clin 57:75–89

Schmidt-Ullrich R, Wazer DE, Tercilla O (1989) Tumor margin assessment as a guide to optimal conservation surgery and irradiation in early stage breast carcinoma. Int J Radiat Oncol Biol Phys 17:733–738

Schwartz GF, Patchefsky SA, Feig SA et al (1980) Clinically occult breast cancer. Multicentricity and implications for treatment. Ann Surg 191:8–12

Silverstein MJ, Lagios MD, Craig PH et al (1996) A prognostic index for ductal carcinoma in situ of the breast. Cancer 77:2267–2274

Sim LS, Hendriks JH, Fook-Chong SM (2004) Breast ultrasound in women with familial risk of breast. Ann Acad Med Singapore 33:600–606

Smith KL, Robson ME (2006) Update on hereditary breast cancer. Curr Oncol Rep 8:14–21. Review

Soderstrom CE, Harms SE, Copit DS et al (1996) Three-dimensional RODEO breast MR imaging of lesions containing ductal carcinoma in situ. Radiology 201(2):427–432

Solin LJ, Fowble BL, Schultz DJ et al (1990) The detection of local recurrence after definitive irradiation for early stage carcinoma of the breast. An analysis of the results of breast biopsies performed in previously irradiated breasts. Cancer 65:2497–2502

Stomper PC, Recht A, Berenberg AL et al (1987) Mammographic detection of recurrent cancer in the irradiated breast. Am J Roentgenol 148:39–43

Stomper P, Connolly J (1992) Ductal carcinoma in situ of the breast:correlation between mammographic calcification and tumor subtype. Am J Roentgenol 159:483–485

Stomper PC, Herman S, Klippenstein DL et al (1995) Suspect breast lesions: findings at dynamic gadolinium-enhanced MR imaging correlated with mammographic and pathologic features. Radiology 197:387–395

Stoutjesdijk MJ, Boetes C, Jager GJ et al (2001) Magnetic resonance imaging and mammography in women with a hereditary risk of breast cancer. J Natl Cancer Inst 93:1095–1102

Tilanus-Linthorst MM, Obdeijn IM, Bartels KC et al (2000) First experiences in screening women at high risk for breast cancer with MR imaging. Breast Cancer Res Treat 63:53–60

Trecate G, Tess JD, Vergnaghi D et al (2002) Breast microcalcifications studied with 3D contrast-enhanced high-field magnetic resonance imaging: more accuracy in the diagnosis of breast cancer. Tumori 88(3):224–233

Trecate G, Vergnaghi D, Manoukian S et al (2006) MRI in the early detection of breast cancer in women with high genetic risk. Tumori 92:517–523

Veronesi U, Saccozzi R, DelVecchio M et al (1981) Comparison radical mastectomy with quadrantectomy, axillary dissection, and radiation therapy in patients with small cancer of the breast. N Engl J Med 305:6–11

Viehweg P, Lampe D, Buchmann J et al (2000) In situ and minimally invasive breast cancer: morphologic and kinetic features on contrast-enhanced MR imaging. MAGMA 11(3):129–137

Warner E, Plewes DB, Shumak RS et al (2001) Comparison of breast magnetic resonance imaging, mammography, and ultrasound for surveillance of women at high risk for hereditary breast cancer. J Clin Oncol 19:3524–3531

Weidner N, Semple JP, Welch WR, Folkman J (1991) Tumor angiogenesis and metastasis: correlation in invasive breast carcinoma. N Engl Med 324:1–8

Westerhof JP, Fischer U, Moritz JD et al (1998) MR imaging of mammographically detected clustered microcalcifications: is there any value? Radiology 207(3):675–681

Winchester D, Cox J (1992) Standards for breast conservation treatment. Cancer J Clin 42:134–162

Zuiani C, Francescutti GE, Londero V, Zunnui I, Bazzocchi M (2002) Ductal carcinoma in situ: is there a role for MRI? J Exp Clin Cancer Res 21:89–95

PET Imaging of Breast Cancer Molecular Biomarkers

11

Elisabetta Brugola, Andreas K. Buck, Luca Tagliabue, Sven N. Reske, and Giovanni Lucignani

CONTENTS

Abstract

Cancer produces major biochemical changes in the cell's energy metabolism, altering utilization of glucose and other substrates, protein synthesis and expression of receptors and antigens. Tumor growth also leads to hypoxia, with heterogeneity in blood flow owing to focal necrosis, neoangiogenesis, as well as disruption of transport mechanisms of substrates across cell membranes and other physiological boundaries. Molecular changes result in cell cycle dysfunction, altered apoptosis and cell differentiation, neovascularization, and tumor cell migration and invasion. Understanding tumorigenesis is crucial for developing molecular therapeutic targets that can overcome current therapeutic limitations. As our understanding of the molecular nature of cancer improves, better methods are being developed to monitor cancer progression and regression in response to treatment. Insights from research into disease-specific biochemical processes have advanced the development of molecular biomarkers as targets for molecular imaging.

A biomarker can be defined as a measurable variable of a molecular, biological or functional process that can also be used as a measure of pharmacologic response to treatment. Biomarker imaging reflects endogenous molecular/genetic processes in normal and pathologic tissues, making it a particularly attractive technique to obtain molecular information that can be rapidly translated into clinically useful information. Biomarkers have proven highly useful for identifying malignant lesions and staging disease extent. In some cases, they can also be used as sensitive indicators of treatment response. Complementary to biopsy and circulating biomarkers assay, biomarker imaging is applied to stage patients and to assess therapeutic response repeatedly in single lesions, as well as to evaluate the global tumor burden at any stage of disease. Many potential imaging targets have been discovered through research in modern genomics and proteomics.

11.1 The Basis of Diagnostic Procedures in Breast Cancer

Biochemical and histological changes, along with their macroscopic anatomical effects, can be assessed with a variety of different non-invasive imaging tools: X-ray computed tomography (CT), magnetic resonance imaging (MRI), magnetic resonance spectroscopy (MRS), positron emission tomography (PET) and single photon emission computed tomography (SPECT). Anatomical imaging (CT and MRI) defines tumor size and site and invasion into surrounding structures, while functional imaging (MRS, PET, SPECT) is better suited for characterizing a tumor's biological properties.

The identification of a tumoral mass and the assessment of its size and degree of vascularization are best achieved with CT and MRI, while functional imaging provides additional information crucial for tumor classification, differential diagnosis and follow-up. Thus, molecular and functional imaging plays a key role in diagnosis, prognosis, therapy monitoring and follow-up of most cancers.

The goals of diagnostic procedures in oncology include: primary diagnosis, ideally obviating the need for biopsy; planning of biopsy and surgical resection; radiation therapy planning for target volume definition; evaluation for chemotherapy in selected cases and experimental therapies; post-treatment re-evaluation. When clinical signs and symptoms raise suspicion of a tumor, the first diagnostic evaluation is based on radiologic imaging. When the diagnosis of cancer is highly suspicious, the type of tumor and its grade of malignancy need to be characterized, as morphologic imaging alone is not specific enough to fully identify the nature of the cancer. The gold standard for diagnosis is histopathological evaluation. However, because of tumor heterogeneity, even biopsy does not always hit the site of highest malignancy that would best define the tumor grade. Hence, histological evaluation yields a minimum grading that does not always reflect the real grade of the tumor. In this situation, non-invasive molecular imaging techniques can be applied to characterize the more subtle tissue differences and enable successful targeting of the biopsy to the site of highest malignancy.

11.2 PET in Breast Cancer

PET permits the assessment of biomarkers characteristic of a neoplastic cell or related to its activity or its environment. The cellular biomarkers of breast cancer reveal changes in glucose metabolism, amino acid transport and protein synthesis, DNA synthesis and cell proliferation, receptor expression (epidermal growth factor receptor, estrogen and progesterone receptors), and induction of apoptosis. Variations in tumor blood flow, vascular permeability and neoangiogenesis, along with hypoxia, are, instead, biological processes that take place in the tissues surrounding the cancer. The oncological biomarker most commonly assessed with PET is [^{18}F]2-deoxy-2-fluoro-d-glucose ([^{18}F]FDG) uptake. PET with [^{18}F]FDG is currently used for tissue characterization and to derive helpful information for patient staging, prognosis, treatment planning and monitoring. With [^{18}F]FDG-PET, benign breast tumors can be differentiated from malignant ones (Avril et al. 1996, 2001), and metastases detected in patients with locally advanced and/or lymph node spread of disease (Schirrmeister et al. 2001). PET with [^{18}F]FDG is complementary to conventional methods for assessing breast cancer patients. There are various applications of [^{18}F]FDG in tumor assessment. Prior to treatment, PET scan with [^{18}F]FDG is a useful part of the diagnostic workup of suspected tumors and metastases as it may identify focal hypermetabolic abnormalities.

11.2.1 Cellular and Molecular Correlates of FDG Uptake in Breast Cancer

[^{18}F]FDG differs from glucose only in the replacement of the hydroxyl group on the second carbon atom by radioactive fluorine. Glucose and [^{18}F]FDG share the same saturable carriers between blood and tissue, and [^{18}F]FDG competes with glucose for hexokinase. Since [^{18}F]FDG-6-phosphate is trapped in cells in proportion to the glucose metabolic rate, its accumulation can be detected by PET. Furthermore, glucose utilization in neoplasms is altered in comparison with normal tissue. In vitro tumor cells have a high rate of glucose degradation into lactic acid even in the presence of oxygen (Warburg 1924). In vitro studies indicate that FDG uptake is determined mainly by the number of viable tumor cells (Higashi et al. 1993). Similarly, FDG uptake in breast cancer correlates well with the number of viable cancer cells in vivo (Brown et al. 1995; Bos et al. 2002). While necrotic or fibrotic tissue may reduce tracer uptake, the presence of inflammatory cells potentially increases [^{18}F]FDG accumulation (Bos et al. 2002, Kubota et al. 1990) and there is a percentage of FDG uptake that is related to non-tumoral tissue (Kubota et al. 1992; Hatanaka 1974) (Table 11.1).

Alterations in glucose transport in experimental cancer cells is related to an increased metabolism and an increased number of existing glucose transporters (Hatanaka 1974). Activation of the gene encoding the synthesis of glucose transporter Glut1 is a major early marker of malignant transformation. [^{18}F]FDG uptake into malignant cells results from the increased expression of glucose transporter molecules and from glycolysis. The molecular mechanism of [^{18}F]FDG accumulation within cells has been investigated in vitro and in vivo. FDG enters the cell by the same membrane transport mechanism as glucose. Phosphorylation by hexokinase is a rate-limiting step reaction because, unlike glucose-6-phosphate, [^{18}F]FDG-6-phosphate is not a substrate of glucose-6-phosphate isomerase and does not undergo further metabolism in the glucose pathway, so that [^{18}F]FDG remains entrapped within the cells. Increased glucose utilization in breast cancer is caused by the overexpression of membrane glucose transporters, especially Glut-1 and Glut-3 (Bos et al. 2002; Maschauer et al. 2004; Reske et al. 1997; Brown and Wahl 1993), and increased hexokinase activity (Bos et al. 2002; Rempel et al. 1996). Moreover, levels of glucose-6-phosphatase can also affect the rate of glucose utilization (Caraco et al. 2000). What remains to be determined is which of these steps is the most important rate limiting in [^{18}F]FDG uptake in breast cancer. The overexpression of Glut-1 in nearly all human cancers has led to speculation that glucose metabolism is predominantly regulated by glucose transporters. Overexpression of Glut-1 has also been reported as a common feature of breast cancer that contributes to increased [^{18}F]FDG uptake (Bos et al. 2002;Brown and Wahl 1993;Brown et al. 1996). The phosphorylation step appears to be rate-determining in the uptake of FDG in breast cancer (Torizuka et al. 1998). A significant correlation has been found between [^{18}F]FDG uptake and hexokinase I, but not hexokinase II and III expression (Bos et al. 2002; Mathupala et al. 2001; Brown et al. 2002).

Table 11.1. Biological correlates of FDG uptake in breast cancer

Variable	Correlation	References
Histology ductal	+++	Avril et al. 2001; Bos et al. 2002; Crippa et al. 1998; Buck et al. 2002
Histology lobular	+	Avril et al. 2001; Bos et al. 2002; Crippa et al. 1998; Buck et al. 2002
Viable tumor cells	+++	Higashi et al. 1993; Brown et al. 1995; Bos et al. 2002
Tumor grading	+	Bos et al. 2002; Crippa et al. 1998; Adler et al. 1993
Glut-1 expression	+	Bos et al. 2002; Maschauer et al. 2004; Reske et al. 1997; Brown and Wahl 1993; Brown et al. 1996
Hexokinase I expression	++	Bos et al. 2002; Rempel et al. 1996
Proliferation fraction (Ki-67, MAI)	+	Bos et al. 2002; Dettmar et al. 1997; Keshgegian and Cnaan 1995; Barnard et al. 1987; Crippa et al. 1998; Buck et al. 2002
Microvessel density	+++	Bos et al. 2002; Buck et al. 2002
Lymphocitic infiltrate	++	Bos et al. 2002
p53 expression	+	Crippa et al. 1998; Buck et al. 2002; Smith et al. 2006
Axillary lymph node status	NS	Avril et al. 2001; Crippa et al. 1998; Buck et al. 2002; Crowe et al. 1994
Tumor size	NS	Avril et al. 2001; Crippa et al. 1998; Crowe et al. 1994
Estrogen receptor status	NS	Avril et al. 2001; Dehdashti et al. 1995; Crippa et al. 1998; Buck et al. 2002; Crowe et al. 1994
Progesterone receptor status	NS	Avril et al. 2001; Crippa et al. 1998; Buck et al. 2002; Crowe et al. 1994
HIF-1 α	NS	Bos et al. 2002
VEGF	NS	Bos et al. 2002
c-erb B-2	NS	Buck et al. 2002

NS, non-significant/controversial

11.2.2 [^{18}F]FDG Data Analysis

By fitting the data of [^{18}F]FDG accumulation in a region of interest in a dynamic study, three constants may be derived: the glucose transport from blood to tumor, the reverse transport from tumor to blood and the phosphorylation of glucose. Quantitative assessment of glucose metabolism with PET, based on this model, is considered highly reproducible, but cumbersome. However, doubt has been raised as to the usefulness of quantitation or even semiquantitation in a clinical setting, where simple visual assessment of tracer accumulation by an experienced reader or measurement of the radioactivity distribution ratio between tumor and normal tissue has proven sufficient in most cases. Semiquantitative analysis of solid cancer [^{18}F]FDG uptake is a recognized standard method in evaluating cancer lesions: standard [^{18}F]FDG uptake values (SUVs) of breast lesions are higher in malignant (SUV=4.5) than in benign lesions (SUV=1.0) (Dehdashti et al. 1995). Furthermore, there is a significant difference in SUVs between dense and non-dense normal breast. However, the maximum SUV in dense breasts is largely below the threshold of 2.5, a widely used cut-off value for malignancy. Menopausal status and age do not significantly affect the [^{18}F]FDG cancer uptake (Kumar et al. 2006).

11.2.3 Relationship between [^{18}F]FDG Uptake and Molecular Markers of Malignancy

Because the grade of tumor malignancy is a crucial variable, different studies have focused on the relationship between the grade of malignancy and the rate of [^{18}F]FDG uptake. Anaplasia is considered a determinant factor for the elevated uptake of [^{18}F]FDG. Accordingly, PET has been proposed as a tool to guide biopsy in the high metabolic area, where sampling is most likely to provide diagnostic results. In the early postoperative period, [^{18}F]FDG-PET can be used to differentiate residual tumor from the effect of surgery. A decline in tumoral uptake of [^{18}F]FDG weeks or months after therapy is suggestive of a good response to treatment, indicating either a reduction in the number of viable cells or in the metabolism of damaged cells. After treatment, [^{18}F]FDG may differentiate recurrence from other therapy-related changes. Ki-67, a marker of cell proliferation, is a nuclear antigen expressed in the G1, G2 and S phases of the cell cycle (Dettmar et al. 1997). Determination of Ki-67 by immunohistochemistry is currently employed to predict clinical outcome in breast cancer (Keshgegian and Cnaan 1995; Barnard et al. 1987). The mean value of Ki-67-positive cells in lobular breast cancer ranges between 0 and 35%. Far fewer Ki-67-positive nuclei are found in the lobular than in the ductal breast cancer subtype. This difference is shown by the significant correlation between [^{18}F]FDG uptake and Ki-67 expression in ductal breast cancer (Avril et al. 2001), whereas no correlation between the two has been observed in lobular cancer. A significant correlation between [^{18}F]FDG uptake and the mitotic activity index has also been described (Bos et al. 2002), further confirming a relationship between proliferation and glucose metabolism (Crippa et al. 1998). The thymidine labeling index (TLI) was used for determining proliferative activity in the tumoral S-phase fraction, but no correlation between the TLI and the SUV was found. Why the results of determining tumor proliferation with Ki-67 and with TLI differed might be explained by the hypothesis for increased glucose consumption during the G1, G2 and S phases of the cell cycle. However, the weak correlation coefficient indicates that only 40% of tumoral [^{18}F]FDG uptake is related to proliferative activity.

Mutations and overexpression of tumor suppressor gene p53 can be frequently observed in malignant breast tumors (Barbareschi 1996). Overexpression of p53 is thought to reflect tumor aggressiveness and to be indicative of a lower survival rate (Barbareschi 1996; Alred et al. 1993; Overgaard et al. 2000). Few studies have correlated p53 expression in breast cancer with [^{18}F]FDG uptake (Buck et al. 2002; Crippa et al. 1998), so far, but available data suggest that abrogation of p53 in breast cancer is associated with specific changes in glucose metabolism detected by PET (Smith et al. 2006). Overexpression of c-erbB-2 has also been suggested as an independent prognostic marker (Pich et al. 2000; Rudolph et al. 2001). However, no significant correlation was found between tumoral [^{18}F]FDG uptake and c-erbB-2 expression (Buck et al. 2002). Because of the limited data available, no final conclusion can be drawn about possible correlations between p53 or c-erbB-2 expression and [^{18}F]FDG uptake.

Another important question is the relationship between histological subtype and [^{18}F]FDG uptake in breast cancer. In ductal or lobular carcinoma in situ (DCIS or LCIS), tumor cells are located within the terminal duct lobular unit and adjacent ducts and have not yet broken through the basal membrane: high-resolution [^{18}F]FDG PET with compression positron emission mammography (PEM) has been reported as highly accurate in depicting primary breast cancer (Berg et al. 2006). Invasive ductal breast cancer is the most common tumor entity, accounting for 80% of all breast carcinomas, whereas invasive lobular carcinoma is diagnosed less frequently (10–20%) (Masood and Chiao 1998). Tumor to background ratio (TBR) is another possible index for grading breast cancer malignancy. In ductal breast cancer, a mean of 17.3 (range 1.6–122.7) was observed. In lobular breast cancer, the mean TBR was 6.5 and significantly lower (range 1.4–22.7) (Avril et al. 2001; Bos et al. 2002; Crippa et al. 1998; Buck et al. 2002). This finding can be explained by a lower tumor cell density, a low level of Glut-1 expression and a decreased proliferation rate (Bos et al. 2002). The lower [^{18}F]FDG uptake in lobular carcinoma may also account for decreased detection rates on [^{18}F]FDG PET: up to two-thirds of lobular breast cancers are false-negative (Avril et al. 2000). False-negative PET results are based on tumor size and tumor grade as independent factors: cancer dimension (≤10 mm) and/or low grade of malignancy are a possible explanation for false-negative FDG-PET results (Kumar et al. 2006).

Accurate determination of tumor stage and prognosis is necessary for assessing a patient's individual risk of developing recurrent disease. It has recently been reported that prognosis may be estimated with [^{18}F]FDG PET (Oshida et al. 1998). Axillary nodal status (N+, node positive; N–, node negative), size of the primary tumor, tumor grading and estrogen and progesterone receptor status are established clinical and biological prognostic markers (Hayes et al. 2001). A variety of additional prognostic markers and parameters potentially predicting therapeutic outcome are currently under investigation, including expression of oncogenes and tumor suppressor genes (c-erbB-2, p53, bcl-2, c-myc), plasminogen activator (uPA) and plasminogen activator inhibitor (PAI-1), adhesion molecules (integrins, CD 44), proliferation markers (S-phase fraction, Ki-67 expression) and DNA ploidy (Loprinzi and Thome 2001; MacGrogan et al. 1996; Kumar et al. 2006) . Despite this variety of biological markers, few parameters have been demonstrated to be clearly associated with prognosis in breast cancer. The prognostic significance of detectable tumor cells in bone marrow or axillary lymph nodes is also controversial (Gebauer et al. 2003; den Bakker et al. 2002).

The most important clinical prognostic markers are axillary nodal status and primary tumor size. The high specificity of PET imaging indicates that patients who have a PET-positive axilla should undergo axillary lymph node dissection rather than a sentinel node biopsy (SNB) for axillary staging. By contrast, [^{18}F]FDG-PET showed poor sensitivity in detecting axillary metastases, thus confirming the need for SNB in those instances where PET is negative in the axilla (Veronesi et al. 2007). It has been shown that [^{18}F]FDG uptake in the primary tumor is not significantly different in patients with axillary lymph node involvement compared to nodal negative patients (Buck et al. 2002). Also, there was no correlation between tumor size and [^{18}F]FDG uptake. A tendency towards lower [^{18}F]FDG uptake in differentiated cancer was demonstrated in tumor grading (Adler et al. 1993). However, this finding was again not statistically significant (Buck et al. 2002). [^{18}F]FDG uptake in grade 3 carcinomas (SUV=6.2) was significantly higher than in grade 1–2 carcinomas (SUV=4.9) (Crippa et al. 1998), and a correlation between tumor grade and [^{18}F]FDG uptake in soft tissue metastases from breast cancer has been reported as well (Crowe et al. 1994).

Besides these uses, there is an increasing need to measure treatment efficacy as soon as possible after initiation because, with so many potential effective treatments to choose from, early identification of therapy ineffectiveness is important. [^{18}F]FDG-PET is currently used for treatment monitoring. But relatively little is known about the expression of key genes and proteins involved in glycolysis shortly after chemotherapy: it has been proven that after therapy (doxorubicin and 5-fluorouracil, two commonly used agents) the relationship between [^{18}F]FDG uptake and viable cell number can be uncoupled, with transient declines in [^{18}F]FDG uptake in excess of the decline in cell number despite increased Glut-1 mRNA levels. This transient effect has potential implications for the interpretation of [^{18}F]FDG studies, especially soon after treatment is initiated (Engles et al. 2006). However, [^{18}F]FDG remains a generally valid marker of viable cell number after cancer chemotherapy and an aid to differentiate responders from non responders early in the course of therapy.

11.2.4 Radiotracers for Imaging Breast Cancer Other than [^{18}F]FDG

A series of peptides other than FDG have been optimized with respect to endogenous analogues with regard to in vivo stability, affinity, binding specificity, unspecific uptake and excretion (Table 11.2).

The most direct measure of tumor growth and proliferation is the rate of DNA synthesis. Because thymidine is present in DNA, but not in RNA, many tracer approaches to measuring tumor growth against the rate of DNA synthesis are based on a labeled form of thymidine. The most widely used compound for this purpose is [^{18}F]fluoro-L-thymidine ([^{18}F]FLT) (Grierson and Shields 2000; Shields et al. 1998; Buck et al. 2002). This tracer is a marker for thymidine kinase activity and for cellular proliferation, potentially making it a more accurate predictor of the long-term effect of chemotherapy on tumor viability. Thymidine is incorporated into DNA; in the tumor it serves as a specific marker of cell growth. [^{18}F]FLT-PET correlates strongly with the Ki-67 labeling index in breast cancer (Kenny

Table 11.2. Radiopharmaceuticals for imaging specific characteristics of breast cancer

Radiopharmaceutical	Biomarker	References
[^{18}F]FDG (2-deoxy-2-fluoro-d-glucose)	Glucose metabolism	Avril et al. 1996, 2001; Schirrmeister et al. 2001; Warburg 1924; Higashi et al. 1993; Brown et al. 1995; Bos et al. 2002; Kubota et al. 1990, 1992 ; Hatanaka 1974; Maschauer et al. 2004; Reske et al. 1997; Brown and Wahl 1993; Rempel et al. 1996; Caraco et al. 2000; Brown et al. 1996; Torizuka et al. 1998; Mathupala et al. 2001; Brown et al. 2002; Dehdashti et al. 1995; Kumar et al. 2006; Dettmar et al. 1997; Keshgegian and Cnaan 1995; Barnard et al. 1987; Crippa et al. 1998; Barbareschi 1996; Alred et al. 1993; Overgaard et al. 2000; Buck et al. 2002; Smith et al. 2006; Pich et al. 2000; Rudolph et al. 2001; Berg et al. 2006; Masood and Chiao 1998; Avril et al. 2000; Kumar et al. 2006; Oshida et al. 1998; Hayes et al. 2001; Loprinzi and Thome 2001; MacGrogan et al. 1996; Gebauer et al. 2003; den Bakker et al. 2002; Veronesi et al. 2007; Adler et al. 1993; Crowe et al. 1994; Engles et al. 2006; Clavo et al. 1995; Burgman et al. 2001; Pedersen et al. 2001; Bos et al. 2001
[^{11}C]methionine	Amino acid metabolism, protein synthesis	Isselbacher 1972; Kubota et al. 1995; Leskinen-Kallio et al. 1991; Jansson et al. 1995
[^{18}F]FES(16-fluoro-17-estradiol)	Hormone receptor expression	Wester 2007; McGuire et al. 1991; Mortimer et al. 2001; Linden et al. 2006
[^{18}F]FLT(fluoro-L-thymidine)	Proliferative activity	Grierson and Shields 2000; Shields et al. 1998; Kenny et al. 2005, 2007; Cobben et al. 2002; Been et al. 2006; Pio et al. 2006
[^{18}F]Annexin V	Apoptosis	Yagle et al. 2005
[^{18}F]MISO (fluoromisonidazole)	Hypoxia	Bos et al. 2001; Rajendran et al. 2005
[^{18}F]FETA (fluoroetanidazole)	Hypoxia	Barthel et al. 2004
[^{18}F]FAZA (fluoroazomycin arabinoside)	Hypoxia	Piert et al. 2005
[^{64}Cu]ATSM (diacetyl-bis-N(4)-methylthiosemicarbazone)	Hypoxia	Rajendran et al. 2005
[^{18}F]Galacto-RGD	Angiogenesis	Hanahan and Folkman 1996; Hasan et al. 2002; Weidner et al. 1991; Wolf et al. 2004; Beer et al. 2006
[^{11}C] Iressa	Signal transduction processes	Hanahan and Folkman 1996; Hasan et al. 2002; Weidner et al. 1991; Wolf et al. 2004; Wang et al. 2006
[1^{5}O]H_2O	Perfusion	Beaney et al. 1984; Wilson et al. 1992; Zasadny et al. 2003

et al. 2005, 2007). Breast cancer and large axillary lymph-node metastases can be visualized with [^{18}F]FLT and PET (Cobben et al. 2002; Been et al. 2006). Radiotracers specifically reflecting proliferative activity may be suitable for evaluating treatment response: it has been shown that a 10-min [^{18}F]FLT-PET scan acquired 2 weeks after the end of the first course of chemotherapy is useful for predicting the longer-term efficacy of therapy regimens (Been et al. 2006; Pio et al. 2006). Imaging with radiolabeled amino acids visualizes protein synthesis and amino acid transport phenomena, which are accelerated in tumors (Isselbacher 1972). Because the uptake of amino acids in macrophages and other inflammatory cells is low, these tracers might be more tumor specific than [^{18}F]FDG for assessing abnormal tissue. In principle, the use of carbon-11 methionine obviates many of the problems related to the tumor/non-tumor uptake ratio that are encountered with [^{18}F]FDG, and it overcomes the difficulty in differentiating tumors from other pathologies that may cause abnormal [^{18}F]FDG uptake, i.e., infection, radiation necrosis and edema (Kubota et al. 1995). For this reason, [^{11}C]methionine PET has been used to image primary breast cancer and for treatment monitoring. Accumulation of this tracer may correlate with the proliferation rate of breast carcinoma. However, methionine uptake is not exclusively related to malignancy (Leskinen-Kallio et al. 1991; Jansson et al. 1995).

Receptor agonists have been shown to be more suitable tracers than antagonists: intracellular accumulation of the ligand in endosomal and lysosomal compartments due to internalization of the receptor agonist complex usually results in high target-to-background ratios. Radiolabeled antagonists, on the other hand, because they lack this ability of receptor-mediated internalization, have not been counted as promising tracers in oncology (Wester 2007). Estrogen receptor (ER) expression in breast cancer is an indicator of prognosis and predicts the likelihood of response to antiestrogen therapy. PET imaging of ER expression provides a new method for evaluating the status of breast cancer in either primary tumor or metastatic lesions. 16-[^{18}F]fluoro-17-estradiol ([^{18}F]FES) is an estrogen receptor substrate that can be utilized for specific receptor imaging with PET (McGuire et al. 1991; Mortimer et al. 2001). A significant correlation between [^{18}F]FES uptake in tumors and respective ER expression was demonstrated (McGuire et al. 1991). Additionally, a significant reduction in lesional [^{18}F]FES uptake was demonstrated in patients receiving antiestrogen therapy (Mortimer et al. 2001). However, receptor-negative tumors could not be visualized with [^{18}F]FES and PET. Since this approach does not target estrogen-negative tumors, this agent can predict response to hormonal therapy and may help guide treatment selection (Linden et al. 2006). Studies using [^{18}F]FES-PET have shown heterogeneous [^{18}F]FES uptake within the same tumor and between different metastatic lesions. This method can also be useful in patients with recurrent metastatic cancer where tissue sampling at all sites is not feasible (Wester 2007).

Apoptosis plays an important role in cancer biology, its etiology and clinical treatment. Cells deficient in apoptotic response can potentially become tumorigenic. Radiotherapy and chemotherapy generally kill tumor cells by inducing apoptosis (programed cell death). Thus, a probe that non-invasively measures apoptosis in cancer patients could have an important role in clinical oncology. Annexin V is a 36-kDa protein that binds with high affinity to phosphatidylserine lipids in the cell membrane. Because one of the earliest measurable events in apoptosis is the eversion of phosphatidylserine from the inner membrane leaflet to the outer cell surface, annexin V has proven useful for detecting the earliest stages of apoptosis. Apoptosis-detecting radioligands are ^{18}F-Annexin V, ^{64}Cu-Annexin V, ^{67}Ga e, ^{68}Ga-Dota-Annexin V (Yagle et al. 2005).

11.2.5 Breast Tumor Cell Environment and Role of PET

Hypoxia, an important variable in the regulation of cancer growth and development, is a resistance factor for radiotherapy; it promotes tumor aggressiveness via genomic changes that produce resistance to a variety of therapies by either remodeling tumor vasculature or inducing direct phenotypic changes in the tumor cells themselves. Spontaneous necrosis suggests the presence of hypoxic regions that are radioresistant. It has been found that cancer overexpresses vascular endothelial growth factor (VEGF) and other stress-related proteins or signaling molecules such as IL-1, TNF-alpha or TGF-beta. It has recently been suggested that hypoxia increases the uptake of [^{18}F]FDG through activation of the glycolytic pathway (Clavo et al. 1995; Burgman et al. 2001). Glut-1 transporters are twofold upregulated in hypoxic breast cancer cells (Burgman et al. 2001). Hypoxia causes upregulation of transcription factor HIF-1alpha (hypoxia inducible factor-1), which is overexpressed in invasive breast cancer (Pedersen et al. 2001) and has been demonstrated to induce glycolysis, angiogenesis and erythropoiesis (Bos et al. 2001). However, a significant correlation between HIF-1alpha protein expression and [^{18}F]FDG uptake in breast cancer has not been shown (Bos et al. 2002). A possible explanation might be that HIF-1 mediated upregulation of Glut-1 is more important for glucose metabolism than upregulation of HIF-1 itself. Although hypoxia probably contributes to increased rates of glycolysis and upregulation of Glut transporters, this cannot be inferred from [^{18}F]FDG uptake alone. One of the most widely used PET agents is [^{18}F]fluoromisonidazole ([^{18}F]MISO), a hypoxia agent for in vivo imaging with PET. [^{18}F]FMISO is not retained in non-hypoxic tissues, and high-grade lesion uptake of [^{18}F]FMISO is frequently heterogeneous and incompletely overlaps with [^{18}F]FDG uptake. A new clinical PET marker of tumor hypoxia is [^{18}F]fluoroetanidazole ([^{18}F]FETA): tumors are sufficiently visualized by PET within 30–60 min, reflecting a higher percentage of pO_2 values <1 mmHg, lower vessel density and higher radiobiological hypoxic fraction of tumors (Barthel et al. 2004). Another hypoxia tracer is [^{18}F]fluoroazomycin arabinoside ([^{18}F]FAZA): In all tumor models tested so far this tracer displayed significantly higher tumor-to-muscle and tumor-to-blood ratios than [^{18}F]MISO, indicating faster clearance from normal tissues and superior biokinetics (Piert et al. 2005). ^{64}Cu-diacetyl-bis-N(4)-methylthiosemicarbazone ([^{64}Cu]ATSM) is another hypoxia tracer that shows the best contrast early after injection, but these images are confounded by blood flow and their mechanism of localization is one step removed from intracellular oxygen concentration. [^{18}F]MISO images show less contrast than those of Cu-ATSM because of the lipophilicity and slower clearance of [^{18}F]MISO. But attempts to increase the rate of clearance led to tracers whose distribution is contaminated by blood flow effects (Rajendran et al. 2005). Tumor hypoxia measured by PET is highly predictive of patient outcome; patients with hypoxia demonstrated by PET had considerably earlier tumor relapse or progression. In this way, PET may suggest alternative therapeutic strategies in tumors resistant to standard treatment and it may direct patients to locoregional therapy and/or agents selective for hypoxic tissue (Wester 2007).

Solid tumors can grow to more than 1–2 mm only when supplied with sufficient oxygen and blood by newly formed blood vessels: this angiogenic switch is also the basis for the invasive growth of carcinomas and metastasis (Hanahan and Folkman 1996). Clinical studies report a significant correlation between microvessel density and tumoral [^{18}F]FDG uptake (Bos et al. 2002, Oshida et al. 1998): microvessel density turned out to be an indicator of aggressiveness (Hasan et al. 2002) and an independent predictor of prognosis in breast cancer (Weidner et al. 1991). For this reason, neoangiogenesis has been investigated as a key step in tumorigenesis and as a target for cancer therapy. Overexpressed in breast cancer, VEGF is an endothelial cytokine that stimulates proliferation and migration of vascular-derived endothelial cells. A 936C > T polymorphism in the gene for VEGF has been associated with VEGF plasma levels and breast cancer risk: VEGF CC, CT and TT genotypes were found in many patients with cancer, and VEGF genotype was significantly associated with [^{18}F]FDG uptake scores (Wolf et al. 2004). Integrin alpha(v)beta 3 plays a key role in angiogenesis and tumor cell metastasis: [^{18}F]Galacto-RGD is a new, highly alpha(v)beta selective tracer for PET, and its uptake correlates with the expression of this integrin (significant correlations between SUV and TBR with immunohistochemical staining intensity, as well as with microvessel density) (Beer et al. 2006). SUV in tumors ranged from 1.2 to 9.0. Tumor-to-blood and tumor-to-muscle ratios increased over time, with peak ratios of approximately 3 and 8 at 70 min after injection (Wester 2007). Another new tracer is [^{11}C]Iressa (Gefitinib), an imaging agent for EGFR-TK involved in cell signal transduction processes critical to cancer cell proliferation, apoptosis, repair and angiogenesis (Wang et al. 2006).

The first study of breast cancer imaging with PET evaluated tumor blood flow and oxygen extraction in nine patients using a [^{15}O]oxygen steady-state inhalation technique. Furthermore, in this series the regional blood flow was measured by means of ^{11}C-labeled carbon monoxide. Regional blood flow in the tumors was reported to be significantly higher than in the surrounding normal tissue (Beaney et al. 1984). Blood flow in breast cancer can also be measured by [^{15}O]H_2O PET and has been reported to be five to six times higher than that in normal tissue (Wilson et al. 1992). Recently, a strong correlation of tumoral blood flow as measured by [^{15}O]H_2O PET and [^{18}F]FDG uptake has been observed (Zasadny et al. 2003).

11.3 Conclusions

[^{18}F]FDG-PET offers the unique advantage of assessing tumor metabolism and has been used for defining prognosis in many types of cancer. [^{18}F]FDG is particularly useful in localizing occult primary tumors or for staging disease when metastases might be missed. The interpretation of [^{18}F]FDG signals can be confounded by tumor flare of inflammation following the treatment of certain tumor types, whereas cell proliferation tracers such as [^{18}F]FLT are more sensitive than [^{18}F]FDG to the effects of cytostatic therapy. Determining receptor status by PET allows non-invasive, in-vivo correlation with treatment benefit, albeit initially validated by correlating it with ex vivo histology. Moreover, the technique might be more reliable than biopsy because of heterogeneity within and across tumor masses. The multimodal combination of PET and CT provides metabolic assessment with optimal spatial resolution.

The aim is to develop and evaluate new biomarkers for imaging that target specific molecules (DNA, mRNA, proteins) or activated enzyme systems in specific signal transduction pathways. Although a direct limit to biomarker imaging strategies is the need to develop a specific probe for each molecular target, validate its sensitivity and specificity, and then use the probe in specific applications before it can be introduced into clinical routine (Blasberg 2007), the advantage of this approach is the development of a biomarker specific for each targeted therapy useful for clinical application for cancer treatment individual monitoring.

Multidimensional imaging adds precision, whereas multimodal imaging adds quantification of metabolic activity or receptor status. PET allows non-invasive quantitative studies of various biologic processes in tumoral tissues. Pharmacokinetics of anticancer drugs, therapeutic targets and monitoring of inhibition of these targets can be studied. Furthermore, PET provides various markers to assess tumor response early in the course of therapy.

Reference

Adler LP, Crowe JP, al-Kaisi NK, Sunshine JL (1993) Evaluation of breast masses and axillary lymph nodes with [F-18] 2-deoxy-2-fluoro-d-glucose PET. Radiology 187:743–750

Alred D, Clatk G, Elledge R (1993) Association of p53 protein expression with tumour cell proliferation rate and clinical outcome in node-negative breast cancer. J Natl Cancer Inst 85:200–206

Avril N, Dose J, Janicke F (1996) Metabolic characterization of breast tumours with positron emission tomography using F-18 fluorodeoxyglucose. J Clin Oncol 14:1848–1857

Avril N, Rose CA, Schelling M, Dose J, Kuhn W, Bense S, Weber W, Ziegler S, Graeff H, Schwaiger M (2000) Breast imaging with positron emission tomography and fluorine-18 fluorodeoxyglucose: use and limitations. J Clin Oncol 18:3495–3502

Avril N, Menzel M, Dose J, Schelling M, Weber W, Jänicke F, Nathrath W, Schwaiger M (2001) Glucose metabolism of breast cancer assessed by ^{18}F-FDG PET: histologic and immunohistochemical tissue analysis. J Nucl Med 42:9–16

Barbareschi M (1996) Prognostic value of immunohistochemical expression of p53 in breast carcinomas. A review of the literature involving over 9,000 patients. Appl Immunohistochem 4:106–116

Barnard NJ, Hall PA, Lemoine NR (1987) Proliferative index in breast carcinoma determined in situ by Ki67 immunostaining and its relationship to clinical and pathological variables. J Pathol 152:287–295

Barthel H, Wilson H, Collingridge DR, Brown G, Osman S, Luthra SK, Brady F, Workman P, Price PM, Aboagye EO (2004) In vivo evaluation of [18(F)]fluoroetanidazole as a new marker for imaging tumour hypoxia with positron emission tomography. Br J Cancer 90:2232–2242

Beaney RP, Lammertsma AA, Jones T, McKenzie CG, Halnan KE (1984) Positron emission tomography for in-vivo measurement of regional blood flow, oxygen utilisation, and blood volume in patients with breast carcinoma. Lancet 1:131–134

Been LB, Elsing PH, de Vries J, Cobben DC, Jager PL, Hoekstra HJ, Suurmeijer AJ (2006) Positron emission tomography in patients with breast cancer using (18)F-3-deoxy-3-fluoro-I-thymidine ((18)F-FLT) - a pilot study. Eur J Surg Oncol 32:39–43

Beer AJ, Haubner R, Sarbia M, Goebel M, Luderschmidt S, Grosu AL, Schnell O, Niemeyer M, Kessler H, Wester HJ, Weber WA, Schwaiger M (2006) Positron emission tomography using [18(F)]Galacto-RGD identifies the level of integrin alpha(v)beta 3 expression in man. Clin Cancer Res 12:3942–3949

Berg WA, Weinberg IN, Narayanan D, Lobrano ME, Ross E, Amodei L, Tafra L, Adler LP, Uddo J, Stein W, Levine EA (2006) High-resolution fluorodeoxyglucose positron emission tomography with compression ("positron emission mammography") is highly accurate in depicting primary breast cancer. Breast J 12:309–323

Blasberg RG (2007) Imaging update: new windows, new views. Clin Cancer Res 13:3444–3448 Schirrmeister H, Kühn T, Guhlmann A, Santjohanser C, Hörster T, Nüssle K, Koretz K, Glatting G, Rieber A, Kreienberg R, Buck A, Reske SN (2001) Fluorine-18 2-deoxy-2-fluoro-d-glucose PET in the preoperative staging of breast cancer: comparison with the standard staging procedures. Eur J Nucl Med 28:351–358

Bos R, Zhong H, Hanrahan CF, Mommers EC, Semenza GL, Pinedo HM, Abeloff MD, Simons JW, van Diest PJ, van der Wall E (2001) Levels of hypoxia-inducible factor-1 alpha during breast carcinogenesis. J Natl Cancer Inst 93:309–314

Bos R, van Der Hoeven JJ, van Der Wall E et al (2002) Biologic correlates of (18)fluorodeoxyglucose uptake in human breast cancer measured by positron emission tomography. J Clin Oncol 20:379–387

Brown RS, Wahl RL (1993) Overexpression of Glut-1 glucose transporter in human breast cancer. Animmunohistochemicalstudy. Cancer 72:2979–2985

Brown RS, Leung JY, Fisher SJ, Frey KA, Ethier SP, Wahl RL (1995) Intratumoral distribution of tritiated fluorodeoxyglucose in breast carcinoma: I. Are inflammatory cells important? J Nucl Med 36:1854–1861

Brown RS, Leung JY, Fisher SJ, Frey KA, Ethier SP, Wahl RL (1996) Intratumoral distribution of tritiated-FDG in breast carcinoma: correlation between Glut-1 expression and FDG uptake. J Nucl Med 37:1042–1047

Brown RS, Goodman TM, Zasadny KR, Greenson JK, Wahl RL (2002) Expression of hexokinase II and Glut-1 in untreated human breast cancer. Nucl Med Biol 29:443–453

Buck AK, Schirrmeister H, Kuhn T, Shen C, Kalker T, Kotzerke J, Dankerl A, Glatting G, Reske S, Mattfeldt T (2002) FDG uptake in breast cancer: correlation with biological and clinical prognostic parameters. Eur J Nucl Med Mol Imaging 29:1317–1323

Buck AK, Schirrmeister H, Hetzel M, Von Der Heide M, Halter G, Glatting G, Mattfeldt T, Liewald F, Reske SN, Neumaier B (2002) 3-deoxy-3-[^{18}F]fluorothymidine-positron emission tomography for noninvasive assessment of proliferation in pulmonary nodules. Cancer Res 62:3331–3334

Burgman P, Odonoghue JA, Humm JL, Ling CC (2001) Hypoxia-induced increase in FDG uptake inMCF7cells. J Nucl Med 42:170–175

Caraco C, Aloj L, Chen LY, Chou JY, Eckelman WC (2000) Cellular release of [^{18}F]2-fluoro-2-deoxyglucose as a function of the glucose-6-phosphatase enzyme system. J Biol Chem 275:18489–18494

Clavo AC, Brown RS, Wahl RL. Fluorodeoxyglucose uptake in human cancer cell lines is increased by hypoxia. J Nucl Med 36:1625–1632

Cobben DC, van der Laan BF, Hoekstra HJ, Jager PL, Willemsen AT, Vaalburg W, Suurmeijer AJ, Elsinga PH (2002) Detection of mammary, laryngeal and soft tissue tumors with FLT-PET. J Nucl Med 43:P278

Crippa F, Seregni E, Agresti R, Chiesa C, Pascali C, Bogni A, Decise D, De Sanctis V, Greco M, Daidone MG, Bombardieri E (1998) Association between [^{18}F]fluorodeoxy-glucose uptake and postoperative histopathology, hormone receptor status, thymidine labelling index and p53 in primary breast cancer: a preliminary observation. Eur J Nucl Med 25:1429–1434

Crowe JP Jr, Adler LP, Shenk RR, Sunshine J (1994) Positron emission tomography and breast masses: comparison with clinical, mammographic, and pathological findings. Ann Surg Oncol 1:132–140

Dehdashti F, Mortimer J, Siegel B (1995) Positron tomographic assessment of estrogen receptors in breast cancer: a comparison with FDG-PET and in vitro receptor assays. J Nucl Med 36:1766–1774

den Bakker MA, van Weeszenberg A, de Kanter AY, Beverdam FH, Pritchard C, van der Kwast TH, Menke-Pluymers M (2002) Non-sentinel lymph node involvement in patients with breast cancer and sentinel node micrometastasis; too early to abandon axillary clearance. J Clin Pathol 55:932–935

Dettmar P, Harbeck N, Thommsen C, Pache L, Ziffer P, Fizi K, Janicke F, Nathrath W, Schmitt M, Graeff H, Hofler H (1997) Prognostic impact of proliferation-associated factors MIB1 (Ki-67) and S-phase in node-negative breast cancer. Br J Cancer 75:1525–1533

Engles JM, Quarless SA, Mambo E, Ishimori T, Cho SY, Wahi RL (2006) Stunning and its effect on 3H-FDG uptake and key gene expression in breast cancer cells undergoing chemotherapy. J Nucl Med 47:603–608

Gebauer G, Fehm T, Merkle E, Jaeger W, Mitze M (2003) Micrometastases in axillary lymph nodes and bone marrow oflymph node-negative breast cancer patients–prognostic relevance after 10 years. Anticancer Res 23:4319–4324

Grierson JR, Shields AF (2000) Radiosynthesis of 3-deoxy-3-18F-fluorothymidine: ^{18}F-FLT for imaging of cellular proliferation in vivo. Nucl Med Biol 27:143–156

Hanahan D, Folkman J (1996) Patterns and emerging mechanisms of the angiogenic switch during tumorigenesis. Cell 86:353–364

Hasan J, Byers R, Jayson GC (2002) Intra-tumoural microvessel density in human solid tumours. Br J Cancer 86:1566–1577

Hatanaka M (1974) Transport of sugars in tumor cell membranes. Biochim Biophys Acta 355:77–104

Hayes DF, Isaacs C, Stearns V (2001) Prognostic factors in breast cancer: current and new predictors of metastasis. J Mammary Gland Biol Neoplasia 6:375–392

Higashi K, Clavo AC, Wahl RL (1993) Does FDG uptake measure proliferative activity of human cancer cells? In vitro comparison with DNA flow cytometry and tritiated thymidine uptake. J Nucl Med 34:414–419

Isselbacher KJ (1972) Sugar and amino acid transport by cells in culture – differences between normal and malignant cells. N Engl J Med 286:929–933

Jansson T, Westlin JE, Ahlstrom H, Lilja A, Langstrom B, Bergh J (1995) Positron emission tomography studies in patients with locally advanced and/or metastatic breast cancer: a method for early therapy evaluation? J Clin Oncol 13:1470–1477

Kenny LM, Vigushin DM, Al-Nahhas A, Osman S, Luthra SK, Shousha S, Coombes RC, Aboagye EO (2005) Quantification of cellular proliferation in tumor and normal tissues of patients with breast cancer by [18(F)]fluorothymidine-positron emission tomography imaging: evaluation of analytical methods. Cancer Res 65:10104–10112

KennyLM, CoombesRC, VigushinDM, Al-NahhasA, Shousha S, Aboagye EO (2007) Imaging early changes in proliferation at 1 week post chemotherapy: a pilot study in breast cancer patients with 3-deoxy-3-[(18)F]fluorothymidine positron emission tomography. Eur J Nucl Mol Imaging 34:1339–1347

Keshgegian A, Cnaan A (1995) Proliferation markers in breast carcinoma. Am J Cell Pathol 5:42–49

Kubota K, Matsuzawa T, Fujiwara T et al (1990) Differential diagnosis of lung tumor with positron emission tomography: a prospective study. J Nucl Med 31:1927–1932

Kubota R, Yamada S, Kubota K, Ishiwata K, Tamahashi N, Ido T (1992) Intratumoral distribution of fluorine-18-fluorodeoxyglucose in vivo: high accumulation in macrophages and granulation tissues studied by microautoradiography. J Nucl Med 33:1972–1980

Kubota R, Kubota K, Yamada S et al (1995) Methionine uptake by tumour tissue: a microautioradiographic comparison with FDG. J Nucl Med 36:484–492

Kumar R, Chauhan A, Zhuang H, Chandra P, Schnall M, Alavi A (2006) Clinicopathologic factors associated with false negative FDG-PET in primary breast cancer. Breast Cancer Res Treat 98:267–274

Kumar R, Chauhan A, Zhuang H, Chandra P, Schnall M, Alavi A (2006) Standardized uptake value of normal breast tissue with 2-deoxy-2-[F-18]fluoro-D-: -glucose positron emission tomography: variation with age, breast density and menopausal status. Mol Imaging Biol 8:355–362

Leskinen-Kallio S, Nagren K, Lehikoinen P, Ruotsalainen U, Joensuu H (1991) Uptake of ^{11}C-methionine in breast cancer studied by PET. An association with the size of S-phase fraction. Br J Cancer 64:1121–1124

Linden HM, Stekova SA, Link JM, Gralow JR, Livingston RB, Ellis GK, Petra PH, Peterson LM, Schubert EK, Dunnwald LK, Krohn KA, Mankoff DA (2006) Quantitative fluoroestradiol positron tomography imaging predicts response to endocrine treatment in breast cancer. J Clin Oncol 24:2793–2799

Loprinzi CL, Thome SD (2001) Understanding the utility of adjuvant systemic therapy for primary breast cancer. J Clin Oncol 19:972–979

MacGrogan G, Mauriac L, Durand M, Bonichon F, Trojani M, deMascarel I, Coindre J (1996) Primary chemotherapy in breast invasive carcinoma: predictive value of the immunohistochemical detection of hormonal receptors, p53, c-erbB-2, MIB1, pS2 and GSTπ. Br J Cancer 74:1458–1465

Maschauer S, Prante O, Hoffmann M, Deichen JT, Kuwert T (2004) Characterization of ^{18}F-FDG uptake in human endothelial cells in vitro. J Nucl Med 45:455–460

Masood S, Chiao J (1998) Pathology of breast cancer. In: Taillefer R, Khalkhali I, Waxman AD, Biersack HJ, eds. Radionuclide imaging of the breast. New York: Dekker

Mathupala SP, Rempel A, Pedersen PL (2001) Glucose catabolism in cancer cells: identification and characterization of a marked activation response of the type II hexokinase gene to hypoxicconditions. J Biol Chem 276:43407–43412

McGuire AH, Dehdashti F, Siegel BA, Lyss AP, Brodack JW, Mathias CJ, Mintun MA, Katzenellenbogen JA, Welch MJ (1991) Positron tomographic assessment of 16 alpha-[^{18}F] fluoro-17 beta-estradiol uptake in metastatic breast carcinoma. J Nucl Med 32:1526–1531

Mortimer JE, Dehdashti F, Siegel BA, Trinkaus K, Katzenellenbogen JA, Welch MJ (2001) Metabolic flare: indicator of hormone responsiveness in advanced breast cancer. J Clin Oncol 19:2797–2803

Oshida M, Uno K, Suzuki M et al (1998) Predicting the prognoses of breast carcinoma patients with positron emission tomography using 2-deoxy-2-fluoro[^{18}F]-d-glucose. Cancer 82:2227–2234

Overgaard J, Yilmaz M, Guldberg P, Hansen L, Alsner J (2000) TP53 mutation is an independent prognostic marker for poor outcome in both node-negative and node-positive breast cancer. Acta Oncol 39:327–333

Pedersen MW, Holm S, Lund EL, Hojgaard L, Kristjansen PE (2001) Coregulation of glucose uptake and vascular endothelial growth factor (VEGF) in two small-cell lung cancer (SCLC) sublinesinvivoandinvitro.Neoplasia 3:80–87

Pich A, Margaria E, Chiusa L (2000) Oncogenes and male breast carcinoma: c-erbB-2 and p53 coexpression predicts a poor survival. J Clin Oncol 18:2948–2956

Piert M, Machulla HJ, Picchio M, Reischl G, Ziegler S, Kumar P, Wester HJ, Beck R, McEwan AJ, Wiebe LI, Schwaiger M (2005) Hypoxia-specific tumor imaging with ^{18}F-fluoroazomycin arabinoside. J Nucl Med 46:106–113

Pio BS, Park CK, Pietras R, Hsueh WA, Satyamurthy N, Pegram MD, Czernin J, Phelps ME, Silverman DH (2006) Usefulness of 3-[F-18]fluoro-3-deoxythymidine with positron emission tomography in predicting breast cancer response to therapy. Mol Imaging Biol 8:36–42

Rajendran JG, Krohn KA (2005) Imaging hypoxia and angiogenesis in tumours. Radiol Clin North Am 43:169–187

Reske SN, Grillenberger KG, Glatting G et al (1997) Overexpression of glucose transporter 1 and increased FDG uptake in pancreatic carcinoma. J Nucl Med 38:1344–1348

Rempel A, Mathupala SP, Griffin CA, Hawkins AL, Pedersen PL (1996) Glucose catabolism in cancer cells: amplification of the gene encoding type II hexokinase. Cancer Res 56:2468–2471

Rudolph P, Alm P, Olsson H, Heidebrecht H, Ferno M, Baldetorp B, Parwaresch R (2001) Concurrent overexpression of p53 and c-erbB-2 correlates with accelerated cycling and concomitant poor prognosis in node-negative breast cancer. Hum Pathol 32:311–319

Shields AF, Grierson JR, Dohmen BM et al (1998) Imaging proliferation in vivo with ^{18}F-FLT and positron emission tomography. Nat Med 4:1334–1336

Smith TA, Sharma RI, Thompson AM, Paulin FE (2006) Tumor ^{18}F-FDG incorporation is enhanced by attenuation of P53 function in breast cancer cells in vitro. J Nucl Med 47:1525–1530

Torizuka T, Zasadny KR, Recker B, Wahl RL (1998) Untreated primary lung and breast cancers: correlation between F-18 FDG kinetic rate constants and findings of in vitro studies. Radiology 207:767–774

Veronesi U, De Cicco C, Galimberti VE, Fernandez JR, Rotmensz N, Viale G, Spano G, Luini A, Intra M, Veronesi P, Berrettini A, Paganelli G (2007) A comparative study on the value of FDG-PET and sentinel node biopsy to identify occult axillary metastases. Ann Oncol 18:473–478

Wang JQ, Gao M, Miller KD, Sledge GW, Zheng QH (2006) Synthesis of [11(C)]Iressa as a new potential PET cancere imaging agent for epidermal growth factor receptor tyrosine kinase. Bioorg Med Chem Lett 16:4102–4106

Warburg O (1924) PKNE. Ueber den Stoffwechsel der Carcinomzelle. Biochem Z 152:309–3444

Weidner N, Semple JP, Welch WR, Folkman J (1991) Tumor angiogenesis and metastasis-correlation in invasive breast carcinoma. N Engl J Med 324:1–8

Wester HJ (2007) Nuclear imaging probes: from bench to bedside. Clin Cancer Res 13:3470–3481

Wilson CB, Lammertsma AA, McKenzie CG, Sikora K, Jones T (1992) Measurements of blood flow and exchanging water space in breast tumors using positron emission tomography: a rapid and noninvasive dynamic method. Cancer Res 52:1592–1597

Wolf G, Aigner RM, Schaffler G, Langsenlehner U, renner W, Samonigg H, Yazdani-Bluki B, Krippl P (2004) The 936C>T polymorphism of the gene for vascular endothelial growth factor is associated with ^{18}F-fluorodeoxyglucose uptake. Breast Cancer Res Treat 88:205–208

Yagle KJ, Eary JF, Tait JF, Grierson JR, Link JM, Lewellen B, Gibson DF, Krohn KA (2005) Evaluation of ^{18}F-annexin V as a PET imaging agent in an animal model of apoptosis. J Nucl Med 46:658–666

Zasadny KR, Tatsumi M, Wahl RL (2003) FDG metabolism and uptake versus blood flow in women with untreated primary breast cancers. Eur J Nucl Med Mol Imaging 30:274–280

The Role of FDG-PET for Axillary Lymph Node Staging in Primary Breast Cancer

12

Flavio Crippa, Alberto Gerali, Alessandra Alessi, Roberto Agresti, and Emilio Bombardieri

CONTENTS

Abstract

PET and PET/CT have revealed a good diagnostic accuracy in visualizing both primary cancer and metastatic lesions, and many clinical studies demonstrate that they can compete with the morphological conventional diagnostic modalities mainly in staging, detecting tumor relapses, evaluating tumor response to therapy and giving useful prognostic indications. Data about the usefulness of PET to stage axillary nodes in breast cancer patients are controversial, also considering that another nuclear medicine technique, the sentinel lymph nodes biopsy (SLNB) after localization with lymphoscintigraphy, is very reliable for this indication. It is well known that SLNB today is considered the standard nuclear medicine method for staging axilla. This chapter is focused on the diagnostic potential of PET in studying lymph node axillary metastases that are one the most important prognostic factors affecting the therapeutic strategies. The diagnostic results of the most important clinical trials carried out with FDG-PET in axillary staging of breast cancer patients have been examined and reported. However, the position of FDG-PET in studying the loco-regional lymph nodal involvement still has to be completely evaluated, since the main problem is the absence of long-term prospective studies able to evaluate the outcome of the patients after FDG-PET staging and treated or not with ALND according to FDG negative or positive uptake.

The main reason for the discussions in the field is the limitation of FDG-PET in depicting the small metastases spread to axillary lymph nodes. This lack in sensitivity has become particularly evident since the introduction of very aggressive pathologic techniques with SLNB, such as multi-slice sectioning and immunocytochemistry staining. These approaches have significantly increased the rate of detection of micrometastases shown in the biopsies from the studies on the clinical validation of SLNB and ALND. On the contrary, the detection of micrometastases with FDG-PET is very critical, being limited by the spatial resolution of the PET scanner. Any discussions about this indication for PET in clinical oncology should take into consideration the fact that at present the standard method for staging axilla remains the ALND, which does not entail any intrinsic risk of downstaging the axillary status. The SLNB plays an important role in selecting patients that should undergo ALND due to its high sensitivity, also for micrometastases, even if the SLNB also has a non-negligible false-negative rate in almost all studies.

The combined used of SNLB and FDG-PET is a new strategy that has been recently proposed. According to the conclusions of some recent studies, this means that FDG-PET does not have to be considered as an alternative diagnostic tool instead of SLNB, but in those patients with clinically negative axillary lymph nodes, PET could discriminate patients eligible for ALND from the patients who should undergo SLNB. This is based on the FDG axillary uptake and on the high positive predictive value of PET. Therefore, breast cancer patients with FDG-positive uptake should directly undergo ALND rather than SLNB for axillary staging. On the contrary, those cases without FDG uptake in the axilla should be examined with SLNB in order to select candidates for ALND. This approach of course has to be validated through adequate large prospective studies with a follow-up evaluation, but it is important to stress the fact that in this way it is possible to take advantage of the strength of the two methods.

Probably the role of PET, even in this new clinical perspective, should be reconsidered due to the improvements of the scanner technology, such as with the hybrid system PET/CT or other more sophisticated advances in the detectors and/or dedicated software.

12.1 Background

The role of nuclear medicine in breast cancer has been extensively studied in recent years. The imaging of primary breast cancer and its loco-regional metastases has been investigated at the beginning with scintimammography, without a satisfactory accuracy, in spite of some improvements obtained by SPECT and the recent development of some dedicated breast gamma cameras (Liberman et al. 2003; Hussain and Buscombe 2006; Sampalis et al. 2003; Brem et al. 2002; Schillaci et al. 2005; Rhodes et al. 2005). PET and PET/CT revealed a great diagnostic accuracy in visualizing both primary and metastatic lesions, and a great deal of clinical evidence demonstrates that they can compete with the morphological conventional diagnostic modalities in staging, detecting tumor relapses, evaluating tumor response to therapy and giving useful prognostic indications (Endo et al. 2006; Zangheri et al. 2004; Rodesse et al. 2005).

Data about the usefulness of PET to staging axillary nodes are more controversial, also considering that another nuclear medicine approach, the sentinel lymph node biopsy (SLNB) after localization with lymphoscintigraphy is very reliable for the same indication. For this reason SLNB has been proposed by several authors as a standard nuclear medicine method for staging axilla. This chapter is focused on the diagnostic potential of PET in studying lymph node axillary metastases, which are one of the most important prognostic factors that affects the therapeutic strategies. The imaging of lymph node invasion by a nuclear medicine modality can be carried out also by SPECT with gamma-emitting radiopharmaceuticals using a pinhole collimator; however, this approach, even if successful in some studies published by a few authors, has been overcome by FDG-PET due to the worldwide application of this technology (Schillaci et al. 2002).

12.2 Sentinel Lymph Node Biopsy (SLNB)

The goal of every diagnostic tool to investigate the axillary status is to avoid the axillary node dissection (ALND), which is not curative; it is an invasive method and brings a significant rate of complications (Giuliano et al. 1997). Among nuclear medicine methods the sentinel lymph node biopsy has been extensively studied as an alternative method to routine ALND to detect axillary node status. The conclusions of many clinical studies in the majority of oncological institutions have proposed SLNB as a standard method for axillary lymph node staging in breast cancer patients (Krag et al. 1993). The diagnostic accuracy of SLNB cannot be discussed; lymphoscintigraphy in combination with gamma-probe-guided surgery is feasible everywhere, improves both the staging and the pathological analysis and shows less morbidity than axillary lymph node dissection (Cody 2003; Veronesi et al. 1997). However, at present the protocols for lymphoscintigraphy are different in the various institutions, and several controversies still exist about the size of radiocolloid used, the injected activity, the volume of injection and the site of injection (intratumoral, intraparenchimal, periareolar/subareolar and intradermal/subdermal) (Krag et al. 1993; Cody 2003; Veronesi et al. 1997; Cody and Borgen 1999; Wilhelm et al. 1999; Mariani et al. 2001). In spite of a lot of discussions about the optimal technique that should be carried out, the general thought is that whatever method is used, lymphoscintigraphy followed by intraoperative gamma-probe detection is always able to localize the axillary SLNs. It should be stressed that lymphoscintigraphy can also visualize the internal mammary chain. This happens in 2% of cases when it is performed after subdermal/intradermal injection of radiocolloid, up to 10% or more when the injection is carried out in the tumor mass or when the tumor is located in the inner quadrant (Paganelli et al. 2002; Clarke et al. 2001).

Today SLNB is routinely performed in clinical practice; however, the clinical indications for SLNB nowadays still represent a matter of study. Many oncological and surgical institutions consider SLNB as a standard practice in the treatment of patients with early breast cancer and clinically negative lymph nodes. Other proposals are under evaluation in order to extend and validate its indications since the available data derive mainly from retrospective studies. Some major randomized clinical trials have been designed with the goal to better validate the clinical indications of SLNB. These prospective trials want to give an answer to the three fundamental critical questions about SLNB: (1) Is the predictive power of the axillary status using SLNB the same as using ALND? (b) Does SLNB reduce complications of breast surgery? (3) What is the effect of SLNB on long-term survival and on the local control of the axilla (Sato 2007)? Even if the overall data from these trials are still not completely available and conclusive, the SLNB technique has been adopted as the standard technique by the majority of surgical institutions since the axillary clearance does not have a curative intent, but represents only diagnostic information. The problem is to understand if SLNB is the only reliable method for loco-regional staging of breast cancer or if there is some role for PET, considering its diagnostic performances.

12.3 PET with ^{18}F-Fluorodeoxyglucose (FDG-PET)

FDG-PET in breast cancer was first studied to investigate glucose metabolism. Breast cancer tissues have proved to have particularly avidity for FDG due both to their elevated metabolic rate and the overexpression of some glucose transporters such as GLUT-1 and GLUT-3 (Som et al. 1980; Brown and Wahl 1993; Pauwels et al. 2000). FDG at 40 min after the injection reaches good tumor/background ratio in the tumor (mean value above 10), which leads to a clear visualization of cancer lesions. The relatively long half-life of ^{18}F makes it possible to study the FDG distribution, improving the identification of malignancy (Wahl et al. 1991). Clinical evidence has demonstrated that FDG-PET has a great diagnostic efficacy in staging and restaging breast cancer patients, detecting local or distance recurrences after surgery and assessing the response to the treatment (Bombardieri and Crippa 2001). FDG-PET was demonstrated to be useful also to study and characterize primary breast cancer lesions; however, PET as a diagnostic approach at the first presentation of a breast mass did not show a higher sensitivity than mammography, ultrasonography and RMI, except in some particular situations.

The loco-regional breast cancer staging, and in particular the study of the axillary region, has been an area of a very intensive investigations with FDG-PET since this technique has revealed good capability to depict the lymph node invasion in patients with pathological nodes (Fig. 12.1). This opportunity resulted in great interest, because the preoperative FDG-PET could be considered as the diagnostic modality to select patients who are candidates for ALND or not. The data from the clinical studies immediately showed great differences in the diagnostic sensitivity, which ranged from 60 to 100%. Utech et al. (1996) studied 124 patients with T1-T3 breast cancer before ALND, and PET correctly identified all 44 patients with axillary metastases with an overall sensitivity of 100%. These impressive results were not repeated in other clinical studies, which in different series of patients found a sensitivity ranging from 67 to 92% (Holle et al. 1996; Crowe et al. 1994; Scheidhauer et al. 1996; Dehdashti et al. 1995). Of course many factors determine this variability, first of all the size of the tumor and consequently the probability of metastases and the extension of lymph node invasion. Avril et al. (1996) demonstrated an

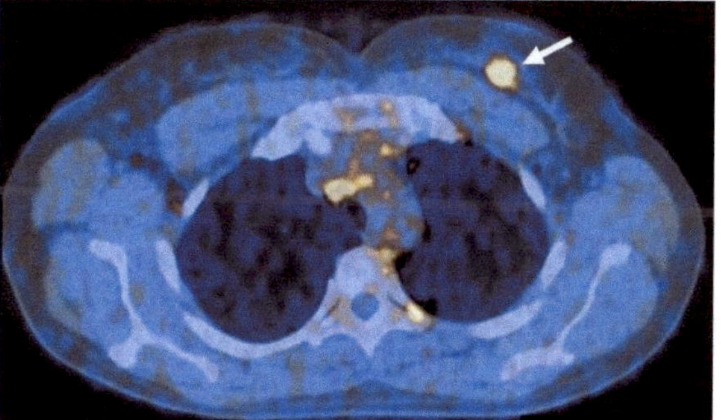
a

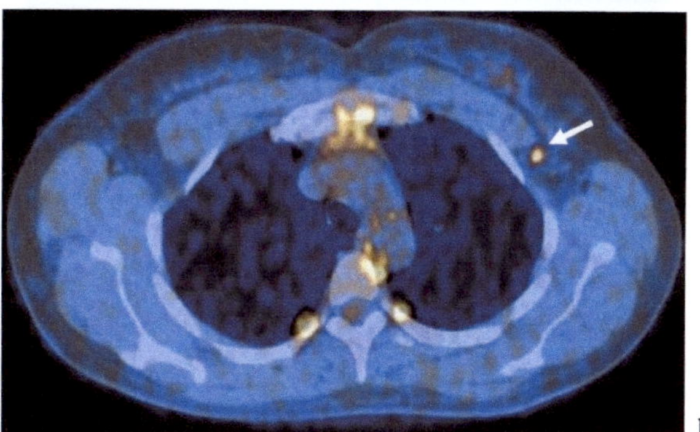
b

Fig. 12.1a,b. PET/CT image (transaxial section) of a breast cancer patient with an intense uptake in the left breast and in the corresponding axillary region. The pathology revealed a ductal infiltrating carcinoma with lymph nodal metastases

overall sensitivity of 79%, which dropped to 33% in a subset of patients with T1 tumors. In an American multicenter and prospective study including a very large series of cases (360 patients), the mean sensitivity and the negative predictive value of FDG-PET were 61% and 76%, respectively (Wahl et al. 2004). As we mentioned above, these very important differences in PET performances might be explained by the different characteristics of the patients studied, such as the prevalence of small and less easily detectable axillary metastases, or the protocols used to reconstruct PET images, or again the pathological method used in depicting lymph nodal metastases that enclose the multi-slice sectioning of the lymph nodes' range and the staining technique ranging from the standard hematoxylin-eosin method to the immunohistochemistry.

At the National Cancer Institute of Milan we performed a large study on breast cancer patients, and we obtained very good results with FDG-PET (Greco et al. 2002). We prospectively studied 167 consecutive breast cancer patients (mean tumor size 21-mm diameter, range 5–50 mm), all non-pre-treated, with tumors T1–T2 scheduled for complete ALND dissection. FDG-PET images were evaluated by nuclear medicine physicians blinded to pathological results, and PET results were compared with pathological findings. The overall sensitivity, specificity and accuracy of PET were 94.4% (PET detected 69 of 72 patients with axillary involvement), 86.3% (PET was negative in 82 out if 95 patients without axillary involvement) and 89.8% (PET gave correct results in 150 out of 167 patients with breast cancer), respectively (Table 12.1). The positive and negative predictive values were 84% (68 out of 81) and 95.3% (82 out of 97), respectively. False-negative results were observed only in a few patients with a low tumor burden or microscopic lymph node metastases. The four false-negative FDG-PET results were three non-palpable and one palpable axillary node; the type of histological involvement was embolic in two cases and partial infiltration in the other two cases. Among the 72 patients with axillary metastases, PET detected three or fewer metastatic nodes in 27 patients (37.5%), about 80% of whom had no clinically palpable axillary lymph nodes. When the PET results were analyzed in relation to the primary tumor size (patients were grouped according to T classification in T1a–b, T1c and T2), the diagnostic accuracy was similar for all groups, with higher sensitivity in patients with larger tumors of 21–50 mm (98%) and higher specificity in patients with tumors of 10 mm or less (87.8%) (Table 12.2). The range for negative predictive values was 93.5 to 97.3% and 54.5 to 94.1% for positive predictive values. Therefore, our data do not exclude using PET for staging axilla. However, it is well known that the limitations of FDG-PET in preoperative axillary staging consist of two critical points: the spatial resolution limits of PET that do not allow detection of lesions under 4–5 mm in diameter and the competition with SLNB, which shows a general sensitivity superior than that of FDG-PET for the smallest metastases. In fact, the role of FDG-PET in the axillary staging of breast cancer has been particularly doubted in some recent studies where immunochemistry and multistep sectioning were used by the pathologist in order to increase the rate of pathological detection of axillary micrometastases (i.e., clusters of malignant cells >0.2 mm to <2.00 mm in diameter). In these studies, including a large number of patients with a microscopic lymph node invasion, FDG-PET proved to have a very poor sensitivity ranging from 20 to 43% (Kelemen et al. 2002; Guller et al. 2002; van der Hoeven et al. 2002; Lovrics et al. 2001).

For these reasons several studies were designed with the goal of comparing FDG-PET versus SLNB in the same patients. At our institute a comparative study between FDG-PET and SLNB in patients with

Table 12.1. Experience of the National Cancer Institute of Milan on FDG-PET diagnostic performances in staging axillary lymph nodes in breast cancer

Diagnostic parameter	N0 (*n* =129)	N1(*n* =39)	Overall (*n*=167)
Sensitivity	92.9% (39/42)	96.7% (29/30)	94.4% (68/72)
Specificity	87.4% (76/87)	75.0% (6/8)	86.3% (83/95)
Accuracy	89.1% (115/129)	92.1% (35/38)	89.8% (150/167)
Positive predictive value	78.0% (39/50)	93.5% (29/31)	84.0% (68/81)
Negative predictive value	96.2% (76/79)	85.7% (6/7)	95.3% (82/86)

Table 12.2. Changes of diagnostic parameters of FDG-PET according to the tumor size of primary breast tumor

Diagnostic parameter	T1 a-b (*n* =48)	T1c (*n* =50)	T2 (*n* =69)
Sensitivity	85.7% (6/7)	87.5% (14/16)	98% (48/49)
Specificity	87.8% (36/41)	85.3% (29/34)	85.0% (17/20)
Accuracy	87.5% (42/48)	86.0 (43/50)	94.2% (65/69)
Positive predictive value	54.5% (6/11)	73.7% (14/19)	94.1% (48/51)
Negative predictive value	97.3 (36/37)	93.5% (29/31)	94.4% (17/18)

T1 breast cancer is ongoing (Agresti et al. 2004). FDG-PET is carried out no later than 48 h before surgery; lymphoscintigraphy is carried out within 6 h before ALDN. Breast surgery is followed by radio-guided SLNB, and ALND is decided in case FDG-PET and/or SLNB is positive. Metastatic involvement of the sentinel node of the other non-sentinel nodes is assessed by histology comparing PET imaging and SLNB. Seventy-one patients have been studied; all patients had pT1 breast cancer with the exception of ten whose tumors were pT2. The average histological tumor size was 15 mm (range 2–25 mm). All lymph nodes detected by lymphoscintigraphy were located in the axillary region, and the detection rate was 100%. All nodes were identified with an intraoperative gamma probe and then examined by pathology. When ALND was performed, an average of ten lymph nodes was removed. Thirty-one of the 71 patients (43%) had nodal metastases; 18 of these 31 patients had only one metastatic node 58%). SLNB gave 6 false-negative results, while FDG-PET failed to detect 11 instances of axillary node involvement (histology described some isolated tumor cells, micro-embolic or pluri-embolic metastases). Only two patients with clear axillary lymph node involvement, one with partial and one with massive involvement, were not identified by FDG-PET. There were three false-positive PET scans. Our preliminary results stress the different sensitivity between FDG-PET and ALNB, especially in the presence of very limited axillary involvement, whereas for metastases exceeding 2 mm in size the sensitivity of the two methods is similar.

Zornoza et al. (2004) evaluated FDG-PET for the detection of lymph node status in 200 breast cancer patients. All patients had a FDG-PET scan, but in a subgroup of 100 patients, FDG-PET was complemented with the detection of the sentinel node when FDG-PET was negative for axillary uptake. The diagnostic sensitivity and specificity of FDG-PET in the diagnosis of axillary involvement were good, equivalent to 84.1 and 97.8%, respectively. Seventeen false-negative cases were described, and the author explained this failure with the low metabolism of breast cancer tissue since a low SUV value was measured in those negative tumors. The discussion on FDG-PET as a diagnostic tool for loco-regional staging has led to the following conclusions. Since the diagnostic specificity of FDG-PET had excellent results, PET should be proposed in substitution of routine SLNB in those cases presenting with axillary uptake. On the contrary, in those patients who had a negative axilla, FDG-PET should be complemented by SLNB.

With a prospective blinded protocol, Lovrics et al. (2004) investigated women with stage I or II breast cancer and compared FDG-PET to SLNB and ALND in staging axilla. The samples of lymph nodes after ALND were stained with standard hematoxylin and eosin staining, while lymph nodes depicted by SLNB were also studied by pathologic techniques able to identify micrometastases. A total of 90 patients were enrolled. PET findings were compared with histology after ALND, and the diagnostic sensitivity was 40%, the positive predictive value 75%. The same figures were similar when compared with positive sentinel node analyzed with standard hematoxylin and eosin staining. A few false-positive scannings were observed. Multiple logistic regression analysis demonstrated that the accuracy of PET was better in patients with high grade and larger tumors. The author's conclusion was that the diagnostic sensitivity of PET is lower than that of SLNB and ALND. On the contrary, PET scanning showed a high specificity and consequently a high positive predictive value. Also this study suggests that PET cannot replace the histological staging in early stage breast cancer. However, the low rate of false-positive findings supports the role of FDG-PET in identifying women who should forego SLNB and require full axillary dissection.

A similar approach was adopted by Gil-Rendo et al. (2006) who evaluated 275 women with breast cancer in order to study the metastatic involvement of axillary lymph nodes by comparing FDG-PET and ALND. In the first group of 150 patients, ALND was performed regardless of the PET results. In a second group of 125 patients, FDG-PET was complemented with SLNB only in those who did not demonstrate any pathological FDG uptake in the axilla. The diagnostic sensitivity and specificity of FDG-PET in detecting axillary involvement were 84.5 and 98.5%, respectively, in the whole series of 275 patients, with only 2 false-positive, but with 22 false-negative results. The high positive predictive value of PET, 98.4%, supports the concept that FDG uptake in the axilla could represent an indicator for full ALND without previous SLNB.

The question whether PET could obviate the necessity for SLNB and for ALND in patients with breast cancer has been recently studied by Kumar et al. (2006). A total of 80 females with breast cancer and clinically negative nodes underwent an FDG-PET and SLNB or ALND for staging the axilla. SLNB and axillary dissection were performed together in 72 patients, while 8 patients had ALND without SLNB. Among these 80 patients, 36 revealed pathologic axillary metastastic involvement. SLNB was positive for metastases in 35 (97%) of 36 patients (29 macrometastases and 7 micrometastases). The false-negative cases at SLNB were due to the fact that lymph nodes were completely replaced by tumor. The FDG-PET determined 16 of 36 patients were true positive (diagnostic sensitivity 44%). Two false-positive studies were described with FDG-PET, resulting in a specificity of 95%. The positive predictive value and accuracy of FDG PET for the detection of axillary lymph node metastases were 89 and 72%, respectively. The statistical analysis revealed that a higher grade of tumor, increased size and number of axillary lymph nodes were significantly associated with positive FDG PET results. This study concluded that FDG PET cannot replace histological staging with SLNB. Therefore, FDG-PET should be considered as a reliable axillary staging only in those patients with larger size, higher grade of tumor and higher number of axillary lymph node. FDG-PET has confirmed its high diagnostic specificity and a good positive predictive value, and for this reason the value of a positive uptake should be considered a highly reliable indicator for the presence of metastatic lymph nodes.

Another important diagnostic study was carried out by Veronesi et al. (2007) who investigated the diagnostic performances of PET compared with SLNB and ALND. The author enrolled 236 patients with breast cancer and clinically negative axilla in the study. FDG PET was carried out before surgery, and SLNB was carried out after identification through lymphoscintigraphy. Patients underwent ALND in cases of positive FDG-PET or positive SNB. The results of PET scan were compared with pathology of SNB and ALND. The clinical results showed that 203 of 236 patients (44%) had metastases in axillary nodes. Sensitivity of FDG-PET scan for detection of axillary lymph nodes metastases in this series was very poor (37%). However, specificity and positive predictive values were acceptable (96% and 88%, respectively), and the figures were similar to those described by other authors in these clinical observations. The conclusions of the author can be summarized as follows: the high specificity of PET imaging supports the indication that patients with FDG-PET-positive axilla should have an ALND rather than a SLNB for axillary staging. In contrast, the poor sensitivity shown by FDG-PET in the detection of axillary metastases supports the need for SLNB in those cases where PET is negative in the axilla.

All of this clinical evidence demonstrates a general lack in sensitivity of FDG-PET in respect to the SLNB, and at present there are no studies in breast cancer that demonstrate that the recent availability of the hybrid system PET/CT can improve the FDG-PET results for axillary staging. From the theoretical point of view PET/CT could enhance PET accuracy for detecting lymph nodal invasion (von Schulthess 2004; Veit et al. 2006). However, until now these kinds of data have been reported in neoplasms other than breast tumors, such as head and neck cancer and esophageal cancer (Yuan et al. 2006; Joeng et al. 2007). Probably we will have to wait until the near future before having an exhaustive evaluation in this area.

On the basis of the observations of the literature on axillary staging, there is a general agreement about the high diagnostic specificity of FDG-PET, despite the well-known occurrence of false-positive results in diagnostic oncology with FDG-PET owing to concomitant inflammatory alteration. Nearly all recent investigations report a false-positive rate ranging from 0–6%, and this is one of the reasons why several authors suggest that patients with FDG-positive uptake should avoid SLNB, and they should be directly addressed to ALND. In this case, FDG-PET can represent an alternative to SLNB.

Another advantage of FDG-PET is its potential to image the abnormal findings that are consistent with supraclavicular or internal lymph nodes metastases (Fig. 12.2). Eubank et al. (2001) found a higher sensitivity of PET versus CT (85 versus 54%) in the detection of mediastinal or internal mammary metastases by means of a retrospective evaluation of 73 patients. Zornosa et al. (2004) in 15 of 200 patients with primary breast cancer visualized abnormal foci of FDG uptake in the internal mammary lymph nodes consistent with metastases. In the study by Gil Rendo et al. (2006), FDG-PET showed pathological uptake in 21 women corresponding to the internal mammary lymph node chain. This issue remains a very critical item, since the difficulty in obtaining histopathological confirmation of PET results precludes estimation of the real contribution of PET in this respect. Besides this, also lymphoscintigraphy, mainly in certain conditions and adopting particular techniques of radiocolloid injection, is able to show some focal uptake corresponding to the internal mammary chain (Paganelli et al. 2002; Clarke et al. 2001). The clinical usefulness of these aspects both for FDG-PET and SLNB still has to be understood.

12.4 Discussion

The position of FDG-PET in studying the loco-regional lymph nodal involvement in breast cancer patients still has to be completely evaluated, since the main problem is the absence of long-term prospective studies able to evaluate the outcome of the patients staged with FDG-PET and treated or not with ALND according to FDG negative or positive uptake (Crippa et al. 2004).

The main reason for this is the limitation of FDG-PET in depicting the spread of small metastases to axillary lymph nodes (van der Hoeven et al. 2002; Barranger et al. 2003). This lack in sensitivity has become particularly evident since the introduction of very aggressive pathologic techniques, such as multi-slice sectioning, immunocytochemistry staining and RT-PCR assay (Viale et al. 2006; Dell'Orto et al. 2006). These approaches have significantly increased the rate of detection of micrometastases shown in the biopsies from the studies on the clinical validation of SLNB and ALND.

It has been well demonstrated, also by our group, that the detection of micrometastases with FDG-PET is very critical, being limited by the spatial resolution of the PET scanner.

In a study carried out on melanoma patients, we observed that the diagnostic sensitivity we obtained for lymph nodal metastases with a PET with a full-ring BGO detector system was 100% for metastases larger than 10 mm, 83% for lesions ranging from 6 and 9 mm, and 23% for localizations smaller than 5 mm (Crippa et al. 2000) (Table 12.3). Also the type of histological involvement of the lymph nodes determines different rates of sensitivity (Table 12.4). These limitations did not affect the sensitivity of FDG-PET in our previous study on axillary staging, probably owing to the low incidence of micrometastases detected by histopathology with hematoxylin-eosin staining, which at that time was the standard method in our institute.

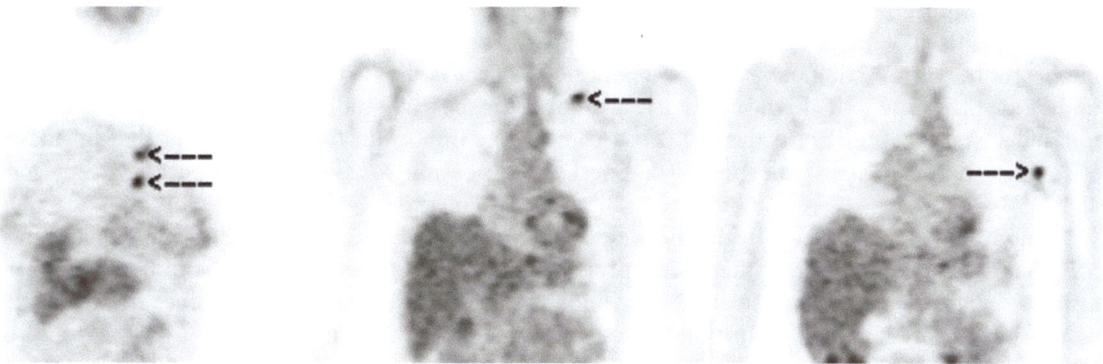

Fig. 12.2. FDG-PET (coronal section) of a breast cancer patient with clear evidence of multiple foci of FDG uptake in the left axillary, supraclavicular and parasternal area. These findings corresponded to lymph node metastatic involvement, confirmed with histology on axillary nodes sample

Table 12.3. Sensitivity of FDG-PET according to the and size of metastases in mm

Size in mm of metastases	Metastases found with histology (no.)	Metastases found by PET no. (%)
≤5	44	10 (23)
6-10	29	24 (83)
11-15	13	13 (100)
16-20	15	15 (100)
21-25	9	9 (100)
>25	4	4 (100)
Total	**114**	**75 (66)**

Table 12.4. Sensitivity of FDG-PET according to the type of metastatic involvement

Type of metastases	Nodes involved histologically (no.)	Nodes involved by FDG-PET no. (%)
Embolic, pluriembolic	11	3 (27)
Partial	48	18 (37.5)
Subtotal	15	14 (93)
Massive	21	21 (100)
Perinodal infiltration	19	19 (100)
Total	**114**	**75 (66)**

On the basis of these indisputable results, many authors have concluded that FDG-PET cannot be routinely used for axillary staging of operable breast cancer. However, any discussion about this indication for PET in clinical oncology should take into consideration the fact that at present the standard method remains the ALND that does not entail an intrinsic risk of down-staging the axillary status. As we have discussed above, the SLNB can play an important role in selecting patients that should not undergo ALND, due to its high sensitivity, also for micrometastases, even if also the SLNB has some false-negative rate in almost all studies (Veronesi et al. 2005).

Combining the different diagnostic value of SNLB and FDG-PET, several interesting proposals to associate the use of both strategies are under discussion. In other terms, according to the conclusions of some recent clinical trials, FDG-PET should not to be considered as an alternative diagnostic tool instead of SLNB, but in those patients with clinically negative axillary lymph nodes PET could select patients eligible for ALND from the patients who should go first to SLNB. This is based on FDG axillary uptake and the high positive predictive value of PET. In other terms, breast cancer patients with FDG-positive uptake should undergo ALND directly rather than a SLNB for axillary staging. On the contrary, those cases without FDG uptake in the axilla should be examined with SLNB in order to select candidates for ALND. This strategy of course has to be validated through adequate large prospective studies with a follow-up evaluation, but it is important to stress the fact that in this way it is possible to take advantage of the strength of the two methods.

Probably the role of PET, even considering this new clinical perspective, has to be reconsidered if some future improvement comes from the scanner technology. We are still waiting for the results of the clinical applications of PET/CT in this area or for other more sophisticated advances in the detector systems and/or dedicated software. Also the combined use of FDG-PET with MRI using ultra-small super paramagnetic iron oxide (USPIO) seems to achieve 100% sensitivity in staging axillary lymph nodes preoperatively (Stadnik et al. 2006). However, in spite of this possible realistic progress, we believe that it should be expected and accepted that a limited number of patients with axillary micrometastases will always remain undetected by any FDG-PET system or combination of tests. Nevertheless, a false-negative FDG-PET result will represent a very small number of lymph node metastases with very limited invasion of the lymphatic structures. Finally, this limitation should be analyzed in relation to the importance of such axillary metastases for the outcome of the patients with breast cancer. There are no definitive data about the role of micrometastes in the natural history of breast cancer. In our institute a prospective non-randomized study was carried out on 401 patients with T1-2N0 breast cancer who had undergone breast surgery without ALND and were monitored with a median follow-up of 5 years. Only 27 (6.7%) patients had axillary recurrence of the disease. This would suggest that only a few axillary micrometasases become clinically evident during such follow-up, and further analysis of these patients revealed that these axillary relapses had no major impact on overall survival (Greco et al. 2000).

However, today the current knowledge in this area seems to give relevance to the combined use of FDG-PET and SLNB, excluding or not the second test on the basis of the presence/absence of the FDG uptake. This means that all patients with small primary tumors and clinically negative axilla should undergo FDG-PET or FDG-PET/CT as preoperative staging, with the goal of sparing the patient SLNB and the eventual following ALND, and have conservative breast surgery. Also patients with larger primary tumors and clinically doubtful or positive axilla should have PET or PET/CT, but in this case with the aim to stage the whole body for disease, searching for metastases. Only a large clinical experience and the evaluation of the outcome of the patients will be able to give a definitive solution about the correct use of this available diagnostic tool.

References

Agresti R, Crippa F, Gerali A et al (2004) Lymph node metastases detection by FDG-PET and sentinel node biopsy in breast cancer patients: comparison of these different approaches. Eur J Nucl Med Mol Imag 31 (Suppl 1):97–102

Avril N, Dose J, Janicke F, Ziegler S et al (1996) Assessment of axillary lymph node involvement in breast cancer patients with positron emission tomography using radiolabeled 2-fluorine-18-fluoro-2-deoxy-D-glucose. J Natl Cancer Inst 88:1204–1209

Barranger E, Grahek D, Antoine M, Montravers F, Talbot JN, Uzan S (2003) Evaluation of fluorodeoxyglucose positron emission tomography in the detection of axillary lymph node metastases in patients with early-stage breast cancer. Ann Surg Oncol 10:622–627

Bombardieri E, Crippa F (2001) PET imaging in breast cancer. Q J Nucl Med 45:245–256

Brem RF, Schoonians JM, Kieper DA et al (2002) High-resolution scintimammography: a pilot study. J Nucl Med 43:909–915

Brown RW, Wahl RL (1993) Overexpression of GLUT-1 glucose transport in human breast cancer: an immunohistochemical study. Cancer 72:2979–2985

Clarke D, Khoni NI, Mansel ER (2001) Sentinel node biopsy in breast cancer. AMLANAC trial. World J Surg 25:819–822

Cody HS 3rd, Borgen PI (1999) State of the art approaches to sentinel node biopsy for biopsy for breast cancer: study design, patient selection, technique, and quality control at Memorial Sloan Kettering Cancer Center. Surg Oncol 8:85–91

Cody HS 3rd (2003) Sentinel lymph node biopsy for breast cancer: does anybody not need one? Ann Surg Oncol 10:1131–1132

Crippa F, Leutner M, Belli F et al (2000) Which kinds of lymph node metastases can FDG PET detect? A clinical study in melanoma. J Nucl Med 41:1491–1494

Crippa F, Gerali A, Alessi A, Agresti R, Bombardieri E (2004) FDG-PET for axillary lymph node staging in primary breast cancer. Eur J Nucl Med Mol Imaging 31:S97–S102

Crowe JP, Adler LP, Shenk RR, Sunshine J (1994) Positron emission tomography and breast masses: comparison with clinical, mammographic, and pathological findings. Ann Surg Oncol 1:132–140

Dehdashti F, Mortimer JE, Siegel BA et al (1995) Positron tomographic assessment of estrogen receptors in breast cancer: comparison with FDG-PET and in vitro receptor assays. J Nucl Med 36:1766–1774

Dell'Orto P, Biasi MO, Del Curto B, Zurrida S, Galimberti V, Viale G (2006) Assessing the status of axillary sentinel lymph nodes of breast carcinoma patients by a real-time quantitative RT-PCR assay for mammaglobin 1 mRNA. Breast Cancer Treat 98:185–190

Endo K, Oriuchi N, Higuchi T, Iida Y, Hanaoka H, Miyakubo M, Ishikita T, Koyama K (2006) PET and PET/CT using ^{18}F-FDG in the diagnosis and management of cancer patients. Int J Clin Oncol 11:286–296

Eubank WB, Mankoff DA, Takasugi J et al (2001) 18Fluorodeoxyglucose positron emission tomography to detect mediastinal or internal mammary metastases in breast cancer. J Clin Oncol 19:3516–3523

Gil-Rendo A, Zornoza G, Garcis-Velloso MJ, Regueira FM, Beorlegui C, Cervera M (2006) Fluorodeoxyglucose positron emission tomography with sentinel lymph node biopsy for evaluation of axillary involvement in breast cancer. Br J Surg 93:707–712

Giuliano AE, Jones RC, Brennan M et al (1997) Sentinel lymphadenectomy and breast cancer. J Clin Oncol 15:2345–2350

Greco M, Agresti R, Cascinelli N et al (2000) Breast cancer patients treated without axillary surgery: clinical implication and biologic analysis. Ann Surg 232:1–7

Greco M, Crippa F, Agresti R et al (2001) Axillary lymph node staging in breast cancer by 2-fluoro-2-deoxy-D-glucose positron emission tomography: clinical evaluation and alternative management. J Natl Cancer Inst 93:630–635

Guller U, Nitzsche EU, Schirp U et al (2002) Selective axillary surgery in breast cancer patients based on positron emission tomography with ^{18}F-fluoro-2-deoxy-D-glucose: not yet! Breast Cancer Res Treat 71:171–173

Holle LH, Trampert L, Lung-Kurt S et al (1996) Investigations of breast tumors with fluorine-18-fluorodeoxyglucose and SPECT. J Nucl Med 37:615–622

Hussain R, Buscombe JR (2006) A meta-analysis of scintimammography: an evidence-based approach to its clinical utility. Nucl Med Commun 27:589–594

Joeng HS, Baek CH, Son YI et al (2007) Use of integrated ^{18}F-FDG/CT to improve the accuracy of initial cervical nodal evaluation in patients with head and neck squamous cell carcinoma. Head Neck 29:203–210

Kelemen PR, Lowe V, Philips N (2002) Positron emission tomography and sentinel lymph node dissection in breast cancer. Clin Breast Cancer 3:73–77

Krag DN, Weaver DL, Alex JC et al (1993) Surgical resection and radiolocalization of the sentinel lymph node in breast cancer using a gamma-probe. Surg Oncol 2:335–340

Kumar R, Zhuang H, Schnall M et al (2006) FDG PET positive lymph nodes are highly predictive of metastasis in breast cancer. NUcl Med Commun 27:231–236

Lovrics P, Chen V, Coates G et al (2001) A prospective study of PET scanning, sentinel node biopsy, and standard axillary dissection for axillary staging in patients with early stage breast cancer. Abstract book 24th Annual Cancer Symposium, Society of Surgical Oncology

Lovrics PJ, Chen V, Coates G et al (2004) A prospective evaluation of positron emission tomography scanning, sentinel lymph node biopsy, and standard axillary dissection for axillary staging in patients with early stage breast cancer. Ann Surg Oncol 11:846–853

Liberman M, Sampalis F, Mulder DS et al (2003) Breast cancer diagnosis by scintimammography: a meta-analysis and review of the literature. Brest Cancer Res Treat 80:115–126

Mariani G, Moresco L, Viale G et al (2001) Radioguided sentinel lymph node biopsy in breast cancer surgery. J Nucl Med 42:1198–1215

Paganelli G, Galimberti V, Trifirò G et al (2002) Internal mammary node lymphoscintigraphy and biopsy in breast cancer. Q J Nucl Med 46:138–144

Pauwels EKJ, Strum EJ, Bombardieri E et al (2000) Positron-emission tomography with (^{18}F) fluorodeoxyglucose. J Cancer Res Clin Oncol 126:549–559

Rhodes DJ, O'Connor MK, Philips SW et al (2005) Molecular breast imaging: a new technique using technetium Tc scintimammography to detect small tumors of the breast. Mayo Clin Proc 80:24–30

Rodesse J, Alberini JL, Wartski M, Gutman F, Collignon MA, Corone C, Pichon MF, Pecking AP (2005) FDG-^{18}fluoro-deoxyglucose-positron emission tomography and breast cancer. Bull Acad Natl Med 189:963–975

Sampalis FS, Denis R, Picard D et al (2003) International prospective evaluation of scintimammography with ^{99m}Tc-sestamibi. Am J Surg 185:544–549

Sato K (2007) Clinical trials for sentinel node biopsy in patients with breast cancer. Breast Cancer 14:31–36

Scheidhauer K, Scharl A, Pietrzyk U et al (1996) Qualitative ^{18}F-FDG positron emission tomography in primary breast cancer: clinical relevance and practicability. Eur J Nucl Med 23:618–623

Schillaci O, Scopinaro F, Spanu A, Donnetti M, Danieli R, Di Luzio E, Madeddu G, David V (2002) Detection of axillary lymph node metastases in breast cancer with Tc-99m tetrofosmin scintimammography. Int J Oncol 20:483–487

Schillaci O, Manni C, Danieli R et al (2005) Tc-99m sestamibi scintimammography with a hybrid SPECT/CT imaging system. Eur J Nucl Med Mol Imaging 32:S128

Som P, Atkins HL, Bandoypadhyay D et al (1980) A fluorinated glucose analog, 2-fluoro-2-deoxy-D-glucose (F18): non-toxic tracer for rapid tumor detection. J Nucl Med 21:670–675

Stadnik TW, Everaert H, Makkat S, Sacré R, Lamote J, Bourgain C (2006) Breast imaging. Preoperative breast cancer staging: comparison of USPIO-enhanced MR imaging and ^{18}F-fluorodeoxyglucose (FDG) positron emission tomography (PET) imaging for axillary lymph node staging-initial findings. Eur Radiol 16:2153–2160

Utech CI, Young CS, Winter PF (1996) Prospective evaluation of fluorine-18 fluorodeoxyglucose positron emission tomography in breast cancer for staging of the axilla related to surgery and immunocytochemistry. Eur J Nucl Med 23:1588–1593

van der Hoeven JJ, Hoekstra OS, Comans EF et al (2002) Determinations of diagnostic performance of F-18 fluorodeoxyglucose positron emission tomography for axillary staging in breast cancer. Ann Surg 236:619–624

Veit P, Ruehm S, Kuehl H, Stergar H, Mueller S, Bockisch A, Antoch G (2006) Lymph node staging with dual-modality PET/CT: enhancing the diagnostic accuracy in oncology. Eur J Radiol 58:383–389

Veronesi U, Paganelli G, Galimberti V et al (1997) Sentinel-node biopsy to avoid AD in breast cancer with clinically negative lymph nodes. Lancet 349:1864–1867

Veronesi U, Galimberti V, Mariani L et al (2005) Sentinel node biopsy in breast cancer: early results in 953 patients with negative sentinel node biopsy and no axillary dissection. Eur J Cancer 41:231–237

Veronesi U, De Cicco C, Galimberti V et al (2007) A comparative study on the value of FDG-PET and sentinel node biopsy to identify occult axillary metastases. Ann Oncol 18:473–478

Viale G, Mastropasqua MG, Maiorano E, Mazzarol G (2006) Pathologic examination of the axillary sentinel lymph nodes in patients with early-stage breast carcinoma: current and resolving controveries on the basis of the European Institute of Oncology experience. Virchows Arch 448:241–247

von Schulthess GK (2004) Positron emission tomography versus positron emission tomography/computed tomography: form "unclear" to "new-clear" medicine. Mol Imaging Biol 6:183–187

Wahl RL, Hutchins GD, Buchsbaum DJ et al (1991) ^{18}F-2-deoxy-2-fluoro-D-glucose (FDG) uptake into human tumor xenografts: feasibility studies for cancer imaging with PET. Cancer 69:349–355

Wilhelm AJ, Mijnhout GS, Franssen EJF (1999) Radiopharmaceutical in sentinel lymph-node detection an overview. Eur J Nucl Med 26:S36–S42

Wahl RL, Siegel BA, Coleman RE, Gatsonis CG (2004) PET Study Group. Prospective muticenter study of axillary nodal staging by positron emission tomography in breast cancer: a report of the staging breast cancer with PET Study Group. J Clin Oncol 22:277–285

Yuan S, Yu Y, Chao KS et al (2006) Additional value of PET/CT over PET in assessment of locoreginal lymph nodes in thoracic esophageal squamous cell cancer. J Nucl Med 47:1255–1259

Zangheri B, Messa C, Picchio M, Gianolli L, Landoni C, Fazio F (2004) PET/CT and breast cancer. Eur J Nucl Med Mol Imaging 31:S135–S142

Zornoza G, Garcia-Velloso MJ, Sola J, Regueira FM, Pina L, Beorlegui C (2004) ^{18}F-FDG PET complemented with sentinel lymph node biopsy in the detection of axillary involvement in breast cancer. Eur J Surg Oncol 30:15–19

Measuring Response to Chemotherapy in Locally Advanced Breast Cancer: Methodological Considerations

13

Nanda C. Krak, Otto S. Hoekstra, and Adriaan A. Lammertsma

CONTENTS

Abstract

In this chapter the findings of response-monitoring studies in breast cancer, using [^{18}F]2-fluoro-2-deoxy-D-glucose (FDG) and positron emission tomography (PET), are summarised. These studies indicate that there is a strong relationship between response and decrease in FDG signal even at an early stage of therapy. The review concentrates on methodological aspects of monitoring response with FDG: timing of serial scans, ROI definition approach, method of quantification, pitfalls of FDG and future directions in functional imaging. For the sake of optimal clinical applicability there now is need to standardise methodology. This is necessary to establish firm cut-off values for discriminating responders from non-responders, which in turn will provide a means for optimal treatment for as many patients as possible.

13.1 Introduction

The diagnosis of locally advanced breast cancer (LABC) is based on characteristics of the primary tumour (larger than 5 cm, inflammatory breast cancer, skin or chest wall involvement) and/or the presence of fixed axillary lymph node metastases (N2/N3). LABC has a relatively poor prognosis, mainly due to the high risk of locoregional recurrence and development of distant metastases. At present, standard treatment consists of neo-adjuvant chemotherapy, usually anthracycline-based, or more recently with taxanes or endocrine therapy (Eltahir et al. 1998; Dixon et al. 2003; Formenti et al. 2003; Hutcheon et al. 2003), followed by mastectomy with axillary lymphadenectomy and irradiation of the chest wall. The aim of such neo-adjuvant systemic therapy is to eliminate occult distant metastases (Pinedo et al. 2000) and to downstage tumour load prior to surgery, rendering previously inoperable breast cancer resectable, and/or to enable breast conserving surgery and sentinel node (SN) biopsy instead of axillary lymph node dissection (Fisher et al. 1998; Breslin et al. 2000; Moneer et al. 2001).

Several studies have shown that complete pathological responses (pCR) in primary tumour and axillary lymph nodes are independent predictors of better (disease free) survival (Honkoop et al. 1998; Kuerer et al. 1998; Machiavelli et al. 1998; Gajdos et al. 2002). In addition, residual tumour in axillary lymph nodes is an independent predictor of locoregional recurrence (Beenken et al. 2003; McIntosh et al. 2003).

Patients who do not achieve pathological response after induction therapy could benefit from prolonged or alternative treatment before surgery. In addition, the option for less radical surgery (such as lumpectomy and SN) depends on presurgical evaluation of clinical response. Clearly there is a need for correct preoperative identification of both responders and non-responders. Clinical examination alone is unreliable for post-therapy evaluation of primary tumour and axilla (Helvie et al. 1996; Herrada et al. 1997). For mammography, ultrasound and MRI results are promising, but pathological determination of tumour specimens remains necessary (Cheung et al. 2003; Delille et al. 2003; Rosen et al. 2003). Usually, clinical evaluation combined with one or more imaging techniques is recommended to increase accuracy. Waiting for changes in tumour volume, morphology, density or vascularity to develop makes follow-up by conventional imaging time consuming, and where cytostatic rather than cytoreductive therapies are concerned, inaccurate.

As an alternative, non-invasive measurement of metabolism rather than anatomy has been explored, in particular by using $[^{18}F]$2-fluoro-2-deoxy-D-glucose (FDG) and serial positron emission tomography (PET). Cellular uptake of glucose is mediated through glucose transporters and hexokinase. Accordingly, biological correlates of FDG uptake have been identified, showing associations of FDG uptake with proliferation rate and density of cells with enhanced glucose transporter/hexokinase activity. It has been shown that intense FDG uptake usually is an adverse prognostic sign (Herholz et al. 1993; Higashi et al. 1993; Oshida et al. 1998; Mankoff et al. 2002; Buchmann et al. 2003; Spaepen et al. 2003). Using FDG to image and monitor glucose metabolism is currently the most common PET application in oncological studies, but with appropriate tracers imaging and quantification of other aspects of tumour biology are possible, such as protein synthesis, regional blood flow, functional hormone status, hypoxia or proliferation. Overall, PET seems a suitable tool for response evaluation and prediction of ultimate pathological response or, patient outcome.

In the following review key aspects of response monitoring are discussed, specifically timing of serial scans, ROI definition approach, method of quantification, pitfalls of FDG and future directions in functional imaging.

13.2 Response Studies and Timing of Scans

In Tables 13.1 and 13.2 data from all LABC response monitoring studies published so far are summarised (Wahl et al. 1993; Bruce et al. 1995; Jansson et al. 1995; Bassa et al. 1996; Schelling et al. 2000; Smith et al. 2000; Tiling et al. 2001; Mankoff et al. 2003; Kim et al. 2004). In Figure 13.1 the results of eight response-monitoring studies are summarised graphically.

Table 13.1. Summary of data from all LABC response monitoring trials published so far using FDG PET

Reference	No. of patient	Clinical tumour stage	Quantification method (acquisition interval, min)	ROI method	Pixel counts
Wahl et al (1993)	11	Stage IIIB or LABC	SUV_W(50–60), NLR, k_3, Patlak	square 16 pixel ROI	Max
Bruce et al (1995)	15	LABC	TNT	Manual	Max
Jansson et al (1995)	16[a]	LABC or stage IV	SUV_W(30–50)	50% isocount contour	Mean
Bassa et al (1996)	16	LABC	SUV_W(40–60)	Pixel-by-pixel color coded	Mean
Smith et al (2000)	30	T3 or LABC	SUV_{BSA}(50–60), Patlak	Manual, whole lesion	Max
Schelling et al (2000)	22	LABC	SUV_W(45–60)	3 circular 15-mm ROIs	Max
Tiling et al (2001)	7	LABC	SUV_W(45–60)	Circular ROI, variable size	Max and mean
Mankoff et al (2003)	35	LABC	Patlak(30–60)	3 circular 15-mm ROIs	Mean
Kim et al (2004)	50	T3 or LABC	SUV_W(>60)	Manual, whole lesion	Max

[a]12 with FDG PET; SUV_W: standard uptake value, normalised for weight; SUV_{BSA}: SUV normalised for body surface area; NLR: non linear regression method; TNT: tumour non-tumour ratio; ROI: region of interest

Table 13.2. Overview of the timing and endpoints used in the nine response monitoring studies listed in Table 13.1

Reference	Baseline PET	PET1 *n*, (cycles)	PET2 *n*, (cycles)	PET3 *n*, (cycles)	PET4 *n*, (cycles)	Tumour response predicted by PET
Wahl et al. (1993)	11	<11a (day 8)	<11 a (1 cycle)	<11 a (2 cycles)	<11 a (3 cycles)	pPR, pCR
Bruce et al. (1995)	15	5 (2 cycles)				pPR
Jansson et al. (1995)	12	7 (1 cycle)	7 (3–4 cycles)			CR
Bassa et al. (1996)	16	13 (1–4 cycles)	14 (pre surgery)			pPR
Smith et al. (2000)	30	28 (1 cycle)	19 (4 cycles)	21 (pre surgery)		pCRmicro/macro
Schelling et al. (2000)	22	14 (1 cycle)	20 (2 cycles)			MRD
Tiling et al. (2001)	7	7 (day 8)	7 (2 cycles)	7 (pre surgery)		cCR, pCR
Mankoff et al. (2003)	35	21 (midway)				pCRmicro/macro
Kim et al. (2004)	50	50 (pre surgery)				pCR

n: no of patients scanned with FDG. [a] Only 47 out of the scheduled 55 scans were performed, but the number of actually performed scans per time point are not specified. CR: clinical response; PR: pathological response; cCR: clinical complete response; pCR: pathological complete response; pCR_{micro}/pCR_{macro}: microscopic/macroscopic pCR; pPR: pathological partial response; MRD: minimal residual disease

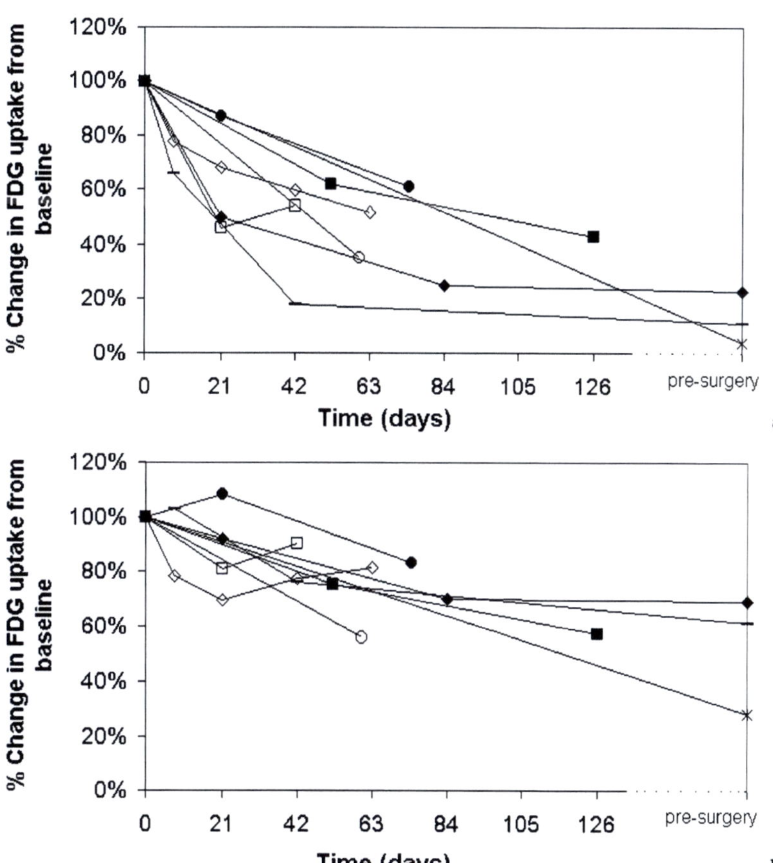

Fig. 13.1a,b. Graphic summary of the results of eight response-monitoring studies

Wahl et al. (1993) scanned 11 women (stage IIIB and localised stage IV) at baseline, after 8 days of chemohormonotherapy and after one, two and three cycles. In responding tumours (partial or complete pathological response) a significant decrease in FDG uptake as early as 8 days after therapy was found. This preceded any decrease in tumour volume as assessed by mammography. Furthermore, only patients with persistently declining FDG uptake achieved complete pathological response (pCR), whilst persistent residual uptake during therapy was a poor prognostic sign.

Bruce et al. (1995) scanned 15 women (LABC) at baseline, but only 5 after 2 cycles of therapy, 4 of whom underwent surgical tumour resection. Using the tumour to non-tumour ratio (TNT) as a semi-quantitative index, a decrease in TNT corresponded with a subsequently demonstrated pathological response.

Jansson et al. (1995) compared ^{11}C-methionine (11 patients) with FDG (12 patients) in the assessment of early response in patients with LABC, locoregrional recurrence and stage IV patients. FDG PET was performed before therapy and after the first and third cycle. Clinical response was determined by palpation and/or imaging (mammography, ultrasonography or computed tomography). A decrease in FDG uptake preceded clinical response and clinical responders demonstrated a continuing decline in FDG uptake.

Bassa et al. (1996) evaluated PET in the assessment of preoperative response of primary (LABC) tumours and axillary lymph nodes. Sixteen LABC patients were scanned at baseline, halfway through therapy and just before surgery. Visual evaluation and standard uptake values (SUV) of PET data were compared with mammography and ultrasound, and correlated with histology and clinical follow-up for up to 3 years. Just before surgery, sensitivity of PET for detection of residual viable tumour in breast and axillary nodes was 75 and 42%, respectively. Corresponding values for mammography were 71 and 71% and for ultrasound 88 and 67%, respectively. Smaller size and less FDG uptake were visible as early as the second study in 11 patients, but no patient achieved pCR. Finally, an elevated SUV just before surgery corresponded with poor clinical outcome.

Smith et al. (2000) performed baseline and three follow-up scans (after one and four courses and after completion of therapy) in 30 LABC patients. After chemotherapy both primary tumours and axillary lymph nodes were evaluated by pathology. Significantly greater reduction in FDG uptake was found in tumours achieving partial or complete microscopic or macroscopic pathological response (pPR, pCRmicro and pCRmacro, respectively) than pathological non-responders. A 20% reduction from baseline FDG uptake after one course of chemotherapy predicted primary tumour pCR (macro and micro combined) with a sensitivity of 90% and a specificity of 74%. Mean decrease in FDG uptake was significantly greater in responding than in non-responding lymph nodes.

Schelling et al. (2000) assessed changes in FDG uptake in 22 LABC patients scanned before therapy and after one and two cycles of chemotherapy. Using a cut-off value of 55% of baseline FDG uptake, minimal residual disease (MRD) (Honkoop et al. 1998) could be predicted with a sensitivity and specificity of 100 and 85%, respectively, after one cycle. The corresponding values after two cycles were 83 and 94%, respectively.

Tiling et al. (2001) performed serial FDG PET scans in seven LABC patients at baseline, after 8 days of therapy, and after the second and final course of chemotherapy. After the second cycle, there was a decline in FDG uptake of more than 60% compared with baseline in three patients with clinical complete response (cCR) or pCR. Small residual tumour (3 mm) identified at pathology could not be visualized with FDG PET.

Mankoff et al. (2003) compared FDG and 15O-water (blood flow) in the assessment of tumour response during therapy, scanning 35 LABC patients before and after 2 months of therapy. The reduction in FDG uptake was larger in pCR patients than in patients with only partial or no response, but the difference was not significant. With blood flow, however, the differences between pathological responders and partial or non-responders were highly significant.

Finally, the largest study so far is by Kim et al. (2004), involving 50 LABC patients who were scanned at baseline and preoperatively after completion of chemotherapy. Response was determined clinically (physical examination, mammography, ultrasound or CT) and pathologically (pCR, pPR, pNR). In patients with pCR the reduction of SUV from baseline was statistically greater than those with pPR or pNR. At a threshold of -79% of baseline, pCR could be differentiated from pPR/pNR with a sensitivity and specificity of 85.2% and 82.6%, respectively.

In summary, even though PET methodology and clinicopathological endpoints are heterogeneous (see Table 13.1 and Fig. 13.1), and despite the lack of a uniform quantitative cut-off point, current data suggest that early decrease in FDG uptake, e.g., after only one course of chemotherapy, can predict pathological response. Furthermore, persistent decline in FDG uptake, demonstrated by serial scans, may also predict (complete) clinical and pathological response. In contrast, persisting focal FDG uptake is likely to be indicative of either only partial pathological response or poor clinical outcome.

13.3 Axillary Lymph Node Evaluation

Only a limited number of studies have looked specifically at response of axillary lymph nodes (ALNs). Smith et al. (2000) found a significantly greater mean decrease in FDG uptake after one cycle of therapy in lymph nodes with pCR_{micro} than in non-responding nodes. Bassa et al. (1996) and Burcombe et al. (2002) reported sensitivities for detecting residual ALN involvement after completion of therapy of 42 and 0%, respectively. Specificity was 100% in both studies.

The low sensitivities for detection of residual axillary tumour activity post-treatment are problematic in a response monitoring setting. In a review on ALN staging with PET, however, Crippa et al. (2004) concluded that a false-negative PET scan generally represented very few and/or very small node metastases.

13.4 Region of Interest Definition

It will be clear that definition of the tumour region of interest (ROI) will be of crucial importance in monitoring tumour uptake of FDG during therapy. In general, partial volume effects should be minimised, as these will reduce the measured tumour signal to a variable degree. This might lead to erroneous results if tumour dimensions change during therapy. Given the variety of ROI methods being used, there appears to be no consensus about the optimal type of ROI for the purpose of monitoring response during therapy. Reproducibility, user-independence and, to a lesser degree, simplicity are important considerations for choosing a ROI method.

Either using the same small square (Wahl et al. 1993) or circular (Schelling et al. 2000) ROI in subsequent scans or using the maximum pixel in a ROI have been proposed as solutions to the above problem. In a recent simulation study comparing several ROI methods (Boellaard et al. 2004), however, it was demonstrated that use of a ROI with fixed dimensions resulted in the poorest estimate of response in small tumours. In many cases, the maximum pixel value within an ROI was a reasonable alternative. If uptake is low (e.g., low injected dose, tumour with low uptake, obese patient), however, significant overestimation of measurements might occur with the use of a maximum pixel ROI (Krak et al. 2005).

Both studies postulated that use of an isocount contour ROI possibly offers the best solution to all requirements for a suitable ROI method (Boellaard et al. 2004).

13.5 Quantitative Measurement of Glucose Metabolism

Over the years, several methods for analysing FDG data have been proposed (Hoekstra et al. 2000). In general, methods can be divided in those requiring a dynamic scanning protocol and those requiring only a static scan. In theory, the first group of methods attempt to measure glucose metabolic rate (MR_{glu}), by using either non-linear regression (NLR) of the operational equation derived from a two-tissue compartment model or Patlak graphical analysis (Patlak et al. 1983). The second group provides measures of FDG uptake that are thought to be an index of MR_{glu} (i.e., semi-quantitative).

All dynamic protocols require arterial input to enable full quantification. For LABC studies, however, the thorax will be in the field of view of the scanner and consequently the required arterial input function can be obtained from the dynamic scan itself rather than from (invasive) arterial sampling. Although, in theory, several large arterial structures can be used for deriving this image derived input function (IDIF), the best results (for FDG) are obtained using the ascending aorta (van der Weerdt et al. 2001; de Geus-Oei et al. 2006). It is important to note that, due to possible spill-over from the myocardium, the left ventricle is less suited for FDG studies.

The two-tissue compartment model was derived from the original autoradiographic method that was developed for measuring MR_{glu} (Sokoloff et al. 1977; Reivich et al. 1979). MR_{glu} is obtained by estimating rate constants (K_1, k_2, k_3 and k_4) depicting exchange between blood and tissue and transport rates between the two tissue compartments. K_1 and k_2 represent rates of forward and reverse capillary glucose transport, respectively, while k_3 and k_4 represent phosphorylation (by hexokinase) and dephosphorylation (by dephosphatase), respectively (Huang et al. 1980; Phelps et al. 1979). The decision to use three or four rate constants is related to the question whether glucose is irreversibly trapped as glucose-6-PO_4 ($k_4 = 0$) or not ($k_4 > 0$). In most tumours the effect of dephosphatase activity is negligible and, therefore, usually three rate constants suffice. For accurate results, however, a blood volume (Vb) term to account for intravascular activity should be included in the model. The rate constants are estimated by non-linear regression of the resulting operational equation (Huang et al. 1980). These rate constants are then used to calculate the net influx constant K_i (of FDG), which is given by:

$$K_i = K_1 \cdot k_3/(k_2 + k_3) \qquad \text{(Eq. 13.1)}$$

Finally, MR_{glu} is calculated using:

$$MR_{glu} = Cglu \cdot K_i/LC \qquad \text{(Eq. 13.2)}$$

Here Cglu is the plasma glucose concentration and the so-called lumped constant (LC) a correction factor that accounts for differences in affinity between FDG and glucose for both glucose transporter and hexokinase.

Because of (potential) biological correlates of the rate constants, use of NLR might provide insight into biological tumour characteristics. The main drawbacks of NLR are the scan time needed together with the relatively complex scanning protocol. In addition, NLR is sensitive to noise and relatively slow, and therefore it is less suited for pixel-by-pixel analyses, precluding the generation of parametric (MR_{glu}) images. Finally, the required LC is largely unknown for tumours outside the central nervous system (Spence et al. 1998; Graham et al. 2002; Wu et al. 2003) and has only been (directly) measured in normal human brain, skeletal muscle, heart and adipose tissue with values ranging from 0.65 to 1.35 (Botker et al. 1997; Virtanen et al. 2001; Selberg et al. 2002).

In Patlak graphical analysis (Patlak et al. 1983) fitting of individual rate constants is replaced by linear regression after transforming (linearising) the data. Here the ratio of tissue concentration to plasma concentration is plotted as a function of "normalised" time (i.e., $\int C_p/C_p$). After a certain equilibration period (usually 10 min or more), the slope of this line equals the net influx constant K_i. After estimating K_i by linear regression of this line, MR_{glu} can again be calculated using Eq. 13.2. The key assumption of the Patlak method is that FDG is irreversibly trapped as FDG-6-PO4 (i.e., $k_4 = 0$). The validity of this assumption has been demonstrated for several tumours (Hoekstra et al. 2002; Krak et al. 2003; Kroep et al. 2003).

Advantages of the Patlak method are a less demanding scanning protocol and less sensitivity to noise. The latter advantage allows for pixel-by-pixel analyses and thus generation of MR_{glu} images. These images might provide insight into tumour heterogeneity, which might be especially important in response studies (with different parts of the tumour responding in a different manner). The main drawback is that no information about individual rate constants can be obtained, i.e., it is not possible to determine whether a change in MR_{glu} is due to glucose transporter or hexokinase changes. Finally, uncertainty in the exact value of the LC also applies to Patlak.

An attempt has been made to improve tumour to non-tumour contrast in Patlak-derived parametric images by applying a threshold to the correlation coefficient of the (linear) regression of pixel K_i values (Zasadny et al. 1996). This approach was taken further in the so-called total lesion evaluation (TLE) method (Wu et al. 1996), in which the concept of metabolic volume was introduced.

In addition, an NLR-derived method, the so-called 6P model (Wu et al. 1995), has been proposed in an effort to correct for possible tumour heterogeneity (i.e., mixture of tumour and relatively normal tissue within a tumour ROI) by using kinetics in a reference (normal tissue) region.

Recently, TLE and 6P methods were compared with NLR for several types of cancer, including breast cancer (Hoekstra et al. 2002; Krak et al. 2003; Kroep et al. 2003). No advantages over standard NLR and Patlak methods were observed. In particular, the 6P method resulted in very noisy data.

13.6 Simplified Clinical Protocols

In general, dynamic protocols are considered to be too time consuming and too complex for routine clinical use. This has resulted in the development of methods that require just a single (static) scan. Most static protocols require no blood sampling, and only provide a semi-quantitative estimate of MR_{glu}.

At present, the standard uptake value (SUV) method is most widely used. This method requires a single scan (e.g., from 50 to 60 min after injection) to measure uptake (concentration) of FDG (C_t), which is then normalised to injected dose (I) and body weight (W) according to:

$$SUV = Ct/(I/W) \quad \text{(Eq. 13.3)}$$

Corrected only for body weight, SUV does not take into account the relatively lower FDG accumulation in fatty tissues. In theory, normalisation to body surface area (BSA) or lean body mass (LBM) should be better (Hoekstra et al. 2000; Erselcan et al. 2002; Shankar et al. 2006), because these normalisations potentially account for the effects of weight loss during therapy on subsequent SUV estimations and because LBM normalisation offers the additional advantage of sex-specific corrections. In practice, different normalisation procedures perform better for different tumours when compared to the 'gold standard' NLR (Hoekstra et al. 2002; Krak et al. 2003; Kroep et al. 2003). The reason for this finding is not clear, but it is probably related to differences in the composition of the various patient groups (gender, patient habitus, fat and non-fatty tissues).

Originally, the EORTC PET Study Group (Young et al. 1999) did not recommend correction for plasma glucose, because of the lack of accuracy of most methods routinely used for glucose measurement. As (corrected) SUV is directly proportional to plasma glucose, an error of 10 to 15% in the latter measurement would compromise the assessment of response by 20 to 30%. Correcting SUV for (variations in) plasma glucose consistently provides better results, i.e., better correlation with NLR (Hoekstra et al. 2002; Krak et al. 2003; Kroep et al. 2003). It is now recommended to correct SUV for plasma glucose using an accurate technique to measure plasma glucose (e.g., the hexokinase method). For large multicentre clinical trials, such a correction could possibly be omitted, provided that serum plasma glucose concentration remains within the reference range.

The main advantages of SUV are its simplicity and the significant reduction in scanning time. The drawbacks are well documented (Keyes et al. 1995; Huang et al. 2000). As SUV is dependent on uptake time, it is very important to keep this fixed. Nevertheless, as plasma clearance of FDG might change due to therapy, a corresponding change in the relationship between SUV and MR_{glu} should be kept in mind (Freedman et al. 2003; Lammertsma et al. 2006).

To reduce sensitivity to plasma clearance, Hunter et al. (1996) proposed an alternative method, the so-called simplified kinetic method (SKM), in which one or a few venous blood samples are taken during the static scan. These samples provide a means to correct for changes in plasma clearance. By assuming that the peak of the (blood) FDG curve can be described by a population mean, the integral of the plasma curve until time of scanning can be calculated for individual studies using these samples. Rather than normalising to injected dose, FDG uptake can now be normalised to the plasma integral, i.e., to the total amount of FDG delivered to the tumour. In theory, this method provides an index of MR_{glu} that is independent of uptake time.

Sadato et al. (1998) introduced a 'SUV-based' method to derive the net influx constant (K_i). In this method a population mean for the plasma curves is used to translate SUV into K_i. The advantage is that units are now compatible with those of MR_{glu}. In essence this method employs a constant scaling factor and therefore it suffers from the same problems and disadvantages as SUV.

Of the single scan methods SKM seems to be the most robust from a methodological point of view. In addition, in several reports it consistently performed better than SUV for different cancers (Graham et al. 2000; Hoekstra et al. 2002; Krak et al. 2003; Kroep et al. 2003). Therefore, if a single scan protocol is used, response studies can be improved by using SKM rather than SUV at the cost of only a few venous blood samples.

13.7 Pitfalls of FDG PET

FDG is not a tumour-specific tracer. In untreated breast cancer, lymphoid infiltration contributes to the tracer signal (Bos et al. 2002). Such infiltration is present in 30% of breast cancers and may vary within a tumour (Pupa et al. 1996; Steele et al. 1985). It is unlikely that this will remain constant during therapy. Known causes for false-positive findings are inflammation and physiological uptake in bowel, muscle and brown adipose tissue (Lind et al. 2004).

In contrast, very small (<1 cm) (Avril et al. 2000), less aggressive tumours and lobular carcinomas show less FDG uptake, which can result in false-negative PET scans. Furthermore, in tumours, marked effects have been observed after neo-adjuvant therapy, including presence of ductal carcinoma in situ (DCIS), cytoplasmic vacuolization, changes in the number of mitoses and localized fibrosis (Honkoop et al. 1997; Moll et al. 1997). In axillary lymph nodes fibrosis, mucin pools and foamy histiocytes have been observed (Newman et al. 2003). It is conceivable that these effects will result in dilution of the FDG signal during therapy.

13.8 Other Tracers and Future Directions

Although FDG is currently the most widely used PET tracer, glucose metabolism reflects only one aspect of tumour biology. In addition, it is not tumour specific (see *Pitfalls*, above). Combinations of FDG with other tracers may offer more insight into tumour biology and/or add new applications to FDG. Mortimer et al. (2001) scanned 40 patients with advanced ER-positive tumours with FDG and the oestrogen analogue 16α-[^{18}F]-17β-fluoroestradiol (FES). After tamoxifen therapy only responding tumours demonstrated a significant hormone-induced rise in FDG uptake. This 'metabolic flare' can thus be an indicator of tumour responsiveness to tamoxifen therapy. Alternatively, one should be aware of this phenomenon if a patient is scanned within 2 weeks of starting a combination of hormone and chemotherapy. Mankoff et al. (2002) scanned 31 LABC patients treated with neo-adjuvant chemotherapy with FDG and $H_2{}^{15}O$ and found a low MR_{glu}/BF ratio to be an independent predictor of pCR and a putative predictor of disease-free survival.

Apart from increased glycolysis, increased proliferation, hypoxia, angiogenesis and alterations in programmed cell death (apoptosis) are also hallmarks of malignancy. There is a trend towards more specific and individualised treatment of breast cancer patients. Immunohistochemical typing of tumours prior to therapy can reveal a certain biological profile (e.g., hormone receptor status, proliferation factors, HER2-status and angiogenesis factors), which may then offer specific targets for therapy. With appropriate tracers, PET allows for imaging and quantification of these targets. In theory, this provides for the ideal situation of giving therapy and monitoring subsequent response using the same target.

An example is the pyrimidine-analogue 3-18F-fluoro-3-deoxythymidine (FLT), which after uptake into the cell is phosphorylated into FLT-5-P by the enzyme thymidine kinase 1 (TK1), the activity of which is principally increased during the S phase of DNA replication. This makes FLT a specific cellular proliferation marker. In a recent study comparing FDG to FLT, Pio et al. (2005) scanned 14 metastatic breast cancer patients at baseline, after one cycle of antiproliferative chemotherapy and after completion of chemotherapy (or 1 year after baseline PET) and found a significant correlation between early change in FLT uptake and late changes (i.e., after completion of therapy) in both CA 27.29 tumour marker levels and tumour size as measured by CT.

Her2 imaging and early response monitoring have been successfully performed in mice bearing BT474 breast tumour xenografts (Smith-Jones et al. 2006).

Tumours may become resistant to chemo-, radio- or hormone therapy as a result of hypoxia (Teicher et al. 1994; Greijer et al. 2005; Kurebayashi et al. 2005). Scanning with ^{18}F-fluoromisonidazole (FMISO) can identify tumours that are intrinsically resistant or become so after therapy (Rajendran et al. 2004; Richin et al. 2006).

Recently, ^{124}I-annexin V has been used to image apoptosis in an animal model of liver apoptosis (Keen et al. 2005). This tracer binds to phosphatidylserine on the surface of apoptotic cells.

Finally, use of radiolabelled drugs has heralded a new phase in the design and development of new drugs or a better understanding of existing drugs by imaging and quantifying drug delivery, (heterogeneity of) distribution and mechanisms of drug resistance (Hendrikse et al. 1999; Aboagye et al. 2000;

Bading et al. 2000), although at present mainly in animal models. By direct measurement of tumour uptake of a radiolabelled chemotherapeutical agent such as ^{11}C-docetaxel (van Tilburg et al. 2004), it should be possible to predict tumour response to this specific treatment and to select responders from non-responders at an early stage of or even prior to treatment. It is conceivable that in the future, testing drug avidity of a tumour prior to treatment through labelled drug imaging will become routine, thereby offering the possibility to provide truly individualised treatment.

13.9 Discussion and Conclusions

From the studies published so far (Table 13.1, Fig. 13.1) the following can be concluded:

1. Accumulated evidence suggests that early changes in FDG uptake, e.g., after a single course of chemotherapy, can predict the ultimate pathological response in primary LABC tumours. Inter-study differences in PET methodology and clinicopathological endpoints, however, impair robust conclusions on the applicability of PET criteria of response. In other words, postulated thresholds for accurate prediction of pathological response, which vary from 20–60% reduction in FDG uptake from baseline (Schelling et al. 2000; Smith et al. 2000; Tiling et al. 2001), still need to be validated in future prospective response-monitoring studies. At the same time it could be argued whether patient outcome should be the endpoint in such future studies, rather than only pathological response.
2. An additional third scan (e.g., after two cycles or halfway through completion of therapy) may be of value in demonstrating either persistent decrease in FDG uptake, thereby improving accuracy of prediction of pathological outcome (Schelling et al. 2000), or persistent or increasing FDG uptake after therapy, indicating poorer clinical or pathological outcome (Wahl et al. 1993; Jansson et al. 1995; Bassa et al. 1996).
3. Although the presence of residual tumour in axillary lymph nodes after chemotherapy is an independent risk factor for locoregional recurrence in LABC (Beenken et al. 2003; McIntosh et al. 2003), data on the accuracy of FDG PET to define axillary status after systemic therapy are relatively scarce and reported post-therapy sensitivity for residual ALN tumour detection quite variable (0–88%) (Bassa et al. 1996; Smith et al. 2000; Burcombe et al. 2002).
4. Definition of ROIs should be automated, user-independent and ideally insensitive to partial volume effects due to therapy-induced changes in tumour dimension. Based on a comprehensive simulation study, there is evidence that a tumour ROI using a percentage threshold of maximum activity, corrected for background activity, is the best ROI method for response-monitoring studies (Boellaard et al. 2004). Small (1.5 cm) fixed ROIs (Schelling et al. 2000; Mankoff et al. 2002) should only be used if tumour size does not fall below 2 cm.
5. Of all methods that can be used for response monitoring in breast cancer, Patlak, SKM and glucose-corrected SUV compare well with the "gold standard" NLR. This is a consistent finding for several tumours (Hoekstra et al. 2002; Krak et al. 2003; Kroep et al. 2003). For new therapeutic agents or when better insight in tumour biology is needed, it is recommended that full quantification be used, either with NLR or Patlak, depending on the specific research question. When the heart is in the field of view the required arterial input function can be obtained from the dynamic scan itself, preferably from the ascending aorta (van der Weerdt et al. 2001; de Geus-Oei et al. 2006), rather than from invasive arterial sampling.
6. Static protocols are more practical for routine use in a busy clinical PET department. Conceptually, SKM is preferable to SUV as it takes individual plasma clearance of FDG into account, making it independent of uptake time and less sensitive to changes in plasma clearance due to therapy. The collection of one to three venous blood samples during scanning seems only a small price to pay for the increased accuracy it provides, especially since correcting SUV for plasma glucose levels require venous blood samples anyway.
7. Although FDG will continue to play an important role in diagnostic and response-monitoring studies, it is to be expected that in the future more specific PET tracers will come into play, assessing more specific tumour processes.

In summary, since 1993, approximately 200 (locally advanced) breast cancer patients have been entered in nine FDG PET studies. Clearly the proof of principle has been well established, namely that there is a strong relationship between decrease in FDG uptake at an early stage of therapy and response. For clinical applications there is now a need to standardise methodology in order to establish firm cut-off values for discriminating between responders and non-responders.

References

Aboagye EO, Price PM (2003) Use of positron emission tomography in anticancer drug development. Invest New Drugs 21:169–181

Avril N, Rose CA, Schelling M et al (2000) Breast imaging with positron emission tomography and fluorine-18 fluorodeoxyglucose: use and limitations. J Clin Oncol 18:3495–3502

Bading JR, Alauddin MM, Fissekis JD et al (2000) Blocking catabolism with eniluracil enhances PET studies of 5-[18F]fluorouracil pharmacokinetics J Nucl Med 2000 41:1714–1724

Bassa P, Kim EE, Inoue T et al (1996) Evaluation of preoperative chemotherapy using PET with fluorine-18-fluorodeoxyglucose in breast cancer. J Nucl Med 37:931–938

Beenken SW, Urist MM, Zhang Y et al (2003) Axillary lymph node status, but not tumor size, predicts locoregional recurrence and overall survival after mastectomy for breast cancer. Ann Surg 237:732–739

Boellaard R, Krak NC, Hoekstra OS et al (2004) Effects of noise, image resolution, and ROI definition on the accuracy of standard uptake values: a simulation study. J Nucl Med 45:1519–1527

Botker HE, Bottcher M, Schmitz O et al (1997) Glucose uptake and lumped constant variability in normal human hearts determined with [18F]fluorodeoxyglucose. J Nucl Cardiol 4:125–132

Bos R, van Der Hoeven JJ, van Der Wall E et al (2002) Biologic correlates of (18)fluorodeoxyglucose uptake in human breast cancer measured by positron emission tomography. J Clin Oncol 20:379–387

Breslin TM, Cohen L, Sahin A et al (2000) Sentinel lymph node biopsy is accurate after neoadjuvant chemotherapy for breast cancer. J Clin Oncol 18:3480–3486

Bruce DM, Evans NT, Heys SD et al (1995) Positron emission tomography: 2-deoxy-2-[18F]-fluoro-D-glucose uptake in locally advanced breast cancers. Eur J Surg Oncol 21:280–283

Buchmann I, Vogg AT, Glatting G et al (2003) [18F]5-fluoro-2-deoxyuridine-PET for imaging of malignant tumors and for measuring tissue proliferation. Cancer Biother Radiopharm 18:327–337

Burcombe RJ, Makris A, Pittam M et al (2002) Evaluation of good clinical response to neoadjuvant chemotherapy in primary breast cancer using [18F]-fluorodeoxyglucose positron emission tomography. Eur J Cancer 38:375–379

Cheung YC, Chen SC, Su MY et al (2003) Monitoring the size and response of locally advanced breast cancers to neoadjuvant chemotherapy (weekly paclitaxel and epirubicin) with serial enhanced MRI. Breast Cancer Res Treat 78:51–58

Crippa F, Gerali A, Alessi A et al (2004) FDG-PET for axillary lymph node staging in primary breast cancer. Eur J Nucl Med Mol Imaging 31:S97–S102

Delille JP, Slanetz PJ, Yeh ED et al (2003) Invasive ductal breast carcinoma response to neoadjuvant chemotherapy: noninvasive monitoring with functional MR imaging pilot study. Radiology 228:63–69

Dixon JM, Jackson J, Renshaw L et al (2003) Neoadjuvant tamoxifen and aromatase inhibitors: comparisons and clinical outcomes. J Steroid Biochem Mol Biol 86:295–299

Eltahir A, Heys SD, Hutcheon AW et al (1998) Treatment of large and locally advanced breast cancers using neoadjuvant chemotherapy. Am J Surg 175:127–132

Erselcan T, Turgut B, Dogan D et al (2002) Lean body mass-based standardized uptake value, derived from a predictive equation, might be misleading in PET studies. Eur J Nucl Med Mol Imaging 29:1630–1638

Fisher B, Bryant J, Wolmark N et al (1998) Effect of preoperative chemotherapy on the outcome of women with operable breast cancer. J Clin Oncol 16:2672–2685

Formenti SC, Volm M, Skinner KA et al (2003) Preoperative twice-weekly paclitaxel with concurrent radiation therapy followed by surgery and postoperative doxorubicin-based chemotherapy in locally advanced breast cancer: a phase I/II trial. J Clin Oncol 21:864–870

Freedman NM, Sundaram SK, Kurdziel K et al (2003) Comparison of SUV and Patlak slope for monitoring of cancer therapy using serial PET scans. Eur J Nucl Med Mol Imaging 30:46–53

Gajdos C, Tartter PI, Estabrook A et al (2002) Relationship of clinical and pathologic response to neoadjuvant chemotherapy and outcome of locally advanced breast cancer. J Surg Oncol 80:4–11

de Geus-Oei LF, Visser EP, Krabbe PF et al (2006) Comparison of image-derived and arterial input functions for estimating the rate of glucose metabolism in therapy-monitoring 18F-FDG PET studies. J Nucl Med 47:945–949

Graham MM, Peterson LM, Hayward RM (2000) Comparison of simplified quantitative analysis of FDG uptake. Nucl Med Biology 27:647–655

Graham MM, Muzi M, Spence AM et al (2002) The FDG lumped constant in normal human brain. J Nucl Med 43:1157–1166

Greijer AE, de Jong MC, Scheffer GL et al (2005) Hypoxia-induced acidification causes mitoxantrone resistance not mediated by drug transporters in human breast cancer cells. Cell Oncol 27:43–49

Herrada J, Iyer RB, Atkinson EN et al (1997) Relative value of physical examination, mammography, and breast sonography in evaluating the size of the primary tumor and regional lymph node metastases in women receiving neoadjuvant chemotherapy for locally advanced breast carcinoma. Clin Cancer Res 3:1565–1569

Helvie MA, Joynt LK, Cody RL et al (1996) Locally advanced breast carcinoma: accuracy of mammography versus clinical examination in the prediction of residual disease after chemotherapy. Radiology 198:327–332

Hendrikse NH, de Vries EG, Eriks-Fluks L et al (1999) A new in vivo method to study P-glycoprotein transport in tumors and the blood-brain barrier. Cancer Res 59:2411–2416

Herholz K, Pietrzyk U, Voges J et al (1993) Correlation of glucose consumption and tumor cell density in astrocytomas. A stereotactic PET study. J Neurosurg 79:853–858

Higashi K, Clavo AC, Wahl RL (1993) Does FDG uptake measure proliferative activity of human cancer cells? In vitro comparison with DNA flow cytometry and tritiated thymidine uptake. J Nucl Med 34:414–419

Hoekstra CJ, Paglianiti I, Hoekstra OS et al (2000) Monitoring response to therapy in cancer using [^{18}F]-2-fluoro-2-deoxy-D-glucose and positron emission tomography: an overview of different analytical methods. Eur J Nucl Med 27:731–743

Hoekstra CJ, Hoekstra OS, Stroobants SG et al (2002) Methods to monitor response to chemotherapy in non-small cell lung cancer with ^{18}F-FDG PET. J Nucl Med 43:1304–1309

Honkoop AH, Pinedo HM, De Jong JS et al (1997) Effects of chemotherapy on pathologic and biologic characteristics of locally advanced breast cancer. Am J Clin Pathol 107:211–218

Honkoop AH, van Diest PJ, de Jong JS et al (1998) Prognostic role of clinical, pathological and biological characteristics in patients with locally advanced breast cancer. Br J Cancer 77:621–626

Huang SC (2000) Anatomy of SUV. Nucl Med Biol 27:643–646

Huang SC, Phelps ME, Hoffman EJ et al (1980) Noninvasive determination of local cerebral metabolic rate of glucose in man. Am J Physiol 238:E69–E82

Hunter GJ, Hamberg LM, Alpert NM et al (1996) Simplified measurement of deoxyglucose utilization rate. J Nucl Med 37:950–955

Hutcheon AW, Heys SD, Sarkar TK (2003) Neoadjuvant docetaxel in locally advanced breast cancer. Breast Cancer Res Treat 79:S19–S24

Jansson T, Westlin JE, Ahlstrom H et al (1995) Positron emission tomography studies in patients with locally advanced and/or metastatic breast cancer: a method for early therapy evaluation? J Clin Oncol 13:1470–1477

Keen HG, Dekker BA, Disley L et al (2005) Imaging apoptosis in vivo using 124I-annexin V and PET. Nucl Med Biol 32:395–402

Keyes JW Jr (1995) SUV: standard uptake or silly useless value? J Nucl Med 36:1836–1839

Kim SJ, Kim SK, Lee ES et al (2004) Predictive value of [^{18}F]FDG PET for pathological response of breast cancer to neo-adjuvant chemotherapy. Ann Oncol 15:1352–1357

Krak NC, Boellaard R, Hoekstra OS et al (2005) Effects of ROI definition and reconstruction method on quantitative outcome and applicability in a response monitoring trial. Eur J Nucl Med Mol Imaging 32:294–301

Krak NC, van der Hoeven JJ, Hoekstra OS et al (2003) Measuring [^{18}F]FDG uptake in breast cancer during chemotherapy: comparison of analytical methods. Eur J Nucl Med Mol Imaging 30:674–681

Kroep JR, Van Groeningen CJ, Cuesta MA (2003) Positron emission tomography using 2-deoxy-2-[^{18}F]-fluoro-D-glucose for response monitoring in locally advanced gastroesophageal cancer; a comparison of different analytical methods. Mol Imaging Biol 5:337–346

Kuerer HM, Newman LA, Buzdar AU et al (1998) Residual metastatic axillary lymph nodes following neoadjuvant chemotherapy predict disease-free survival in patients with locally advanced breast cancer. Am J Surg 176:502–509

Kurebayashi J (2005) Resistance to endocrine therapy in breast cancer. Cancer Chemother Pharmacol 56:S39–S46

Lammertsma AA, Hoekstra CJ, Giaconne G et al (2006) How should we analyse FDG PET studies for monitoring tumour response? Eur J Nucl Med Mol Imaging 33 (Suppl 1):16–21

Lind P, Igerc I, Beyer T et al (2004) Advantages and limitations of FDG PET in the follow-up of breast cancer. Eur J Nucl Med Mol Imaging 31:S125–S134

Machiavelli MR, Romero AO, Perez JE et al (1998) Prognostic significance of pathological response of primary tumor and metastatic axillary lymph nodes after neoadjuvant chemotherapy for locally advanced breast carcinoma. Cancer J Sci Am 4:125–131

Mankoff DA, Dunnwald LK, Gralow JR et al (2002) Blood flow and metabolism in locally advanced breast cancer: relationship to response to therapy. J Nucl Med 43:500–509

Mankoff DA, Dunnwald LK, Gralow JR et al (2003) Changes in blood flow and metabolism in locally advanced breast cancer treated with neoadjuvant chemotherapy. J Nucl Med 44:1806–1814

McIntosh SA, Ogston KN, Payne S et al (2003) Local recurrence in patients with large and locally advanced breast cancer treated with primary chemotherapy. Am J Surg 185:525–531

Moll UM, Chumas J (1997) Morphologic effects of neoadjuvant chemotherapy in locally advanced breast cancer. Pathol Res Pract 193:187–196

Moneer M, Ismael S, Khaled H et al (2001) A new surgical strategy for breast conservation in locally advanced breast cancer that achieves a good locoregional control rate: preliminary report. Breast 10:220–224

Mortimer JE, Dehdashti F, Siegel BA et al (2001) Metabolic flare: indicator of hormone responsiveness in advanced breast cancer. J Clin Oncol 19:2797–2803

Newman LA, Pernick NL, Adsay V et al (2003) Histopathologic evidence of tumor regression in the axillary lymph nodes of patients treated with preoperative chemotherapy correlates with breast cancer outcome. Ann Surg Oncol 10:734–739

Oshida M et al, Uno K, Suzuki M et al (1998) Predicting the prognoses of breast carcinoma patients with positron emission tomography using 2-deoxy-2-fluoro[^{18}F]-D-glucose. Cancer 82:2227–2234

Patlak CS, Blasberg RG, Fenstermacher JD (1983) Graphical evaluation of blood-to-brain transfer constants from multiple-time uptake data. J Cereb Blood Flow Metab 3:1–7

Phelps ME, Huang SC, Hoffman EJ et al (1979) Tomographic measurement of local cerebral glucose metabolic rate in humans with (F-18)2-fluoro-2-deoxy-D-glucose: validation of method. Ann Neurol 6:371–388

Pinedo HM, de Gruijl TD, van Der Wall E et al (2000) Biological concepts of prolonged neoadjuvant treatment plus GM-CSF in locally advanced tumors. Oncologist 5:497–500

Pio BS, Park CK, Pietras R et al (2006) Usefulness of 3'-[F-18]fluoro-3'-deoxythymidine with positron emission tomography in predicting breast cancer response to therapy. Mol Imaging Biol 8:36–42

Pupa SM, Bufalino R, Invernizzi AM et al (1996) Macrophage infiltrate and prognosis in c-erbB-2-overexpressing breast carcinomas. J Clin Oncol 14:85–94

Rajendran JG, Mankoff DA, O'Sullivan F et al (2004) Hypoxia and glucose metabolism in malignant tumors: evaluation by [^{18}F]fluoromisonidazole and [^{18}F]fluorodeoxyglucose positron emission tomography imaging. Clin Cancer Res 10:2245–2252

Reivich M, Kuhl D, Wolf A, Greenberg J et al (1979) The [^{18}F]fluorodeoxyglucose method for the measurement of local cerebral glucose utilization in man. Circ Res 44:127–137

Rischin D, Hicks RJ, Fisher R et al (2006) Prognostic significance of [^{18}F]-misonidazole positron emission tomography-detected tumor hypoxia in patients with advanced head and neck cancer randomly assigned to chemoradiation with or without tirapazamine: a substudy of Trans-Tasman Radiation Oncology Group Study 98.02. J Clin Oncol 24:2098–2104

Rosen EL, Blackwell KL, Baker JA et al (2003) Accuracy of MRI in the detection of residual breast cancer after neoadjuvant chemotherapy. AJR Am J Roentgenol 181:1275–1282

Sadato N, Tsuchida T, Nakaumra S et al (1998) Non-invasive estimation of the net influx constant using the standardized uptake value for quantification of FDG uptake of tumours. Eur J Nucl Med 25:559–564

Schelling M, Avril N, Nahrig J et al (2000) Positron emission tomography using [^{18}F]fluorodeoxyglucose for monitoring primary chemotherapy in breast cancer. J Clin Oncol 18:1689–1695

Selberg O, Muller MJ, van den Hoff J et al (2002) Use of positron emission tomography for the assessment of skeletal muscle glucose metabolism. Nutrition 18:323–328

Shankar LK, Hoffman JM, Bacharach S et al (2006) Consensus recommendations for the use of ^{18}F-FDG PET as an indicator of therapeutic response in patients in National Cancer Institute trials. J Nucl Med 47:1059–1066

Smith IC, Welch AE, Hutcheon AW et al (2000) Positron emission tomography using [^{18}F]-fluorodeoxy-D-glucose to predict the pathologic response of breast cancer to primary chemotherapy. J Clin Oncol 18:1676–1688

Smith-Jones PM, Solit D, Afroze F et al (2006) Early tumor response to Hsp90 therapy using HER2 PET: comparison with ^{18}F-FDG PET. J Nucl Med 47:793–796

Sokoloff L, Reivich M, Kennedy C et al (1977) The [14C]deoxyglucose method for the measurement of local cerebral glucose utilization: theory, procedure, and normal values in the conscious and anesthetized albino rat. J Neurochem 28:897–916

Spaepen K, Stroobants S, Dupont P et al (2003) [^{18}F]FDG PET monitoring of tumour response to chemotherapy: does [(18)F]FDG uptake correlate with the viable tumour cell fraction? Eur J Nucl Med Mol Imaging 30:682–688

Spence AM, Muzi M, Graham MM et al (1998) Glucose metabolism in human malignant gliomas measured quantitatively with PET, 1-[C-11]glucose and FDG: analysis of the FDG lumped constant. J Nucl Med 39:440–448

Steele RJ, Brown M, Eremin O (1985) Characterisation of macrophages infiltrating human mammary carcinomas. Br J Cancer 51:135–138

Teicher BA (1994) Hypoxia and drug resistance. Cancer Metastasis Rev 13:139–168

van Tilburg EW, Franssen EJF, van der Hoeven JJM et al (2004) Radiosynthesis of [^{11}C]-docetaxel. J Label Compd Radiopharm 47:763–777

Tiling R, Linke R, Untch M et al (2001) ^{18}F-FDG PET and ^{99m}Tc-sestamibi scintimammography for monitoring breast cancer response to neoadjuvant chemotherapy: a comparative study. Eur J Nucl Med 28:711–720

Van der Weerdt AP, Klein LJ, Boellaard R et al (2001) Image-derived input functions for determination of MRglu in cardiac ^{18}F-FDG PET scans. J Nucl Med 42:1622–1629

Virtanen KA, Peltoniemi P, Marjamaki P et al (2001) Human adipose tissue glucose uptake determined using [^{18}F]-fluoro-deoxy-glucose ([^{18}F]FDG) and PET in combination with microdialysis. Diabetologia 44:2171–2179

Wahl RL, Zasadny K, Helvie M et al (1993) Metabolic monitoring of breast cancer chemohormonotherapy using positron emission tomography: initial evaluation. J Clin Oncol 11:2101–2111

Wahl RL, Siegel BA, Coleman RE et al (2004) Prospective multicenter study of axillary nodal staging by positron emission tomography in breast cancer: a report of the staging breast cancer with PET Study Group. J Clin Oncol 22:277–285

Wu HM, Huang SC, Choi Y et al (1995) A modeling method to improve quantitation of fluorodeoxyglucose uptake in heterogeneous tumor tissue. J Nucl Med 36:297–306

Wu HM, Hoh CK, Huang SC et al (1996) Quantification of serial tumor glucose metabolism. J Nucl Med 37:506–513

Wu HM, Bergsneider M, Glenn TC et al (2003) Measurement of the global lumped constant for 2-deoxy-2-[^{18}F]fluoro-D-glucose in normal human brain using [15O]water and 2-deoxy-2-[^{18}F]fluoro-D-glucose positron emission tomography imaging. A method with validation based on multiple methodologies. Mol Imaging Biol 5:32–41

Young H, Baum R, Cremerius U et al (1999) Measurement of clinical and subclinical tumour response using [^{18}F]-fluoredeoxyglucose and positron emisson tomography: review and 1999 EORTC recommendations. Eur J Cancer 35:1773–1782

Zasadny KR, Wahl RL (1996) Enhanced FDG-PET tumor imaging with correlation-coefficient filtered influx-constant images. J Nucl Med 37:371–374

FDG-PET in Monitoring Therapy of Breast Cancer

14

Hans-Jürgen Biersack, Hans Bender, and Holger Palmedo

CONTENTS

Abstract

Fluorine-18-fluorodeoxyglucose positron emission tomography (FDG-PET) has been used successfully for the staging and re-staging of breast cancer. Another significant indication is the evaluation of therapy response. There are only few data on FDG-PET in breast cancer after radiation therapy. The same holds true for chemotherapy. Only the therapy response in locally advanced breast cancer after chemotherapy has been investigated thoroughly. Histopathologic response could be predicted with an accuracy of 88–91% after the first and second course of therapy. A quantitative evaluation is of course a prerequisite when FDG-PET is used for therapy monitoring. Only few studies have focussed on hormone therapy. Here, a flare phenomenon with increasing SUVs after initiation of tamoxifen therapy has been observed. More prospective multicenter trials will be needed to make FDG-PET a powerful tool in monitoring chemotherapy in breast cancer.

Whole body imaging with fluorine-18 deoxyglucose PET (FDG-PET) has gained widespread acceptance for the staging and restaging of breast cancer (Biersack et at. 2001; Kostakoglu and Goldsmith 2003; Grahek et al. 2004). Another significant indication for FDG-PET is the evaluation of therapy response. Above that the proof of viability of tumour tissue after termination of chemotherapy is another indication for PET. The evaluation of therapy response is usually done by CT, sonography or MRI (Biersack and Palmedo 2003). These imaging procedures allow the detection of changes of the tumour size or volume. Because the majority of cells within a tumour mass are in a resting state, reduction of tumour volume requires time and might be masked by unspecific effects (edema as a result of necrosis). In contrast, cellular uptake of FDG is a function of cell viability and seems to be associated with the increased cell turnover. Animal models have shown that, after therapy, the amount of tumour FDG uptake reflects the number of viable tumour cells present (Haberkorn et al. 1987).

Already in 1989, Minn et al. (1989) studied patients with breast cancer before and after therapy using FDG-PET. Even using a planar gamma camera equipped with thick lead collimators, they could show that increasing FDG uptake over time was associated with tumour progression. These data make evident that new cumbersome sophisticated FDG imaging procedures may further increase the diagnostic significance of FDG-PET in therapy monitoring.

14.1 FDG-PET before and after Radiotherapy

PET scans before, during and after treatment may provide information that is useful for managing patients undergoing radiation therapy (Lowe 2003; Kumar and Alavi 2004; Zangheri et al. 2004). A pre-treatment PET study allows not only to evaluate metabolic tumour activity, but also treatment planning. The overlay of the PET image onto the CT allows the target to be hit precisely, even in CT negative findings (Bockisch et al. 2003). The high occurrence of recurrences within the primary target volume in some tumours necessitates a dose escalation to improve the probability of tumour control. However, radiotoxicity to healthy tissue limits its strategy. Therefore, there is a need to increase the dose in the target volume. Because of the biological effect, this is only possible by reducing the irradiated volume. As a consequence, as safety margins are to be reduced, the extent of the disease has to be determined more precisely. PET adds valuable information in this context. The PET findings can be translated into morphologic coordinates only by the fusion of PET and CT as is realized with PET-CT. PET data are utilized directly by mapping accurately into the spatial coordinate system of the treatment planning system. Thus, treatment planning using PET gives reliable estimates of the tumour volume and improves isodose tumour coverage (Lowe 2003). PET during radiation therapy may cause some problems in so far as radiotherapy may induce early acute inflammatory hypermetabolism that can be confused with tumour hypermetabolism. In addition, it has been concluded that an early decrease in FDG uptake does not necessarily indicate a good prognosis. This phenomenon highlights the need for a detailed time course and treatment response parameter evaluation as the FDG uptake may be influenced by a variety of metabolic changes that may be unrelated to tumour response.

Immediately after completion of radiation therapy, PET may demonstrate continued uptake in the periphery of the tumour. This FDG accumulation was found to correlate pathologically with the formation of a fibrous pseudocapsule rather than residual disease (Lowe 2003; Jones et al. 1996). In cases where more than 90% of tumour cells were killed, such residual hypermetabolism was seen, but was usually found to be less pronounced than the pretreatment PET.

Radiotherapy response will of course be associated with reduction in tumour size. Complete response is generally felt to be the only standard for indicating tumour control. A partial response is considered to be a radiotherapeutic failure in most cases (Lowe 2003). The definition of complete response can be problematic as complete disappearance of the tumour may only occur rarely, and more commonly residual tissue, whether it be scar or residual tumour, can remain (Fig. 14.1).

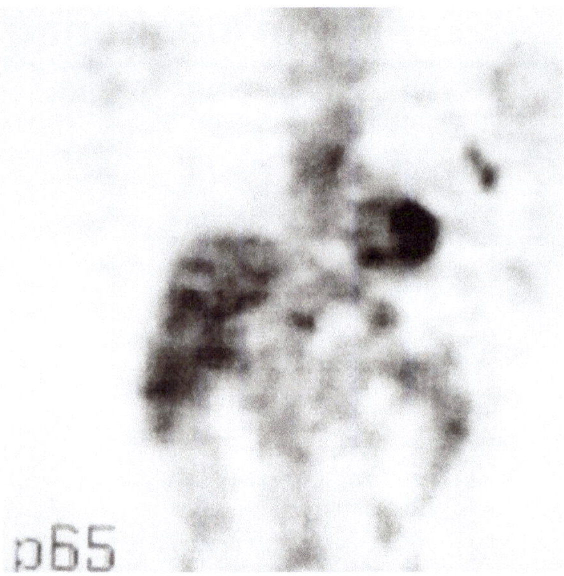

Fig. 14.1. FDG-PET after radiation therapy of breast cancer: positive PET due left axilla to tumour recurrence

PET has been used to assess the therapeutic response to radiation therapy. FDG-PET can identify changes in glucose uptake after treatment and may prove to be a better indicator of a favourable response of therapy (Lowe 2003). However, it may be important to differentiate between a decrease in FDG uptake and the complete absence of FDG uptake. Posttreatment normalization of FDG uptake will probably be a good prognostic sign. Usually, a PET tumour complete response will be predictive of improved survival (Lowe 2003).

A major problem of post-radiation therapy PET is that normal tissues can manifest radiotherapy toxicity to different degrees. Some tissues will demonstrate toxicity in a few days. These tissues are bone marrow, gonads, lymph nodes, salivary glands, gastrointestinal tract, larynx and skin. Other tissues demonstrate radiation damage in weeks to months, and some examples are lung, liver, kidney, spinal cord and brain (Lowe 2003). Because of these effects, significantly increased FDG uptake can be seen in selected soft tissue regions that are irradiated. Data suggest that radiotherapy may induce early acute inflammatory hypermetabolism on PET that is likely related to healing of tissues damaged by radiation (Lowe 2003). This effect will of course depend on the radiosensitivity of the normal tissue being irradiated. For example, increased FDG uptake may be found at 12–16 months after treatment. Some studies showed that normal tissue activity inflammatory responses are at maximum at about 6 months, but can be seen for at least 1 year (Lowe 2003). A study by Jones et al. (1996) showed that immediately following radiation, a hypermetabolic pseudo capsule can be seen that may appear to falsely represent tumour, at least in sarcoma. Lowe (2003) suggests that a fair compromise may be to recommend PET imaging 4–6 months after completion of radiation, if possible. This would allow for assessment of early recurrence and probably give high accuracy of treatment assessment. If inflammatory hypermetabolism is confusing, a follow-up scan may be required to see if the activity diminishes over time.

There are only very few data available on FDG-PET after radiotherapy of breast cancer. Minn et al. (1989) studied ten patients with breast cancer before and after therapy (systemic therapy alone in seven and in combination with radiotherapy in three patients) and showed that an increased FDG uptake in breast cancer over time is a sign of tumour progression. There are no other reports dealing with radiotherapy. These data make evident that a lot of work is ahead of us to evaluate the usefulness of PET after radio- or radiochemotherapy.

Tumour hypoxia has been established as a resistance factor for radiotherapy, and it has been suggested that it promotes tumour aggressiveness and resistance to different treatment modalities (Eubank and Mankoff 2005). Some data suggest that up to 30% of larger or more advanced breast cancers exhibit severe hypoxia at least in parts of the cancer. Although hypoxia may contribute to increased rates of glycolyses, it could not be proven that hypoxia could be simply predicted by FDG uptake. Thus, PET agents specifically designed to image tumour hypoxia have been tested for hypoxia imaging, and especially for (F-18)-fluoromisodinazole, its ability to image hypoxia has been proven (Rasey et al. 1989).

14.2 Chemotherapy and PET

The prediction of response to therapy after its completion has been addressed by several authors. In a retrospective study of 61 patients, Vranjesevic et al. (2002) compared the value of FDG-PET with conventional imaging to predict outcome in breast cancer patients who had previously undergone primary therapy. FDG-PET was more accurate than conventional imaging for predicting outcome, with positive and negative predictive values of 93% und 84% (FDG-PET) versus 85% and 59% (conventional imaging). Prognostic accuracy of FDG-PET reached 90%. Jansson et al. (1995) performed FDG studies before and after three or four courses of polychemotherapy. Eight of the 12 clinical responders had a significant decrease in tracer uptake at the first PET scan performed 6–13 days after the first polychemotherapy course, and these reductions were further augmented after the third or fourth course and corresponded to the conventional therapy evaluation with other imaging procedures. These data show that PET may be able to detect therapy response even 1 week after the beginning of therapy. Similar data had already been published in 1993 by Wahl et al. (1993) who also could show that already at day 8 of the first cycle of chemotherapy a response could be documented. Gennari et al. (2000) investigated 13 patients with metastatic breast cancer who were referred for treatment protocols with gemcitabine/epirubicin/paclitaxel or epirubicin/paclitaxel chemotherapy regimens. All metastatic sites were visualised on the baseline FDG-PET scan. Nine patients were available for final evaluation. In the six patients who seemed to respond to treatment, median SUV was 7.65 at baseline, 5.7 at day 8 after the first course and 1.2 at the end of the courses. Three patients had stable disease and showed no significant decrease in tumour glucose SUV compared to the baseline level.

In a small series of patients, Tiling et al. (2001) performed FDG-PET (in addition to Tc-99m MIBI) before and after neoadjuvant chemotherapy. All three patients with complete remission showed decreasing FDG as early as 8 days after therapy. Three patients had partial remission and presented with persisting focal FDG uptake. One non-responder remained unchanged during chemotherapy. Tiling et al. (2001) could also show that increased tracer uptake after the first cycle did not exclude a partial tumour response. Only after the second chemotherapeutic cycle FDG-PET (and MIBI imaging) was able to distinguish between complete and partial/no response.

Krak et al. (2003) performed studies in 20 women with locally advanced (n=10) or metastasized (n=10) breast cancer. Follow-up PET scans were obtained after 8 days and after one, three and six courses of chemotherapy. Mathematical models were used for measurement of FDG uptake. It turned out that SUV was the least accurate procedure in predicting changes in FDG uptake over time during therapy. The authors propose a quantitative evaluation procedure including Patlak graphical analyses, SUV and a kinetic procedure.

Eubank and Mankoff (2005) again focussed on the evaluation of therapy response. Smith et al. (2000) showed by quantitative methods that a significant reduction of axillary nodule FDG uptake after neoadjuvant chemotherapy can predict complete microscopic pathologic response. Here it has to be noted that axillary nodule response to therapy might be an important marker for prognosis since nodule disease reflects the presence of occult disseminated disease.

In a retrospective study, Staffort et al. (2002) evaluated the response of skeletal metastases to therapy using serial FDG-PET. These authors found a strong correlation between the quantitative change in FDG SUV and overall clinical assessment of response and change in tumour markers.

Again, it is evident that PET shows potential for evaluation of chemotherapy in breast cancer (Figs. 14.2, 14.3). However, all presented studies lack significant numbers of patients. We strongly believe that only multicentre trials may solve this problem.

14.3 Monitoring of Primary Chemotherapy in Locally Advanced Breast Cancer (LABC)

While – as has already been mentioned – data on FDG-PET in radio- and chemotherapy in general are scarce, some valid data are available regarding the monitoring of primary chemotherapy. An important advantage of primary chemotherapy in breast cancer is that it can increase the rate of breast-conserving surgery by preoperatively reducing tumour volume (Fisher et al. 1997).

Neoadjuvant chemotherapy has been used in patients with LABC to improve primary tumour resectibility, including the use of breast-conserving surgery and assess in vivo response to selected chemotherapy (Eubank and Mankoff 2005).

Because of the excellent results of this procedure, chemotherapy before definitive surgical therapy (neoadjuvant, primary or induction chemotherapy) has also been applied to the treatment of lower-stage breast cancer. Recent trials reported clinical response rates greater than 70%, but only in a small fraction of patients a macroscopic complete response to therapy had been achieved (Booser and Hortobagyi 1992). In patients with macroscopic complete response a significantly better prognoses than in patients presenting with residual tumour after com-

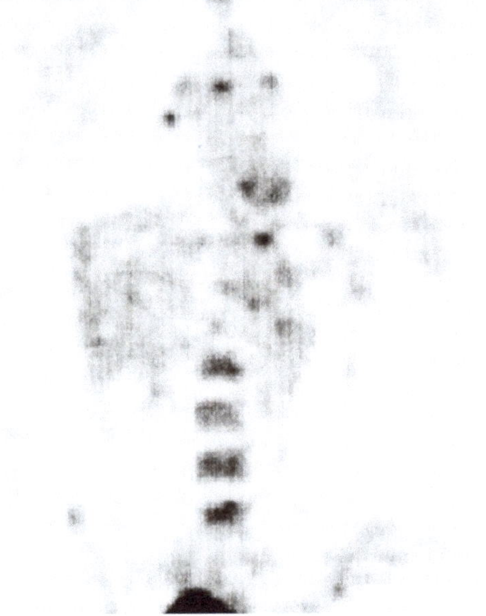
a

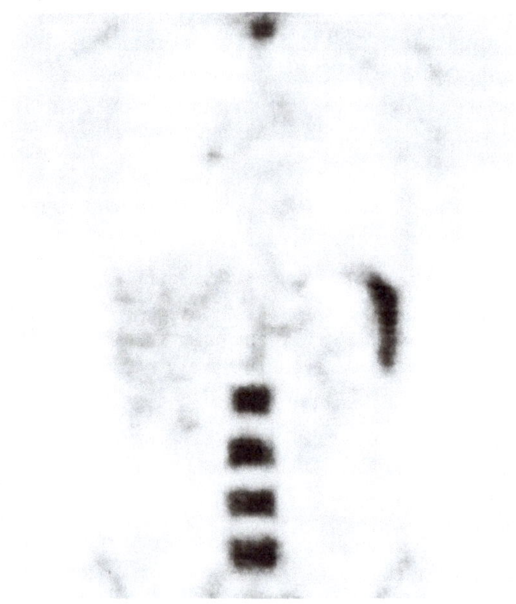
b

Fig. 14.2a,b. FDG-PET before and after chemotherapy: multiple mediastinal lymph node metastases before therapy (**a**); reduction of metastases in number and activity after therapy (**b**) (Biersack et al. 2001)

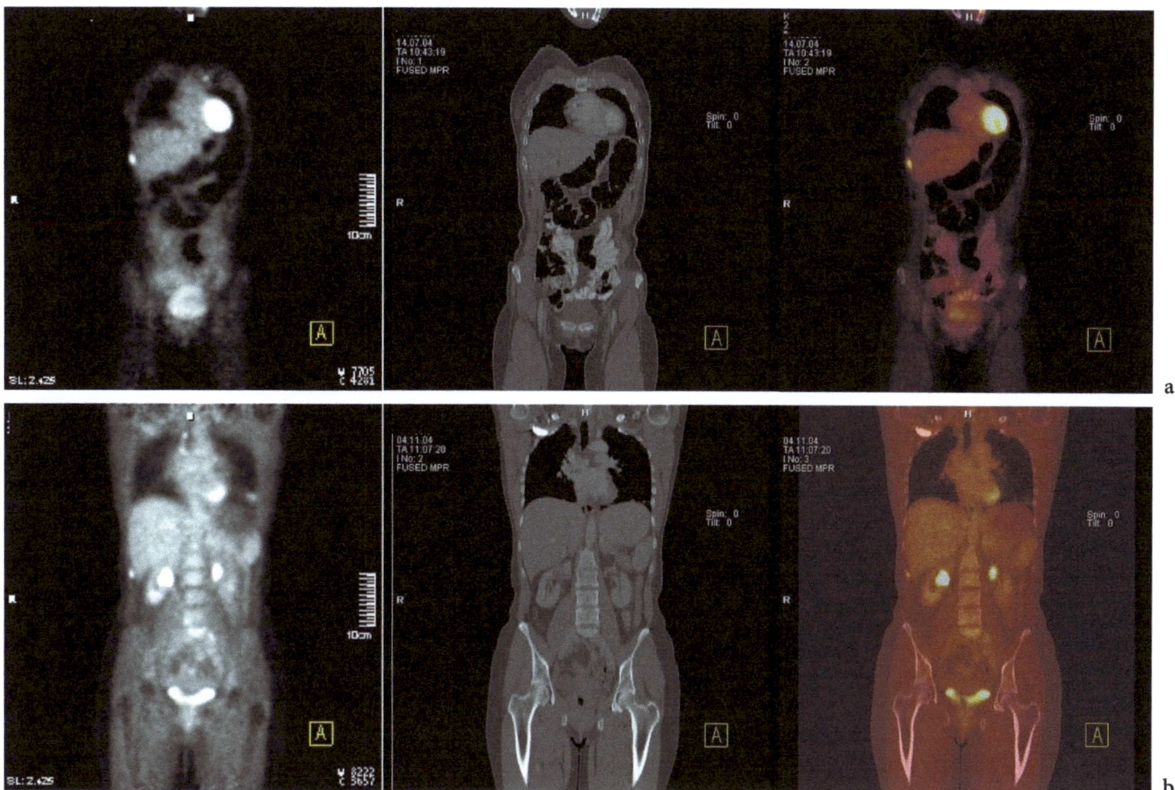

Fig. 14.3a,b. FDG-PET/CT before (**a**) and after (**b**) chemotherapy: **a,b** rib metastasis (right thorax) responds to therapy; however, a new rib metastasis can be seen under therapy, again right thorax (**b**)

pletion of chemotherapy has been observed (Machiavelli 1998). Furthermore, patients with minimal residual disease had significantly higher disease-free and overall survival rates compared to patients with gross residual disease. Partial or complete regression proven by histopathologic tissue analysis is achieved in only 20–30% of patients (Chollet et al. 1997). From these data it is evident that clinical response does not necessarily reflect histopathologic response. Thus, tumour markers may be used to determine the therapeutic effect until definitive breast surgery is performed. Considering the side effects of primary chemotherapy, there is a need for early therapy monitoring to identify non-responding patients. Imaging procedures such as mammography, ultrasonography and MRI have been used for evaluating tumour size in relation to response to therapy. As has been shown before, tumour shrinkage as evidenced by morphologic imaging does not reflect response to therapy, which causes a certain delay between initiation of therapy and proof of tumour response. In addition, these procedures do not allow differentiation between viable tumour tissue and fibrotic scar tissue (Vinnicombe et al. 1996). Although clinical evaluation and tumour markers might be useful for this purpose, they have not yet been applied in larger patient populations (Mankoff et al. 2002).

For these reasons, nuclear medicine procedures offer opportunities for the evaluation of the success of chemotherapy. Tiling et al. have used Tc-99m sestamibi imaging – in addition to FDG-PET – for the evaluation of therapy success (Tiling et al. 2001). Furthermore, this procedure offers the opportunity to detect multi-drug resistance (Palmedo 2002).

One of the factors that may influence responses to systemic chemotherapy is tumour perfusion (Sagar et al. 1993), which may of course be evaluated by 15 O-water PET (Mankoff et al. 1999). Good perfusion is crucial for the delivery of chemotherapy to the tumour cell (Chollet et al. 1997). Tumours with low perfusion may be hypoxic, and hypoxia has been related to aggressive tumour behaviour and poor response to chemotherapy (Teicher 1994). Mankoff et al. (2003) have thus estimated changes in blood flow and metabolism in locally advanced breast cancer treated with neoadjuvant chemotherapy. Additionally, FDG has been used for calculating the metabolic rate. Both parameters were used for attempting to predict the outcome by a baseline study alone (Mankoff et al. 2003). A second procedure offered by nuclear medicine is FDG-PET, which has previously been shown to be beneficial in monitoring the response to chemotherapy (Wahl et al. 1993; Smith et al. 2000; Teicher 1994; Bassa et al. 1996; Schelling et al. 2000; Weber et al. 2002). The experiences with FDG-PET are encouraging, but somewhat controversial. Despite these drawbacks, FDG-PET allows prediction of the response to chemotherapy in LABC even shortly after the onset of the therapy. Thus, FDG-PET is expected to be useful for reducing the costs of cytotoxic therapy and the unnecessary side effects of chemotherapy, which are not useful. These economic and clinical advantages will certainly outweigh the expense of PET. A prerequisite for monitoring therapy response is, of course, a quantification of PET data. Wahl et al. (1993) were the first to use FDG-PET for metabolic monitoring of breast cancer chemohormonotherapy. Bassa et al. (1996) presented the first data concerning FDG-PET studies in 16 patients with LABC. All patients had PET studies before chemotherapy, 13 patients between the end of the first cycle and at the midpoint of chemotherapy, and 14 patients before surgery. Visual diagnoses and SUVs of PET scans were compared with pathology findings at surgery and with the results of mammography, ultrasonography or both, which were performed before chemotherapy and before local surgery for residual disease. Each patient's clinical course was monitored for up to 3 years. Sensitivity (in general) for detection of pathologically proven primary lesions was 100% for FDG-PET, and sensitivity for detection of initial nodal involvement was 77%. Sensitivity for the detection of residual primary tumour was 75%, and sensitivity for detection of residual nodal involvement was 41.6%. Clinical improvement of primary lesions was seen in all patients, improvement with smaller size and less FDG uptake as early as at the second study in 69%. Mean SUV values decreased significantly. These data were extended by Schelling et al. (2000) and Smith et al. (2000). Usually, SUVs are used for quantification of PET. Because a tumour shrinks during response, the placement of regions of interest (ROIs) is crucial. It has been proposed that circular ROIs with a diameter of 1.5 cm should be placed (Schelling et al. 2000). This procedure has been chosen to reduce partial volume effects, which play a substantial role if ROI is placed visually around the entire tumour and tumour size changes after the baseline study (Sagar et al. 1993). Smith et al. (2000) have used a cumbersome protocol in performing a time-consuming dynamic imaging study and collecting sequential arterial blood samples. The influx constant was calculated for each voxel of the image resulting in a parametric map of FDG uptake. The dose to uptake ratio (DUR) was also calculated for each voxel from the final frame of the dynamic data. It has also been proposed to calculate the metabolic rate of FDG using the tracer influx constant K_i (ml/min/g), resulting in units of micromoles per minute per 100 gram.

All quantitative FDG protocols require constant glucose levels; thus, the glucose level has to be determined before injection. The follow-up data also have to be normalized to the blood glucose level. Most studies have focussed on serial PET scans. Mankoff et al. (2002) attempted to predict the outcome by a baseline study alone. However, they combined both ^{15}O and FDG-PET in one study.

Bender et al. (1999) have shown that at least in non-resectable liver metastases of colorectal cancer early identification of non-responders is possible. Smith et al. (2000) obtained four PET scans: at baseline, before the second and fifth doses of chemotherapy, and shortly before surgical excision of the primary tumour and axillary lymph nodes. Schelling et al. (2000) used a protocol including a PET scan 10 days after the first course and 9 days after the second course of chemotherapy in addition to the baseline study. Mankoff et al. (2003) added to the previous protocol a follow-up scan after 2 months of chemotherapy. The results of these studies may be summarised as follows: Smith et al. concluded that the decrease in FDG uptake is a marker of tumour response (Smith et al. 2000). They concluded that FDG-PET imaging of primary metastatic breast cancer after a single course of chemotherapy may be of value in predicting pathologic treatment response with a sensitivity of 90% and a specificity of 74%. However, in metastatic lesions this effect could not be observed. The mean pre-treatment FDG uptake values of the lesions that achieved a microscopic complete pathologic response were significantly higher than those from less responsive lesions. Schelling et al. (2000) also correctly identified responders by follow-up PET, with a sensitivity of 100% and a specificity of 85%. A threshold was set by an SUV decrease below 55% of the baseline scan. At this threshold, histopathologic response could be predicted with an accuracy of 88% and 91%, respectively, after the first and second course of therapy.

In contrast to these results, Mankoff et al. (2003) did not find differences between responders and non-responders using FDG-PET alone. Using water PET, the change in blood flow after 2 months of therapy predicted disease-free and overall survival. While cumbersome techniques such as a combination of FDG with water PET imaging may be restricted to research, FDG-PET alone has to be recommended for predicting response to chemotherapy in LABC in a clinical setting. The estimation of SUVs (in defined circular ROIs) should be recommended for clinical purposes. These SUVs will not be hampered by partial volume and tumour shrinkage effects. The SUVs of baseline and follow-up investigation should be normalised to the blood glucose level. With the increasing availability of clinical PET, the use of this powerful technology for monitoring primary chemotherapy is expected to become routine.

14.4 FDG-PET during Hormone Therapy

Some researchers have used ^{18}F-labelled estradiole (McGuire et al. 1991) and other radiolabelled estrogens and progestins (Jonson and Welch 1998) as well as fluoro-tamoxifen (Inoue et al. 1996). In 1999, Dehdashti et al. (1999) performed fluoro-estradiole and FDG-PET before and 7–10 days after initiation of tamoxifen therapy. The PET results were correlated with follow-up evaluation and continued until the patient became unresponsive to hormone therapy (3–24 months). There were seven responders and four non-responders. With respect to FDG, it could be proven that none of the responders had a clinical flare reaction, but all demonstrated metabolic flare with the mean standard deviation increase in tumour SUVs of 1.4 ± 0.7. No evidence for flare was noted in the non-responders. The findings of a metabolic flare by FDG-PET early after institution of tamoxifen treatment appeared to predict responsiveness to antiestrogen therapy in patients with receptor-positive breast cancer. To our knowledge the flare phenomenon has never been observed after chemotherapy. If hormono-chemotherapy is performed, this finding should be kept in mind.

In another study, Mortimer et al. (2001) have again described a "metabolic flare".

14.5 Conclusion

Although FDG-PET has been used as tracer in many entities of tumours after radiation and chemotherapy, data in breast cancer are still scarce. The only indication where valid data are obtainable is the monitoring of primary chemotherapy in locally advanced breast cancer. Here, it could be proven that the FDG uptake is reduced even after the first cycle of chemotherapy. Quantitative evaluation of the data is a prerequisite. The estimation of SUVs in defined circular ROIs of approximately 1.5-cm diameter is recommended for clinical purposes. These SUVs will not be hampered by partial volume and tumour shrinkage effects. The SUVs of baseline and follow-up investigations have to be normalised to the blood glucose level. Whenever hormone therapy (tamoxifen) is being performed, one should keep in mind that a metabolic flare phenomenon with an increase in tumour SUVs for FDG has been observed in responders. Another problem that should be addressed is secondary effects such as neovascularisation and inflammatory cell infiltration, which may lead to changes in tumour blood flow and may mask tumour response. However, these changes will be observed mainly after radiation therapy and not after chemotherapy in breast cancer.

References

Bassa P, Kim EE, Inoue T et al (1996) Evaluation of preoperative chemotherapy using PET with fluorine-18-fluorodeoxyglucose in breast cancer. J Nucl Med 37: 931–938.

Bender H, Bangard M, Metten N et al (1999) Possible role of FDG-PET in the early prediction of therapy outcome in liver metastases of colorectal cancer. Hybridoma 18:87–91

Biersack HJ, Palmedo H, Bender H, Krause T (2001) Nuclear medicine and breast cancer. In: Freeman LM (ed) Nuclear medicine annual 2001. Philadelphia, Lippincott Williams & Wilkens, pp 69–108

Biersack HJ, Palmedo H (2003) Locally advanced breast cancer: Is PET useful for monitoring primary chemotherapy? J Nucl Med 44:1815–1817

Bockisch A, Freudenberg L, Antoch G, Müller S (2004) PET/CT: Clinical considerations. In: Oehr P, Biersack HJ, Coleman RE (eds) PET and PET-CT in oncology. Berlin Heidelberg New York, Springer, pp 101–125

Booser DJ, Hortobagyi GN (1992) Treatment of locally advanced breast cancer. Semin Oncol 19:278–285

Chollet P, Charrier S, Brain E et al (1997) Clinical and pathological response to primary chemotherapy in operable breast cancer. Eur J Cancer 3:862–866

Dehdashti F, Flanagan FL, Mortimer JE et al (1999) Positron emission tomographic assessment of „metabolic flare“ to predict response of metastatic breast cancer to antiestrogen therapy. Eur J Nucl Med 26:51–56

Eubank WB, Mankoff DA (2005) Evolving role of positron emission tomography in breast cancer imaging. Semin Nucl Med 2:84–99

Fisher B, Brown A, Mamounas E et al (1997) Effect of preoperative chemotherapy on local-regional disease in women with operable breast cancer: Findings from National Surgical Adjuvant Breast and Bowel Project B-18. J Clin Oncol 15:2483–2493

Gennari A, Donati S, Salvadori B et al (2000) Role of 2-(^{18}F)-fluorodeoxyglucose (FDG) positron emission tomography (PET) in the early assessment of response to chemotherapy in metastatic breast cancer patients. Clin Breast Cancer 1:156–161

Grahek D, Montravers F, Kerrou K, Aide N, Lotz JP, Talbot JN (2004) (^{18}F)FDG in recurrent breast cancer: Diagnostic perfomances, clinical impact and relevance of induced changes in management. Eur J Nucl Med Mol Imaging 31:179–188

Haberkorn U, Reinhardt M, Strauss LG (1987) Metabolic design of combination therapy: Use of enhanced fluorodeoxyglucose uptake caused by chemotherapy. J Nucl Med 33:1981–1987

Inoue T, Kim EE, Wallace S et al (1996) Positron emission tomography using (^{18}F) fluoro-tamoxifen to evaluate therapeutic responses in patients with breast cancer: Preliminary study. Cancer Biother Radiopharm 11:235–245

Kostakoglu L, Goldsmith SJ (2003) ^{18}F-FDG-PET evaluation of the response to therapy for lymphoma and for breast, lung and colorectal carcinoma. J Nucl Med 44:224–239

Minn H, Soini I (1989) (^{18}F)Fluorodeoxyglucose scintigraphy in diagnosis and follow-up of treatment in advanced breast cancer. Eur J Nucl Med Mol Imaging 15:61–66

Lowe VJ (2004) PET in radiotherapy. In: Oehr P, Biersack HJ, Coleman RE (eds) PET and PET-CT in oncology. Berlin Heidelberg New York, Springer, pp 303–308

Jansson T, Westlin JE, Ahlstrom H et al (1995) Positron emission tomography studies in patients with locally advanced and/or metastatic breast cancer: a method for early therapy evaluation? J Clin Oncol 13:1470–1477

Jones DN, McCowage GW, Soestman HD et al (1996) Monitoring of neoadjuvant therapy response of soft-tissue and musculoskeletal sarcoma using fluorine-18-FDG-PET. J Nucl Med 37:1438–1444

Jonson SD, Welch MJ (1998) PET imaging of breast cancer with fluorine-18 radiolabelled estrogens and progrestins. Q J Nucl Med 42:8–17

Krak NC, van der Hoeven JJ, Hoekstra OS et al (2003) Measuring (^{18}F) FDG uptake in breast cancer during chemotherapy: comparison of analytical methods. Eur J Nucl Med Mol Imaging 30:674–681

Kumar R, Alavi A (2004) Fluorodeoxyglucose-PET in the management of breast cancer. Radiol Clin North Am 6:1113–1122

Machiavelli M, Romero A, Pérez K et al (1998) Prognostic significance of pathological response of primary tumor and metastatic axillary lymph nodes after neoadjuvant chemotherapy for locally advanced breast carcinoma. Cancer J Sci Am 4:125–131

Mankoff DA, Dunnwald LK, Gralow JR et al (1999) Monitoring the response of patients with locally advanced breast carcinoma to neoadjuvant chemotherapy using (Technetium-99m)-sestamibi scintimammography. Cancer 85:2410–2423

Mankoff DA, Dunnwald LK, Gralow JR et al (2002) Blood flow and metabolism in locally advanced breast cancer: Relationship to response to therapy. J Nucl Med 43:500–509

Mankoff DA, Dunnwald LK, Gralow JR et al (2003) Changes in blood flow and metabolism in locally advanced breast cancer (LABC) treated with neo-adjuvant chemotherapy. J Nucl Med 44:1806–1814

McGuire AH, Dehdashti F, Siegel BA et al (1991) Positron tomographic assessment of 16-(^{18}F)fluoro-17-estradiol uptake in metastatic breast carcinoma. J Nucl Med 32:1526–1531

Mortimer JE, Dedashti F, Siegel BA et al (2001) Metabolic flare: Indicator of hormone responsiveness in advanced breast cancer. J Clin Oncol 19:2797–2803

Palmedo H (2002) What can we expect from MDR breast cancer imaging with sestamibi? J Nucl Med 43:526–529

Rasey JX, Koh W, Grieason JR et al (1989) Radiolabelled fluoromisodinazole as an imaging agent for tumor hypoxia. Int J Radiat Oncol Biol Phys 17:985–991

Sagar SM, Klassen GA, Barclay KD, Aldrich JE (1993) Antitumor treatment: Tumor blood flow-measurement and manipulation for therapeutic gain. Cancer Treat Rev 19:299–349

Schelling M, Avril N, Nährig J et al (2000) Positron emission tomography using (^{18}F) fluorodeoxyglucose for monitoring primary chemotherapy in breast cancer. J Clin Oncol 18:1689–1695

Smith TC, Welch AE, Hutcheon AW et al (2000) Positron emission tomography using (^{18}F) -fluorodeoxy-D-glucose to predict the pathologic response of breast cancer to primary chemotherapy. J Clin Oncol 18:1676–1688

Stafford SE, Agraloff JR, Schubert EK et al (2002) Use of serial FDG-PET to measure the response of bone dominant breast cancer to therapy. Acta Radiol 9:913–921

Teicher BA (1994) Hypoxia and drug resistance. Cancer Metastasis Rev 13:139–168

Tiling R, Linke R, Untch M et al (2001) ^{18}F-FDG-PET and ^{99m}Tc-Sestamibi scintimammography for monitoring breast cancer response to neoadjuvant chemotherapy: A comparative study. Eur J Nucl Med Mol Imaging 28:711–720

Vinnicombe SJ, MacVicar AD, Guy RL et al (1996) Primary breast cancer: Mammographic changes after neoadjuvant chemotherapy, with pathologic correlation. Radiology 198:333–340

Vranjesevic D, Filmont JE, Meta J et al (2002) Whole body (^{18}F)-FDG-PET and conventional imaging for predicting outcome in previously treated breast cancer patients. J Nucl Med 43:325–329

Wahl RL, Zasadny K, Helvie M et al (1993) Metabolic monitoring of breast cancer chemo-hormonotherapy using positron emission tomography: Initial evaluation. J Clin Oncol 11:2101–2111

Weber WA, Schwaiger M, Avril N (2002) Quantitative assessment of tumor metabolism using FDG-PET imaging. Nucl Med Biol 27:683–687

Wilson CBJH, Lammertsma AA, McKienzie CG, Sikora K, Johns T (1992) Measurement of blood flow and exchanging water space in breast tumors using positron emission tomography: A rapid and non-invasive dynamic method. Cancer Res 52:1592–1597

Zangheri B, Messa C, Picchio M et al (2004) PET/CT and breast cancer. Eur J Nucl Med Mol Imaging 1:112–117

FDG-PET and Tumour Marker Tests for the Diagnosis of Breast Cancer*

15

Emilio Bombardieri, Alessandra Alessi, Federica Pallotti, Gianluca Serafini, Nicola Mazzuca, Ettore Seregni, and Flavio Crippa

CONTENTS

Abstract

Circulating tumour markers for breast cancer can be classified in different groups: mucins such as CA 15.3, CA 27.29 and CA 549, carcinoembryonic antigen (CEA), cytokeratins (TPA, TPs, Cyfra 21.1), enzymes (LDH), hormones and their subunits. All of them have been proposed over the years for the diagnosis and monitoring of breast cancer at different stages. It is well known that tumour marker tests lack in sensitivity at the earliest stage of cancer and also in specificity. False-negative results are rare in patients with advanced disease and metastases; on the contrary they are most frequent in the first stages. Besides this, false-positive results can be due to different non-malignant conditions. At present CA 15.3 is the most widely used tumour marker in breast cancer patients. Its use follows the general concepts everywhere accepted for mucinic markers: the CA 15.3 test is not useful in screening and early diagnosis; it has an established role in the diagnosis of recurrences; it has an established role in therapy monitoring, alone or in association with other diagnostic tools; it is still under study as a predictor of response to therapy. Several international guidelines help physicians in using tumour markers giving practical recommendations for the appropriate interpretation of circulating tumour markers. CEA and cytokeratins markers are so far less specific than mucinic markers; therefore, they are sometimes tested for evaluating breast cancer patients.

The association of tumour marker tests with a diagnostic imaging modality such as FDG-PET today is of great interest, because sometimes the patients present with a tumour marker increase and do not show clinical symptoms or signs of cancer, or on the contrary some others subjects present with some doubtful symptoms or signs of cancer, and the association with a biochemical test for malignancy can be helpful to make the final diagnosis. FDG-PET is known as a metabolic imaging modality, that, contrary to radiological techniques, reveals cancer not on the basis of morphology like the radiological methods, but because of the uptake and/or processing of a radioactive tracer in cancer tissue. The visualization of cancer by PET depends on the viability and activity of the tumour, and this requirement is very close to the function of synthesis and secretion of tumour markers as products of cell metabolism. One can say that FDG-PET and tumour marker tests describe cancer activities in different ways, and their diagnostic added value takes advantage of this combination.

This chapter overviews the results of the association of FDG-PET with elevated or progressively increasing tumour markers. Tumour-marker-guided PET has demonstrated a diagnostic effectiveness in detecting cancer lesions with variable sensitivity, both at presentation (staging) and during the follow-up (discovery of relapses, metastases and re-staging). It is well known that tumour marker increase

*The authors have written this paper on behalf of the Group of Immunometric Assays of the Italian Association of Nuclear Medicine and Molecular Imaging (AIMN).

is a reliable signal of the presence of occult disease, and this suspicion can be explored by FDG-PET. For this reason some authors have proposed that whole body PET may become the method of choice for the assessment of asymptomatic patients with elevated tumour marker levels. The recent development of hybrid systems, allowing the concomitant examination of the patient by combining PET with CT, has increased the accuracy of diagnostic imaging, and several papers support the evidence that PET/CT is able to add incremental diagnostic confidence to PET and detects more lesions than CT or PET alone. A discussion is still open about the question if FDG-PET or PET/CT can substitute the entire battery of tests routinely used for staging breast cancer or detecting relapse in all breast cancer patients. At present, it is very difficult to draw a final conclusion, since one should consider the cost of the test, the non-complete availability of this examination in all clinical centres, and the problem of the limited sensitivity of PET in early stages, which is not able to rule out the microscopic metastases. There is still a need for further prospective clinical trials for evaluating the impact of this approach on patient management and survival, according to the different risk groups. However, in spite of several controversies in this field, there is no doubt that the association of tumour marker tests with PET or PET/CT seems to provide useful information, and this approach is indicated, mainly in the follow-up of patients at risk, in re-staging patients with symptoms and in evaluating the response to treatments.

15.1 Background

The definition of tumour markers includes different substances that are secreted by the cancer cells in the blood stream and can be interpreted as a biochemical signal of the presence and of the growth of a malignant tumour (Seregni et al. 1999). The measurement of these substances, usually performed by immunoradiometric assays, offers functional information about the clinical evolution of the disease, and its most important role consists in the diagnosis of metastases and the evaluation of response to treatment (Bombardieri 1998).

These substances for breast cancer can be divided in different groups: (1) mucins (mucin-associated antigens such as CA 15.3, CA 27.29 and CA 549); (2) carcinoembryonic antigen (CEA); (3) cytokeratins (TPA, TPs, Cyfra 21.1); (4) enzymes (LDH); (5) hormones and their subunits (HCG). All of them have been proposed over the years for the diagnosis and monitoring of breast cancer at different stages (Seregni et al. 2004).

Mucinic markers, CEA and cytokeratins are not strictly specific for breast cancer, such as other tumour markers (PSA, thyroglobulin, hormones, etc., that correlate with histology), and at the same time they are not specific for breast cancer, since they can be associated with other neoplastic conditions and are often increased in several non-malignant conditions. False-positive results can be due to some inflammatory situations, autoimmune diseases, chronic liver diseases and also some physiological situations.

It is well known that tumour markers are not always elevated in the presence of cancer, since their increase over the cut-off levels is associated with the mass and the growth of the tumour. This means that the smallest tumours at the first stages of disease are not frequently associated with a significant increase of marker levels. Therefore, false-negative results are rare in patients with advanced disease and metastases; on the contrary they are most frequent in the first stages. This is a reason why tumour markers are not recommended for screening cancer, except in some particular conditions, for some tissue-specific markers and in the group at high-risk of disease (Gion et al. 1993).

Among the wide spectrum of the circulating tumour markers developed for clinical use in oncology, those that obtained the major attention from the oncologists were CA 15.3, CEA and cytokeratins (Hayes et al. 1985, 1986; Berling et al. 1990; Benchimol et al. 1989; Steiner and Roop 1988; Nagle 1988). At present CA 15.3 is the most widely used tumour marker in breast cancer patients; other similar mucins have been studied, namely MCA and CA 549, but they have had limited clinical applications. Their use follows the general concepts everywhere accepted for mucinic markers: (1) the CA 15.3 test is not useful in the screening and early diagnosis; (2) some studies suggest that the elevated levels of CA 15.3 can have a role as an independent prognostic factor; (3) CA 15.3 has an established role in the diagnosis of recurrences; (4) CA 15.3 has an established role in therapy monitoring, alone or in association with other diagnostic tools; (5) CA 15.3 is still under study as a predictor of response to therapy (Seregni et al. 2004). There are several international guidelines that help physicians in using tumour markers, and the recommendations for the appropriate use of circulating tumour markers in breast cancer patients are included (Bast et al. 2001; Basuyan et al. 2000; Cheung et al. 2000; Duffy 2001; Sturgeon 2002; Duffy 2006).

The association of the tumour marker test with a diagnostic imaging modality such as FDG-PET is of great interest because sometimes the patients present with some tumour marker increase and do not show clinical symptoms or signs of cancer, or on the contrary some other subjects present with some doubtful symptoms or signs of cancer, and the association with a biochemical test for malignancy can be helpful to make the final diagnosis. This is particularly true for those tumour markers with a good tissue specificity such as thyroglobulin (TG) in thyroid cancer, prostate-specific antigen (PSA) in prostate cancer, chromogranin A (CgA) in neuroendocrine tumours, alpha fetoprotein (AFP) in endodermal sinus tumours and hepatoblastomas, and human chorion gonadotropin (HCG) in tumour deriving from trophoblast, since these substances give an additional specific indication about the tissue of production (Ugrinska et al. 2002). Even if the mucinic tumour markers, such as CA.15.3, CA 125 and CA 19.9, do not show the optimal tissue specificity, their clinical use has been validated in association with breast cancer, ovarian cancer and gastrointestinal cancer, respectively, and therefore at present they are considered as tumour markers preferentially associated with these histotypes. CEA and cytokeratin markers are so far less specific than mucinic markers; therefore, they are currently tested for the diagnosis of many tumours, including breast cancer.

On the other hand, FDG-PET is known as a metabolic imaging modality that, contrary to radiological techniques, reveals cancer not on the basis of morphology like the radiological methods, but because of the uptake and/or processing of a radioactive tracer by cancer tissue (Delbeke et al. 2004). Therefore, the visualization of cancer by PET depends on many variables. For this reason the viability and activity of the tumour are essential, and this requirement is very close to the function of synthesis and secretion of tumour markers as products of cell metabolism (Rohren et al. 2004). One can say that FDG-PET and tumour marker tests describe some cancer activities in different ways, and their diagnostic added value takes advantage of these two different dynamic mechanisms.

15.2 Screening and Diagnosis of Early Cancer

At present there are no tumour markers that are useful for screening or early diagnosis of breast cancer. In fact the diagnostic accuracy of tumour marker tests is limited by the low sensitivity in early-stage disease and by the lack of specificity. For the CA 15.3 assays, different studies have demonstrated that the diagnostic sensitivity is about 10–15% in patients at stage I, 20–15% in patients at stage II and 30–50% in patients at stage III. The rate of false-negative results is very relevant. Besides this, one should consider that a certain number of false-positive results can be observed in patients with benign breast pathology, hepatic diseases and autoimmune diseases.

It is generally known that FDG-PET in the diagnosis of primary breast cancer has shown a satisfactory sensitivity only for tumours >0.8 cm in size that are palpable with a high probability of malignancy. It is well known that these cancers can be easily visualized by other diagnostic modalities; some of them (like digital mammography, MRI) have very high resolution limits, around 2 mm in diameter. The major factors limiting the accuracy of PET are the physical detection limits of the available scanners and also the different rate of utilization of glucose by the breast tissue (Bender et al. 1998; Avril et al. 1996). On the contrary some false-positive uptakes have been observed in different benign disease such as fibroadenoma, severe fibrocystic mastopathy, ductal ectasia and tubular angiomyoepitelioma (Palmedo et al. 1997; Avril et al. 2000; Scheidhauer et al. 2004). The association of a tumour marker test for the diagnosis of small primary breast cancer does not improve the diagnostic accuracy significantly, since a negative CA 15.3 test cannot exclude the presence breast cancer, and a positive CA 15.3 test is not sufficient to confirm malignancy.

The screening of breast cancer does not have to be proposed by a diagnostic imaging modality with a relatively low sensitivity for the small tumours. In the recent literature there is only one paper that evaluates FDG-PET in cancer screening on a large series of asymptomatic subjects. This study has been carried out by Shen et al. (2003) on 1,283 patients who underwent FDG-PET with the additional information coming from the measurement of circulating tumour markers. The final diagnosis in those subjects with positive FDG-PET was confirmed by other imaging modalities or pathological findings, while cases with negative FDG-PET were evaluated with a follow-up of at least 6 months. A total of 18 subjects (1.4%) had cancer, and FDG-PET showed pathological uptake in 15 (1.2%). The three false-negative cases included one hepatoma (with high serum levels of AFP 129.6 ng/ml), one prostate cancer (with high serum levels of PSA 25.1 ng/ml) and one breast cancer (with CA 15.3 and CEA under the normal cut-off levels). The false-positive FDG-PET studies resulted in 24 (1.9%); however, none had abnormal levels of tumour markers. In spite of the conclusions of the author about the potential of tumour marker tests in reducing the rate of false-negative and false-positive results in cancer screening, this kind of study should not be encouraged because of the low positive predictive value of PET in the healthy population, the cost of the program and the poor clinical impact of the results.

15.3 Diagnosis of Loco-Regional and Distant Metastases at Tumour Presentation

The best sensitivity of the tumour marker test is found in metastatic disease, since the elevation of circulating levels is related to tumour mass. The most widely accepted indication of FDG-PET is the diagnosis of metastases, with PET being a whole body test that allows the depiction of metastases in the lymph nodes, bone and visceral organs. Many clinical studies have demonstrated that FDG-PET in breast cancer staging is able to discover a significant number of metastases that would have been missed or incorrectly diagnosed by CT, US, MRI and also by bone scintigraphy, which is still widely used in breast cancer. The recent availability of the hybrid system PET/CT has led to registering better performances when compared with PET or CT alone, and these new instruments have improved the diagnostic accuracy in several situations (Zangheri et al. 2004; Adler and Bakale 2001).

The incidence of loco-regional metastases is related to the size of primary breast cancer. Only 5% of patients with primary tumour <1 cm in diameter has axillary lymph node involvement; this rate increases to 25% in patients with primary tumour from 1 to 2 cm in diameter. The involvement of the internal mammary chain is around 30% in T1-T2 patients with tumours located in the internal quadrant, and this frequency reaches 30–50% in patients with T3 tumours. The presence of distant metastases defines stage IV; the frequency of the topographic distribution of metastases in bone is 70–80%, in lung 65%, in liver 60% and in brain 25%. Other sites are the ovary up to 45%, thyroid 20%, kidney 15% and gastrointestinal organs 20%. It goes without saying that the diagnosis of metastases is very important because it obviously affects the prognosis and can modify the therapy. The diagnostic modalities to image metastases currently adopted in the clinical practice are: (1) for loco-regional metastases lymphoscintigraphy with sentinel lymph node biopsy (SLNB), scintimammography or FDG-PET, mammography, US and RMI; (2) for distant metastases chest X-rays, US, CT, bone scintigraphy and FDG-PET.

The diagnostic performances of the conventional radiological modalities show some limitations, mainly in depicting lymph node metastases or studying breast lesions in areas with anatomical distortions or alteration due to dense breast, previous surgery, radiotherapy or breast implants. However some of them (mammography, US and MRI) are considered the standard methods to study breast tumours. Lymphoscintigraphy with sentinel node biopsy has been shown to be the best diagnostic modality to stage the loco-regional lymph node invasion, since its sensitivity is very high in depicting also the microscopic localisations (Krag et al. 1993; Cody 2003; Veronesi et al. 1997). Even this technique until now has not been completely standardised; it has been adopted by a wide number of surgical institutions and represents the routine approach in patients with small breast cancer mass (<2 cm in diameter) and clinically negative lymph nodes, in order to avoid the axillary lymph node dissection (ALND), which still remains the reference method for staging axillary nodes. Scintimammography with ^{99m}Tc sestamibi has lower diagnostic sensitivity than SLNB, even if some authors, using single photon emission computerised tomography (SPECT) and special collimators, have obtained very satisfactory results (Sampalis et al. 2003; Liberman et al. 2003; Brem et al. 2002; Schillaci et al. 2002, 2005). FDG-PET is much more successful than scintimammography for loco-regional staging. This has been demonstrated by the many studies describing excellent results mainly in terms of a high specificity and good positive predictive value (Greco et al. 2001; Agresti et al. 2004; Zornoza et al. 2004; Lovrics et al. 2004). Therefore, in spite of its variable diagnostic sensitivity, ranging from 60% to 90% in different series published,

FDG-PET should not be considered as an alternative tool to SLNB, but it can be proposed for patients with non-palpable lymph nodes to select patients who should directly undergo ALND (with positive axillary FDG uptake) from those who should previously undergo SLNB (with negative FDG axillary uptake) prior to receiving ALND or not (Veronesi et al. 2007; Gil-Rendo et al. 2006). There are no studies about the association of tumour marker tests and SLNB or FDG-PET for loco-regional staging, since the frequency of high levels of breast cancer tumour markers in these early stages is very low, and the clinical indication deriving from tumour marker measurements has no clinical value.

Schirrmeister et al. (2001) studied the value of FDG-PET as a staging procedure on 89 breast cancer patients at tumour presentation and compared PET with other conventional methods (chest X-ray, liver US and bone scintigraphy) for depicting distant metastases. In six patients FDG-PET showed distant metastases, and the accuracy of PET resulted in being higher than conventional methods, irrespective of metastatic localisations. Another study confirmed the superior sensitivity of FDG-PET in visualising distant metastases when it was compared to the association of chest X-rays, US and bone scintigraphy (Dose et al. 2002). Different authors found that FDG-PET for the diagnosis of bone metastases had sensitivity comparable to that of bone scintigraphy, but the specificity was so far better, with the advantage of also being able to image metastases in soft tissues (Ohta et al. 2001; Yang et al. 2002).

To summarise the general thought about the use of whole body PET as a single staging modality in primary breast cancer, one should say that we do not see any important clinical advantages in the first stages of disease (I and II), due to the low incidence of metastases. The use of FDG-PET or PET/CT in our opinion could be justified only in patients with T3–T4 tumours, palpable lymph nodes and high risk of distant metastases. Besides this, a critical issue about the association of the CA 15.3 test with PET at cancer presentation consists of the evidence that low levels of CA 15.3 do not exclude metastases and elevated levels are not able to determine the cancer extent with accuracy. Therefore, the combination of tumour marker tests with PET should not be recommended as the standard examination in patients with primary breast cancer. In addition, on this subject there are not adequate prospective trials to evaluate the clinical impact of these procedures.

15.4 Diagnosis of Relapses and Metastases

In patients treated with surgery, loco-regional and distant metastases occur in 35% of cases within 10 years of surgery (Voogd et al. 2001). The follow-up of the patients is intended to make a diagnosis of cancer recurrence, with the goal to treat metastases at the earliest stage of development. Different kinds of follow-up approaches have been proposed: only clinical control in asymptomatic patients, intensive and aggressive periodic examinations with a battery of imaging and biochemical tests in asymptomatic patients, diagnostic tests only in presence of symptoms, etc. However at present no differences in survival rates have been demonstrated among the different groups of asymptomatic patients undergoing different follow-up regimens (Danforth et al. 2002).

In spite of this evidence, it is clear that the correct identification of the localisation of metastases affects the choice of therapy and can contribute to optimising the treatment. Local metastases, isolated metastases and lymph node metastases can be treated with surgery or radiation therapy. Distant or multiple metastases should be treated with chemotherapy, hormone therapy, immunotherapy or high-dose chemotherapy with bone marrow stem cell transplantation according to the different prognostic factors.

Siggelkoff et al. published a recent good overview of the diagnostic value of FDG-PET guided by a tumour marker increase, and he discussed the results published in different papers (Siggelkow et al. 2004) (Table 15.1).

Lonneaux et al. studied 39 breast cancer patients with FDG-PET; 34 were included because of asymptomatic tumour marker increase (Lonneux et al. 2000). PET findings were confirmed by other imaging modalities of biopsy. PET depicted 37 out of 39 sites in 31 out of 33 patients with recurrences. PET missed one loco-regional recurrence, and one patient developed a peritoneal carcinomatosis 6 months after a negative PET. False-positive PET corresponded to lung infections, arthrosis and a synthetic implant.

Pecking et al. obtained similar results on 132 patients, treated for breast cancer, all presenting an isolated increase of CA 15.3 test without any other evidence of disease. One hundred nineteen patients were eligible for correlation (Pecking et al. 2001). PET was performed by means of a PET camera. Positive

PET scans were obtained in 106 patients, including 89 with a single lesion and 17 with more than one lesion. The overall sensitivity in identifying occult lesions resulted in 93.6% and the positive predictive value was 96.2%. The smallest lesion detect by PET was a lymph node metastasis sized 6 mm in diameter. PET was able to localize tumours in 85.7% of cases suspected for clinically occult metastatic disease on the basis of an increase of tumour marker levels.

Suarez et al. studied 45 women with histological diagnosis of breast cancer who underwent a tumour-guided whole-body PET (Suarez et al. 2002). All patients were in remission without any signs of relapses except for a progressive increase of CA 15.3 or CEA. FDG-PET results were controlled by pathology when possible, by other conventional imaging methods and by clinical follow-up. PET findings were evaluated in 38 patients: 27 resulted positive. Among these 27 positive patients 24 were true positive and 3 true negative. Tumour-marker-guided PET was able to discover three unknown neoplasms not visualised by other modalities. The diagnostic performances of tumour-marker-guided PET per patient resulted as follows: sensitivity 92%, specificity 75% and accuracy 87%.

Liu et al. evaluated 30 patients with suspected recurrent breast cancer and asymptomatic tumour marker increase (CA 15.3 or CEA), but negative or equivocal other imaging modality results (Liu et al. 2002). The final diagnosis of recurrent breast cancer was established by biopsy or clinical follow-up. Among the 30 patients the final diagnosis of recurrent breast cancer was established in 38 sites in 28 patients. Pet accurately detected 35 out of 38 sites in 25 out of 28 patients with recurrence. The diagnostic sensitivity and accuracy of FDG-PET in patients with suspected recurrent breast cancer and asymptomatically elevated tumour marker levels were 96% and 90%, respectively.

Kamel et al. (2003) evaluated FDG-PET in 60 patients with suspected local recurrence. In 25 patients the elevation of CA 15.3 was compared with PET results. Disease relapse was proven in 40 patients on the basis of histology and follow-up. Additionally in three patients a second cancer was diagnosed with (in one case) and without (in two cases) concomitant disease relapse. PET missed local recurrences in three patients and was false positive in four. In patient-based analysis PET sensitivity, specificity and accuracy for loco-regional recurrence were 89%, 84% and 87%, while for distant metastases they were 100%, 97% and 98%, respectively. The author concluded that FDG-PET was more sensitive than serum tumour marker CA 15.3 in detecting relapsed breast cancer.

Table 15.1. Results of tumour marker-guided FDG-PET in different studies on breast cancer

Author (year and ref.)	No. of patients studied	Diagnostic sensitivity	Diagnostic specificity	Remarks
Lonneaux et al. 2000	39	93%	–	PET missed only a locoregional recurrence and a peritoneal carcinosis
Pecking et al. 2001	132	93.6%	–	
Suarez et al. 2002	45	92%	75%	Clinical management was modified in patients with unsuspected primary or tumour relapse
Liu et al. 2002	30	25/28* 35/38°	90%	Demonstrated an impact in patient management
Kamel et al. 2003	35	89%	84%	PET was more sensitive than serum tumour markers in detecting relapses
Siggelkoff et al. 2003	35	80.6%	97.6%	PET had impact on staging and management in case of suspicion and in follow-up setting
Radan et al. 2007	47	90%* 99%°	71%* 72°	PET/CT led to changing clinical management in 51% of patients

*Patient-based analysis; °lesion-based analysis

Siggelkoff et al. studied 35 patients suspected of having recurrent disease or elevated tumour markers (Siggelkow et al. 2003). Depending on the region of suspicion, conventional imaging included chest X-ray, MRI, CT and US. All patients had at least a period of 12 months of follow-up. In patients examined because of elevated tumour marker CA 15.3, PET was able to detect recurrence or metastatic disease in six of the eight patients (sensitivity 75%). PET missed three tumour sites in three patients: two supraclavicular lymph node metastases and one lung metastasis. The overall sensitivity and specificity for PET on the whole series of patients were 80.6% and 97.6, respectively.

The role of PET/CT in the follow-up of patients who presented with elevated levels of tumour markers has been recently studied by Radan et al. (2006). Forty-seven consecutive FDG/PET studies of 46 women with a history of breast cancer presented with elevated levels of tumour markers and were retrospectively evaluated. PET/CT results were confirmed by pathology, further imaging and follow-up (mean 17.2 months). Changes in further management were recorded. Thirty (65%) patients had tumour recurrence and 16 (35%) patients showed no further evidence of disease. The performance indices of PET/CT for recurrent breast cancer in 47 studies on patient-based analysis obtained on overall sensitivity, specificity and accuracy of 90%, 71% and 83%, respectively. The site-based analysis gave a sensitivity, specificity and accuracy of 99%, 72% and 96%, respectively. PET/CT was compared with contrast-enhanced CT and had better diagnostic performances. PET/CT also had an impact on patient management in 24 cases (51%).

15.5 Some Problems in the Interpretation of the Marker Level Test during Follow-Up

Circulating tumour markers can be considered elevated when their blood concentration is higher than a conventional analytical cut-off. This is currently established for each tumour marker in correspondence with the 95th centile of the concentrations measured in a population of healthy subjects. Therefore it is generally accepted in the clinical practice that 5% of the normal population has tumour marker levels higher than the threshold of normality, usually because of the effect of several physiological variables, or the presence of some benign pathologies that can cause false-positive results. Using the common immunoradiometric assays, the cut-off for CA 15.3 is approximately 35 mU/ml, for CEA it is 5 ng/ml, and for TPA it is 70 U/l. This knowledge is very important for the clinical interpretation of these laboratory tests. Another relevant issue for tumour marker interpretation lies in the meaning of the absolute concentrations of the tumour marker that are related to tumour mass and therefore to tumour stage. In fact the highest levels of tumour makers can be found mainly in patients with advanced disease and in the presence of large or multiple metastatic lesions, and this is the reason why the positive predictive value of the tumour marker tests is more reliable when the concentrations are very high.

Besides this, in recent years great importance has been given to the dynamic behaviour of the tumour marker levels. In other terms the changes observed during the time assume more clinical value than the isolated single measurements. In the presence of a progressive increase of tumour marker concentration in patients treated for breast cancer who are clinically tumour free, there is a very strong likelihood of a concomitant occult tumour growth determining the rising levels in the blood stream. It has been demonstrated that the progressive elevations of mucinic tumour markers, even under the cut-off, can anticipate the discovery of the tumour relapses some months before (Chan et al. 1997). In this field there are also non-concordant opinions supported by clinical studies (Nakamura et al. 2005).

The analysis of the progressive changes of tumour marker levels of course should take into account the physiological individual variability of serum levels and also the analytical coefficient of variations (CV) existing among laboratory assays. A general agreement among pathologists accepts as significant the progressive changes of circulating tumour marker, when the registered increase results in being at least two times superior to two CVs (around 20%) when compared to the levels of the previous test. Therefore, in the presence of any asymptomatic patient already treated for cancer, and with occasional elevated high levels of CA 15.3, the clinical experience suggests repeating the same measurement at least two times every month in order to confirm that this serum abnormality is really related to a cancer growth or evolution. According to this thought some authors have considered the rate of marker increase, the marker doubling time and the association of marker levels with doubling time (Soletormos et al. 2004; Aide et al. 2007). Aide et al. (2007) demonstrated that the probability of depicting breast cancer recurrence is influenced by the CA 15.3 marker levels and marker level doubling time.

The patient-based sensitivity of CA 15.3 results in the depiction of metastases in the follow-up in the literature ranges from 33% to 78% and specificity from 60% to 90% (Gion et al. 2002, 1995). As already mentioned above, much clinical evidence indicates that the tumour marker tests have low efficacy in detecting early breast cancer relapse (Kokko et al. 2002; Valenzuela et al. 2003; Molina et al. 2005). In order to define which group of patients should undergo serial measurements of tumour markers during follow-up, Ravaioli et al. identified two groups of patients: patients stage pT1-3, N0-1 and patients stage pT4, N2 (Ravaioli et al. 2002). The second series of patients should be considered as high-risk metastases and tumour marker measurements can be recommended, as the rate of detection resulted in up to 11% of the population. The highest sensitivity of CA 15.3 in case of disease progression has been shown in the presence of bone and liver metastases and multiple metastatic sites (Molina et al. 1999). On the contrary tumour marker tests do not seem appropriate in low-risk groups due to the very poor diagnostic sensitivity of the assays.

In spite of the open controversies in this area, the general opinion is that no breast cancer tumour marker either as an isolated value or as a dynamic measurement is sufficient for the oncologists to decide on a cancer treatment. Laboratory data should always be confirmed by other diagnostic positive findings such as diagnostic imaging or pathology. The combined used of FDG-PET with breast cancer tumour marker tests provides this opportunity with several points of strength and some limitations (Table 15.2).

15.6 Conclusions

The data reported in this overview agree on the evidence that FDG-PET carried out in the presence of elevated or progressively increasing tumour markers has demonstrated a diagnostic effectiveness in detecting cancer lesions with variable sensitivity, both at presentation (staging) and during the follow-up (discovery of relapses, metastases and re-staging) (Santiago et al. 2006). It is well known that tumour marker increase is a reliable signal of the presence of occult disease, and this is a suspicion that can be explored by FDG-PET. Therefore, some authors have proposed that whole body PET may become the method of choice for the assessment of asymptomatic patients with elevated tumour marker levels (Ugrinska et al. 2002; Siggelkow et al. 2004; Trampal et al. 2000) (Fig. 15.1).

Table 15.2. Advantages and limitations of FDG-PET for the diagnosis of breast cancer recurrences and metastatic disease (*)

	Added value	Limitations
Diagnosis of metastatic disease at tumour presentation	PET seems more accurate than conventional imaging in the diagnosis of metastatic disease at cancer presentation (except for loco-regional lymph node invasion)	PET usefulness is related to the stage of disease. The sensitivity of tumour markers is very low at early stages. Tumour marker tests are not recommended at tumour presentation in low-risk patients.
Detection of recurrent disease	Sufficient sensitivity of PET in depiction of loco-regional recurrences (few data available). High accuracy (around 90%) for the detection of metastatic disease.	Inadequate detection by PET of anatomical details. PET/CT overcomes this problem and increases the diagnostic accuracy.
Unclear elevation of tumour markers in asymptomatic patients during follow-up	High sensitivity (more than 90%) for the detection of occult recurrence in asymptomatic patients with a progressive increase of tumour marker levels	Some false-negative results in breast cancer with low metabolism (lobular carcinoma). Additional diagnostic conventional confirmatory methods sometimes are necessary

(From Siggelkow et al., modified)

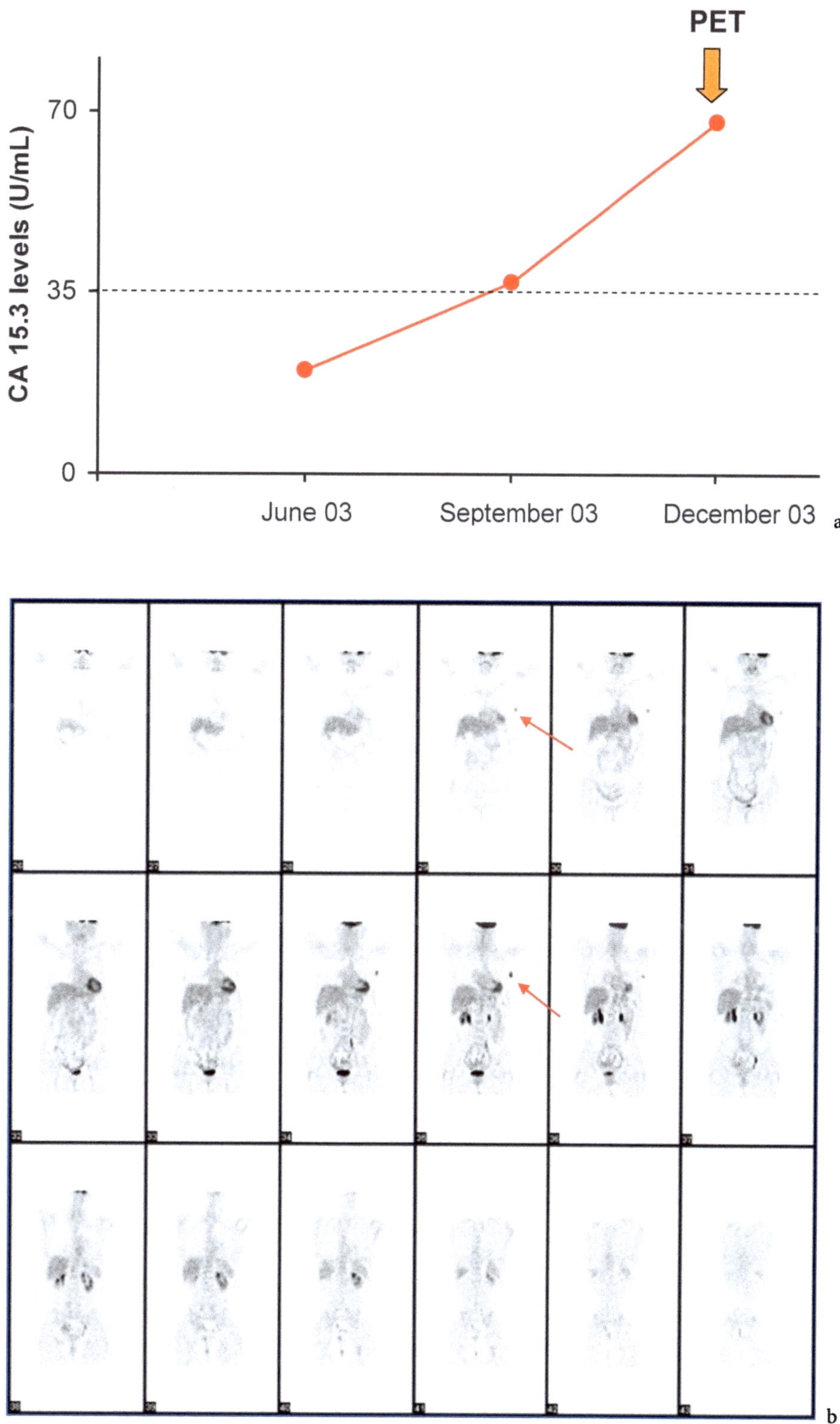

Fig. 15.1. a Progressive increase of CA 15.3 levels in a women with previous history of tumorectomy presenting with axillary adenopathy. Diagnostic imaging was performed after some months on the basis of a progressive increase of CA 15.3. **b** PET imaging showing focal uptakes in the axillary region and in the left breast. Pathological analysis demonstrated infiltrating ductal carcinoma of the breast with lymph nodal metastases

The recent development of hybrid systems, allowing the concomitant examination of the patient by combining PET with CT, has increased the accuracy of diagnostic imaging, and several papers support the evidence that PET/CT is able to add incremental diagnostic confidence to PET and accurately detects more lesions than CT or PET alone (Tatsumi et al. 2006). This is also the reason why recently the discussion has been renewed about the possible role of PET/CT also for screening breast, prostate and lung cancers, even if the clinical and statistical relevance of the occasionally detected cancers is likely to justify large screening efforts with these imaging modalities (Schoder and Gonen 2007).

Besides this, the controversial question if FDG-PET or PET/CT can substitute the entire battery of tests routinely used for staging breast cancer or detecting relapse in all breast cancer patients remains unsolved. There is a need for perspective clinical trials for evaluating the impact of this approach on patient management and survival, according to the different risk groups. At present it is very difficult to draw a final conclusion, since one should consider the high cost of the test, the incomplete availability of this kind of examinations in all clinical centres, and the problem of the sensitivity of PET in early stages that is not able to rule out the microscopic metastases. On the contrary tumour-marker-guided PET or PET/CT seems to work better in the follow-up of patients at risk, in re-staging patients with symptoms and in evaluating the response to treatments.

Acknowledgements

The authors are grateful to Ms. Rita Filieri for her help in preparing the material for this manuscript.

Reference

Adler LP, Bakale G (2001) Positron emission tomography imaging. In: Khalkali I, Maublant JC, Goldsmith SJ (eds) Nuclear oncology. Diagnosis and therapy. Lippincott Williams & Wilkins, Philadelphia 289–295

Agresti R, Crippa F, Gerali A et al (2004) Lymph node metastases detection by FDG-PET and sentinel node biopsy in breast cancer patients: comparison of these different approaches. ESSOI Congress

Aide N, Huchet V, Switsers O et al (2007) Influence of CA 15-3 blood level and doubling time on diagnostic performances of ^{18}F-FDG PET in breast cancer patients with occult recurrence. Nucl Med Commun 28:267–272

Avril N, Dose J, Janicke F et al (1996) Metabolic characterization of breast tumours with positron emission tomography using F-18 fluorodeoxyglucose. J Clin Oncol 14:1848–1857

Avril N, Scheidhauer K, Kuhun W (2000) Breast cancer. In: Helmut J, Wieler R, Coleman E (eds) PET in clinical oncology. Springer, New York, 355–372

Bast RC, Ravdin P, Hayes DF et al (2001) American Society of Clinical Oncology Tumor Markers Expert Panel. J Clin Oncol 19:1865–1878

Basuyau JP, Blanc-Vincent MP, Bidart JM et al (2003) Summary report of the standards, options and recommendations for the use of serum tumour markers on breast cancer: 2000. Br J Cancer 89:32–34

Benchimol S. Fuks A, Jothy S, Beauchemin N, Shirota K, Stanner C (1989) Carcinoembryonic antigen, a human tumor marker, functions as a intercellular adhesion molecule. Cell 57:327–334

Bender H, Palmedo H, Biersack HJ (1998) Breast imaging with positron emission tomography. In: Taillefer R, Khalkhali I, Waxman AD, Biersack HJ (eds) Radionuclide imaging of the breast. Marcel Dekker, New York, 147–175

Berling B, Kolbinger F, Gruntert F et al (1990) Molecular cloning of a carcinoembryonic antigen (CEA)-gene family member expressed in leukocytes of chronic myeloid leukaemia patients and bone marrow. Cancer Res 50:6534–6539

Bombardieri E (1998) Tumor markers. In: Masson (ed) Handbook of medical oncology. Parigi, Barcellona, Messico, Milan, 145–159

Brem RF, Schoonians JM, Kieper DA et al (2002) High-resolution scintimammography: a pilot study. J Nucl Med 43:909–915

Chan DW, Beveridge RA, Muss H et al (1997) Use of Truquant BR radioimmunoassay for early detection of breast cancer recurrence in patients with stage II and stage III disease. J Clin Oncol 15:2322–2328

Cheung KL, Graves CRL, Robertson JFR (2000) Tumour marker measurements in the diagnosis and monitoring of breast cancer. Cancer Treat Rev 26:91–102

Cody HS 3rd (2003) Sentinel lymph node biopsy for breast cancer: does anybody not need one? Ann Surg Oncol 10:1131–1132

Danforth DN Jr, Aloj L, Carrasquillo JA et al (2002) The role of ^{18}F-FDG-PET in the local/regional evaluation of women with breast cancer. Breast Cancer Res Treat 75:135–146

Delbeke D, Martin WH (2004) Metabolic imaging with FDG: a primer. Cancer J 10:201–213

Dose J, Bleckmann S, Bachmann S et al (2002) Comparison of fluorodeoxyglucose positron emission tomography and conventional diagnosis procedures for the detection of distant metastases in breast cancer patients. Nucl Med Commun 23:857–864

Duffy MJ (2001) Biochemical markers in breast cancer: which ones are clinically useful? Clin Biochem 34:347–352

Duffy MJ (2006) Serum tumor markers in breast cancer: are they of clinical value? Clin Chem 52:345–351

Gil-Rendo A, Zorzona G, Garcia-Velloso MJ, Regueira FM, Beorlegui C, Cervera M (2006) Fluorodeoxyglucose positron emission tomography with sentinel lymph node biopsy for evaluation of axillary involvement in breast cancer. Br J Surg 93:707–712

Gion M, Barioli P, Mione R et al (1995) Tumor markers in breast cancer follow-up: a potentially useful parameter still awaiting definitive assessment. Forza Operativa Nazionale sul Carcinoma Mammario (FONCaM) Ann Oncol 6:31–35

Gion M, Boracchi P, Dittadi R et al (2002) Prognostic role of serum CA 15.3 in 362 node-negative breast cancer. An old player for a new game. Eur J Cancer 38:1181–1188

Gion M, Mione R, Bruscagni G (1993) Clinical use of tumor markers, current strategies for decision making. In: Ballesta A, Torre GC, Bombardieri E, Gion M, Molina R. Updating on tumor markers in tissues and in biological fluids. Minerva Medica, Torino, 179–202

Greco M, Crippa F, Agresti R et al (2001) Axillary lymph node staging in breast cancer by 2-fluoro-2-deoxy-D-glucose positron emission tomography: clinical evaluation and alternative management. J Natl Cancer Inst 93:630–635

Hayes D, Sekine H, Ohao T et al (1985) Use of murine monoclonal antibody for detection of circulating plasma DF3 antigen levels in breast cancer patients. J Clin Invest 75:1671–1678

Hayes DF, Zurawski VR, Kufe DW (1986) Comparison of circulating CA 15.3 and carcinoembryonic antigen levels in patients with breast cancer. J Clin Oncol 10:1542–1550

Kamel EM, Wyss MT, Fehr ML, von Schulthess GK, Goerres GW (2003) ^{18}F-fluorodeoxyglucose positron emission tomography in patients with suspected recurrence of breast cancer. J Cancer Res Clin Oncol 129:147–153

Kokko R, Holli K, Hakama M (2002) CA 15-3 in the follow-up of localised breast cancer: a prospective study. Eur J Cancer 38:1189–1193

Krag DN, Weaver DL, Alex JC et al (1993) Surgical resection and radiolocalization of the sentinel lymph node in breast cancer using a gamma-probe. Surg Oncol 2:335–340

Liberman M, Sampalis F, Mulder DS et al (2003) Breast cancer diagnosis by scintimammography: a meta-analysis and review of the literature. Breast Cancer Res Treat 80:115–126

Liu CS, Shen YY, Lin CC, Yen RF, Kao CH (2002) Clinical impact of ^{18}F-FDG PET in patients with suspected recurrent breast cancer based on asymptomatically elevated tumor marker serum levels: a preliminary report. Jpn J Clin Oncol 32:244–247

Lonneux M, Borbath I, Berlìere M, Kirkove C, Pauwels S (2000) The place of whole body PET FDG for the diagnosis of distant recurrence of breast cancer. Clin Positron Imaging 3:45–49

Lovrics PJ, Chen V, Coates G et al (2004) A prospective evaluation of positron emission tomography scanning, sentinel lymph node biopsy, and standard axillary dissection for axillary staging in patients with early stage breast cancer. Ann Surg Oncol 11:846–853

Molina R, Barak V, van Dalen A et al (2005) Tumor markers in breast cancer–European Group on Tumour Markers recommendations. Tumour Biol 26:281–293

Molina R, Jo J, Filella X et al (1999) C-erbB-2, CEA and CA 15.3 serum levels in the early diagnosis of recurrence of breast cancer patients. Anticancer Res 19:2551–2555

Nagle R (1988) Intermediate filaments: a review of the basic biology. Am J Surg Pathol 12:4–16

Nakamura T, Kimura T, Umehara Y et al (2005) Periodic measurement of serum carcinombryonic antigen and carbohydrate antigen 15-3 levels as postoperative surveillance after breast cancer surgery. Surg Today 35:19–21

Ohta M, Tokuda Y, Suzuki Y et al (2001) Whole body PET for the evaluation of bony metastases in patients with breast cancer: comparison with 99Tcm-MDP bone scintigraphy. Nucl Med Commun 22:875–879

Palmedo H, Bender H, Grunwald F et al (1997) Comparison of fluorine-18 fluorodeoxyglucose positron emission tomography and technetium-99m methoxysobutylisonitrile scintimammography in the detection of breast tumours. Eur J Nucl Med 24:1138–1145

Pecking AP, Mechelany-Corone C, Bertrand-Kermorgant F et al (2001) Detection of occult disease in breast cancer using fluorodeoxyglucose camera-based positron emission tomography. Clin Breast Cancer 2:229–234

Radan L, Ben-Haim S, Bar-Shalom R, Guralnik L, Isreal O (2006) The role of FDG-PET/CT in suspected recurrence of breast cancer. Cancer 107:2545–2551

Ravaioli A, Pasini G, Polselli A et al (2002) Staging of breast cancer: new recommended standard procedure. Breast Cancer Res Treat 72:53–60

Rohren EM, Turkington TG, Coleman RE (2004) Clinical applications of PET in oncology. Radiology 231:305–332

Sampalis FS, Denis R, Picard D et al (2003) International prospective evaluation of scintimammography with ^{99m}Tc-sestamibi. Am J Surg 185:544–549

Santiago JF, Gonen M, Yeung H, Macapinlac H, Larson S (2006) A retrospective analysis of the impact of ^{18}F-FDG PET scans on clinical management of 133 breast cancer patients. Q J Nucl Med Mol Imaging 50:61–67

Scheidhauer K, Walter C, Seeman MD (2004) FDG PET and other imaging modalities in the primary diagnosis of suspicious breast lesions. Eur J Nucl Med Mol Imaging 31:S170–S179

Schillaci O, Manni C, Danieli R et al (2005) Tc-99m sestamibi scintimammography with a hybrid SPECT/CT imaging system. Eur J Nucl Med Mol Imaging 32:S128

Schillaci O, Scopinaro F, Spanu A et al (2002) Detection of axillary lymph node metastases in breast cancer with Tc-99m tetrofosmin scintimammography. Int J Oncol 20:483–487

Schirrmeister H, Kuhn T, Guhlmann A et al (2001) Fluorine-18 2-deoxy-2-fluoro-D-glucose PET in the preoperative staging of breast cancer: comparison with the standard staging procedures. Eur J Nucl Med 28:351–358

Schoder H, Gonen M (2007) Screening for cancer with PET and PET/CT: potential and limitations. J Nucl Med 48: S4–S18

Seregni E, Bombardieri E (1999) Tumor markers in oncology. In: Aktolun C, Tauxe WN (eds) Nuclear oncology. Springer, Berlin Heidelberg New York, 415–432

Seregni E, Coli A, Mazzuca N (2004) Circulating tumour markers in breast cancer. Eur J Nucl Med Mol Imaging 31:S15–S22

Shen YY, Su CT, Chen GJ, Chen YK, Liao AC, Tsai FS (2003) The value of ^{18}F-fluorodeoxyglucose positron emission tomography with the additional help of tumor markers in cancer screening. Neoplasma 50:217–221

Siggelkow W, Rath W, Buell U, Zimny M (2004) FDG PET and tumour markers in the diagnosis of recurrent and metastatic breast cancer. Eur J Nucl Med Mol Imaging 31:S118–S124

Siggelkow W, Zimny M, Faridi A, Petzold K, Buell U, Rath W (2003) The value of positron emission tomography in the follow-up for breast cancer. Anticancer Res 23:1859–1867

Soletormos G, Nielsen D, Schioler V, Mouridsen H, Dombernowsky P (2004) Monitoring different stages of breast cancer using tumour markers CA 15-3, CEA and TPA. Eur J Cancer 40:481–486

Steiner PM, Roop DR (1988) Molecular and cellular biology of intermediate filaments. Ann Rev Biochem 57:593–625

Sturgeon C (2002) Practice guidelines for tumor marker use in the clinic. Clin Chem 48:1151–1159

Suarez M, Perez-Castejon MJ, Jimenez A, Domper M, Ruiz G, Montz R, Carreras JL (2002) Early diagnosis of recurrent breast cancer with FDG-PET in patients with progressive elevation of serum tumor markers. Q J Nucl Med 46:113–121

Tatsumi M, Cohade C, Mourtzikos KA, Fishman EK, Wahl RL (2006) Initial experience with FDG-PET/CT in the evaluation of breast cancer. Eur J Nucl Med Mol Imaging 33:254–262

Trampal C, Maldonado A, Sancho Cuesta F et al (2000) Role of the positron emission tomography (PET) in suspected tumor recurrence when there are increased serum tumor markers. Rev Esp Med Nucl 19:279–287

Ugrinska A, Bombardieri E, Stokkel MP, Crippa F, Pauwels EK (2002) Circulating tumor markers and nuclear medicine imaging modalities: breast, prostate and ovarian cancer. Q J Nucl Med 46:88–104

Valenzuela P, Mateos S, Tello E, Lopez-Bueno MJ, Garrido N, Gaspar MJ (2003) The contribution of the CEA marker to CA 15.3 in the follow-up of breast cancer. Eur J Gynaecol Oncol 24:60–62

Veronesi U, De Cicco C, Galimberti V et al (2007) A comparative study on the value of FDG-PET and sentinel node biopsy to identify occult axillary metastases. Ann Oncol 18:473–478

Veronesi U., Paganelli G, Galimberti V et al (1997) Sentinel-node biopsy to avoid AD in breast cancer with clinically negative lymph nodes. Lancet 349:1864–1867

Voogd AC, Nielsen M, Peterse JL et al (2001) Breast Cancer Cooperative Group of the European Organization for Research and Treatment of Cancer. Differences in risk factors for local and distant recurrence after breast-conserving therapy or mastectomy for stage I and II breast cancer: pooled results of two large European randomized trials. J Clin Oncol 19:1688–1697

Yang SN, Liang JA, Lin FJ, Kao CH, Lin CC, Lee CC (2002) Comparing whole body ^{18}F-2-deoxyglucose positron emission tomography and technetium-99m methylene diphosphonate bone scan to detect bone metastases in patients with breast cancer. J Cancer Res Clin Oncol 128:325–328

Zangheri B, Messa C, Picchio M et al (2004) PET/CT and breast cancer. Eur J Nucl Med Mol Imaging 31:S135–S142

Zornoza G, Garcia-Velloso MJ, Sola J, Regueira FM, Pina L, Beorlegui C (2004) ^{18}F-FDG PET complemented with sentinel lymph node biopsy in the detection of axillary involvement in breast cancer. Eur J Surg Oncol 30:15–19

Advantages and Limitations of FDG PET in the Follow-Up of Breast Cancer

16

Peter Lind, Isabel Igerc, Thomas Beyer, Abdul Jalil Nordin,
Peter Reinprecht, and Klaus Hausegger

CONTENTS

Abstract

F-18 FDG PET in breast cancer was evaluated for the characterization of primary breast tumors, lymph node staging and the follow-up of patients after surgery, chemotherapy and/or external radiotherapy. Despite the low sensitivity and moderate specificity of FDG PET in the initial detection and characterization of breast cancer and the low lesion-based sensitivity for lymph node staging, the results from using FDG PET in re-staging breast cancer patients are very promising.

A major advantage of FDG PET imaging compared to conventional imaging is to screen the entire patient for local recurrence, lymph node metastases and distant metastases during a single whole-body examination using a single injection of activity with a reported average sensitivity and specificity of 96% and 77%, respectively. In most studies the sensitivity of FDG PET is higher than that of a combination of conventional imaging methods.

Limitations of FDG PET in the follow-up of breast cancer patients include the relatively low detection rate of bone metastases, especially in case of sclerotic subtype, and the relatively high rate of false-positive results. The rather low specificity of FDG PET can be improved/increased by utilizing combined anatomical-molecular imaging techniques, such as a PET/CT tomograph. First results using PET/CT imaging in the follow-up of breast cancer patients demonstrate increased specificity compared to FDG PET alone. Both imaging modalities, however, offer the detection of recurrent and metastatic breast cancer disease at an early stage and thus continue to demonstrate the efficacy of molecular imaging in patient management, despite the limited therapeutic options in recurrent and metastatic breast cancer.

16.1 Introduction

Breast cancer is the most prominent cancer and the second most prominent cause of mortality in women. In recent years the incidence of breast cancer has increased to 102 per 100,000 per year. Early diagnosis and accurate follow-up of these patients is important for efficient patient management. Standard imaging techniques include radiological examinations, such as X-ray mammography, ultrasonography (US), computed tomography (CT) and magnetic resonance imaging (MRI). Nuclear medicine techniques also play an increasing role in diagnosing and staging breast cancer. In the past only bone scintigraphy was used for follow-up of women with breast cancer to detect bone metastases at an early stage (Cook and

Fogelman 1999). More than 10 years ago immunoscintigraphy became available with the introduction of monoclonal antibodies against CEA and other antigens expressed in breast cancer (e.g., 170H.82). However, with only a moderate sensitivity and with the development of human anti-mouse antibodies immunoscintigrapy was not introduced in routine follow-up of breast cancer (Lind et al. 1991, 1997). In the early 1990s kationic complexes such as Tc-99m tetrofosmin or sestamibi became available and were used in breast cancer patients with reasonable success in detecting primary and recurrent disease (Lind et al. 1996; Spanu et al. 2003). At the same time F-18-fluoro-2-deoxy-D-glucose positron emission tomography (FDG-PET) was introduced in clinical oncology, and the first results were discussed also for breast cancer (Wahl et al. 1991).

Since then FDG-PET was shown to be an effective and accurate imaging technique for a variety of diagnostic oncology tasks in breast cancer, lymph node staging, staging and restaging of recurrent and metastatic disease, and for monitoring treatment (Flanagan et al. 1998; Avril et al. 1999; Bombardieri and Grippa 2001; Czerin 2002). However, FDG-PET is of limited value in the characterization of primary breast lesions due to its moderate sensitivity that is lower than that of MRI (Heinisch et al. 2003). This technique has demonstrated its value in the detection of breast cancer especially in case of dense breasts or breast implants because of the low sensitivity of X-ray mammography. FDG-PET imaging is superior to conventional imaging techniques since it allows for accurate detection of lymph node involvement in the axilla and in the internal mammary nodes (Alder et al. 1993; Hathaway et al. 1999; Goerres 2003). However, neither the number of involved lymph nodes nor the presence or absence of micrometastatic disease can be determined sufficiently with FDG-PET alone (Hathaway et al. 1999). Although the Third German Consensus Conference defined staging and restaging in recurrent and metastatic breast cancer as a class 2 and 3 indication only (Reske and Kotzerke 2001), there is recent evidence that these patients still may benefit from an FDG-PET examination, since no other imaging modality can demonstrate either the absence or the extent of the disease within a single investigation. This overview discusses the advantages and limitations of FDG-PET imaging in the follow-up of breast cancer. We describe the technical considerations of PET and PET/CT imaging briefly and point out potential advantages of using PET/CT for this particular imaging scenario. Multiple literature reviews revealed that FDG PET is also a useful tool for detecting small breast tumors but most lesions have been larger than 1 cm (Adler and Wahl 1995; Rigo et al. 1996). Yasuda et al. reported smaller breast cancer less than 1 cm as also detectable on FDG PET in an asymptomatic individual who was initially missed during the conventional method of screening breast cancers (Yasuda et al. 1999). Other reports of FDG PET depicting breast cancers less than 1 cm were also documented in other articles (Crippa et al. 1998; Schneiderhauer et al. 1996).

16.2 Technical Considerations and Acquisition Protocols for FDG-PET and FDG-PET/CT Imaging

16.2.1 Whole-Body FDG Imaging Using PET

The methodology of PET imaging in breast cancer is based primarily on the ability of PET to detect, visualize and quantify extensive disease by means of whole-body FDG studies (Hoh et al. 1993). Careful patient preparation (Hamblen and Lowe 2003) and choice of imaging parameters are paramount for an accurate diagnosis. Minn and Soini (1989) presented the first results of using FDG imaging in breast cancer in 1989. Most of the studies conducted since then have employed 2D emission scanning mostly in conjunction with a separate transmission scan for attenuation correction (Kamel et al. 2003; Liu et al. 2002; Eubank et al. 2002; Hathaway et al. 1999). It is well known that attenuation correction is required for a quantitative assessment of tumor response to therapy and for accurate lesion localization (Wahl 1999; Coleman 2001).

In the lack of comprehensive PET imaging standards for breast cancer patients we have performed a literature search on Ovid for publications between 1989 and 2004 on the following keywords: breast cancer, glucose and positron. The resulting 201 citations were reviewed for methodological aspects on PET imaging, such as total FDG activity administered, emission and transmission scan time, patient positioning, image review and additional scans. The range of acquisition parameters is given in Table 16.1, which also contains the recommendations for standardized PET imaging of breast cancer, as suggested by Avril et al. (2000) and Palmedo et al. (2003) for comparison.

An important methodological aspect of PET imaging in breast cancer is to ensure that the activity is injected in the arm vein contralateral to the suspected breast lesion in order to avoid artificial tracer retention in the ipsilateral axilla. Whole-body PET examinations with BGO- and NaI-based PET tomographs typically last for 45 min or longer, and therefore patients are positioned head first supine with the arms close to the trunk. Most reports (Table 16.1) indicate an average FDG activity of 375 MBq that is administered 40–60 min prior to the emission scan, although Boerner et al. showed that by prolonging the uptake time to 90 min lesion detectability of breast lesions is improved (Boerner et al. 1999). Emission scans were performed in 2D whole-body mode in the majority of studies over up to eight bed positions with an individual scan time of as short as 4 min (Kamel et al. 2003; Langsteger et al. 2002) and as long as 10 min (Baslaim et al. 2003) per bed position. Attenuation correction by means of measured rod-source transmission scans was also performed in most studies. There have been reports on dynamic emission scanning (Smith et al. 2000; Yang et al. 2001), albeit the axial imaging range was limited to one or two bed positions covering the breast and the axilla.

16.2.2 Dedicated Breast Exams in Prone Position

While the supine position is adequate for general whole-body imaging, the search for small lesions in the breast and the axilla mandates high signal-to-noise imaging situations. In addition the breasts are compressed and deformed in the supine position, which makes it difficult to register the PET images of that area with complementary MRI images (Pietrzyk et al. 1995; Pietrzyk 2003). Complementary

Table 16.1. Range of acquisition parameters for PET imaging protocols for breast cancer as determined from a Medline search of publications between 1989 and 2004. For comparison the recommendations by Avril et al. (1999) and Palmedo et al. (2003) are given in the right column

Parameter	Review of 1989–2004	Recommendations
Patient preparation	Fasted for ~7 h	Fasted for >6 h
FDG activity [MBq]	~ 375 (190–630)	300–400, contra-lateral arm vein
Uptake time [min]	40–60 (min 30, max 90)	45–60, up to 90
Whole-body and/or dedicated breast scan	WB and dedicated breast scans are equally frequent	WB + breast
Whole body		
Patient positioning	Supine in most cases	Supine
Attenuation correction?	Yes	
Emission acquisition mode	Mostly 2D	
Em/Tx scan time [min]	4–10/2–10	
Image reconstruction	Filtered back-proj, iterative	
Breast scan		
Patient positioning	Prone	Prone with the arms at the side (Avril et al. 2000) or raised (Palmedo 2003)
Attenuation correction?	yes	Yes
Em/Tx scan time [min] per bed position	2 beds of 4–15 min/10 min	10–15 in 2D (Palmedo 2003) 15–20 in 2D (Avril 2000), 5–10 min in 3D (Palmedo 2003), 3–5 min for TX (Avril 2000), >1.5 10e6 counts/slice
Image reconstruction	Iterative	Iterative 4 iter, 8 subsets
Image interpretation (Visual, SUV)	Visual and SUV	Visual and SUV

MRI can be used to substitute the lack of anatomical information of the PET images with high-resolution anatomical information of a very high soft tissue contrast in the breast (Hathaway et al. 1999). Several groups have suggested acquiring an independent PET scan in prone position with the breast hanging and the arms at the side or raised above the head to increase the quality of the PET imaging results in the breast region (Avril et al. 2000). This dedicated breast examination sometimes replaces the whole-body PET imaging session (Dose et al. 2002; Krak et al. 2003), but frequently is complementary (Goerres et al. 2003; Langsteger et al. 2002; Brix et al. 2001).

16.2.3 3D-PET and Emission Scan Time

Other aspects of PET imaging to increase patient comfort as well as to potentially increase the accuracy of the diagnosis include the introduction of faster PET scintillation detectors (LSO, GSO) in fully 3D PET and PET/CT tomographs. Lartizien et al. (2002) discussed the benefits of 3D-PET imaging in terms of noise characteristics of whole-body acquisitions, although not specifically for a dedicated breast exam. Palmedo et al. (2003) discuss the benefit of a 3D emission protocol in breast cancer imaging for reducing the total scan time, which seems particularly beneficial in dedicated breast imaging situations with the patient in prone position. Using LSO-based 3D-PET technology, for example, a patient-weight adjusted emission scan time of 1–2 min per bed position can be used for routine whole-body imaging, as discussed by Halpern et al. (2003). GSO-based PET systems also allow for a significant reduction in emission scan time (Muehllehner et al. 2002), and thus prone scans for dedicated breast examinations seem feasible within 5–10 min for two bed positions including the transmission scan for absolute tracer quantification.

16.2.4 PET/CT Systems

Further reduction in total scan time can be achieved by employing a combined PET/CT system (Townsend et al. 2004) in substitution of the dedicated PET scan. Dual-modality PET/CT tomographs allow almost simultaneous acquisition of anatomical (CT) and molecular (PET) information without moving the patient off and on the table in between exams. The CT transmission information can be used not only for an anatomical localization and radiological assessment of lesions, but also for attenuation correction of the complementary emission data (Kinahan et al. 2003). Since the X-ray CT tube is equivalent to a high-flux transmission source (Zaidi and Hasegawa 2003), transmission scan times per bed position are reduced to a few seconds. Total PET/CT imaging times are thus reduced by 30% (Schulthess 2000), assuming an optimized emission/transmission scan time partition (Holm et al. 1996; Beyer et al. 1997).

In our experience (Beyer et al. 2004; Antoch et al. 2004), PET/CT scanning of the breast and axilla is feasible in routine diagnostic oncology (Fig. 16.1), although prospective studies to estimate the diagnostic accuracy of PET/CT in breast cancer are still needed. When a dedicated PET/CT exam of the breast is performed in addition to the whole-body PET/CT examination, total patient exposure should be accounted for by optimizing the co-axial imaging range and by modulating the X-ray tube current (Tack et al. 2003). We hypothesize that the availability of full set of CT images from a combined PET/CT exam will be helpful in the registration of the molecular information with anatomical information from high-contrast MRT, when available, and for subsequent follow-up.

16.2.5 Alternative Developments for Dedicated Breast Imaging Devices

Since the early 1990s alternative hardware concepts have been proposed that seek to take advantage of the high specificity of PET imaging relative to mammography, while improving the sensitivity of PET by increasing the image resolution and system sensitivity relative to standard whole-body PET tomography designs. By moving the detectors closer to the object of interest (breast), image blurring is reduced and spatial resolution is improved. The efficiency of the detection system is also increased because a greater solid angle is subtended. Thompson et al. first presented a feasibility study for a positron emission mammography (PEM) device in 1994 (Thompson et al. 1994). The anticipated device consisted of two detector arrays of BGO, and simulations showed that the efficiency of the proposed PET design was about ten times that of a conventional brain scanner and that spatial resolution of about 2 mm should be possible. It was also foreseen to place this device in a

Fig. 16.1a–c. PET/CT imaging of breast cancer patients. When patients are positioned head first supine the breasts appear condensed (**a**) with average CT attenuation values on the order of 47 HU (*L*, lesion) and -88 HU (*B*, background). In prone position (**b**) lesion-to-background ratios in the mamma decrease slightly (*L*: 40 HU, *B*: -96 HU), but visual contrast is improved somewhat due to the elongation of the mamma. PET/CT examinations in prone position over 1 (**c**, sagittal images) or 2 bed positions are feasible when the patient is positioned on low-density support structures (e.g., vacuum lock bags, MedTec, USA) with the mamma hanging freely and with the arms raised above the head and resting on the cranial support. (Data from University Hospital Essen, Germany)

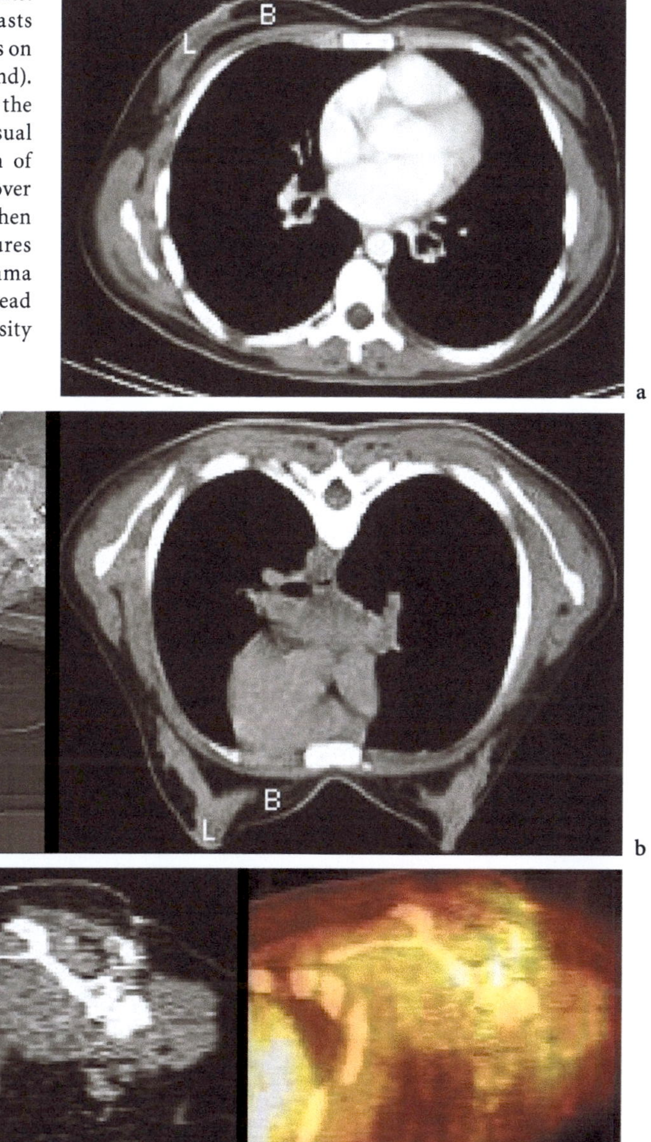

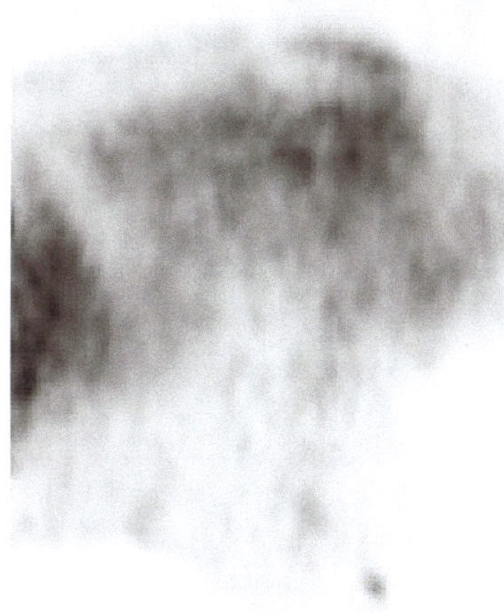

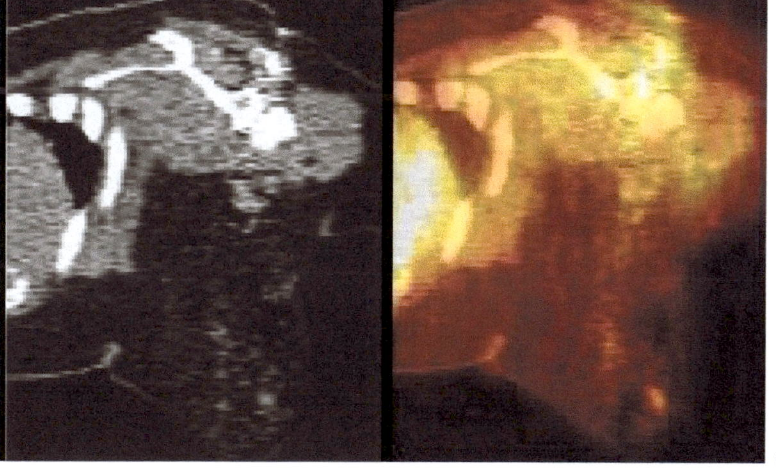

conventional mammography unit. The breast would be positioned in between the two horizontal detector arrays for the PET system, and the top array would be removed to give way to the X-ray tube during the mammography measurement without moving the breast. Weinberg et al. (1996) presented first results, and Murthy et al. (2000) were able to demonstrate the advantages of combined focal-plane emission tomography and mammography in 14 patients. Without going into detail, other groups have developed the idea of a dedicated, dual-modality functional/anatomical breast imaging platform further by incorporating alternative PET detector arrays (Doshi et al. 2000; Freifelder and Karp 1997) or by proposing the incorporation into a stereotatactic biopsy table (Raylman et al. 2001).

Thus, dedicated PET imaging devices in combination with mammography, or separate, appear to substitute a number of performance disadvantages of standard whole-body PET tomographs. Nevertheless, whole-body PET tomographs are more widely available and continue to play the dominant role in diagnostic PET imaging for the diagnosis and follow-up of breast cancer. Dedicated PET and PEM systems, however, have the potential of playing a major role in dedicated examinations of the breasts (and possibly the axilla), particularly when a combination of molecular and anatomical information is desirable (screening), or when registration with morphological information is crucial for the assessment of inconclusive findings.

16.3 Advantages of FDG PET in the Follow-Up of Breast Cancer

A number of imaging examinations such as X-ray mammography, US, CT, MRI and bone scans are performed frequently during the follow-up of breast cancer patients. In contrast to morphological imaging, which aims at detecting primary, recurrent and metastatic disease based on observable differences or changes in density and size, PET is a molecular imaging technique sensitive to functional or metabolic changes tissues. Since functional changes precede anatomical changes FDG-PET has the potential to detect viable tumor tissue early through its elevated glucose metabolism in comparison to surrounding normal tissues (Warburg et al. 1924). For a single injection of a given amount of FDG PET imaging can be performed in whole-body mode, which allows screening the entire patient from head to toe for re-/staging of the full body (Hoh et al. 1993). While there are an extensive number of reports available on the characterization of primary breast lesion and lymph node staging, only few studies discuss the use of FDG-PET in recurrent and metastatic disease.

For recurrent breast cancer and assessment of loco-regional lymph node metastases, FDG-PET was compared mainly with MRI. Hathaway et al. compared FDG-PET and MRI in ten patients with clinical suspicion of recurrent loco-regional breast cancer (1999). Nine patients had evidence of loco-regional metastases from breast cancer. MRI was diagnostic in five and indeterminate in four patients. FDG-avid tumor was identified in all nine patients. In a similar study Goerres et al. (2003) compared FDG-PET and MRI in 32 patients with suspicious loco-regional recurrence, chest wall recurrence or suspicion of secondary tumor on the contralateral side. Sensitivity, specificity and accuracy were 79%, 94% and 88% for MRI, respectively, compared to 100%, 72% and 84% for FDG-PET, respectively. In five patients (15%) PET detected metastases outside of the axial field-of-view of the MRI.

In a retrospective study Moon et al. (1998) investigated 57 patients using FDG-PET with clinical suspicion of recurrent or metastatic disease after a history of breast cancer. On a patient basis they reported a sensitivity and specificity of 93% and 79%, respectively. On a lesion basis sensitivity was only 85%, which was explained by the low sensitivity of detecting bone metastases. Similar results were also found at our department (Gallowitsch et al. 2003) and by others (Kamel et al. 2003; Dose et al. 2002). In a retrospective study of 62 patients after surgical resection of breast cancer, we have compared FDG-PET with conventional imaging, including X-ray mammography, US, CT, MRI and bone scans (Gallwitsch et al. 2003). Patient-based sensitivity, specificity, NPV, PPV and accuracy were 97%, 82%, 92%, 87% and 90%, respectively. For comparison, the corresponding values for conventional imaging were 84%, 60%, 75%, 73% and 74%, respectively. Similar to the study by Moon et al. (1998), the lesion-based sensitivity was much lower due to the low sensitivity in detecting bone metastases (57%). This can be explained by the fact that sclerotic lesion are visualized less well than osteolytic or mixed osteoplastic/osteolytic metastases. Bender et al. compared the diagnostic accuracy of CT and MRI with that of whole-body FDG-PET in 75 patients with suspected recurrent or metastatic disease (Bender et al. 1997). PET imaging correctly identified 28/29 patients with lymph node metastases (97%), 5/6 patients with lung metastases (83%) and 2 patients with liver metastases. In contrast to other authors and our experience, bone metastases were detected in all patients (15/15). FDG-PET detected eight lymph node and seven bone metastases that were not detected by CT or MRI. Suarez et al. (2002) performed FDG-PET studies in 45 patients with increased tumor markers (CEA and/or Ca 15–3) in case of clinical remission and no sign of relapse in conventional imaging. FDG-PET was evaluated in 38/45 patients. PET was positive in 27 patients (24 true positive and 3 false positive); PET was negative in 11 patients (9 true negative, 2 false negative). Tumor marker-guided FDG-PET resulted in a sensitivity, specificity, PPV and NPV of 92%, 75%, 89% and 82%, respectively. A similarly high sensitivity of 96% was found by Liu et al. (2002) for tumor marker guided FDG-PET in restaging of breast cancer. In a meta-analysis of FDG-PET for the evaluation of breast cancer recurrence and metastases from Isasi et al. (2005) including 18 studies, 16 studies reported patient-based data, two studies reported lesion-based data, and five studies reported both. Among the studies with patient-based data, the median sensitivity was 92.7%, ranging from 56 to 100%, and the specificity was 81.6%, varying from 0 to 100%. A summary of sensitivities, specificities, PPVs, NPVs and accuracies of FDG-PET in restaging breast cancer is given in Table 16.2. Figure 16.2 visualizes recurrence of breast cancer in the thoracic wall and in multiple lymph node metastases as detected by FDG-PET. Smith et al. (2000) found in their study that [^{18}F]-FDG PET may be a useful method in predicting pathologic breast cancer response to a variety of chemotherapy agents at an early stage in a treatment regimen. This method is also a useful tool for semi-quantitative PET assessment of [^{18}F]-FDG uptake to predict the pathologic response of metastatic tumor within axillary lymph nodes after a single dose of primary chemotherapy. These findings, together with the primary tumor response in the FDG PET study, may be clinically relevant if PET is to be used as a routine method of predicting cancer response to therapy. Several other recent reports have suggested that axillary lymph node status demonstrated changes during the course of a primary chemotherapy regimen, and this change may be of considerable value in determining prognostic significance. Thus, the results of this study indicate that PET may be used before and during a chemotherapy regimen to assess the status of locoregional lymph nodes during treatment (Fisher et al. 1998; Kuerer et al. 1999; Mamounas 1999).

Table 16.2. Sensitivity, specificity, positive predictive value (PPV), negative predictive value (NPV) and accuracy [%] of FDG-PET in the follow-up of breast cancer

	Year	Patients	Sensitivity	Specificity	PPV	NPV	Accuracy
Goerres	2003	32	100	72	–	–	84
Gallowitsch	2003	62	97	82	87	96	90
Suarez	2002	45	92	75	82	89	87
Moon	1998	57	93	79	–	–	–
Average			94	77	85	93	87

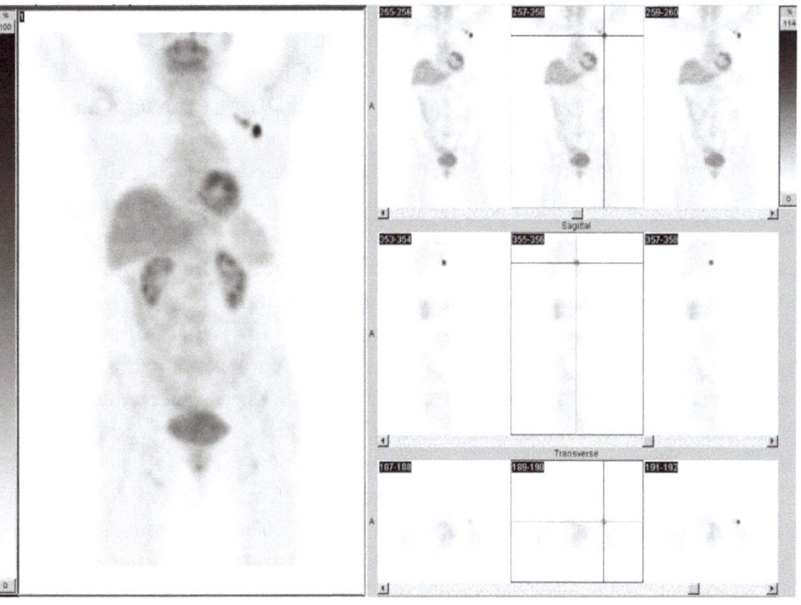

Fig. 16.2. A 62-year-old female after breast surgery and axillary lymph node dissection due to breast cancer on the *left side*. A thoracic wall recurrence was treated by surgery followed by external radiation and chemotherapy. A follow-up CT detected a nodular lesion on the lateral rim of the pectoralis muscle. FDG-PET demonstrated three areas with circumscribed uptake-suspicious for recurrent disease. All lesions were confirmed by histology

16.4 Limitations of PET in the Follow-Up of Breast Cancer

The major limitation for the widespread acceptance of FDG-PET is the lack of appreciation that PET imaging is given by the government and healthcare providers in a number of European countries. For example, as of today PET is not reimbursed in Germany and Austria. Irrespective of the outcome of the restaging procedures of breast cancer therapeutic options are limited in case metastatic breast cancer has been detected, although novel therapy concepts using taxanes, aromatase inhibitors and anti-erb-B2 receptor antibodies demonstrate encouraging results. By comparison molecular imaging has a higher accuracy and detects recurrent and metastatic disease earlier than conventional imaging, which translates into earlier and likely more efficient treatment.

Additional methodological limitations can be divided into false-negative results because of sclerotic bone lesions and interpretation pitfalls in physiologic tracer distributions. While soft tissue and organ metastases are detected with higher sensitivity and accuracy by FDG-PET compared to conventional imaging, the detection of bone metastases by FDG-PET depends primarily on the subtype (osteolytic or osteoplastic) of a metastasis. The lesion-based sensitivity for FDG-PET in recurrent breast cancer is significantly lower than the patient-based sensitivity due to the lower detection rate of bone metastases (Moon et al. 1998; Gallowitsch et al. 2003). When comparing FDG-PET to conventional bone scintigraphy in patients with skeletal metastases from breast cancer, Cook et al. (1998) reported that more bone metastases were reported with FDG-PET. However, in a subgroup of patients with osteoblastic lesions, bone metastases frequently remained undetected in FDG-PET. Therefore, FDG-PET must be combined with bone scans using either Tc-99m-labeled diphosphates or F-18 PET, in case it should substitute conventional imaging techniques. Nakai et al. (2005) performed a study regarding the diagnosis of osteoblastic bone metastases in 89 patients with breast cancer by comparing FDG-PET with bone scintigraphy. The bone metastases were classified by multi-slice CT into four subtypes: osteoblastic, osteolytic, mixed and invisible. The visualization rate of bone scintigraphy/FDG-PET was 100%/55.6% for the blastic type, 70.0%/100.0% for the lytic type, 84.2%/94.7% for the mixed type and 25.0%/87.5% for the invisible type, which means once again that FDG PET suffers from limitations in depicting metastasis of the osteoblastic type. This means that on bone scintigraphy increased accumulation in blastic metastases is usually observed owing to an osteoblastic bone reaction to cancer cells; however, the cause of the decreased and absent, respectively, FDG uptake by osteoblastic bone metastases on FDG-PET is largely unknown (Person et al. 2003).

A general limitation of FDG-PET is the number of false-positive results due to interpretative pitfalls and the non-specificity of FDG that lead to specificities that rarely exceed 80%. Apart from the known areas and organs with physiological uptake, the causes for interpretative pitfalls (e.g., intense focal FDG uptake) may be divided into (1) granulomatous and infectious diseases, (2) muscle activity, (3) brown fat and (4) and bowel activity. The reason for the intense FDG uptake in the lung and mediastinum (1) may be tuberculosis and sarcoidosis. Sometimes other infectious diseases may cause focal uptake patterns, especially in lymph nodes, which reduce the specificity for staging and restaging of breast cancer. In most cases longitudinal F-18 FDG uptake in dense muscles (2) (e.g., musculus sternocleidomastoideus) does not represent an interpretative problem. However, intense focal uptake is seen sometimes within the muscle, or at the insertions of the muscle, thus mimicking bone or soft tissue metastases. This uptake pattern is most frequently observed in head and neck muscles, but also in the diaphragm.

With the introduction of PET/CT it became evident that some FDG uptake patterns in the cervical region were caused by fatty tissue in the neck region (Hany et al. 2002) rather than muscle activity. Rousseau et al. (2006) performed a study regarding brown fat and analyzed 163 PET images in 33 female breast cancer patients receiving neoadjuvant chemotherapy. Seventy-four PET/scans (45%) revealed abnormal uptake in the supraclavicular area. There was no significant relationship between abnormal FDG uptake and outdoor temperature, age or time interval between chemotherapy and PET. Abnormal FDG uptake in the neck seemed to predominantly occur in patients with a low body mass index. In our experience circumscribed FDG uptake may also be observed in the paracardial fat, which may also lead to false-positive interpretations without morphological correlation (Fig. 16.3). Similar to longitudinal muscle uptake, bowel-shaped FDG uptake does not cause problems for the interpretation of the PET images (4). However, sometimes there is intense focal uptake in the bowel, which may cause false-positive results. A combination of PET and CT might be helpful, but negative oral CT contrast is needed for proper bowel distension. The issue of false-negative and false-positive interpretations with FDG-PET in the follow-up of breast cancer leads to the question whether combined PET/CT may increase specificity and, if so, is there is an impact for the therapeutic management of breast cancer patients. Yang et al. (2001) carried out a study and found that the intraoperative frozen biopsy result of sentinel lymph node detection was superior to preoperative PET in determining the diagnostic accuracy of axillary lymph node metastases. The detectability of breast cancer by PET does not depend solely on tumor size. A study using transplantable tumors showed that the principal sites of FDG uptake are viable cancer cells and that the degree of FDG uptake depends on tumor cellularity (Brown et al. 1995). Another report by Carter et al. (1989) stated that the tumor size was closely related to the nodal metastasis and, as a result, a smaller tumor has a lesser metastatic rate and smaller number of metastatic nodes. Also, if the node is smaller than the resolution power of PET, it could not be identified by PET scan. False-positive PET findings may occur in inflammatory lesions, and the specificity has not been fully determined in a large number of benign lesions, including fibrocystic diseases and fibroadenomas.

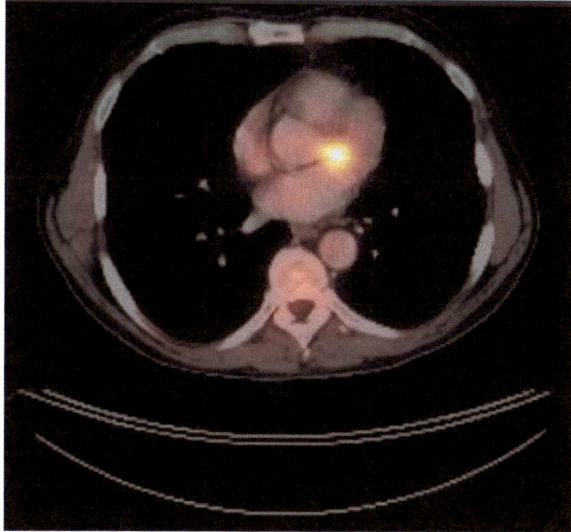

Fig. 16.3. Fused PET/CT of a 54-year-old female referred for restaging of breast cancer after a slight increase of Ca 15-3. A circumscribed FDG uptake in the FDG-PET correlated with paracardial fat in the combined PET/CT image. No other pathology was found in this patient

16.5 Is There an Advantage Using PET/CT?

Up to now few PET/CT studies have been performed concerning the value of combined PET/CT in the follow-up of breast cancer patients. In general the problem of FDG-PET is that an exact localization of an area with increased FDG uptake is often very difficult. The combination of metabolic and morphologic imaging within the same position of the patient following image fusion should be advantageous in terms of an exact localization of lesions and, in turn, reducing any interpretative pitfalls.

Therefore, PET/CT can improve both sensitivity, as is the case for mildly hypermetabolic lesions, and specificity due to accurate localization of hypermetabolic foci to normal tissues, such as brown fat, muscle, bowel and others.

In a retrospective study by Tatsumi et al. (2005) with 75 patients with known breast cancer, the FDG PET/CT was compared with PET alone. In 69 of the 75 patients PET/CT and CT findings were compared regarding lesion characterization and staging. PET/CT added incremental diagnostic confidence to PET in 60% of patients and in more than 50% of regions with increased FDG uptake. In the comparison of PET/CT and CT findings PET/CT demonstrated a significantly better accuracy than CT ($P<0.05$). This initial evaluation suggests that PET/CT is preferable to PET or CT in the diagnosis of breast cancer.

Fueger et al. (2005) investigated the added diagnostic value of PET/CT over PET for restaging of breast cancer patients. Fifty-eight female patients were included in the study. PET/CT tended to improve the restaging accuracy when compared to PET alone by slightly raising both sensitivity and specificity. The difference, however, did not reach statistical significance.

In a first series of 50 PET/CT patients at the Department of Nuclear Medicine in Klagenfurt, we were able to show that the combination of PET/CT provided additional (albeit not always relevant for assessing the primary disease) information in 78% compared to each modality alone. In 10% of patients the combination of PET/CT led to a change in patient management (Igerc et al. 2003). In contrast, PET/CT was able to reduce false-positive results and pitfalls in 32% of all patients (lesion-based) (Kumnig et al. 2003). This was due mainly to localization of FDG uptake in the bowel, muscles, inflammatory processes, cavity of the uterus and brown fat tissue

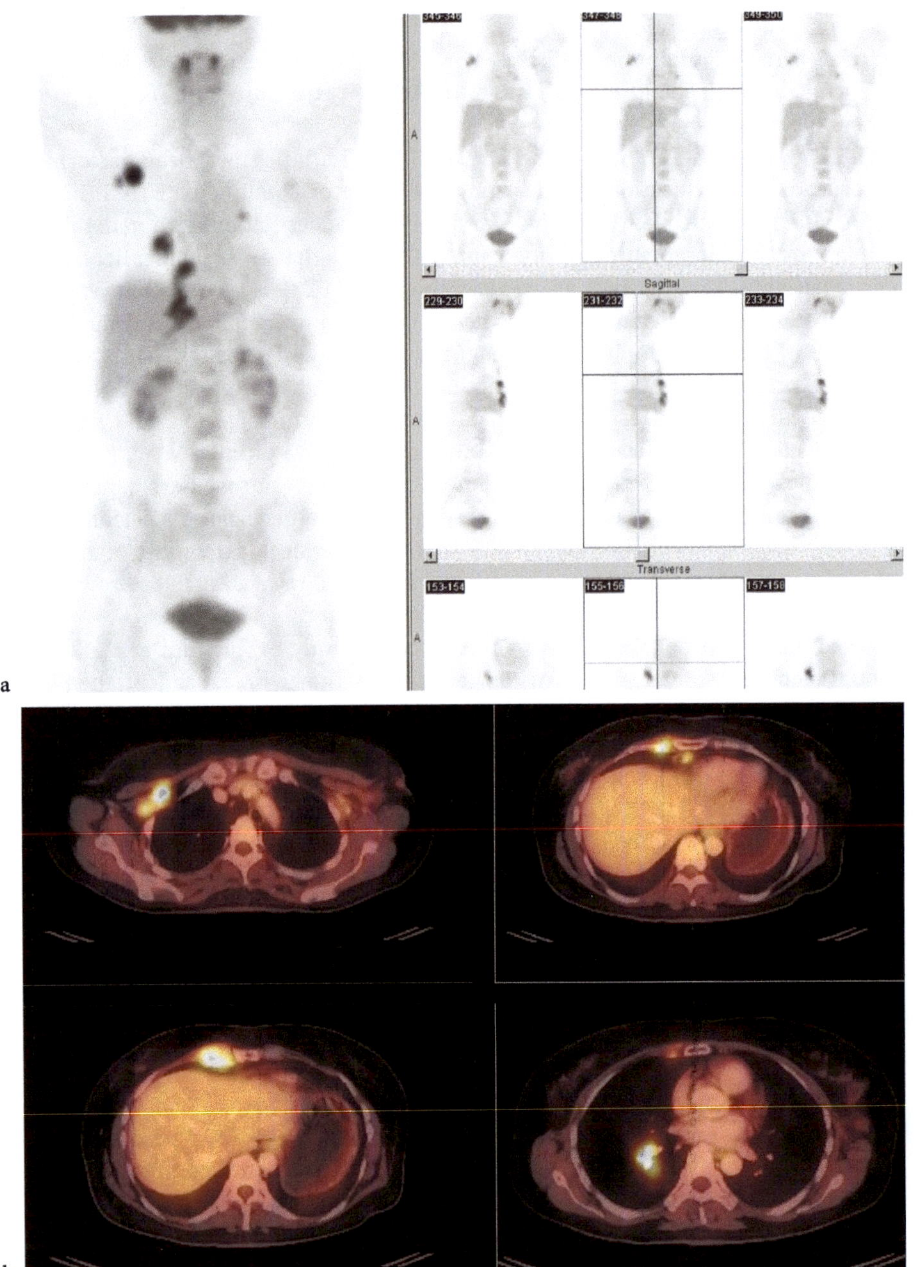

Fig. 16.4a,b. A 43-year-old female after breast surgery and axillary lymph node dissection due to breast cancer in 1998 on the *right side.* Follow-up CT demonstrated a lesion in the right lower lobe of the lung. FDG PET showed FDG uptake in the lung lesion, but also several areas with circumscribed FDG uptake in the right axilla, left hilus, in the ventral lower mediastinum and several sternal and parasternal bone metastases (**a**). PET/CT was able to exactly localize the FDG PET-positive lesions (**b**)

(Figs. 16.4, 16.5). The exact localization of increased FDG uptake within fatty tissue in the neck and upper mediastinal region is important to avoid false-positive interpretation in lymph node metastases (Kumnig et al. 2003). In a study by Buck et al. (2003) 78 patients with a history of breast cancer underwent a PET/CT exam for restaging after a rise in tumor markers or recurrent disease was suspected from clinical follow-up. Malignant lesions were detected by means of the PET/CT in 77% of patients. In 36% of the patients FDG-PET/CT led to a change of the therapeutic management.

From August 2003 to January 2004 our department (Klagenfurt) examined 41 patients with a history of breast cancer and suspected recurrence using FDG-PET/CT (biograph LSO duo, Siemens Medical Solutions, Erlangen, Germany). FDG-PET detected malignant lesion in 22/41 patients (54%). Five patients had local recurrence (two additional distant metastases), seven patients lymph node metastases (five additional distant metastases), ten patients bone metastases including seven patients with metastases in various locations including lung, soft tissue, adrenal gland (Fig. 16.6, Fig. 16.7). Patient-based sensitivity and specificity of FDG-PET/CT was 96% and 89%, respectively. While the sensitivity was similar to our previous study using FDG-PET alone, the specificity was significantly higher for PET/CT. However, there were still some false-positive results. In one patient an inflammatory fibrinoid local lesion was reported, and in another patient FDG uptake within the thoracic wall early after external radiation was interpreted as positive. In patients with multiple bone metastases not all bone lesions demonstrated increased FDG uptake, which was explained by the well-known phenomenon that sclerotic metastases are visualized better using bone scintigraphy than FDG-PET.

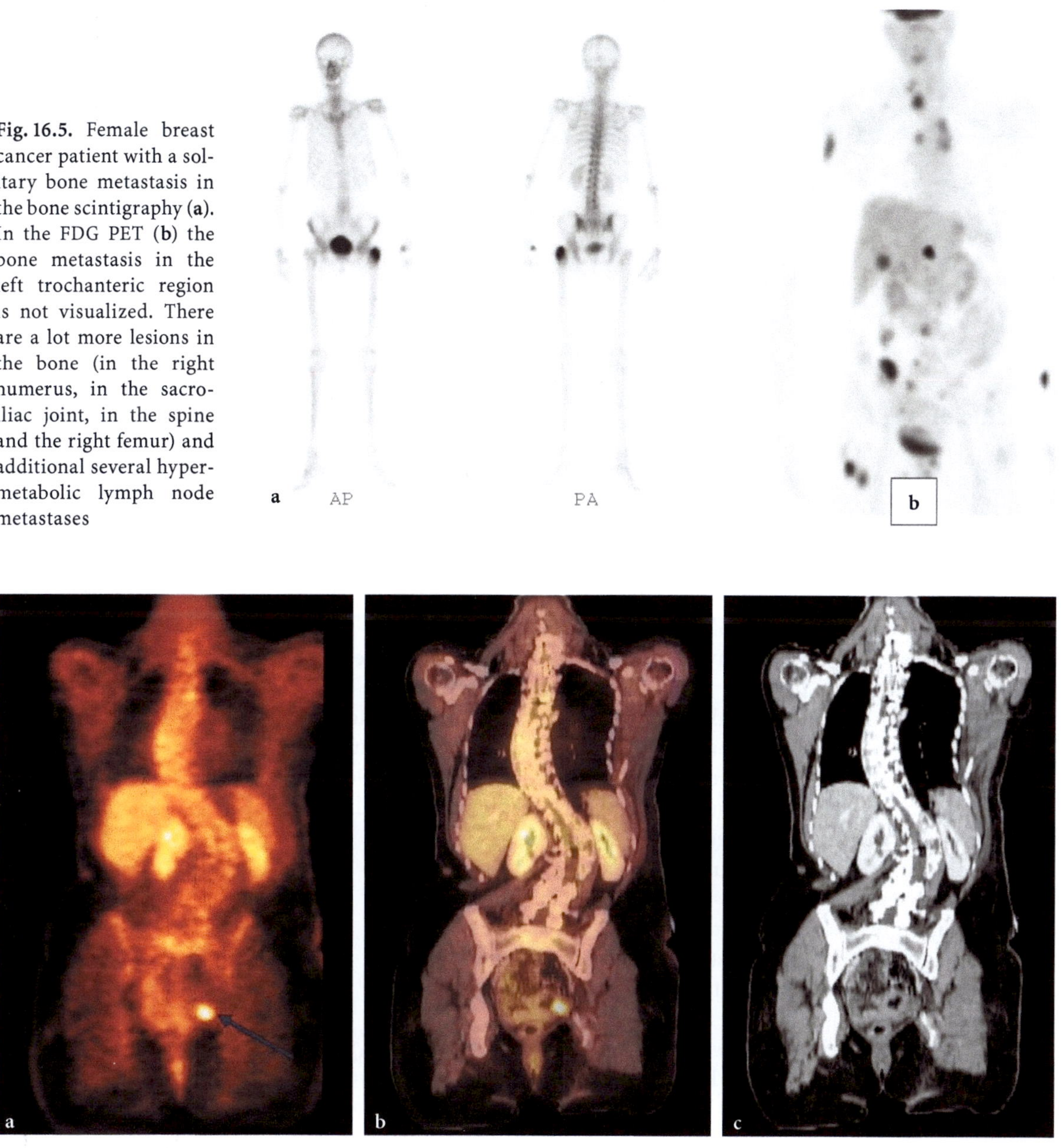

Fig. 16.5. Female breast cancer patient with a solitary bone metastasis in the bone scintigraphy (**a**). In the FDG PET (**b**) the bone metastasis in the left trochanteric region is not visualized. There are a lot more lesions in the bone (in the right humerus, in the sacroiliac joint, in the spine and the right femur) and additional several hypermetabolic lymph node metastases

Fig. 16.6a–c. A 43-year-old female with ductal invasive breast cancer diagnosed in 2003. In the PET images there is a focal FDG uptake in the pelvis, suggesting a lymph node or bone metastasis. The combined PET/CT localizes the FDG spot into bowel activity and therefor reduces false positive results

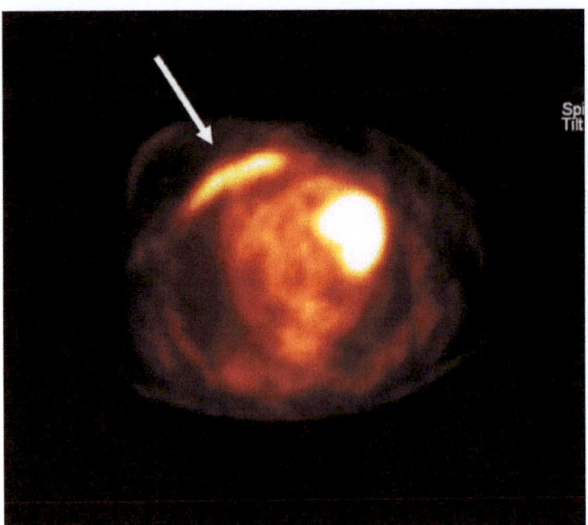

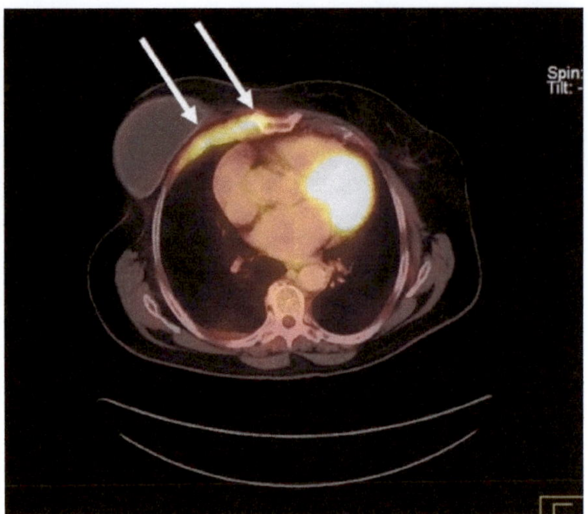

Fig. 16.7. A 68-year-old female with ductal invasive breast cancer diagnosed in 1987 and increasing Ca 15-3 level. PET demonstrates diffusely increased FDG uptake due to local recurrence. PET/CT reveals additional osseous infiltration of the sternum

16.6 Conclusion

There is increasing evidence that FDG-PET has an important role in the follow-up of breast cancer patients. Several studies have demonstrated that whole-body FDG-PET is superior to conventional imaging in detecting recurrent and metastatic disease from breast cancer. A major strength of FDG-PET is that recurrent disease, lymph node involvement or distant metastases can be detected at an early stage when metabolic changes precede and dominate morphological changes or anatomical alterations. Therefore, FDG-PET should be performed as early as possible in case of any suspicion of recurrence or metastases, i.e., slightly increased tumor markers or any clinical suspicion of recurrent disease. As patient-based sensitivity of FDG-PET is very high for detecting recurrent and metastatic disease, it is a reliable imaging technique for restaging breast cancer. However, due low detectability of sclerotic and mixed sclerotic/osteolytic bone metastases FDG-PET results in a somewhat low lesion-based sensitivity. Furthermore, specificity is limited due to the non-specificity of FDG, which has been discussed in the literature before. Therefore, FDG uptake in granulomatous disease, inflammation, post-therapeutic repair processes, muscles and brown fat tissue may lead potentially to false-positive results. With the introduction of combined PET/CT tomographs and subsequently combined anatomical and metabolic interpretation false-positive readings are expected to be reduced, and overall accuracy of diagnosis is increased. Assuming that restaging of breast cancer is a sensible pre-requisite for breast cancer patient management, FDG-PET/CT appears to be the imaging modality of choice.

Acknowledgements

We would like to thank Dr. Lutz S. Freudenberg (Department of Nuclear Medicine, University Hospital Essen, Essen, Germany) for helpful discussions and for providing the materials for Figure 16.1.

References

Adler DD, Wahl RL (1995) New methods for imaging the breast: techniques, findings and potential. Am J Roentgenol 164:19–30

Adler LP, Crowe JP, Al-Kaisi NK, Sunshine JL (1993) Evaluation of breast masses and axillary lymph nodes with [F-18] 2-deoxy-2-fluoro-D-glucose PET. Radiology 187:743–750

Antoch G, Freudenberg LS, Beyer T, Bockisch A, Debatin JF (2004) To enhance or not to enhance? ^{18}F-FDG and CT contrast agents in dual-modality ^{18}F-0FDG PET/CT. J Nucl Med 45(Suppl 1):56S–65S

Avril N, Scheidhauer K, Kuhn W (2000) Dual-modality PET/CT imaging for clinical oncology using a single tomograph. In: Wieler HJ and Coleman RE (eds) PET in clinical oncology. Springer: Darmstadt. 355–371

Avril N, Schelling M, Dose J, Weber W, Schwaiger M (1999) Utility of PET in breast cancer. Clin Pos Imag 2:261–271

Baslaim M, Bakheet S, Bakheet R, Ezzat A, El-Foudeh M, Tulbah A (2003) 18-Fluorodeoxyglucose-positron emission tomography in inflammatory breast cancer. World J Surg 27:1099–1104

Bender H, Kirst J, Palmedo H (1997) Value of ^{18}fluorodeoxyglucose positron emission tomography in the staging of recurrent breast cancer. Anticancer Res 17(3B):1687–1692

Beyer T, Antoch G, Freudenberg TS, Egelhof T, Müller SP (2004) Considerations on FDG-PET/CT imaging protocols. J Nucl Med 45(suppl 1):25S–35S

Beyer T, Kinahan PE, Townsend DW (1997) Optimization of emission and transmission scan duration in 3D whole-body PET. IEEE Transactions in Nuclear Science 44:2400–2407

Boerner A, Weckesser M, Herzog H, Schmitz T, Audretsch W, Nitz U, Bender H, Mueller-Gaertner H (1999) Optimal scan time for fluorine-18 fluorodeoxyglucose positron emission tomography in breast cancer. Eur J Nucl Med 26(3):226–230

Bombardieri E, Grippa F (2001) PET imaging in breast cancer. Q J Nucl Med 43:245–256

Brix G, Henze M, Knopp N, Lucht R, Doll J, Junkermann H, Hawighorst H, Haberkorn U (2001) Comparison of pharmacokinetic MRI and [^{18}F] fluorodeoxyglucose PET in the diagnosis of breast cancer: initial experience. Eur Rad 11(10):2058–2070

Brown RS, Leung JY, Fisher SJ, Frey KA, Ethier SP, Wahl RL (1995) Intratumoral distribution of tritiated fluorodeoxyglucose in breast carcinoma: I. Are inflammatory cells important? J Nucl Med 36:1854–1861

Buck A, Wahl A, Eicher U, Blumstein N, Schirrmeister H, Helms G, Glattnig G, Neumaier B, Reske S (2003) Combined morphological and functional imaging with FDG-PET/CT for restaging breast cancer–impact on patient management. J Nucl Med 44S:78P

Carter CL, Allen C, Henson DE (1989) Relation of tumor size, lymph node status and survival in 24,740 breast cancer cases. Cancer 63:181–187

Coleman RE (2001) Is quantitation necessary for oncological PET studies? Eur J Nucl Med 29:133–135

Cook G, Houston S, Rubens R, Maisey M, Fogelman I (1998) Detection of bone metastases in breast cancer by F-18 FDG PET: differing metabolic activity in osteoblastic and osteolytic lesions. J Clin Oncol 16:3375–3379

Cook G, Fogelman I (1999) Skeletal metastases from breast cancer: imaging with nuclear medicine. Semin Nucl Med 29:69–79

Crippa F, Seregni E, Agresti R et al (1998) Association between [^{18}F]fluorodeoxyglucose uptake and postoperative histopathology, hormone receptor status, thymidine labelling index and p53 in primary breast cancer: a preliminary observation. Eur J Nucl Med 25:1429–1434

Czernin J (2002) FDG PET in breast cancer: A different view of its clinical use. Mol Imag Biol 4:35–45

Dose J, Bleckmann C, Bachmann S, Bohuslavizki K, Berger J, Habermann C, Jänicke F (2002) Comparison of fluorodeoxyglucose positron emission tomography and "conventional diagnostic procedures" for the detection of distant metastases in breast cancer patients. Nucl Med Commun 23:857–864

Doshi NK, Shao Y, Silverman RW, Cherry SR (2000) Design and evaluation of an LSO PET detector for breast cancer imaging. Med Phys 27:1535–1543

Eubank WB, Mankoff DA, Vesselle HJ, Eary JF, Schubert EK, Dunnwald LK, Lindsley SK, Gralow JR, Austin-Seymour MM, Ellis GK, Livingston RB (2002) Detection of locoregional and distant recurrences in breast cancer patients by using FDG PET. Radiographics 22:5–17

Fisher B, Bryant J, Wolmark N et al (1998) Effect of preoperative chemotherapy on the outcome of women with operable breast cancer. J Clin Oncol 16:2672–2685

Flanagan F, Dehdashti F, Siegel B (1998) PET in breast cancer. Semin Nucl Med 28:290–302

Freifelder R, Karp J (1997) Dedicated PET scanners for breast imaging. Phys Med Biol 42:2463–2480

Fueger BJ, Weber WA, Quon A, Crawford TL, Allen-Auerbach MS, Halpern BS, Ratib O, Phelps ME, Czernin J () Performance of 2-deoxy-2-[F-18]fluoro-D-glucose positron emission tomography and integrated PET/CT in restaged breast cancer patients. Mol Imaging Biol 7:369–376

Gallowitsch H, Kresnik E, Gasser J, Kumnig G, Igerc I, Mikosch P, Lind P (2003) F-18 fluorodeoxyglucose positron-emission tomography in the diagnosis of tumor recurrence and metastases in the follow up of patients with breast carcinoma: a comparison to conventional imaging. Invest Radiol 38:250–256

Goerres G, Michel S, Fehr M, Kaim A, Steinert H, Seifert B, Schulthess Gv, Kubik-Huch R (2003) Follow-up of women with breast cancer: comparison between MRI and FDG PET. Eur Radiol 13:1635–1644

Halpern B, Dahlbom M, Waldherr C, Quon A, Schiepers C, Silverman D, Ratib O, Czernin J (2003) A new time-saving whole-body protocol for PET/CT imaging. Mol Imaging Biol 5:182

Hamblen SM, Lowe VJ (2003) Clinical ^{18}F-FDG oncology patient preparation techniques. J Nucl Med Technol 31:3–10

Hany TF, Gharepapagh E, Kamel EM, Buck A, Himms-Hagen J, von Schulthess GK (2002) Brown adipose tissue: a factor to consider in symmetrical tracer uptake in the neck and upper chest region. Eur J Nucl Med Mol Imaging 29:1393–1398

Hathaway P, Mankoff D, Maravilla K, Austin-Seymour M, Gralow J, Cortese A, Hayes C, Moe R (1999) Value of combined FDG PET and MRI imaging in the evaluation of suspected recurrent local-regional breast cancer: preliminary results. Radiology 210:807–814

Heinisch M, Gallowitsch H, Mikosch P, Kresnik E, Kumnig G, Gomez I, Lind P, Umschaden H, Gasser J, Forsthuber E (2003) Comparison of FDG PET and dynamic contrast enhanced MRI in the evaluation of suggestive breast lesions. Breast 12:7–22

Hoh CK, Hawkins RA, Glaspy JA, Dahlbom M, Tse NY, Hoffman EJ, Schiepers C, Choi Y, Rege S, Nitzsche E, Maddahi J, Phelps ME (1993) Cancer detection with whole-body PET using 2-[^{18}F]fluoro-2-deoxy-D-glucose. J Comp Assist Tomo 17:582–589

Holm S, Toft P, Jensen M (1996) Estimation of the noise contributions from blank, transmission and emission scans in PET. IEEE Transactions on Nuclear Sciences 43:2285–2291

Igerc I, Gallowitsch H, Kumnig G, Reinprecht P, Gomez I, Kresnik E, Matschnig S, Hausegger K, Lind P (2003) Clinical performance of PET/CT in oncological patients: Impact on diagnostic accuracy and patient management. Nucl Med 42:A181

Isasi CR, Moadel RM, Blaufox MD (2005) A meta-analysis of FDG-PET for the evaluation of breast cancer recurrence and metastases. Breast Cancer Res Treat 90:105–112

Kamel E, Wyss M, Fehr M, Schulthess Gv, Goerres W (2003) [^{18}F]-Fluorodeoxyglucose positron emission tomography in patients with suspected recurrence of breast cancer. J Cancer Res Clin Oncol 129:147–153

Kinahan P, Hasegawa B, Beyer T (2003) X-ray based attenuation correction for PET/CT scanners. Semin Nucl Med 33:166–179

Krak NC, Hoeven JJvd, Hoekstra OS, Twisk JW, Wall EVD, Lammertsma AA (2003) Measuring [^{18}F]FDG uptake in breast cancer during chemotherapy: comparison of analytical methods. Eur J Nucl Med Mol Imaging 30:674–681

Kuerer HM, Sahin A, Hunt KK et al (1999) Incidence and impact of documented eradication of breast cancer axillary lymph node metastases before surgery in patients treated with neoadjuvant chemotherapy. Ann Surg 230:72–78

Kumnig G, Igerc I, Gallowitsch H, Reinprecht P, Kresnik E, Lind P, Hausegger K (2003) Impact of combined PET/CT imaging in reducing false positive results in FDG PET. Nucl Med 42:A166

Langsteger W, Jorg L, Tausch C, Heinisch M, Wieser B, Rechberger E, Panholzer P, Sega W, Aufschnaiter M (2002) The value of F-18 fluorodeoxyglucose in positron emission tomography diagnosis of breast carcinoma [German]. Wiener Medizinische Wochenschrift 152:255–258

Lartizien C, Comtat C, Kinahan PE, Ferreira N, Bendriem B, Trebossen R (2002) Optimization of injected dose based on noise equivalent count rates for 2- and 3-dimensional whole-body PET. J Nucl Med 43:1268–1278

Lind P, Gallowitsch H, Kogler D, Kresnik E, Mikosch P, Gomez I (1996) Tc-99m Tetrofosmin mammoscintigraphy: A prospective study in primary breast lesions. Nucl Med 35:225–229

Lind P, Gallowitsch H, Mikosch P, Kresnik E, Gomez I, Oman J, Dinges H, Boniface G (1997) Radioimmunoscintigraphy with Tc99m labelled monoclonal antibody 170H.82 in suspected primary recurrent, or metastatic breast cancer. Clin Nucl Med 22:30–34

Lind P, Smola M, Lechner P, Ratschek M, Klima G, Költringer P, Steindorfer P, Eber O (1991) The immunoscintigraphic use of Tc-99m labelled monoclonal anti-CEA antibody (BW 431/26) in patients with suspected primary, recurrent and metastatic breast cancer. Int J Cancer 47:865–869

Liu C, Shen Y, Lin C, Yen R, Kao C (2002) Clinical impact of [(^{18})F] FDG PET in patients with suspected recurrent breast cancer based on asymptomatically elevated tumor marker serum levels: a preliminary study. Jpn J Clin Oncol 32:244–247

Mamounas EP (1999) Overview of National Surgical Adjuvant Breast Project neoadjuvant chemotherapy studies. Semin Oncol 25:31–35

Minn H, Soini I (1989) F-18 fluoroddeoxyglucose scintigraphy in diagnosis and follow-up of treatment in advanced breast cancer. Eur J Nucl Med Mol Imaging 15:61–66

Moon DH, Maddahi J, Silverman DHS, Glaspy JA, Phelps ME, Hoh CK (1998) Accuracy of whole-body fluorine-18-FDG PET for the detection of recurrent or metastatic breast carcinoma. J Nucl Med 39:431–435

Muehllehner G, Karp K, Surti S (2002) Design considerations for PET scanners. Q J Nucl Med 46:16–23

Murthy K, Aznar M, Thompson CJ, Loutfi A, Lisbona R, Gagnon JH (2000) Results of preliminary clinical trials of the positron emission mammography system PEM-I: A dedicated breast imaging system producing glucose metabolic images using FDG. J Nucl Med 41:1851–1858

Nakai T, Okuyama C, Kubota T, Yamada K, Ushijima Y, Taniike K, Suzuki T, Nishimura T (2005) Pitfalls of FDG-PET for the diagnosis of osteoblastic bone metastases in patients with breast cancer. Eur J Nucl Med Mol Imaging 32:1253–1258

Palmedo H (2003) Breast cancer. In: PET and PET/CT in Clinical Oncology. P Oehr, H-J Biersack and E Coleman, Editors. Springer: Heidelberg. 167–178

Person JJ, Kransdorf MJ, O'Connor MI (2003) Diagnosis of occult bone metastases: positron emission tomography. Clin Orthop (415 Suppl):S120–128

Pietrzyk U, Scheidhauer K, Scharl A, Schuster A, Schicha H (1995) Presurgical visualization of primary breast carcinoma with PET emission and transmission imaging. J Nucl Med 36:1882–1884

Pietrzyk U (2003) Fortschritte in der Bildfusion medizinischer Bilddaten aus PET, SPET, CT und MRT. Der Nuklearmediziner 26:235–244

Raylman RR, Majewski S, Weisenberger AG, Popov V, Wojcik R, Kross B, Schreiman JS, Bishop HA (2001) Positron emission mammography-guided breast biopsy. J Nucl Med 42:960–966

Reske SN and Kotzerke J (2001) FDG-PET for clinical use. Results of the 3rd German Interdisciplinary Consensus Conference, "Onko-PET III", 21 July and 19 September 2000. Eur J Nucl Med 28:1707–1723

Rigo P, Paulus P, Kaschten BJ, Hustinx R, Bury T, Jerusalem G et al (1996) Oncological application of positron emission tomography with fluorine-18 fluorodeoxyglucose. Eur J Nucl Med 23:1641–1674

Rousseau C, Bourbouloux E, Campion L, Fleury N, Bridji B, Chatal JF, Resche I, Campone M (2006) Brown fat in breast cancer patients: analysis of serial (^{18})F-FDG PET/CT scans. Eur J Nucl Med Mol Imaging 33:785–791

Scheidhauer K, Scharl A, Pietrzyk U, Wagner R, Göhring U-J, Schomäcker K et al (1996) Qualitative [^{18}F]FDG positron emission tomography in primary breast cancer: clinical relevance and practicability. Eur J Nucl Med 23:618–623

Smith I, Welch A, Hutcheon A, Miller I, Payne S, Chilcott F, Waikar S, Whitaker T, Ah-See A, Eremin O, Heys S, Gilbert F, Sharp P (2000) Positron emission tomography using [(^{18})F]-fluorodeoxy-D-glucose to predict the pathologic response of breast cancer to primary chemotherapy. J Clin Oncol 18:1676–1688

Spanu A, Farris A, Schillaci O, Chessa F, Solinas M, Falchi A, Madi G, Nuvoli S, Madeddu G (2003) The usefulness of Tc-99m tetrofosmin scintigraphy in patients with breast cancer recurrences. Nucl Med Commun 24:145–154

Suarez M, Perez-Castejon M, Jimenez A, Domper M, Ruiz G, Carreras J (2002) Early diagnosis of recurrent breast cancer with FDG PET in patients with progressive elevation of serum tumor markers. Q J Nucl Med 46:113–121

Tack D, De Maertelaer V, Gevenois PA (2003) Dose reduction in multidetector CT using attenuation-based online tube current modulation. Am J Roentgenol 181:331–334

Tatsumi M, Cohade C, Mourtzikos KA, Fishman EK, Wahl RL (2006) Initial experience with FDG-PET/CT in the evaluation of breast cancer. Eur J Nucl Med Mol Imaging 33:254–262

Thompson CJ, Murthy K, Weinberg IN, Mako F (1994) Feasibility study for positron emission mammography. Med Phys 21:529–538

Townsend D, Carney JP, Yap JT, Hall NC (2004) PET/CT today and tomorrow. J Nucl Med 45(suppl 1):4S–14S

von Schulthess GK (2000) Cost considerations regarding an integrated CT-PET system. Eur Rad 10(suppl 3):S377–S380

Wahl R, Cody R, Hutchins G, Mudgett E (1991) Positron emission tomography scanning of primary and metastatic breast cancer with radioloabeled glucose analoque 2-deoxy-2(^{18}F)fluoro-D-glucose. N Engl J Med 324:200

Wahl RL (1999) To AC or not to AC: That is the question. J Nucl Med 40:2025–2028

Warburg O, Posener K, Negelein E (1924) The metabolism of cancer cells. Biochem Zeitschrift 152:129–169

Weinberg I, Majewski S, Weisenberger A, Markowitz A, Aloj L, Majewski L, Danforth D, Mulshine J, Cowan K, Zujewski J, Chow C, Jones E, Chang V, Berg W, Frank J (1996) Preliminary results for positron emission mammography: real-time functional breast imaging in a conventional mammography gantry. Eur J Nucl Med 23:804–806

Yang H, Nam SJ, Lee TS, Lee HK, Jung SH, Kim BT (2001) Japanese comparison of intraoperative frozen section analysis of sentinel node with preoperative positron emission tomography in the diagnosis of axillary lymph node status in breast cancer patients. Japan J Clin Oncol 31:1–6

Yasuda S, Kubota M, Tajima T, Tajima T, Umemura S, Fujii H, Takahashi W, Ide M, Shohtsu A (1999) A small breast cancer detected by PET. Japan J Clin Oncol 29:387–389

Zaidi H, Hasegawa B (2003) Determination of the attenuation map in emission tomography. J Nucl Med 44:291–315

PET/CT and Breast Cancer

17

Maria Picchio, Cristina Messa, Barbara Zangheri, Claudio Landoni, Luigi Gianolli, and Ferruccio Fazio

CONTENTS

Abstract

During the last decade, the application of positron emission tomography (PET) has remarkably improved the management of cancer patients. The radiotracer most widely used in clinical practice is the glucose analogue 2-[^{18}F]-fluoro-2-deoxy-D-glucose (FDG). FDG-PET is showing increasing usefulness in the distinction between malignant and benign lesions, in disease staging, re-staging and therapy planning. Due to the lack of precise anatomic landmarks, PET may present limitations in lesion localization. In contrast, PET/computed tomography (CT), by directly combining functional and morphological aspects, provides more reliable anatomical details. The main advantage of combined PET/CT imaging is, in fact, its ability to accurately correlate abnormal metabolic changes detected on PET imaging to anatomic structures defined at CT imaging (Townsend 2001).

With this chapter, the impact in breast cancer diagnosis of PET/CT will be evaluated and compared with PET alone, visually correlated with morphologic imaging obtained in a separate session.

17.1 PET/CT or PET Alone?

In principle, clinical applications of PET/CT in oncology are those of PET, i.e., diagnosis, staging, restaging and follow-up of a wide number of malignancies, including breast cancer.

The integrated PET/CT system consists of a CT and PET scanner assembled together. This combined system has some advantages over CT alone, as functional information is added to morphological data, and over PET alone, mainly due to better accuracy in localizing pathological areas of tracer uptake and to a shorter image acquisition time. In the PET/CT system, the CT scan is used for attenuation correction of PET emission images. By using the CT scan instead of PET transmission scan, a gain in time (more than 10 min/patient) is obtained, even when segmentation techniques are used (Bettinardi et al. 1999). A shorter acquisition time allows a better compliance of the patient, improving patient comfort and reducing possible artifacts due to movements.

According to the literature, the PET/CT system is more accurate for tumor staging than either PET alone or CT alone (Vansteenkiste et al. 1998; Kluetz et al. 2000). Antoch et al. (2003) evaluated the accuracy of PET/CT in lung cancer in comparison to PET alone and to CT showing a change in tumor stage in 26% of patients when compared to PET alone and in 30% when compared to CT. Pelosi et al. (2004), in a retrospective study conducted on 210 neoplastic patients, showed that PET/CT improves the diagnostic accuracy in lesion localization compared to the combination of PET and morphologic imaging, the number of lesions with an uncertain localization being lower by using PET/CT (3.4%) than by using PET and separate morphological imaging (15.3%). These data are in agreement with other studies where a lower rate of lesions with uncertain localization was found using PET/CT with respect to PET alone. Hany et al. (2002) reported that 21% of all lesions detected by PET were classified as undecided, whereas an additional 9% of lesions could have been properly classified when using PET/CT. Lardinois et al. (2003) showed that PET/CT provided additional information in 41% of patients who underwent staging or re-staging evaluation for non-small cell lung cancer. Furthermore, they found a better diagnostic accuracy of PET/CT in comparison with PET alone, CT alone and visual correlation of PET and CT. Bar-Shalom et al. (2003) reported that PET/CT provided additional information over the separate interpretation of PET and CT in 49% in their series of patients.

The major conclusion of all these studies is the superiority of PET/CT compared to PET alone in the detection of recurrence or metastatic disease in patients with high suspicion of disease, but negative morphological imaging studies.

Breast cancer represents the most frequent disease in women and the second cause of cancer death in western countries. Breast cancer is often curable, when diagnosed in an early stage. Currently, diagnostic procedures for both primary staging and re-staging include mammary echography, mammography, magnetic resonance (MR) imaging, thorax CT and bone scan scintigraphy (Jemal et al. 2003).

Published experience reporting the role of PET in breast cancer is now extensive, and populations mainly include primary breast cancer, recurrent and metastatic disease, axillary nodal metastases and monitoring response to therapy (Santiago et al. 2006). However, only few PET/CT studies have been performed (Buck et al. 2003; Tatsumi et al. 2003; Fueger et al. 2005; Tatsumi et al. 2006). Recently, the added diagnostic value of PET/CT over PET in re-staging patients with breast cancer has been established. The reported sensitivity, specificity and accuracy are 94%, 84% and 98%, respectively, for PET/CT vs. 85%, 72% and 79%, respectively, for PET (Fueger et al. 2005).

In general, the principal applications of PET in breast cancer are disease re-staging and treatment monitoring (Fueger et al. 2005; Tatsumi et al. 2006; Avril et al. 2000; Bombardieri et al. 2003; Leung 2002). However, other possible indications are preoperative staging and primary diagnosis (Santiago et al. 2006; Tatsumi et al. 2006; Avril et al. 1999, 2000; Bombardieri et al. 2001, 2003; Leung 2002; Mankoff et al. 2003; Crippa et al. 1998; Wahl et al. 2004; Landheer et al. 2005; Tran et al. 2005). PET/CT clinical applications vs. PET alone for all these indications will be reviewed. In addition, as for the relevant role of PET/CT in radiotherapy (RT), the possible use of PET/CT in that field will also be evaluated.

17.2 Re-Staging and Follow-Up

Local or regional recurrence after initial diagnosis and treatment of breast cancer occurs in 7–30% of patients (Santiago et al. 2006). Follow-up examinations for early detection of local recurrence are thus required. However, the conventional imaging modalities usually performed, such as mammography, CT and MR imaging, may present limitations in distinguishing between anatomical modifications induced by therapy and relapse of disease (Moore et al. 1990; Goerres et. al. 2003). In contrast to morphological imaging, assessment of disease with FDG-PET is made on functional rather than anatomical criteria. FDG-PET is, in fact, a method based on the increased glucose metabolism of malignant tumor tissue. In recurrent or metastatic breast cancer FDG-PET shows a high diagnostic accuracy (Santiago et al. 2006; Moon et al. 1998). One of most important prognostic factors for recurrence in breast cancer is the axillary lymph node involvement. In fact, a number of studies have focused on PET accuracy in axillary staging, and the reported sensitivity and specificity ranged between 85% and 100% and between 66% and 100%, respectively (Santiago et al. 2006).

PET/CT has been shown to be superior to PET alone in re-staging disease of patients previously treated for various tumors, including breast cancer (Fueger et al. 2005), particularly in those cases where the only indicator of recurrence of disease is a rise of serum tumor markers such as CA 15-3 (Suarez et al. 2002). In those cases, PET/CT may allow an earlier diagnosis and a prompt treatment of disease. When compared to PET alone, PET/CT has been reported to improve the accuracy by raising both sensitivity and specificity (Fueger et al. 2005). In general, as previously reported, the advantages of PET/CT are mainly due to the improved anatomical localization of hypermetabolic foci. As for sensitivity, the addition of CT may help in correctly defining doubtful hypermetabolic PET lesions. In addition, one of the most common causes of PET false-negative findings is the presence of sclerotic bone metastases. It is well known that PET may detect lytic bone metastases with a high accuracy. However, PET sensitivity in detecting osteoblastc lesions is limited. This limitation may be overcome by PET/CT as CT may properly detect sclerotic bone lesions with an accuracy even higher than that of conventional radiography. As for specificity, the morphological information provided by CT allows the correct anatomical localization of normal tissue, such as brown fat, muscle and bowel that may represent PET false-positive lesions. The information derived by CT may also improve specificity in cases such as fatty necrosis and artificially focal FDG uptake due to low count statistics that may wrongly be interpreted as false-positive results at PET (Fueger et al. 2005). Conversely, the limited specificity of PET due to increased metabolic activity of inflammatory tissue may be only partially overcome by PET/CT. In fact, enlarged inflammatory lymph nodes may have a positive result at PET such as at PET/CT.

A suggestion that PET/CT could provide more accurate diagnosis in re-staging breast cancer can be extrapolated by the work of Pelosi et al. (2004). Out of the 210 patients recruited, 40 were affected by previously treated breast cancer and examined by PET/CT (n=19) or PET with morphological imaging (n=21). In the 19 PET/CT patients, 45/47 (96%) lesions were correctly localized. The remaining two lesions with uncertain localization, both located in the mediastinum, could be referred to either lymph node or pleura. In the 21 patients studied by PET only, 58/63 (92%) lesions could be correctly localized with separate morphological imaging. Of the remaining five, four were located in the thorax and could be referred either to bone or soft tissue, and either to lymph node or lung. In the remaining one, located in the abdomen, the focal FDG uptake could be referred either to lymph node or physiological urinary/intestinal uptake. Additional studies in breast cancer and PET/CT have yielded similar results (Fueger et al. 2005; Quon and Gambhir 2005). In particular, Fueger et al. (2005) recently suggested that integrated PET/CT presents a higher accuracy than PET alone in re-staging breast cancer patients, even if only marginally (P=0.059).

PET is a whole body study and provides an effective and convenient method for assessing multiple sites of the body at one time. In patients who have a newly diagnosed recurrence, PET may be useful in identifying additional sites of disease not detected by conventional imaging modalities. This is particularly important in patients who have a local recurrence, as a regional disease may be treated with curative intent. Weir et al. (2005) recently described the capability of PET to detect additional distant metastases in 30% of patients studied, thus providing relevant information for management decisions.

Examples of PET/CT images in re-staging patients with local recurrence (Fig. 17.1) and distant metastases (Fig. 17.2) are reported.

In conclusion, the utility of using PET/CT in restaging and in establishing the correct management of breast cancer patients is evident both in early restaging of patients after primary treatment and in follow-up. In particular, PET appears particularly valuable in the evaluation of patients who are suspected of having a tumor recurrence and to exclude multifocal or distant sites of malignancy in patients who appear to have an isolated, potentially curable, local recurrence (Weir et al. 2005).

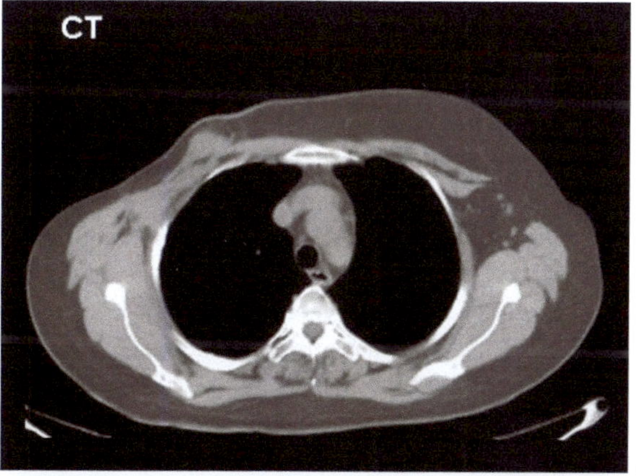

a

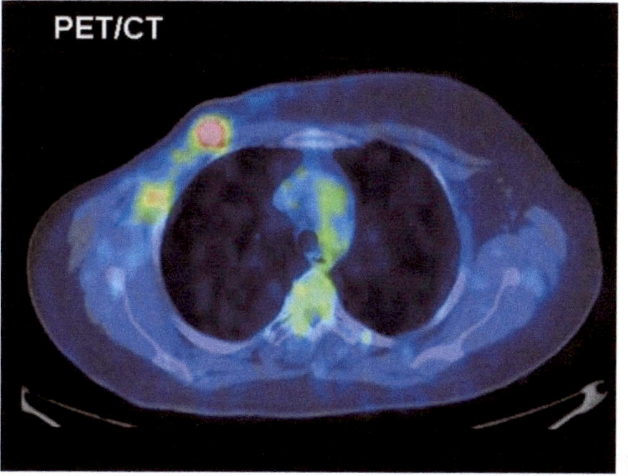

b

Fig. 17.1a,b. Patient surgically treated for breast cancer: recurrences in the left mammary region were detected by PET/CT during follow-up

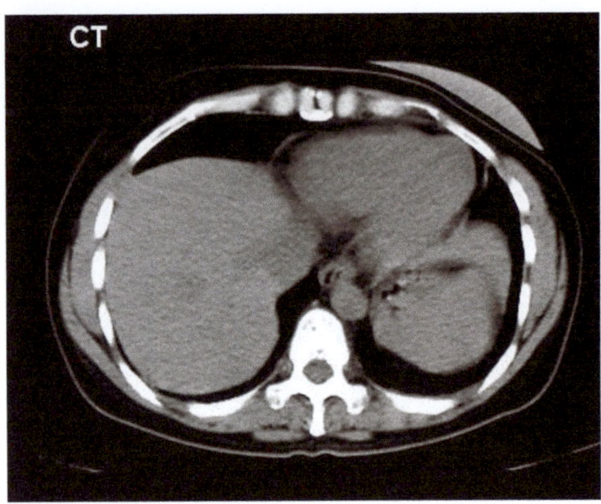

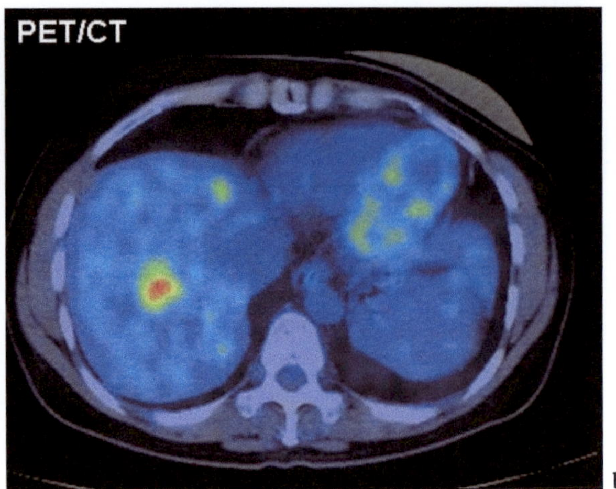

a b

Fig. 17.2a,b. Patient surgically treated for breast cancer and presenting an increasing serum marker value: a single liver metastasis was detected by PET/CT

17.3 Treatment Monitoring

One of the most challenging aspects in cancer imaging is the assessment of therapy response. Traditionally, response is determined at the end of treatment by measuring changes in tumor size, assessed by CT or MR imaging. The early diagnosis of a relapse is an important issue, as it ensures a fast therapeutic reaction. However, after treatment, morphological imaging may fail in differentiating between viable tumor tissue and either fibrotic or necrotic tissue. In contrast to morphological imaging techniques, PET is a functional imaging modality that allows the visualization and the quantitative calculation of regional glucose metabolism within the body. As PET may detect the increased metabolic rate, the assessment of the presence of viable tumor tissue is possible independently on morphological criteria. The use of FDG-PET in monitoring tumor response to chemotherapy is gaining increasing interest. Its role in the assessment of response at the end of chemotherapeutic treatment has been established in different neoplasms, including breast cancer (Baum and Przetak 2001). In particular, in patients with locally advanced breast cancer, PET may provide important prognostic information regarding disease-free and overall survival (Avril et al. 1999; Stafford et al. 2002). Since PET imaging seems to be highly useful for monitoring therapeutic effects earlier than any other imaging procedure actually available, the early identification of non-responders would significantly improve patient management by reducing ineffective therapies, preventing side effects, reducing delay in initiating a more effective treatment and minimizing the costs. The possibility to predict response during the early phases of treatment is a major challenge in oncology, in particular for the recent clinical introduction of individualized treatment regimens that require improved early risk stratification. Several studies have shown the prognostic value of FDG-PET after the first cycles of chemotherapy in different cancers (Stafford et al. 2002; Dose et al. 2005). In particular, in breast cancer, PET may differentiate responding and non-responding patients as early as after the first cycle of chemotherapy. The FDG standardized uptake value (SUV) is considered the most widely prognostic factor for assessing the response in breast cancer, even in the early phases of treatment (Tran et al. 2005). As an example, a good correlation between SUV changes and clinical response was described by Stafford et al. (2002). Although these studies involved a relatively small number of patients, there is evidence that PET may be used for early therapy evaluation of patients with breast cancer (Quon and Gambhir 2005), in particular in patients with bone-dominant metastatic disease, and in those with locally advanced breast cancer undergoing primary chemotherapy (Weir et al. 2005).

On the basis of the already mentioned advantages of PET/CT compared to PET alone, PET/CT is supposed to further improve the accuracy in the evaluation of treatment response by directly defining metabolic and morphologic changes.

17.4 Preoperative Staging

Preoperative staging of breast cancer is extremely important as it influences the treatment decision. In particular, the evaluation of local staging is an indicator of prognosis and a relevant factor to determine the choice of surgical treatment, which can include the axillary dissection or not (Quon and Gambhir 2005; Sloka et al. 2005). Since conventional morphological imaging modalities cannot accurately detect axillary lymph nodal metastases, patients with advanced breast cancer routinely undergo lymphoscintigraphy, axillary lymph node dissection and histological examination. However, the axillary dissection procedure is still controversial as no clear survival advantages on its routine use have been reported. In addition, this procedure is associated with a high incidence of morbidities (Quon and Gambhir 2005; Sloka et al. 2005). Therefore, the role of FDG-PET in the evaluation of axillary lymph node status has been largely assessed (Crippa et al. 1998; Wahl et al. 2004; Avril et al. 1999; Quon and Gambhir 2005; Utech et al. 1996). In a prospective study on 124 patients, preoperative FDG-PET showed a sensitivity and a specificity in detecting metastatic axillary lymph nodes of 100% and 64%, respectively (Utech et al. 1996). More recently, an overall sensitivity, specificity and accuracy of 88%, 92% and 89%, respectively, have been reported (Quon and Gambhir 2005). Wahl et al. (2004), in a prospective study on 360 women with primary breast cancer, showed that PET, performed before surgery, may frequently miss small metastases in the axilla, thus suggesting that detection of micro-metastases and small tumor-infiltrated lymph nodes is limited by the currently achievable spatial resolution of PET imaging. Sensitivity in lymph-node detection is mainly related to primary tumor size: PET sensitivity rises from 79% to 94% if only large tumors (>2 cm) are considered (Avril et al. 1996). Although high values of PET sensitivity have been reported (Quon and Gambhir 2005; Utech et al. 1996), the general opinion is that FDG-PET is not sufficiently accurate in axillary lymph-node staging, mainly due to the unfeasibility of PET in detecting micro-metastatic disease. In addition, when metastatic lymph nodes are detected, PET imaging does not allow the determination of the number of neoplastic lymph nodes, which is important for subsequent therapy strategy. Conversely, PET may be highly predictive for nodal tumor involvement when multiple intense foci of tracer uptake are identified. Wahl el al. (2004) suggest that axillary node dissection may be omitted in patients with highly positive PET. Except for these cases, PET is not yet sensitive enough to replace axillary lymph node dissection as a staging method for the axilla (Wahl et al. 2004; Quon and Gambhir 2005; Weir et al. 2005).

If the role of PET in axillary status evaluation is still controversial, many studies have consistently demonstrated that FDG-PET is superior to CT in the detection of internal mammary and mediastinal lymph nodal metastases (Quon and Gambhir 2005; Bellon et al. 2004). The reported values of sensitivity, specificity and accuracy are 85%, 90% and 88%, respectively, for PET vs. 54%, 85% and 73%, respectively, for CT (Quon and Gambhir 2005; Eubank et al. 2001; Wu and Gambhir 2003). PET/CT could further improve the staging of breast cancer patients in the detection of metastases of the internal mammary node chain. In our own clinical experience with PET/CT, the finding of pathological focal uptake in the region of the internal mammary chain appears to be more frequent than when using PET alone (Fig. 17.3). This could be due to the higher localization accuracy of PET/CT vs. PET, which allows the detection of lesions previously disregarded as non-specific uptakes.

In breast cancer patients, PET has also proved effective in detecting distant lesions (Quon and Gambhir 2005). In fact, as previously reported, with FDG-PET being a whole body technique, it provides additional information on all body regions, including lymph nodes, liver, lung, bone and bone marrow, and it may detect distant metastases that are not detected by conventional methods. Several investigators have shown that in the evaluation of distant metastases, PET is relatively sensitive, reporting values between 84% and 93%, and presenting a negative predictive value higher than 90% (Quon and Gambhir 2005). Thus, it could be suggested to include FDG-PET in the preoperative work-up of mammary carcinomas, particularly in patients with high risk of metastatic disease. Conversely, specificity and positive predictive values are not quite as high, being in the range of 55% to 86% and 82%, respectively. These values are mainly due to the presence of possible false-positive findings, including physiological muscle and FDG bowel uptake (Quon and Gambhir 2005). PET/CT may overcome those limitations, but only preliminary analyses are currently available. Wang et al. (2003) reported the results of PET/CT in staging breast cancer patients, including 15 patients with lesion size ranging between 3.1–8.0 mm. They described values of sensitivity, specificity and accuracy in the diagnosis of primary tumor of 93%, 91% and 100%, respectively, and in detecting lymph-node metastases of 80%, 90% and 87%, respectively. They suggested that PET/CT diagnosis of both primary tumor and axillary lymph-node involvement is more accurate than that of mammography, ultrasound and PET alone, due to the combination of the metabolic information provided by PET and the high spatial resolution of CT. In a recent study on 75 patients with known breast cancer (Tatsumi et al. 2006), comparing PET/CT with PET and CT alone, PET/CT was suggested to add incremental diagnostic confidence to PET in more than 50% of patients and to accurately detect more neoplastic regions than CT did. This preliminary evaluation suggests that PET/CT is preferable to PET and CT in the diagnosis of breast cancer. In addition, PET/CT reduces the number of equivocal interpretations (Lardinois et al. 2003) and increases reader confidence (Fueger et al. 2005). As for bone metastases, PET is known to be superior to bone scintigraphy in the detection of osteolytic lesions, but inferior in the detection of osteoblastic lesions (Abe et al. 2005). As previously reported, the use of PET/CT may help in the detection of sclerotic bone lesions. In fact, even if negative by PET, those lesions may be readily identified on CT images. In addition, PET/CT can reliably assign normal or pathological tissues areas of mild hyperglicotic activity (Fueger et al. 2005).

Although the prevalence of distant metastases increases with the stage of the primary tumor at diagnosis, the diagnosis of distant metastases at the screening examinations in women who are asymptomatic is relatively uncommon (Weir et al. 2005). Weir et al. (2005) reported that unsuspected distant metastases may be detected in 5% of asymptomatic patients by PET at the time of primary diagnosis. Therefore, a PET scan is unlikely to be useful as a screening test for distant metastases at the time of initial diagnosis in patients with early stage breast cancer.

The impact of PET on clinical management in breast cancer patients was evaluated by Yap et al. (2001), showing a change of the clinical staging in 36% of patients and of the clinical management in 60%, with a change in treatment strategy, mainly due to the detection of a higher number of distant metastases by PET.

Although encouraging, PET/CT studies do not yet allow the evaluation of its possible impact in staging breast cancer of small size (<3 cm). At least for several years the main limitation of PET/CT spatial resolution will not be solved, and lesions smaller than 1 cm will remain difficult to detect.

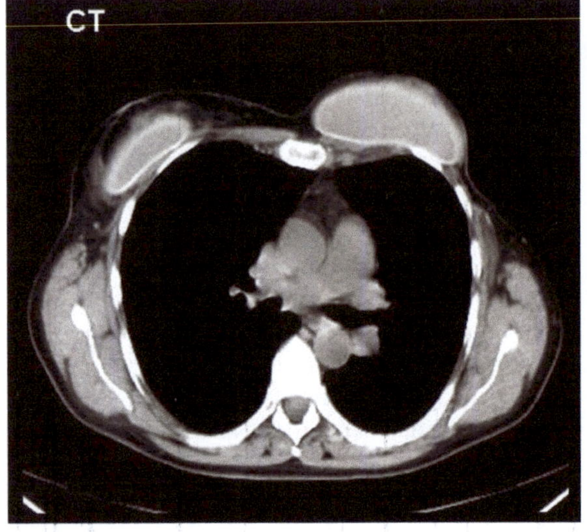

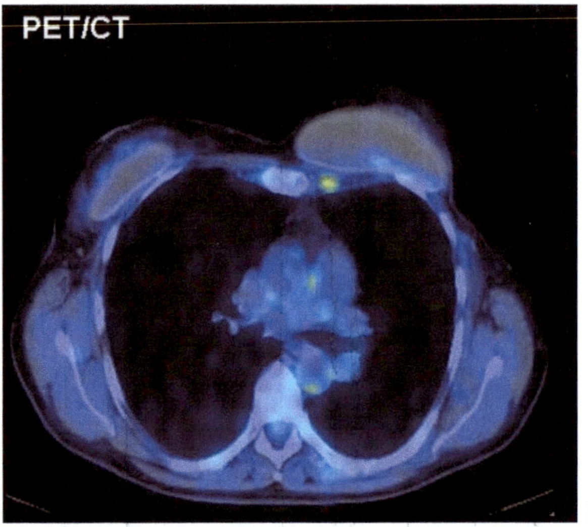

Fig. 17.3a,b. Patient with breast cancer: a metastasis in a lymph node of the left internal mammary chain was detected by PET/CT

17.5 Diagnosis of Primary Tumor

As a result of better screening procedures, the mortality rate for breast cancer is declining. However, the incidence of breast cancer continues to rise (Sloka et al. 2005). At present, the diagnosis of primary breast cancer is principally based on mammography. However, this technique has a low specificity, and about 10% of breast carcinomas cannot be identified by mammography, even if palpable (>1 cm in diameter) (Tabar et al. 1987; Kopans 1992; Bird et al. 1992). To overcome this limitation, other diagnostic techniques such as ultrasounds and MR imaging are being used. Ultrasound specificity is reported to be superior to that of mammography, especially in distinguishing solid and cystic lesions (Jackson 1995). MR imaging presents a sensitivity higher than 90%, but its specificity is lower than that of mammography (Friedrich 1998). In conclusion, the combination of these examinations is not sufficiently conclusive to significantly reduce invasive diagnostic procedures in the primary diagnosis of breast cancer.

Several investigations have been conducted to assess the role of FDG-PET in detecting primary breast cancer and in distinguishing malignant from benign disease. FDG-PET has yielded encouraging results showing a diagnostic sensitivity ranging between 80% and 96% and a specificity between 83% and 100% (Avril et al. 1996; Crowe et al. 1994; Scheidhauer et al. 1996; Tse et al. 1992; Buck et al. 2002). Non-invasive breast cancer has been only deficiently imaged by FDG-PET, and the majority of PET research studies have been performed on patients with invasive breast cancer (Quon and Gambhir 2005). The overall sensitivity, specificity and accuracy of PET in the detection of primary invasive breast cancer are 90%, 92% and 93%, respectively (Wu and Gambhir 2003).

Because of limitations in spatial resolution, PET is not recommended for lesions smaller than 1 cm in diameter. With the newest PET/CT system having a spatial resolution as good as 4 mm, the detection of smaller lesions may be partially improved (Quon et Gambhir 2005). Moreover, PET imaging accuracy is affected by tumor histology. Invasive breast cancer includes multiple histologic types mainly represented by ductal and lobular carcinomas. Infiltrating ductal carcinoma has a higher level of FDG uptake and therefore is detected at a significantly higher sensitivity than infiltrating lobular breast cancer (Quon et Gambhir 2005). In addition, the identification of non-invasive cancer such as carcinoma in situ can be missed by using FDG-PET (Wahl et al. 2004). As for specificity, overall values are relatively high, but false-positive findings may occur in inflammatory tissues and in some benign conditions such as fibroadenoma (Weir et al. 2005).

Although the dual system PET/CT solves the problem of lesion localization, the high cost and the limit in spatial resolution discourage the application of FDG-PET data in the screening and in the diagnosis of primary tumor. A possible role of PET/CT in the primary diagnosis of breast cancer could be the selection of patients with dense breast where mammography presents a low sensitivity (Weir et al. 2005). Finally, a new PET scanner utilizing a small gantry size specifically designed for breast imaging is being developed, and it could significantly increase the spatial resolution and sensitivity of the method (Weir et al. 2005).

17.6 PET/CT and Radiotherapy

PET/CT can be successfully used in radiotherapy at different steps, including (1) patients selection by correct staging disease, (2) target volume and treatment planning definition by evaluating biological target volumes (BTV) and (3) evaluation of RT biological effect by monitoring the disease.

As for patient staging and selection, PET accuracy in staging patients with cancer has been largely explored, showing to be higher than CT or MR in many tumors. The use of integrated PET/CT systems has further improved the diagnostic accuracy of PET (Wechalekar et al. 2005). As an example, in lung cancer, Lardinois et al. (2003) showed that PET/CT may provide additional information in 41% of patients compared with PET and CT viewed side-by-side. In particular, they reported an overall diagnostic accuracy of PET/CT for tumor (T) staging of 88% and for node (N) staging of 81%. In addition, unsuspected metastases were found by PET in 16% of patients (Lardinois et al. 2003). In general, unsuspected metastases are found by PET and PET/CT in approximately 20% of patients. The high accuracy of PET/CT for N and M staging will certainly have an impact on RT treatment by reducing the number of diagnostic investigations in patients who are candidates for radical RT and by excluding subjects from radical RT when unsuspected metastases are detected. This is particularly important as the most proper treatments can be proposed and ineffective treatments may be avoided.

The role of PET in oncology is mainly focused on assessing lymph node and distant metastases rather than determining tumor extension and its relationship with surrounding tissues. However, PET/CT is changing such roles by integrating the information on tumor morphology provided by CT with those on its metabolism and, particularly, on the number of neoplastic viable cells. For modern radiotherapy, precise and accurate target delineation is an important step to achieve the delivery of a tumoricidal dose of radiation, sparing adjacent normal tissue.

Recently, the use of functional imaging to obtain an accurate biological delineation of the BTV has been proposed, and PET/CT has been described to be successfully used in RT to define the target volume and the treatment planning. The introduction of functional imaging into RT planning provides different information that may positively influence the treatment itself. In particular, PET/CT can reveal targets that are not detected by CT/MR morphological imaging; it can detect additional regions outside the tumor volume defined by CT/MR imaging or it can reduce the probability of malignancy of regions whose appearance at CT/MR imaging is 'uncertain' (e.g., atelectasic areas). In addition, functional imaging may show foci with increased biological activity within sub-regions of the tumor volume determined by CT/MR imaging. Sub-regions of the tumor may be selectively targeted at the molecular level. Of particular interest is the use of specific tracers studying specific biological parameters such as those for tumor hypoxia, angiogenesis and apoptosis. The identification of sub-regions of the tumor with specific biological behavior may be particularly relevant to obtain tumor-specific therapies (Grosu et al. 2005).

PET/CT has been described to significantly change treatment planning (22% to 64% changes in planning treatment volume – PTV) in a significant number of patients (22% to 100%) (Messa et al. 2005; Paulino et al. 2005; Nestle et al. 2005; Yaremko et al. 2005). Such modifications are due to changes in both N and M, but also in T staging. The use of the most recent PET/CT technology with improved image quality (sensitivity, spatial resolution, lesion detectability) combined with the use of the integrated information from PET and CT with or without contrast media are expected to further improve the detection rate of tumor extension, lymph nodal and distant metastases as well as the specificity of the signal, thus reducing the number of diagnostic investigations in patients who are candidates for radical RT.

As for monitoring the disease, response to RT treatment may be evaluated by PET when a persistent tissue mass is shown by morphological imaging by differentiating between viable tumor tissue and scar. However, after RT, PET may result falsely positive as radiation-induced inflammation accumulates with FDG. In fact, it has been frequently recommended that PET should not be performed until several months after the end of RT treatment. Nevertheless, as emphasized by Weber (2005), there is a surprising lack of data to support this recommendation. No data are currently available on the role of PET in predicting early response after RT in breast cancer patients. However, recent data on lung cancer patients (Erdi et al. 2000) are very promising, and the use of PET during RT or the early phases after treatment could be further implemented also in other neoplasms.

References

Abe K, Sasaki M, Kuwabara Y et al (2005) Comparison of ^{18}FDG-PET with ^{99m}Tc-HMDP scintigraphy for the detection of bone metastases in patients with breast cancer. Ann Nucl Med 19:573–579

Antoch G, Stattus J, Nemat AT, Marnitz S, Beyer T, Kuehl H et al (2003) Non-small cell lung cancer: dual modality PET/CT in preoperative staging. Radiology 229:526–533

Avril N, Dose J, Janicke F et al (1996) Assessment of axillary lymph node involvement in breast cancer patients with positron emission tomography using radiolabeled 2-(fluorine-18)-fluoro-2-deoxy-D-glucose. J Natl Cancer Inst 88:1204–1209

Avril N, Dose J, Janicke F et al (1996) Metabolic characterization of breast tumors with positron emission tomography using F-18 fluorodeoxyglucose. J Clin Oncol 14:1848–1857

Avril N, Rose CA, Schelling M et al (2000) Breast imaging positron emission tomography and fluor-18 fluorodeoxyglucose: use and limitations. J Clin Oncol 18:3495–3502

Avril N, Schelling M, Dose J, Weber WA, Schwaiger M (1999) Utility of PET in breast cancer. Clin Positron Imaging2:261–271

Bar-Shalom R, Yefremov N, Guralnik L, Gaitini D, Frenkel A, Kuten A et al (2003) Clinical performance of PET/CT in evaluation of cancer: additional value for diagnostic imaging and patient management. J Nucl Med 44:1200–1209

Baum RP, Przetak C (2001) Evaluation of therapy response in breast and ovarian cancer patients by positron emission tomography (PET). Q J Nucl Med 45:257–268

Bellon JR, Livingston RB, Eubank WB et al (2004) Evaluation of the internal mammary lymph nodes by FDG-PET in locally advanced breast cancer (LABC). Am J Clin Oncol 27:407–410

Bettinardi V, Pagani E, Gilardi MC et al (1999) An automatic classification technique for attenuation correction in positron emission tomography. Eur J Nucl Med 26:447–458

Bird RE, Wallace TW, Yankaskas BC (1992) Analysis of cancer missed at screening mammography. Radiology 184:613–617

Bombardieri E, Aktolun C, Baum RP, Bishof-Delaloye A, Buscombe J, Chatal JF et al (2003) FDG-PET: procedure guidelines for tumor imaging. Eur J Nucl Med Mol Imaging 30:115–124

Bombardieri E, Crippa F, Baio SM, Peeters BAM, Greco M, Pauwels EKJ (2001) Nuclear medicine advances in breast cancer imaging. Tumori 87:277–287

Buck A, Schirrmeister H, Kuhn T et al (2002) FDG uptake in breast cancer: correlation with biological and clinical prognostic parameters. Eur J Nucl Med Mol Imaging 29:1317–1323

Buck A, Wahl A, Eicher U (2003) Combined morphological and functional imaging with FDG PET/CT for restaging breast cancer: impact on patient management. J Nucl Med 44:78P

Crippa F, Agresti R, Seregni E, Greco M, Pascali C, Bogni A et al (1998) Prospective evaluation of fluorine-18-FDG PET in presurgical staging of the axilla in breast cancer. J Nucl Med 39:4–8

Crowe JP Jr, Adler LP, Shenk RR, Sunshine J (1994) Positron emission tomography and breast masses: comparison with clinical, mammographic, and pathological findings. Ann Surg Oncol 1:132–140

Dose Schwarz J, Bader M, Jenicke L, Hemminger G, Janicke F, Avril N (2005) Early prediction of response to chemotherapy in metastatic breast cancer using sequential ^{18}F-FDG PET. J Nucl Med 46:1144–1150

Erdi YE, Macapinlac H, Rosenzweig KE et al (2000) Use of PET to monitor the response of lung cancer to radiation treatment. Eur J Nucl Med 27:861–866

Eubank WB, Mankoff DA, Takasugi J et al (2001) 18-fluorodeoxyglucose positron emission tomography to detect mediastinal or internal mammary metastases in breast cancer. J Clin Oncol 19:3516–3523

Friedrich M (1998) MRI of the breast: state of the art. Eur Radiol 8:707–725

Fueger BJ, Weber WA, Quon A et al (2005) Performance of 2-deoxy-2-[F-18]fluoro-D-glucose positron emission tomography and integrated PET/CT in restaged breast cancer patients. Mol Imaging Biol 7:369–376

Goerres GW, Michel SC, Fehr MK, Kaim AH, Steinert HC, Seifert B et al. Follow-up of women with breast cancer: comparison between MRI and FDG PET. Eur Radiol 13:1635–1644

Grosu AL, Piert M, Weber WA et al (2005) Positron emission tomography for radiation treatment planning. Strahlenther Onkol 181:483–499

Hany TF, Steinert HC, Goerres GW, Buck A, von Schulthess GK (2002) PET diagnostic accuracy: improvement with in-line PET/CT system: initial results. Radiology 225:575–581

Jackson VP (1995) The current role of ultrasonography in breast imaging. Radiol Clin North Am 33:305–311

Jemal A, Murray T, Samuels A, Ghafford A, Ward E, Thun MJ (2003) Cancer statistics. CA Cancer J Clin 53:5–26

Kluetz PG, Meltzer CC, Villemagne VL et al (2000) Combined PET/CT imaging in oncology: impact in patient management. Clin Pos Imag 3:223–230

Kopans DB (1992) The positive predictive value of mammography. Am J Roentgenol 158:521–526

Landheer ML, Steffens MG, Klinkenbijl JH, Westenberg AH, Oyen WJ (2005) Value of fluorodeoxyglucose positron emission tomography in women with breast cancer. Br J Surg 92:1363–1367

Lardinois D, Weder W, Hany TF, Kamel EM, Korom S, Seifert B et al (2003) Staging of non-small-cell lung cancer with integrated positron-emission tomography and computed tomography. N Engl J Med 348:2500–2507

Leung JWT (2002) New modalities in breast imaging: digital mammography, positron emission tomography, and sestamibi scintimammography. Radiol Clin N Am 40:467–482

Mankoff DA, Dunnwald LK, Kinahan P (2003) Are we ready for dedicated breast imaging approaches? J Nucl Med 44:594–595

Messa C, Ceresoli GL, Rizzo G et al (2005) Feasibility of [^{18}F]FDG-PET and coregistered CT on clinical target volume definition of advanced non-small cell lung cancer. Q J Nucl Med Mol Imaging 49:259–266

Moon DH, Maddahi J, Siverman DH, Glaspy JA, Phelps ME, Hoh CK (1998) Accuracy of whole-body fluorine-18-FDG PET for the detection of recurrent or metastatic breast carcinoma. J Nucl Med 16:3375–3379

Moore NR, Dixon AK, Wheeler TK, Freer CE, Hall LD, Sims C (1990) Axillary fibrosis or recurrent tumor: an MRI study in breast cancer. Clin Radiol 42:42–46

Nestle U, Kremp S, Schaefer-Schuler A et al (2005) Comparison of different methods for delineation of ^{18}F-FDG PET-positive tissue for target volume definition in radiotherapy of patients with non-small cell lung cancer. J Nucl Med 46:1342–1348

Paulino AC, Koshy M, Howell R, Schuster D, Davis LW (2005) Comparison of CT- and FDG-PET-defined gross tumor volume in intensity-modulated radiotherapy for head-and-neck cancer. Int J Radiat Oncol Biol Phys 61:1385–1392

Pelosi E, Messa C, Sironi S, Picchio M, Landoni C, Bettinardi V, Gianolli L, Del Maschio A, Gilardi MC, Fazio F (2004) Value of integrated PET/CT for lesion localization in cancer patients: a comparative study. Eur J Nucl Med Mol Imaging 31:932–939

Quon A, Gambhir SS (2005) FDG-PET and beyond: molecular breast cancer imaging. J Clin Oncol 10:1664–1673

Santiago JF, Gonen M, Yeung H, Macapinlac H, Larson S (2006) A retrospective analysis of the impact of ^{18}F-FDG PET scans on clinical management of 133 breast cancer patients. Q J Nucl Med Mol Imaging 50:61–67

Scheidhauer K, Scharl A, Pietrzyk U et al (1996) Qualitative FDG positron emission tomography in primary breast cancer: clinical relevance and practicability. Eur J Nucl Med 23:618–623

Sloka JS, Hollett PD, Mathews M (2005) Cost-effectiveness of positron emission tomography in breast cancer. Mol Imaging Biol 7:351–360

Stafford SE, Gralow JR, Schubert EK et al (2002) Use of serial FDG PET to measure the response of bone-dominant breast cancer to therapy. Acad Radiol 9:913–921

Suarez M, Perez-Castejon MJ, Jimenez A, Domper M, Ruiz G, Montz R, Carreras JL (2002) Early diagnosis of recurrent breast cancer with FDG-PET in patients' progressive elevation of serum tumor markers. Q J Nucl Med 46:113–121

Tabar L, Duffy SW, Krusemo UB (1987) Detection method, tumor size and node metastasis in breast cancer diagnosed during a trial of breast cancer screening. Eur J Cancer Clin Oncol 23:959–962

Tatsumi M, Cohade C, Mourtzikos K, Wahl R (2003) Initial experience with FDG PET/CT in the evaluation of breast cancer. J Nucl Med 44:394P

Tatsumi M, Cohade C, Mourtzikos KA, Fishman EK, Wahl RL (2006) Initial experience with FDG-PET/CT in the evaluation of breast cancer. Eur J Nucl Med Mol Imaging 33:254–262

Townsend DW (2001) A combined PET/CT scanner: the choices. J Nucl Med 42:533–534

Tran A, Pio BS, Khatibi B, Czernin J, Phelps ME, Silverman DH (2005) ^{18}F-FDG PET for staging breast cancer in patients with inner-quadrant versus outer-quadrant tumors: comparison with long-term clinical outcome. J Nucl Med 46:1455–1459

Tse NY, Hoh CK, Hawkins RA et al (1992) The application of positron emission tomographic imaging with fluorodeoxyglucose to the evaluation of breast disease. Ann Surg 216:27–34

Utech CI, Young CS, Winter PF (1996) Prospective evaluation of fluorine-18fluorodeoxyglucose positron emission tomography in breast cancer for staging the axilla related to surgery and immunocytochemistry. Eur J Nucl Med 23:1588–1593

Vansteenkiste JF, Stroobants SG, Dupont PJ et al (1998) FDG-PET scan in potentially operable non-small cell lung cancer: do anatometabolic PET/CT fusion images improve the localization of regional lymph node metastasis? The Leuven Lung Cancer Group. Eur J Nucl Med 25:1495–1501

Wahl RL, Siegel BA, Coleman RE, Gatsonis CG (2004) Prospective multicenter study of axillary nodal staging by positron emission tomography in breast cancer: a report of re-staging breast cancer with PET study group. J Clin Oncol 22:277–285

Wang Y, Yu J, Liu J, Tong Z, Sun X, Yang G (2003) PET/CT in the diagnosis of both primary breast cancer and axillary lymph node metastasis: initial experience. J Rad Oncol 57:362–363

Weber WA (2005) PET for response assessment in oncology: radiotherapy and chemotherapy. Br J Radiol 15:2651–2657

Wechalekar K, Sharma B, Cook G (2005) PET/CT in oncology--a major advance. Clin Radiol 60:1143–1155

Weir L, Worsley D, Bernstein V (2005) The value of FDG positron emission tomography in the management of patients with breast cancer. Breast J 11:204–209

Wu D, Gambhir SS (2003) Positron emission tomography in diagnosis and management of invasive breast cancer: Current status and future perspectives. Clin Breast Cancer 4:S55–S63

Yap CS, Seltzer A, Schiepers C et al (2001) Impact of whole-body ^{18}F-FDG PET on staging and managing patients with breast cancer: the referring physician's perspective. J Nucl Med 42:1334–1337

Yaremko B, Riauka T, Robinson D, Murray B, McEwan A, Roa W (2005) Threshold modification for tumor imaging in non-small-cell lung cancer using positron emission tomography. Nucl Med Commun 26:433–440

Current Role of Bone Scan with Phosphonates in the Follow-Up of Breast Cancer

18

Lorenzo Maffioli, Luigia Florimonte, Luca Pagani, Ivana Butti, and Isabel Roca

CONTENTS

Abstract

Bone scintigraphy with radiolabelled phosphonates shows a high sensitivity in detecting breast cancer metastases. For this reason it has been considered the most useful tool for early diagnosing and monitoring the metastatic spread of breast cancer. In the past years, there has been wide debate on its impact on survival time, morbidity and quality of life. The results of some studies on the asymptomatic patients during follow-up have led to the adoption of an almost minimalist policy for breast cancer surveillance including only a few procedures (breast self-examination, history, physical examination, patient education on symptoms, and abdomen ultrasonography). The routine use of additional tests, such as tumour markers, chest X-rays, bone scintigraphy, and computed tomography (CT), has not been recommended, except in those cases with clinical suspicion or in patients at high risk of metastases. On the other hand, the early diagnosis of bone involvement may reduce the risk of skeletal-related events, thus leading to a significant improvement in quality of life and opening the options of the new therapy choices in order to plan more aggressive systemic treatments whose efficacy could have impact even on survival. Besides this, the recent development of nuclear medicine modalities, the evolution of PET and PET/CT systems has brought new elements of discussion in this area, since at present the depiction of skeletal metastases can be carried out with ^{99m}Tc-phosphonates and also with ^{18}F-PET, ^{18}F-FDG-PET, and ^{18}F-FDG-PET/CT . Therefore, the clinical problem today is not only when and whether bone scans should be used, but the question has also become which diagnostic modality can be used? In our opinion the choice of the modality has to consider different general and local factors such as the diagnostic accuracy, the availability, the economic costs, and so on. The most important issue is that every new diagnostic approach should be validated by large randomised prospective clinical trials with the goal to measure the effective impact on the course of the disease and on patient management. Nowadays, we do not have a sufficient amount of this kind of data, in spite of much clinical evidence that demonstrates the excellent sensitivity of bone scintigraphy in discovering skeletal metastases.

18.1 Physiopathology of Metastatic Breast Cancer

Metastatic bone disease is frequent in patients with advanced (and/or node-positive) breast cancer (Goldhirsch 1997; Kamby and Senegelov 1997). Osteolytic bone lesions are quite common in breast cancer, due to the predominant activity of the osteoclasts. After the diagnosis of bony metastases, the mean survival time generally ranges from 2 to 3 years (Martin and Moseley 2000). In this period they suffer from significant cumulative osseous morbidity and discomfort, mainly due to skeletal-related events, such as pathologic fracture, spinal cord compression, occurrence of bone pain (that requires palliative radiation therapy, radiometabolic treatments and surgery to bone) or hypercalcemia (Hortobagyi et al. 1998; Cook and Major 2001). Vertebrae are the most common site of spread, followed by the ribs, skull and proximal long bones (Mundy 1995), even if peripheral metastases account for 7% of cases (Corcoran et al. 1976).

18.1.1 Vessels and Metastases

Bone metastases result from hematogenous dissemination of cancer cells associated with complex interaction between metastatic cells and tissue. Batson et al. (1940) first described the evidence of a venous connection between vertebral veins and systemic circulation. Their model is representative of a network of longitudinal and valveless vessels, forming anastomoses with sinusoidal structures of the vertebral marrow and epidural venous channels. The absence of valves in these venous plexuses allows a double direction of the blood flow dependently upon the changes in hemodynamic pressure arising from the normal daily activity.

Other studies suggest that this network could involve other vascular districts. From this point of view, one could imagine the existence of a link between Batson's system and azygos and hemi-azygos systems and the internal mammary system, by means of thoracic wall veins (i.e., lateral and intercostals veins). This could explain the spread from breast cancer to bone (Morgan-Parkes 1995). A particular site of dissemination is the sternum: its involvement can result from local dissemination from a pathologic internal mammary chain (O'Sullivan and Cook 2002).

18.1.2 Natural History of the Disease

Valagussa et al. (1978) demonstrated that in most patients with axillary lymph-node involvement there is a progressive increase in the frequency of bone metastases during the first 10 years after mastectomy. Starting from an initial occurrence rate of 8.9% at 3 years, this value rises up to 11.2% at 5 years, and up to 14.4% at 10 years. So, as previously stated, skeleton is the most frequent site of metastatic spread from breast cancer. Bones are often involved by metastatic spread in about 5–10% of patients in the first stages. In advanced diseases, bone metastases may be detected in up to 70% of cases at autopsy (Coleman and Rubens 1987).

The Danish Breast Cancer Group demonstrated that this rate is still higher if one considers the distribution at the time of the first recurrence. In a population of 1,259 patients, they found that the bone metastases are present in one third of cases (Kamby 1990).

This can explain the interest in bone scintigraphy in the follow-up of breast cancer. In fact, even if the role of bone scintigraphy in the follow-up of breast cancer is still a matter of controversy, its role in every nuclear medicine department is of primary importance for oncological purposes. This evidence should suggest to the clinician to perform bone scan in the follow-up of women not only with advanced, but also with early breast cancer.

18.2 Bone Scintigraphy

Large clinical trials demonstrated that this procedure is very sensitive and, in skilled hands, can be also very specific. The adoption of technical guidelines can help in producing high quality images (Bombardieri 2003). Crippa and coworkers (1993) carried out a 10-year follow-up study involving 260 patients with 1,971 scans. They demonstrated that, in a dedicated center (such as the National Cancer Institute of Milan), bone scan shows a sensitivity of 98.2%, a specificity of 95.2% and a positive predictive value of 72.8%, while the negative predictive value approximates 100% (99.8%) (Table 18.1). This specificity is, obviously, increased, when the "pre-test" probability increases (e.g., in case of onset of bone pain). In a meta-analysis by Hamaoka et al. (2004), a combination of level II and level III evidence indicates that the detection rates of bone scan for skeletal metastases increase with the stage (Wickerham et al. 1984; Coleman et al. 1988; Kunkler et al. 1985; Khansur et al. 1987; Brar et al. 1993; Yeh 1995; Samant and Ganguly 1999; Koizumi et al. 2001) (Table 18.2).

Table 18.1. Characteristics of bone scintigraphy in the follow-up of breast cancer (from Crippa and coworkers, 1993, modified)

	%
Sensitivity	98.2
Specificity	95.2
Accuracy	95.5
Positive predictive value	72.8
Negative predictive value	99.8

Table 18.2. Detection rate of bone metastases by bone scintigraphy in breast cancer (from Hamaoka et al. 2004, modified)

STAGE	%
I	0.82
II	2.55
III	16.75
IV	40.52

In order to improve the specificity of the scintigraphy, in selected cases, a SPET study should be acquired in addition to the standard whole body scan. In fact, when a solitary doubtful uptake of the tracer is detected in correspondence with a vertebra, a SPET study of this area can result in particular usefulness. Keeping in mind the particular arterovenous vertebral anatomy, it is clear that the part of the vertebral body most frequently involved by metastasis is the posterior (Algra et al. 1992). Twenty to 50% of solitary spine lesions are due to metastatic dissemination, and 30–50% of patients do not present symptoms. These rates demonstrate that the only clinical analysis is inadequate to diagnose the presence of bone metastases. In a recent paper, Savelli et al. (2001) underlined the added value of bone SPET in solitary spine lesions, in order to differentiate degenerative disease from malignancy, obtaining results similar to those obtained by MRI studies (Fig. 18.1). However, MRI could be more effective in the early diagnosis of distant metastases. This is due to the following facts: (1) metastases often originate from red marrow, (2) MRI can visualize the cortical involvement and (3) scintigraphic evidence depends on the cortical infiltration that happens after the localization of disease into the red marrow. There is no doubt that, due to diffusion, high costs and the long time for a whole body study, MRI cannot be routinely used as a standard procedure for follow-up. Similar considerations can be made for CT and PET scans (www.senologia.it/foncam/). In particular, F-18 FDG PET (as discussed elsewhere in this issue), even if it is characterized by higher specificity and allows detection of both bone and visceral disease, still presents high costs and a relative geographic availability. Therefore, these procedures are used only as third level procedures when other investigations are not able to produce a final diagnosis.

It should be noted that (as discussed elsewhere in this book) FDG-PET is, in general, superior to bone scan in detecting skeletal metastases (Bury et al. 1998). However, the detection rate varies depending on the type of lesions (Table 18.3; Fig. 18.2) (Nakai et al. 2005).

This is due to the fact that Tc99m-MDP accumulation represents the osteoblastic reaction to cancer cells. The lack of ^{18}F-FDG uptake has been postulated by Nakai et al. (2005) to be related to the increased bone matrix and reduced cell density due to the osteoblastic proliferation.

The aim of follow-up in breast cancer patients is addressed to early detection and treating relapses and metastases. It is believed by both patients and clinicians that if a metastasis is detected when the tumor mass is small, there is a higher probability of obtaining a better control of the disease and a longer survival time. Under these conditions, an early diagnosis of tumor metastasis can allow an early treatment and, consequently, a better quality of life. The extent and site of disease at recurrence influences the response to treatment and determines possible changes in therapy planning. Some authors, however, believe that this is true for recurrent localized disease, and it does not seem to be true for established metastatic disease (Loprinzi et al. 2003). Improved survival is dependent on the time of diagnosis of recurrence (early diagnosis of disease), sites of metastases and the most adequate treatment (based

Table 18.3. Detection rate of metastases with bone scan or FDG PET (from Nakai et al 2005, modified)

CT type	BS	FDG-PET
Blastic	100%	55.6%
Lytic	70%	100%
Mixed	84.2%	94.7%
Invisible	25%	87.5%

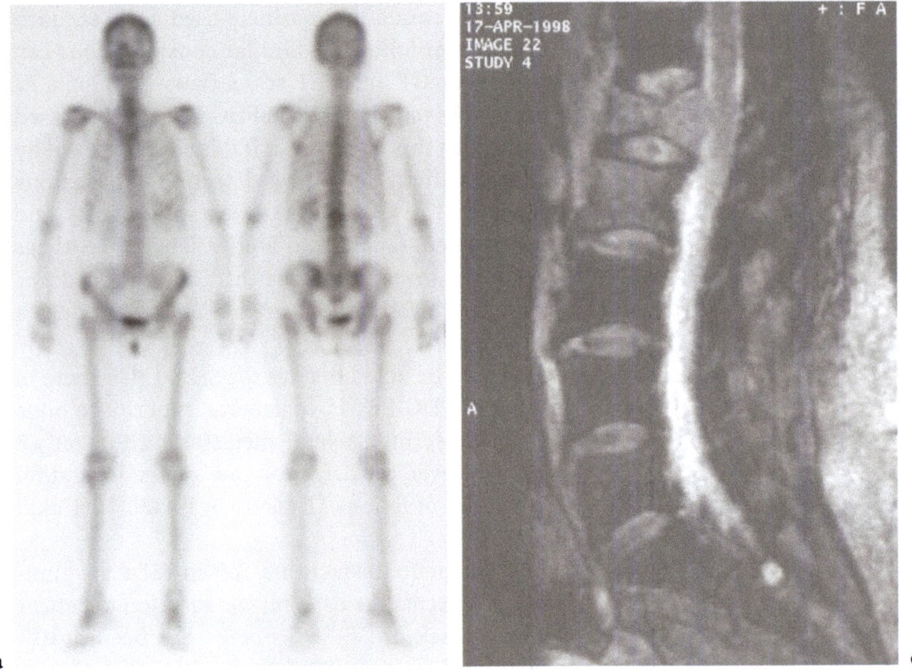

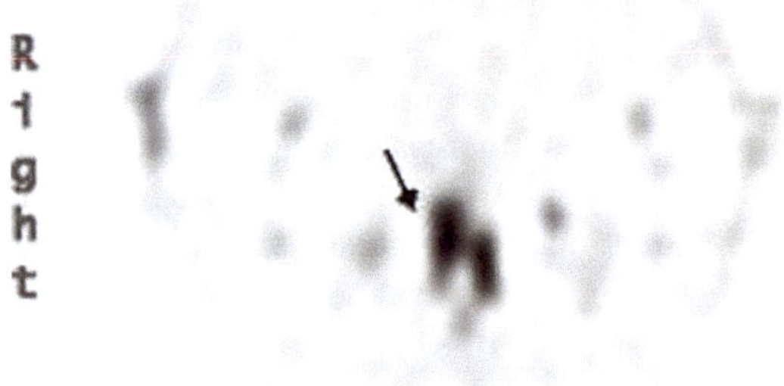

Fig. 18.1a–c. Some papers report that bone SPECT can improve the specificity of the scintigraphy (Savelli et al 2001). In this figure total body scan (**a**) shows an area of doubtful uptake in a lumbar vertebra, while the SPECT (**b**) indicates a pathologic accumulation of the tracer in the posterior part of the vertebral body and pedicles, as confirmed by MRI (**c**)

on site, extent, receptor status and several other variables) (Cocconi 1994). Furthermore, it has to be remembered that several patients may have asymptomatic lesions (59% of positive scans) (Crippa et al. 1993), and the scintigraphic diagnosis may precede radiological evidence by several months. This aspect is well known, because the bisphosphonate uptake depends upon the local blood flow and osteoblastic activity: therefore, the events evaluated and detectable by bone scan are the causes of the epiphenomena revealed by X-rays.

Moreover, the time on study and rate of occurrence of skeletal-related events (as stated above) in large series of patients are extremely variable.

An aid in the early diagnosis of tumor relapse can be the association of serum marker (such as CA 15–3) to bone scan, as reported in a study carried out in 864 patients at the National Cancer Institute of Milan. They demonstrated that the circulating levels of the marker are proportional to the number of metastases. The positive predictive value of the double test is greater than that of each test (Crippa et al. 1992).

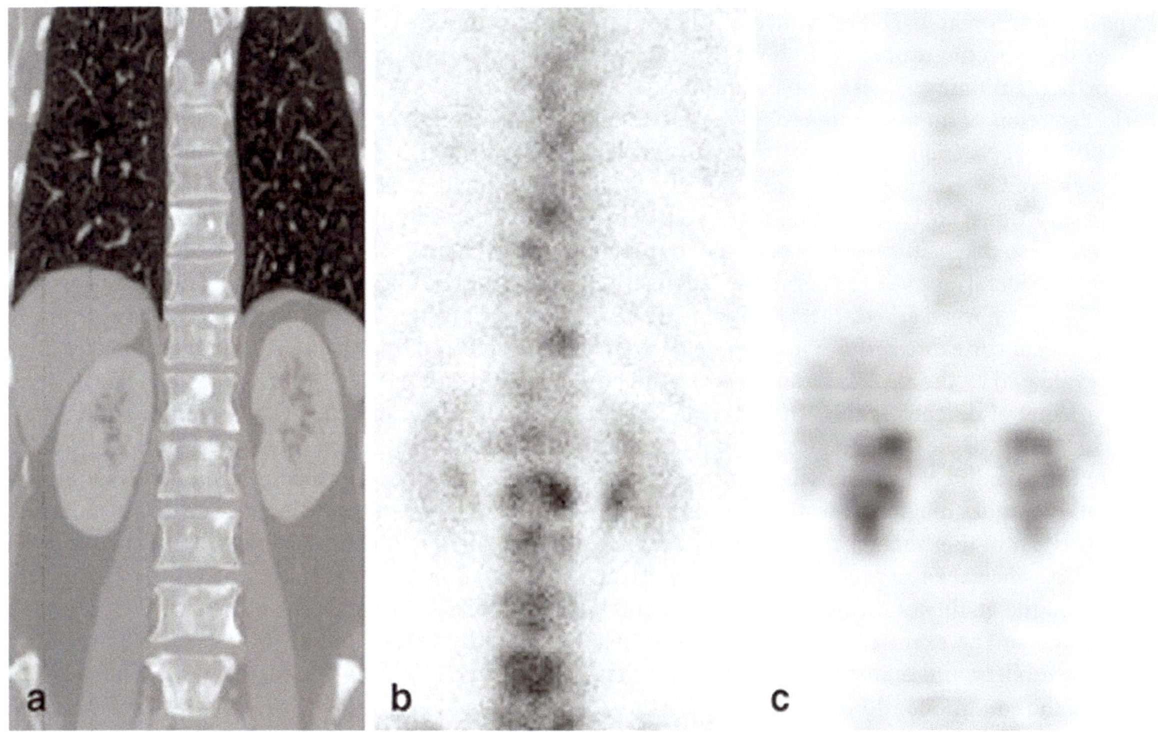

Fig. 18.2a–c. Some studies demonstrated that bone scan is superior to FDG-PET in detecting osteoblastic bone metastases. In this figure (from Nakai et al.2005) the CT scan in a 75-year-old female with bone metastases from breast cancer shows sclerotic areas in multiple vertebral bodies (**a**). Posterior view of a bone scan shows increased uptake in correspondence of these areas (**b**), whereas no pathological uptake of FDG is present in the PET study (**c**)

A similar study, performed in patients with equivocal bone scan, showed that CA 15.3-CEA-TPA determination has high value in revealing patients with bone metastases or at high risk of developing clinically evident bone metastases (Nicolini et al. 1999). More recently, Rajic et al. (2005) compared bone scan with CA 15.3 and the alkaline phosphatase serum level in 129 patients with breast cancer. They concluded that bone scans cannot be replaced by tumor markers because they did not correlate with the number of metastases. Thus, the determination of serum tumor markers alone cannot overcome the need to perform bone scans in order to detect skeletal involvement early (Bombardieri et al. 1997; Younsi et al. 1997).

18.3 A Minimalist Policy and the Guidelines

Since the early 1990s great debate has involved the oncology community regarding the intensity of the follow-up of patients with breast cancer. In the same issue of JAMA two papers explained the pros and cons of a minimalist policy for these patients (Schapira and Urban 1991; Wertheimer 1991). Against the minimalism there was the old position of the clinician that reflected the need for a wide study of the patient regardless of economic constraints. On the other hand, some important studies clearly demonstrated that an intensive follow-up does not improve the survival of patients with early breast cancer. They showed that there is no difference between detection of symptomatic and asymptomatic skeletal metastases, and there is no impact on the prognosis (at least after a follow-up period of 5 years) (Rosselli del Turco 1994). Moreover, the GIVIO study (Interdisciplinary Group for Cancer Care Evaluation) demonstrated that there is no difference in 5-year mortality between a large group of patients submitted to an "intensive" and another identical group submitted to a "minimalist" policy. It is to be noted that an intensive follow-up (bone scan every 6 months) can detect more bone metastases than does clinical follow-up alone (84 vs.

53 patients at 5 years). The relevance of the results of two retrospective studies with level III evidence is worth mentioning. These papers indicate that early detection of an asymptomatic bone metastasis allows a 14% improvement of overall survival at 4 years and 10% at 5 years (Komaki et al. 1979; Tomin and Donegan 1987). The GIVIO study demonstrated also that neither quality of life nor psychological considerations were better in the "intensive" group. Anyway, when asked, 70% of patients treated for breast cancer expressed the need to be periodically evaluated by the clinician and to be re-studied with a panel of diagnostic tests that included bone scan regardless of the presence of symptoms. From a psychological point of view, it is obvious that when a patient undergoes diagnostic tests (e.g., bone scan), she has a fear of the "sentence", but the reassurance that arises when the test proves negative is of great impact on the quality of life of the patient. A doubtful finding of the exam can be a problem. It can generate anxiety and fear until a further test that clarifies the condition is done. In order to minimize patient's anxiety and reduce the number (and costs) of additional testing, the nuclear physician should be, in some cases, more definitive in diagnosing the abnormality detected on the bone scan. Finally, in most cases, the same clinician needs the support of some examinations when in doubt (the GIVIO Investigators 1994).

So, to be realistic, a completely minimalist follow-up protocol cannot be carried out in clinical practice, even if also the last version of the American Society of Clinical Oncology (ASCO) guidelines strongly suggests reducing the procedures to be performed during follow-up to the minimum (www.asco.org). Concerning bone scan, ASCO guidelines that aim to determine an effective, evidence-based, postoperative surveillance strategy for the detection and treatment of recurrent breast cancer state that "the data are insufficient to suggest the routine use of bone scans" (Smith et al. 1999).

The ASCO guidelines have been made on the basis of the evidence. However, it is a common feeling that, at least in Europe, these guidelines are in practice not completely implemented, and, except for some very early breast cancer, the bone scan is routinely used in clinical practice for the staging and the surveillance of breast cancer.

The lack of evidence of usefulness of the bone scan is mainly due to an analysis performed on studies carried out regardless of a specific consideration of the impact of some diagnostic tools, such as scintigraphy, on the management of the patient. Since scintigraphy is characterized by high sensitivity, and, in skilled hands, high specificity, there is no reason to exclude it from the body of tests to be performed during the follow-up. To exclude bone scan from the follow-up test, one should admit that there is an inability of the clinician to effectively treat overt metastatic breast cancer. And this concept could be underlined by the statement that once the patients develop metastases they are essentially incurable and that the instrumental follow-up does not allow an earlier detection of metastases and does not affect the cure rate (Schapira and Urban 1991). These statements are based on the difficulty to establish the improvement in survival for patients with recurrent or metastatic disease, despite the important advances in supportive care and the introduction of several new antineoplastic or hormonal drugs. Fortunately, something has changed in the last years. Overall breast cancer mortality has been decreasing (-3.2% per year) from 1995 to 1999 (Jemal et al. 2003), and there is evidence that the prognosis for patients with recurrent or metastatic breast cancer is improving (Giordano et al. 2004).

Recently, the Swedish Cancer Registry reported the epidemiologic results from a comprehensive study of cancer survival in Sweden across 4 decades (1960–1998). The paper demonstrated that the expectation of life for a person diagnosed with cancer today is greatly longer than that of one diagnosed during the mid-1960s. The survival of patients affected by breast cancer improved during the 1990s (even if this period was shorter than that observed for patients with other tumors). The natural development of cancer, as well as the measures to fight the disease, can be long processes, which need rather long follow-up. The newest therapies determined a general improvement in survival and in disease control. Therefore, longer follow-up periods than the traditional 5 years are generally needed to evaluate the trend in survival. In particular for some tumors, such as breast cancer, 15–20 years after diagnosis seems to be an appropriate time for epidemiological purposes (Talbäck et al. 2003). Probably, this time is too long for a clinical follow-up, but today a 5-year period is to be considered a period too short to evaluate the impact of some procedures in the survival and quality of life. In this context, it is obvious that bone scans cannot be abandoned and are to be used to survey the state of bone in these patients.

18.4 Economic Considerations

The widespread economic restrictions in the western countries are one of the most important constraints to the extensive use of follow-up in medicine. Cost/benefits ratios and, more generally, cost effectiveness analyses are becoming a usual tools for the physicians. Therefore, it has to be taken into account whether a patient should undergo a medical procedure (in particular when the a priori probability of a positive test is low). When the reader faces the statements of a guideline that emphasizes the relevance of the economic problems, he/she should consider that, most often, several parameters can vary country by country. Thus, the social impact of the implementation of a procedure in the work up of the patient may be different and should be calculated for each individual region. To better explain this point, many readers can appreciate and agree with the paper by Wikenheiser and Silberstein (1996). However, in this study, the analysis was made in the USA, considering a cost of a total body scan of about 600€, but in many countries the cost is much lower (e.g., about 150€ in Italy and 90€ in Spain-Public Health Service). The same considerations can be valid considering, step by step, the cost of the physician, structure and, eventually, social impact of a delayed or missed diagnosis (Drummond et al. 1992). In fact, recently Hortobagyi demonstrated that patients with bone metastases who showed one skeletal complication had a higher probability to develop a clustering phenomenon with many events occurring closely in time (Hortobagyi et al. 1998; Major et al. 2002). However, the compliance with guidelines produces a reduction of the risk of over-prescriptions (Simon et al. 1996; Mille et al 2000). Therefore, these aspects are worthy of further investigations, with particular attention to the impact of bone scans in early and in advanced breast cancer, in order to integrate these results into the development of appropriate guidelines (Williams 1994).

18.5 New Trends and Bone Scan

Over the years many new therapies have been approved that can palliate metastatic breast cancer. With the introduction of these new drugs over the past years, post-recurrence treatment has changed; the survival and the quality of life of these patients have improved.

If there is an early diagnosis of bone metastasis, early aggressive treatments are possible and, to avoid skeletal-related events (SRE), treatment with bisphosphonate is indicated (Grenberg et al. 1996; Nieto et al. 2002; Hortobagyi et al. 1996; Hortobagyi 2002; Chen et al. 2003; Lipton 2003). Bisphosponates inhibit the osteoclast activity and reduce bone resorption (Riccardi et al. 2003). Moreover, the effect of bisphosphonates is hypothesized to be additive to the effect of antineoplastic drugs as adjuvant therapy. In fact, bisphosphonates can reduce the release of growth factors from microfoci of bone destruction: with this mechanism they could reduce bone absorption and decrease stimuli of micrometastatic breast cancer (Kanis 1995; Nemoto et al. 1987).

The International (Ludwig) Breast Cancer Study Group found, in a large series of patients (6,792), the incidence of bone metastases is higher in subjects with 4+ nodes positives (Colleoni et al. 2000). Among these, the cumulative incidence of bone metastases as first metastases was 12.2% after randomization and 26.8% at 10 years. If one considers the onset of bone metastases at any time as a possible target for therapy with bisphosphonates, the cumulative incidence raises up to 14.9% at 2 years and 40.8% at 10 years. However, also in node-negative patients the number of bone metastases is not negligible (202 of 1,275 patients). The ASCO Guidelines on the role of bisphosphonates in breast cancer conclude that this treatment is indicated in order to reduce skeletal complications (pathologic fractures, spinal cord compression and hypercalcemia) and their treatment (with surgery or radiation) for women with evidence of lytic lesions. Bisphosphonate as an adjuvant treatment is not recommended. Moreover, the ASCO suggests not to start bisphosphonates in patients with only non-osseous metastases, despite a high risk for future bone metastasis. The evaluation of the role of this treatment as an adjuvant setting in preventing bone metastases and to better determine their cost-benefit consequences are worthy of further research (Hillner et al. 2000). The ASCO, in these guidelines, states that to start the therapy with bisphosphonates it is necessary not only to have an abnormal bone scan, but also the evidence of a lytic lesion demonstrated by CT or MRI (even if the plain X-ray is normal). There is a general feeling reflected in the literature that leads some authors to raise criticism on the specificity of bone scans in detecting bone metastases (Hamaoka et al. 2004). The main drawback mentioned is the possible increase of osseous turnover by other diseases (trauma, arthritis, metabolic bone disease, osteomyelitis and osteoporosis). This aspect must be overcome. Based on widely adopted guidelines (e.g., SNM or EANM guidelines), it is mandatory to collect the most complete clinical information before any diagnostic procedure. An anamnestic report of a bone fracture or infection cannot be missed, and it is easy to interpret the scintigram. Similarly, arthritis is a focal process involving an articulation: this site is rarely involved in neoplastic dissemination, and in doubtful cases, a SPECT can be effective in the diagnosis, as previously discussed (e.g., a single hot-spot). Moreover, the recent introduction of hybrid cameras (SPECT-CT) can lead to a substantial diagnostic improvement. The data obtainable by single- or multi-slice diagnostic CT, integrated with a SPECT gamma-camera, are valuable not only for attenuation correction, but also as anatomic landmarks of scintigraphic findings coupled with a detailed morphology of the lesion (Even-Sapir 2005; Keidar et al. 2003).

A particular improvement could be achieved in case of small lesions when bone metastasis is near to physiologic uptake sites. It is our opinion that if this can be correct in some cases, it cannot be the rule due to the good characteristics of sensitivity and specificity of the scintigraphy in skilled hands.

In any event, for patients with high risk of skeletal involvement and/or bone pain, bone scintigraphy seems to continue to play an important role in selecting patients for further specific therapies, thereby reducing the risk of (and the cost for) skeletal-related events (Plunkett et al. 2000).

Another indication for bone scan is before radiometabolic treatment (as discussed in other parts of this issue) with radio-labeled bisphosphonates.

In this case, bone scan usefulness goes beyond the consolidated role to demonstrate the presence of osteoblastic metastases. In a favorable future of nuclear medicine therapies, correlation studies on efficacy or toxicity of a radiometabolic treatment will be based on the adsorbed dose rather than administered activity (Fig. 18.3).

The introduction of ICRU Report 67 (2001) "Absorbed dose specification in nuclear medicine" states: "The absorbed dose is used to correlate radiation-induced biological and clinical effects and is thus a fundamental quantity in radiation therapy, nuclear medicine and radiation protection." Then, with the need for treatment optimization, "patient specific dosimetry should be performed when radioactivity is administered for therapeutic purposes."

Moreover, it has to be pointed out that the Euratom Directive 43/97 on patient radioprotection stated that (article 4, comma 2) "for all medical exposure of individuals for radiotherapeutic purposes...ex-

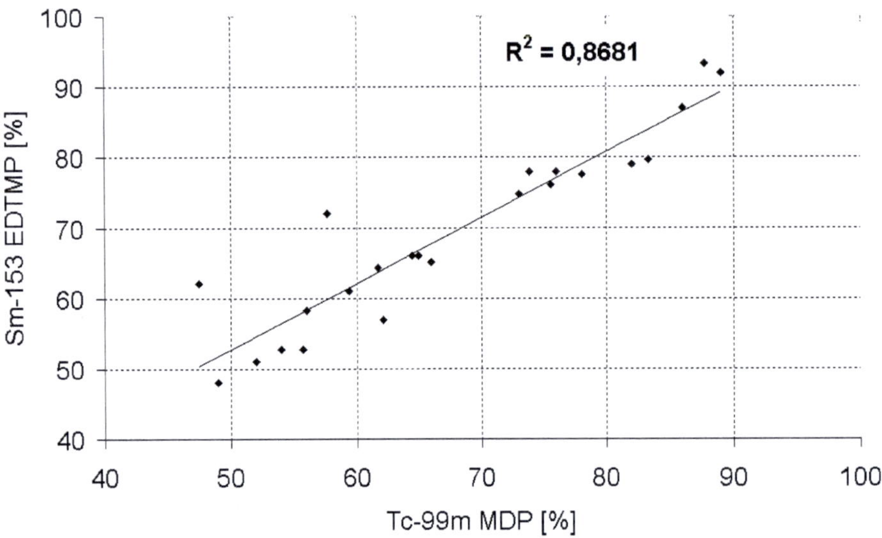

Fig. 18.3. Correlation between ^{99m}Tc-MDP and ^{153}Sm-EDTMP uptake in patients with bone metastases

posures of target volumes shall be individually planned; taking into account that doses of non-target volumes and tissues shall be as low as reasonably achievable and consistent with the intended radiotherapeutic purpose of the exposure."

In the treatments of painful bone metastases, efficacy and toxicity correlation studies should be done with dose to metastases and red marrow, respectively. The red marrow dose is proportional to skeletal uptake. Therefore, a provisional study to estimate skeletal and metastases uptakes of the radiolabeled bisphosphonates used in therapy allows the personalization of the radiometabolic treatment.

Some recent studies (Graham et al. 1999; Israel et al 2000; Kendler et al 2004), demonstrate that skeletal metabolisms of ^{186}Re-HEDP and ^{153}Sm-EDTMP are similar to that of technetium-99m-labeled bone scanning agents, such as MDP and HDP. These studies underline also the existence of a correlation between mielotoxicity and red marrow dose and efficacy and dose to metastases, emphasizing the great potentiality of bone scanning in treatment optimization.

A simple method to calculate red marrow dose in order to personalize ^{153}Sm-EDTMP administration is described in a recent work of Maffioli et al. (2005) performed in patients with bone pain from metastatic cancer.

Bone scintigraphy with ^{99m}Tc-Medronate (MDP) was routinely performed to verify the correspondence between bone pain and the presence of an increased uptake of the tracer into metastases within 1 month prior to radiometabolic treatment.

Additional early (10 min p.i.) and delayed (6 h p.i.) whole body scans were acquired with a double-headed gamma camera in order to evaluate the skeletal uptake and personalize the radioactive amount of ^{153}Sm-EDTMP for the treatment.

On the bases of the MDP skeletal uptake (Ut), the injected activity of Samarium was calculated in order not to exceed the 2-Gy red marrow dose constraint with this equation:

$$A(MBq)=(2\ Gy * 848.17\ MBq/Gy)/Ut$$

After therapeutic administration of ^{153}Sm-EDTMP, a double total body scan, 10 min and 24 h p.i., was performed to calculate EDTMP skeletal uptake (Us).

As shown in Table 18.4, the difference between Us and Ut was less then 5% in all patients but two. In these two cases, the error was higher than 20%. These subjects were the only two patients with a concomitant therapy based on zoledronate infusion. The remaining subjects had no third generation bisphosphonate treatment ongoing.

These data demonstrate that a double MDP scan is an appropriate and simple approach to preview Samarium skeletal uptake and, subsequently, the red marrow dose. However, particular attention must be made to concomitant third-generation bisphosphonate therapies that could impair bone uptake.

18.6 Conclusions

Bone scan represents a diagnostic procedure characterized by very high accuracy in the detection of skeletal metastases from breast cancer. Its role has been crucial for an early detection of metastatic dissemination to bone. At present, international clinical guidelines and some trials limit its use in the follow-up of asymptomatic early breast cancer, due to a lack of evidence of clinical impact (on survival, prognosis and quality of life) of this procedure (and others) in these patients. Bone scan has to be performed in patients with bone pain, in advanced breast cancer and whenever an osseous involvement is suspected, in order to minimize the risk of skeletal-related events. A new role can be played in planning new treatments (particularly with pamidronate, zoledronate, other bisphosphonates or new antineoplastic drugs). Furthermore, a scintigraphic follow-up of patients during treatment can be indicated in order to evaluate the response to conventional anti-neoplastic or hormonal therapy (even if, rather rarely and early after treatment, a flare phenomenon can occur) (Koizumi et al. 1999; Vogel et al. 1995; Cook and Fogelman 2001). Another indication of bone scan is prior radiometabolic treatment (as discussed in other parts of this issue) with radiolabeled bisphosphonates. Eventually, since this nuclear medicine technology can precede the radiological evidence of a metastasis, we would like to encourage the oncologist to proceed with more aggressive therapies on the basis of the only positive scintigraphy.

In conclusion, the clinical usefulness of bone scintigraphy has to be re-evaluated, possibly with large randomized prospective trials that could elucidate these aspects.

Table 18.4. Comparison between ^{99m}Tc-MDP and ^{153}Sm-EDTMP uptake in patients with bone metastases

Pt.	Age	Zoledronate	Ut%	Us%	%err Tc vs Sm
1	58	No	49.0%	48.0%	2.1%
2	67	Yes	47.5%	62.0%	-23.4%
3	73	Yes	57.6%	72.0%	-20.0%
4	67	No	82.0%	79.0%	3.8%
5	62	No	76.0%	78.0%	-2.6%
6	69	No	65.0%	66.0%	-1.5%
7	57	No	61.7%	64.3%	-4.0%
8	69	No	86.0%	87.0%	-1.1%
9	68	No	89.0%	92.0%	-3.3%
10	65	No	52.0%	51.0%	2.0%
11	68	No	73.0%	74.8%	-2.4%
12	44	No	54.0%	52.8%	2.3%
13	71	No	64.5%	66.0%	-2.3%
14	64	No	78.1%	77.5%	0.8%
15	70	No	56.0%	58.2%	-3.8%
16	58	No	75.6%	76.1%	-0.7%
Global mean			66.7%	69.0%	-3.4%
Mean without pts. 2 and 3			70.4%	71.1%	-1.0%

References

Algra PR, Heimans JH, Valk J, Nauta JJ, Lachniet M, Van Kooten B (1992) Do metastases in vertebrae begin in the body or the pedicles? AJR 158:1275–1279

Batson OV (1940) Function of vertebral veins and their role in spread and metastases. Ann Surg 112:138–149

Bombardieri E, Aktolun C, Baum RP, Bishof-Delaloye A, Buscombe J, Chatal JF, Maffioli L, Moncayo R, Mortelmans L, Reske SN (2003) Bone scintigraphy procedure guidelines for tumour imaging. Eur J Nucl Med Mol Imaging 30:BP99–BP106

Bombardieri E, Martinetti A, Miceli R, Mariani L, Castellani MR, Seregni E (1997) Can bone metabolism markers be adopted as an alternative to scintigraphic imaging in monitoring bone metastases from breast cancer? Eur J Nucl Med 24:1349–1355

Brar HS, Sisley JF, Johnson RH Jr (1993) Value of pre-operative bone and liver scans and alkaline phosphatase in the evaluation of breast cancer patients. Am J Surg 165:221–223

Bury T, Barreto A, Daenen F, Berthelemy N, Ghaya B, Rigo P (1998) Fluorine-18 deoxyglucose positron emission tomography for the detection of bone metastases in patients with non-small cell lung cancer. Eur J Nucl Med 25:1244–1247

Chen HHW, Su WC, Guo HR, Lee BF, Su WR, Wu PS, Chiu NT (2003) Clinical significance and outcome of one or two rib lesions on bone scans in breast cancer patients without metastases. Nucl Med Comm 24:1167–1174

Cocconi G (1994) Follow-up of patients with breast cancer (letter). JAMA 272:1657–1658

Coleman RE, Rubens RD, Fogelman I (1988) Reappraisal of the baseline bone scan in breast cancer J Nucl Med 29:1045–1049

Coleman SJ, Rubens RD (1987) The clinical course of bone metastasis from breast cancer. Br J Cancer 55: 61–66

Colleoni M, O'Neill A, Goldhirsh A et al for the International (Ludwig) Breast Cancer Group (2000) Identifying breast cancer patients at high risk for bone metastases. J Clin Oncol 18:3925–3935

Cook GJ, Fogelman I (2001) The role of nuclear medicine in monitoring treatment in skeletal malignancy. Sem Nucl Med 31:206–211

Cook RJ, Major P (2001) Methodology for treatment evaluation in patients with cancer metastatic to bone. J Natl Cancer Inst 93:534–538

Corcoran RJ, Thrall JH, Kyle RW, Kaminski RJ, Johnson MC (1976) Solitary abnormalities in bone scans of patients with extraosseous malignancies. Radiology 121(3 pt1):663–667

Crippa F, Bombardieri E, Seregni E, Castellani MR, Gasparini M, Maffioli L, Pizzichetta M, Buraggi GL (1992) Single determination of CA15.3 and bone scintigraphy in the diagnosis of skeletal metastases of breast cancer. J Nucl Biol Med 36:52–55

Crippa F, Seregni E, Agresti R, Bombardieri E, Buraggi GL (1993) Bone scintigraphy in breast cancer: a 10-year follow-up study. J Nucl Biol Med 37:57–61

Drummond MF, Bloom BS, Carrin G et al (1992) Issues in the cross-national assessment of health technology. Int J Technol Assess Health Care 8:671–682

Even-Sapir E (2005) Imaging of malignant bone involvement by morphologic, scintigraphic, and hybrid modalities. J Nucl Med 46:1356–1367

Forza Operativa Nazionale sul Carcinoma Mammario (FONCaM). Linee guida sulla diagnosi, il trattamento e la ribilitazione. In: www.senologia.it/foncam/

Giordano SH, Buzdar AU, Smith TL, Kau S-W, Yang Y, Hortobagyi GN (2004) Is breast cancer survival improving? Trends in survival for patients with recurrent breast cancer diagnosed from 1974 through 2000. Cancer 100:44–52

Goldhirsch A, Gelber RD, Castiglione M, for the Ludwig Breast Cancer Study Group (1997) Relapse of breast cancer after adjuvant treatment in premenopausal and perimenopausal women: Patterns and prognoses. J Clin Oncol ;6:89–97

Graham MC, Scher HI, Liu G-B et al (1999) Rhenium-186-labeled hydroxyethylidene diphosphonate dosimetry and dosing guidelines for the palliation of skeletal metastases from androgen-independent prostate cancer. Clin Can Res 5:1307–1318

Grenberg PA, Hortobagyi GN, Smith TL, Ziegler LD, Frye DK, Buzdar AU (1996) Long-term follow-up of patient with completed remission following combination chemotherapy for metastatic breast cancer. J Clin Oncol 14:2197–2205

Hamaoka T, Madewell JE, Podoloff DA, Hortobagy GN, Ueno NT (2004) Bone imaging in metastatic breast cancer. J Clin Oncol 22:2942–2953

Hillner BE, Ingle JN, Berenson JR, Janjan NA, Albani KS, Lipton A, Yee G, Bierman JS, Chlebowski RT, Pfister DG for the American Society of Clinical Oncology Bisphosphonate Export Panel (2000) American Society of Clinical Oncology guidelines on the role of bisphosphonates in breast cancer. J Clin Oncol 18:1378–1391

Hortobagyi GN, Theriault RL, Lipton A et al (1998) Long-term prevention of skeletal complications of metastatic breast cancer with pamidronate. Protocol 19 Aredia Breast Cancer Study Group. J Clin Oncol 16:2038–2044

Hortobagyi GN, Theriault RL, Porter L et al (1996) Efficacy pamidronate in reducing skeletal complication in patients with breast cancer and lytic bone metastasis. Protocol 19 Aredia Breast Cancer Study Group. N Engl J Med 335:1785–1791

Hortobagyi GN (2002) Can we cure limited metastatic breast cancer? J Clin Oncol 20:620–623

Israel O, Keidar Z, Rubinov R et al (2000) Quantitative bone single-photon emission computed tomography for prediction of pain relief in metastatic bone disease treated with Rhenium-186 etidronate. J Clin Oncol 18:2747–2754

Jemal A, Murray T, Samuels A, Ghafoor A, Ward E, Thun MJ (2003) Cancer statistics, 2003. CA Cancer J Clin 53:5–26

Kamby C (1990) The pattern of metastases in human breast cancer: methodological aspects and influence of prognostic factors. Cancer Treat Rev 17:37–61

Kamby K, Senegelov L (1997) Pattern of dissemination and survival following isolated locoregional recurrence of breast cancer: A prospective study with more than 10 years of follow-up. Breast Cancer Res Treat 45:181–192

Kanis JA (1995) Bone and cancer. Pathophysiology and treatment of metastases. Bone 17:S101–S105

Keidar Z, Israel O, Krausz Y (2003) SPECT/CT in tumor imaging: technical aspects and clinical application. Semin Nucl Med 33:205–218

Kendler D, Donnemiller E, Oberladstätter M, Erler H, Gabriel M, Riccabona G (2004) An individual dosimetric approach to 153Sm-EDTMP therapy for pain palliation in bone metastases in correlation with clinical results. Nucl Med Comm 25:367–373

Khansur T, Haick A, Patel B et al (1987) Evaluation of bone scan as a screening work-up in primary and local-regional recurrence of breast cancer patients. Am J Clin Oncol 10:167–170

Koizumi M, Matsumoto S, Takahashi S, Yamashita T, Ogata E (1999) Bone metabolic markers in the evaluation of bone scan flare phenomenon in bone metastases of breast cancer. Clin Nucl Med 24:15–20

Koizumi M, Yoshimoto M, Kasumi F et al (2001) What do breast cancer patients benefit from staging bone scintigraphy? J Clin Oncol 31:263–269

Komaki R, Donegan W, Manoli R et al (1979) Prognostic value of pre-treatment bone scan in breast carcinoma. Am J Roentgenol 132:877–881

Kunkler IH, Merrick MV, Rodger A (1985) Bone scintigraphy in breast cancer: A 9-year follow-up. Clin Radiol 36:279–282

Lipton A (2003) Bisphosphonates and metastatic breast carcinoma. Cancer 97 (3 Suppl):848–853

Loprinzi CC, Hayes D, Smith T (2003) Doc, shouldn't we be getting some tests? J Clin Oncol 21:108s–111s

Maffioli LS, Butti I, Florimonte L, Pagani L (2005) ^{99m}Tc-MDP double bone scan to predict the bone morrow dose from 153Sm-EDTMP. JNM 46 (Suppl 1):P1122

Major PP, Cook R (2002) Efficacy of bisphosphonates in the management of skeletal complications of bone metastases and selection of clinical endopoints. Am J Clin Oncol 25 (6 Suppl 1):S10–S18

Martin TJ, Moseley JM (2000) Mechanisms in the skeletal complications of breast cancer. Endocrin Relat Cancer 7:271–284

Mille D, Roy T, Carrère M-O, Ray I, Ferdjaoui N, Späth H-M, Chauvin F, Philip T (2000) Economic impact of harmonizing medical practices: compliance with clinical practice guidelines in the follow-up of breast cancer in a French comprehensive cancer center. J Clin Oncol 18:1718–1724

Morgan-Parkes JH (1995) Metastases: mechanism, pathways, and cases. AJR 164:1075–1082

Mundy G (1995) Metastatic bone disease. In: Fogelman I, Editor. Bone remodelling and its disorders. London: Martin Dunitz, p 104–122

Nakai T, Okujama C, Kubota T, Yamada K, Ushijima Y, Taniike K, Suzuky T, Nishimura T (2005) Pitfalls of FDG-PET for the diagnosis of osteoblastic bone metastases in patients with breast cancer Eur J Nucl Med Mol Imaging 32:1253–1258

Nemoto R, Uchida K, Tsutsumi M et al (1987) A model of localized osteolysis induced by the MBT-2 tumor in mice and its responsiveness to etidronate disodium. J Cancer Res Clin Oncol 113:539–543

Nicolini A, Ferrari P, Sagripanti A, Carpi A (1999) The role of tumour markers in predicting skeletal metastases in breast cancer patients with equivocal bone scintigraphy. Br J Cancer 79:1443–1447

Nieto Y, Nawaz S, Jones RB et al (2002) Prognostic model for relapse after high-dose chemotherapy with autologous stem-cell transplantation for stage IV oligometastatic breast cancer. J Clin Oncol 20:707–718

O'Sullivan JM, Cook GJR (2002) A review of the efficacy of bone scanning in prostate and breast cancer. Q J Nucl Med 46:152–159

Plunkett TA, Smith P, Rubens RD (2000) Risk of complications from bone metastases in breast cancer: implications for management. Eur J Cancer 36:476–482

Rajic MP, Bogicevic M, Ilic S, Vlajcovic M, Lilic G, Sekulic V, Lilic B (2005) Comparison of skeletal scintigraphy findings with levels of serum markers Ca15.3 with alkaline phosphatase (ALP) in breast cancer patients. Eur J Nucl Med Mol Imag 32(Suppl 1):P43

Riccardi A, Grasso D, Danova M (2003) Bisphosphonates in oncology: physiopathology bases and clinical activity. Tumori 89:223–236

Rosselli del Turco M, Palli D, Cariddi, Ciatto S, Pacini P, Distante V (1994) Intensive diagnostic follow-up after treatment of primary breast cancer. JAMA 271:1593–1597

Samant R, Ganguly P (1999) Staging investigations in patients with breast cancer: the role of bone scan and liver imaging. Arch Surg 134:551–553

Savelli G, Maffioli L, Maccauro M, De Deckere E, Bombardieri E (2001) Bone scintigraphy and the added value of SPET (single photon emission tomography) in detecting skeletal lesions. Q J Nucl Med 45:27–37

Schapira DV, Urban N (1991) A minimalist policy for breast cancer surveillance. JAMA 265:380–382

Simon MC, Miron S, Severson RK et al (1996) Clinical surveillance of for early stage breast cancer. An analysis of claims data. Breast Cancer Res Treat 40:119–128

Smith TJ, Davidson NE, Schapira DV, Grunfeld E, Muss HB, Vogel VG III , Sommefield MR for the ASCO Breast Cancer Surveillance Expert Panel (1999) American Society of Clinical Oncology 1988 update of recommended breast cancer surveillance guidelines. J Clin Oncol 17:1080–1082

Talbäck M, Stenbeck M, Rosén M, Barlow L, Glimelius B (2003) Cancer survival in Sweden 1960–1998. Acta Oncologica 42(7):637–659

The GIVIO Investigators (1994) Impact of follow-up testing on survival and health related quality of life in breast cancer patients. JAMA 271:1587–1592

Tomin R, Donegan WL (1987) Screening for recurrent breast cancer: its effectiveness and prognostic value J Clin Oncol 5:62–67

Valagussa P, Bonadonna G, Veronesi U (1978) Patterns of relapse and survival following radical mastectomy. Cancer 41:1170–1178

Vogel CL, Schoenfelder J, Shemano I, Hayes DF, Gams RA (1995) Worsening bone scan in the evaluation of antitumor response during hormonal therapy of breast cancer. J Clin Oncol 13:1123–1128

Wertheimer MD (1991) Against minimalism in breast cancer follow-up. JAMA 265:396–397

Wickerham L, Fisher B, Cronin W (1984) The efficacy of bone scanning in the follow-up of patients with operable breast cancer. Breast Cancer Res Treat 4:303–307

Wikenheiser KA, Silberstein EB (1996) Bone scintigraphy screening in stage I-II breast cancer: is it cost effective? Cleve Clin J Med 63:43–47

Williams A (1994) How should information on cost effectiveness influence clinical practice? In: Delamothe T (ed) Outcomes into clinical practice. London: BMJ Publishing Group p 99–107

Yeh KA, Fortunato L, Ridge JA et al (1995) Routine bone scanning in patients with T1 and T2 breast cancer. A waste of money. Ann Surg Oncol 2:319–324

Younsi N, Montravers F, Philippe C, Seddiki M, Uzan S, Izrael V, Talbot JN (1997) CA15.3 and bone scintigraphy in the follow-up of breast cancer. Int J Biol Markers 12:154–157

Progress in the Treatment of Early and Advanced Breast Cancer

19

Valentina Guarneri, Federico Piacentini, and Pier Franco Conte

CONTENTS

Abstract

Breast cancer represents a major health problem with more than 1,000,000 new cases and 370,000 deaths yearly worldwide. In the last decade, in spite of increasing incidence, breast cancer mortality is declining in the majority of developed countries. This is the combined result of better education, widespread screening programs and more efficacious adjuvant treatments.

The better knowledge of breast cancer biology nowadays allows sparing the cosmetic, physical and psychological consequences of radical mastectomy to the majority of breast cancer patients. The sentinel node technique is rapidly expanding and will further reduce the extent and the consequences of surgery.

Several clinical and pathologic factors are used to discriminate among patients at low (<10%), average (10–40%) and high risk of relapse, and international guidelines have been established to help clinicians to choose the appropriate postoperative treatments. Nodal status, tumor size, tumor grade, age and HER2 expression are universally accepted as important factors to define risk categories. Newer factors such as uPA/PAI-1, cyclin-E and other proliferative indices and the gene expression profile are promising and will allow a better discrimination among patients at different risk. Their generalized use is, however, not yet recommended because of lack of reproducibility, necessity of fresh tumor samples, limited data and follow-up. Endocrine manipulation with tamoxifen, ovarian ablation or aromatase inhibitors is the preferred option in case of endocrine-responsive tumors. Tamoxifen administered for 5 years has been considered for many years the standard treatment for postmenopausal patients; tamoxifen plus ovarian ablation is more effective than tamoxifen alone for premenopausal women. Recent data demonstrate that, for postmenopausal patients, the aromatase inhibitors are superior to tamoxifen with a different safety profile. At the present time aromatase inhibitors represent the preferred option for postmenopausal patients.

Chemotherapy is the treatment of choice in case of steroid receptor negative tumors. Polychemotherapy is superior to single agents, and anthracycline-containing regimens are superior to CMF. Six courses of FEC or FAC or the sequential administration of four doses of anthracycline followed by four CMF are the recommended regimens.

New regimens including the taxanes have produced a further improvement in risk reduction and are reasonable therapeutic options. These agents are currently approved for adjuvant therapy in the US and European countries.

Chemotherapy followed by endocrine therapy represents the standard adjuvant treatment of high-risk patients with endocrine responsive tumors. For Her2-neu overexpressing tumors, the addition of trastuzumab, a monoclonal antibody directed against the extra-membrane portion of the Her2 receptor, significantly reduced the risk of recurrence and death.

Primary chemotherapy is increasingly used in the treatment of locally advanced and operable breast cancer. The upfront administration of chemotherapy significantly increases the rate of breast-conserving surgery and allows an in vivo chemosensitivity testing. A proportion of patients achieve a pathologic complete response, and these patients have significantly better long-term outcomes.

Twenty-five to 40% of breast cancer patients eventually develop distant metastases. At this stage the disease is incurable; however, treatments can assure a significant prolongation of survival, symptomatic control and maintenance of quality of life. In case of hormone receptor positivity and in the absence of visceral, life-threatening disease, endocrine manipulation is the treatment of choice. Active treatments include tamoxifen, ovarian ablation, aromatase inhibitors, pure antiestrogens and progestins. Aromatase inhibitors are the most active agents; however, the choice and the sequence of endocrine therapies are also dictated by prior adjuvant treatment. Chemotherapy has to be preferred in case of receptor-negative tumors, acquired resistance to hormones and aggressive visceral disease. Combination regimens are usually associated with higher response rates and sometimes survival prolongation, and this approach should be recommended in young patients with good PS and visceral disease. On the contrary, single agents have a better tolerability profile and should be the treatment of choice when a careful balance between activity and tolerability is needed. In case of Her2-positive tumors, the combination of trastuzumab and chemotherapy is significantly superior to chemotherapy alone both in terms of response rates and survival. Other useful palliative treatments include the bisphosphonates for the control of the metastatic bone disease and radiotherapy for painful bone lesions or local relapses.

19.1 Introduction

Breast cancer represents the most common cancer in women in the world, with more than 1,100,000 new cases and approximately 410,000 deaths each year. In Europe, in the year 1998, there were 210,000 new diagnoses, and about 73,500 women have died because of breast cancer (Ferlay et al. 2004, 1999). However, in the last decade breast cancer mortality has been declining in most Western countries as a consequence of better education, implementation of screening programs and more effective therapies.

In this review we will summarize the state of the art in the management of early and advanced disease and will discuss the more promising research approaches.

19.2 Treatment of Early Disease

19.2.1 Locoregional Treatment

Breast cancer is a systemic disease, and the micrometastatic process can occur early, even independently from lymphatic spread. These biological considerations, earlier diagnosis and the availability of efficacious adjuvant treatments have drastically changed the surgical approach to early breast cancer. Several trials have shown that breast-conserving surgery followed by external radiotherapy produces local control and survival rates equivalent to those produced by radical or modified radical mastectomy (Veronesi et al. 1990; Jacobson et al. 1995; Fisher et al. 2005). Breast-conserving surgery must now be considered the standard surgical procedure for the majority of the patients; it is contraindicated in cases of macroscopic multicentric disease or positivity of surgical margins, and for all conditions exposing the patients to unacceptable risk from radiation therapy, such as early pregnancy, prior radiation therapy and collagenous disease (Kurtz et al. 1990; Park et al. 2000; De Naeyer et al. 1999). Relative contraindications to breast-conserving surgery are: high probability of subsequent breast cancer, as in BRCA1–2 mutation carriers (Pierce et al. 2000), poor cosmetic results, as when there is a high tumor-to-breast ratio, medial lesions or necessity of nipple-areolar complex removal. The extent of surgery can be further reduced with the increasing use of the sentinel node biopsy. Here again, well-designed and conducted trials have shown that in early stage disease, sentinel node biopsy is an accurate predictor of axillary nodal status and allows conservation of the physiological lymphatic drainage with no additional risk of local or systemic failure (Guliano et al. 1997, Krag et al. 1998). Recently published guidelines of the American Society of Clinical Oncology state that sentinel node biopsy is an appropriate alternative to staging axillary node dissection for early breast cancer patients with clinically negative axillary nodes and is associated with less morbidity. It is, however, reinforced that this procedure must be performed by experienced clinicians only (Lyman et al. 2005).

19.2.2 Systemic Treatment

19.2.2.1 Definition of Risk

Adjuvant systemic treatment significantly improves disease-free and overall survival in the majority of breast cancer patients, although the magnitude of the effect is greater in patients at high risk of relapse. Various efforts have been made to identify clinical and pathological factors able to discriminate low- and high-risk patients in order to avoid unnecessary treatments or underestimation of probability of relapse.

At present, internationally recognized prognostic parameters are: age, nodal status, tumor size, histological grade, steroid receptor expression, HER2-neu expression and presence of linfovascular invasion. Newer prognostic factors such as uPA/PAI-1, cyclin-E and other proliferative indices are not yet routinely used, even if there is enough evidence to support their potential role in discriminating between low- and high-risk patients, in particular in cases of node negativity (Spyratos et al. 2002, Lindahle et al. 2004). The impressive advances in the microarray technique now allow the rapid evaluation of thousands of genes with a single procedure. Initial data on the possible usefulness of gene profiling to identify patients at different risk of relapse or different sensitivity to anticancer drugs look very promising (Sorlie et al. 2001, Van de Vijver et al. 2002, Ayers et al. 2004). According to the 2005 Consensus Conference of St. Gallen, node-negative patients are categorized as low risk of relapse in the presence of all the following features: pT ≤2 cm, histologic and/or nuclear grade 1, absence of peritumoral vascular invasion, HER2-neu gene neither overexpressed nor amplified, and age ≥35 years. Patients without lymph node involvement are considered at intermediate risk in the presence of at least one of the following features: pT >2 cm, or grade 2–3 or presence of peritumoral vascular invasion, or HER2-neu gene overexpressed or amplified, or age <35 years; also patients with 1–3 positive lymph nodes are considered at intermediate risk in case of HER2-neu negativity. The high-risk category includes patients with four or more positive lymph nodes, or patients with one to three involved nodes and HER2-neu gene overexpressed or amplified (Goldhirsch et al. 2005).

Patients are also subdivided into three disease responsiveness categories: (1) endocrine responsive, (2) uncertain endocrine responsiveness and (3) endocrine non-responsive. The following sections will briefly summarize treatment options according to risk and responsiveness categories.

1. *Endocrine responsive patients:* This category includes patients whose tumors clearly express estrogen receptors (ER) and progesterone receptors (PgR), and for those it is reliable that the major benefit of disease-free and overall survival derives from endocrine therapy. In case of low-risk patients, hormonal therapy alone is recommended, while no therapy can be considered a reasonable option in case of contraindication to hormonal therapy. In patients with intermediate risk, hormonal therapy alone is considered appropriate as well as the combination of chemotherapy and hormonal therapy. For patients at high risk of relapse, the appropriate treatment is chemotherapy followed by hormonal therapy.
2. *Endocrine response uncertain:* Patients whose tumors have features suggesting uncertainty of endocrine responsiveness, such as low expression of ER, absence of PgR, HER2-neu overexpression or amplification, increased proliferation markers or high expression of uPA/PAI-1 are included in this category. Because any detectable HR is associated with some degree of endocrine responsiveness, these patients are candidates for hormonal therapy; however, the addition of chemotherapy is recommended for all the patients who are at intermediate or high risk of relapse.
3. *Endocrine non-responsive:* In the case of tumors without detectable expression of hormone receptors, chemotherapy alone is the appropriate treatment.

19.2.2.2
Endocrine Therapy

Endocrine options for steroid receptor-expressing tumors include tamoxifen, ovarian ablation/suppression, and, more recently, for postmenopausal women, aromatase inhibitors. Adjuvant tamoxifen has represented the standard of care for both pre- and postmenopausal women over several years. As reported from the last EBCTCG overview, which reported the 15-year recurrence and breast cancer mortality rate combining six meta-analyses of adjuvant chemo and hormonal therapy, 5 years of tamoxifen reduces the annual breast cancer death rate by 31%, irrespective of age, chemotherapy use and expression of PgR. It is also clear that 5 years of tamoxifen treatment are superior to 1 or 2 years; however, the use of tamoxifen beyond 5 years is not recommended because the increasing partial agonist effects on coagulation, the endometrium and breast cancer growth outweigh the possible benefits (EBCTCG 2005, 1998).

Ovarian ablation (OA) was the first example of systemic therapy for breast cancer (Beatson 1898). Permanent OA can be achieved with radiotherapy and surgical oophorectomy, while a temporary ovarian suppression can be achieved with gonadotropin-releasing hormone (Gn-RH) agonists. In patients with ER-positive or unknown tumors and less than 50 years at study entry, OA alone induces an improvement in 15-year survival (59.7% vs. 56.5%, 2p=0.004), and in recurrence-free survival (52.7% vs. 48.4%, 2p=0.00001) (EBCTCG 2005). Some studies have shown that OA is as effective as CMF (cyclophosphamide, methotrexate and 5-fluorouracil) in premenopausal patients with ER-positive tumors (SCTBG 1993, Kaufman et al. 2003; von Minckwitz et al. 2006; Ejertsen et al. 2006); however, there are no data comparing the effect of OA with anthracycline-based regimens. The addition of OA to chemotherapy does not improve survival as compared to CT alone, probably because the effect of chemotherapy by itself on ovarian activity might limit the benefit of ovarian suppression (EBCTCG 1996; Rivkin et al. 1996). In conclusion, OA can be considered an acceptable adjuvant treatment for premenopausal patients with endocrine-responsive tumors in case of contraindication to tamoxifen; if ovarian suppression is achieved with Gn-RH agonists, it should be maintained for at least 2 years even if data on the optimal duration of ovarian suppression are lacking. In intermediate- or high-risk very young patients, or for high-risk premenopausal patients who are not amenorrhoeic following chemotherapy, a combined treatment including tamoxifen and OA is a reasonable therapeutic strategy.

More recently, several large randomized trials have shown superiority of the aromatase inhibitors over tamoxifen in postmenopausal patients with endocrine-responsive tumors. Three different approaches have been tested: the upfront utilization of aromatase inhibitors, the switch to an aromatase inhibitor after 2 to 3 years of tamoxifen and the extended therapy with aromatase inhibitors following 5 years of tamoxifen.

The ATAC trial (Arimidex, Tamoxifen Alone or in Combination) evaluated tamoxifen or anastrozole or the combination of the two drugs for 5 years in more than 9,000 women. Anastrozole has shown a significant reduction in the risk of relapse, while the anastrozole-tamoxifen combination was not better than either agent alone. At a median follow-up of 68 months, the relative risk reduction with anastrozole was 13% (*P*=0.01) and time to recurrence was significantly increased (Baum et al. 2002; Howell et al. 2005).

The switch to aromatase inhibitors following 2 to 3 years of tamoxifen represents another interesting approach. The BIG 1–98 is an ongoing four-arm randomized trial, comparing the upfront treatment with (1) tamoxifen or (2) letrozole for 5 years, (3) tamoxifen for 2 years followed by letrozole for 3 years, or (4) letrozole for 2 years followed by tamoxifen for 3 years. At a median follow-up of 25.8 months, letrozole significantly prolonged DFS as compared with tamoxifen (Thurlimann et al. 2005).

In the IES trial (International Exemestane Study), which is so far the largest such study, switching to exemestane after 2–3 years of tamoxifen improved DFS as compared to 5 years of tamoxifen (Coombes et al. 2004). These results have been recently confirmed after a median follow-up of 58 months, at the last ASCO meeting. In particular, in ER+ or unknown subgroups, exemestane significantly reduces the risk of death (HR 0.83, *P*= 0.05) (Coombes et al. 2006).

A further confirmation of the superior efficacy of aromatase inhibitors comes from an Italian trial (ITA), where patients on adjuvant tamoxifen after 2–3 years were randomized to complete 5 years of tamoxifen or to receive 2–3 years of anastrozole. Here again, anastrozole induced a significant reduction in the risk of relapse (Boccardo et al. 2005).

The results of a meta-analysis including ITA, ARNO 95 and ABCSG 8 trials have shown a survival advantage for switching to anastrozole after 2–3 years of tamoxifen (Jonat et al. 2006). The MA17 trial has explored the role of extended adjuvant therapy with an aromatase inhibitor after tamoxifen. More than 5,000 postmenopausal early breast cancer patients were randomized to letrozole or placebo for 5 years at the completion of 5 years of tamoxifen. The trial was closed prematurely because of a clear benefit in RFS for patients receiving letrozole with a hazard ratio for the letrozole group of 0.57 (P=0.00008) (Goss et al. 2003). The updated results after a median follow-up of 54 months have confirmed the advantages in terms of disease recurrence for letrozole over placebo (Ingle et al. 2006).

In general, as compared to tamoxifen, aromatase inhibitors are better tolerated regarding the risk of endometrial cancer, vaginal discharge, vaginal bleeding and thromboembolic events; on the contrary, these agents are associated with higher incidence of muscle and osteoarticular pain, cardiovascular disorders and fractures.

In summary, these agents have become the treatment of choice for postmenopausal patients with receptor-positive tumors; however, their long-term side effects can be of concern. The best way of administration (upfront, sequentially after or before tamoxifen, for 5 years or lifetime) is still under investigation, and, to date, no comparative trial between the different aromatase inhibitors has been completed.

19.2.2.3 Chemotherapy

The majority of the data on the effects of chemotherapy on the risk of relapse and death derive from the EBCTCB meta-analyses (the Oxford Overviews), which include all randomized adjuvant trials conducted worldwide from 1985 (EBCTCB 1988, 1992, 1998, 2005). In particular, the 1998 overview revealed that poly-chemotherapy yields a significant improvement in both long-term disease-free survival (DFS) and overall survival (OS); the effect is greater in patients younger than 40 years (37% reduction in risk of relapse, 27% reduction in risk of death); however, this advantage remains significant even in patients aged 60–69 (with 18% and 8% reductions, respectively). The benefit derived from systemic chemotherapy is generally not affected by estrogen receptor status, even if the magnitude of the effect is greater for patients younger than 50 years and for hormonal receptor-negative tumors (30% versus 18%).

For patients older than 70 years, no definitive conclusions can be drawn, owing to the limited number of patients included in the studies. Nevertheless, combination chemotherapy remains a valid option for elderly patients with good PS and poor prognostic features in the absence of significant co-morbidities.

CMF administered for six courses over several years has been considered the standard adjuvant treatment; however, due to their clear superiority in the metastatic setting, anthracycline-containing regimens have been extensively studied as adjuvant treatment. According to the 2000 overview, about 6 months of anthracycline-containing regimens (e.g., as FAC or FEC) have shown a moderate, but significant benefit over CMF (recurrence rate ratio 0.89, P=0.001; breast cancer death ratio: 0.84, P<0.00001). The absolute difference in recurrence and mortality is about 3% at 5 years and 4% at 10 years. This benefit seems to be as great for older as for younger women (EBCTCB 2005).

More recently, results from three randomised trials of epirubicin-based chemotherapy have reinforced the superiority of anthracycline over CMF. The NCIC MA 5 trial compared six courses of FEC (5-fluorouracil, epirubicin, cyclophosphamide) versus six courses of CMF and showed that FEC yielded a significant improvement in both 10-year DFS (HR 0.69, P=0.005) and 10-year OS (HR 0.82, P=0.047) (Levine et al. 2005). At the 2003 ASCO meeting, the data of the pre-planned joint efficacy analysis of the NEAT and STCBG BR 9601 trials were presented, showing a significant relapse-free survival and OS advantage for the sequential ECMF (epirubicin plus CMF) over CMF (HR 0.69 for RFS, 0.65 for OS) (Poole et al. 2003). Six courses of FEC (with an epirubicin dose of 100 mg/m^2) or four courses of anthracycline (epirubicin 100 mg/m^2 or doxorubicin 60 mg/m^2) followed by four courses of CMF can be considered the best standard options.

19.2.2.4 Role of Taxanes

The taxanes, which represent the most effective single anticancer agents since the introduction of anthracyclines, have been tested in several randomized trials, exploring both the sequential and concomitant strategies. To date, the results from four large randomized trials are available.

The CALGB 9344 is the largest trial reported to date, with 3,170 node-positive breast cancer patients randomized to receive four courses of AC (cyclophosphamide plus doxorubicin) at different doxorubicin doses, followed by four additional courses of paclitaxel versus no further treatment. The fourth interim analysis, after a median follow-up of 69 months, has shown a significant reduction in both risk of recurrence and death, by 17% and 18%, respectively, in favor of the paclitaxel arm; no difference was reported according to the doxorubicin dose (Henderson et al. 2003).

The NSABP-B28 trial had a similar study design: four AC courses randomly followed by four doses of paclitaxel or no further therapy. The differences in comparison with the CALGB study were the fixed doxorubicin dose, the inclusion of patients at lower risk of relapse and the concomitant administration of tamoxifen to all the patients. This trial enrolled 3,060 node-positive patients between 1995 and 1998. The addition of paclitaxel significantly improved the hazard for a DFS event by 17% (P=0.006), while the improvement in OS was small and not significant (Mamounas et al. 2005).

The MD Anderson Cancer Center trial evaluated eight courses of 5-fluorouracil, doxorubicin and cyclophosphamide (FAC) versus four courses of paclitaxel followed by four courses of FAC (P-FAC) in 524 operable breast cancer patients. At a median follow-up of 60 months, the estimated 4-year DFS was 83% for the FAC arm and 86% for the P-FAC (P: 0.09) (Buzdar et al. 2002). More recently, in the GEICAM 9906 trial, six courses of FEC have been compared to four courses of FEC followed by eight doses of weekly paclitaxel in 1,249 node-positive breast cancer patients, showing a significant improvement in DFS (Martin et al. 2005).

Similar results have been observed with docetaxel: 5 years DFS was improved by three courses of FEC followed by three courses of docetaxel as compared to six courses of FEC, as shown in the PACS01 trial, which enrolled 1,999 patients (Roche et al. 2004). However, in a smaller series by far, the sequential administration of epirubicin, docetaxel and CMF (E→T→CMF) yields only a borderline improvement in DFS as compared to E→CMF (Bianco et al. 2006). In the BCIRG 001 trial, 1,491 node-positive patients were randomized to six courses of FAC or six courses of docetaxel-doxorubicin-cyclophosphamide (TAC). At a median follow-up of 55 months, there was a significant improvement in DFS (HR 0.72, P=0.001) and OS (HR 0.70, P=0.008) for the TAC regimen (Martin et al. 2005b).

In the ECOG 2197 trial, four courses of doxorubicin-docetaxel failed to show any advantage in terms of DFS and OS as compared to AC times four (Goldstein et al. 2005). On the other hand, four courses of docetaxel-cyclophosphamide have shown an improved DFS over four courses of AC (Jones et al. 2005).

A direct comparison of paclitaxel and docetaxel administered weekly or every 3 weeks has been performed in a large four-arm randomized trial. A total of 4,988 patients were randomized to receive four courses of AC followed by: (1) paclitaxel 175 mg/m^2 every 3 weeks times 4; (2) paclitaxel 80 mg/m^2 weekly for 12 weeks; (3) docetaxel 100 mg/m^2 every 3 weeks times 4; (4) docetaxel 80 mg/m^2 weekly for 12 weeks. No differences were observed in DFS comparing taxane or schedule (Sparano et al. 2005).

Currently, taxanes are approved for adjuvant treatment; docetaxel and paclitaxel can be considered equally active, and a taxane-based combination represents to date a reasonable strategy for high-risk patients. A sequential approach might represent a good balance between activity and safety.

19.2.2.5 Dose Dense and High Dose Chemotherapy

Ongoing research aims to increase the efficacy of chemotherapy by exploiting the dose-dense or high-dose concept. Recently, the dose-dense approach was evaluated by the CALGB C9741 Intergroup trial, which compared sequential doxorubicin (A), paclitaxel (T) and cyclophosphamide (C) with concurrent (AC) followed by paclitaxel (T). A total of 1,972 women with axillary node-positive breast cancer were randomized to four arms: (1) sequential regimen every 3 weeks, (2) sequential regimen every 2 weeks plus G-CSF, (3) concurrent regimen every 3 weeks and (4) concurrent regimen every 2 weeks plus G-CSF. At a median follow-up of 6.5 years, dose-dense treatment significantly improves disease-free survival and overall survival rates as compared to the 3-weekly regimens. There was no difference in either DFS or OS between the concurrent and sequential schedules (Hudis et al. 2005). However, when taxanes are not incorporated in the chemotherapy regimen, the results are not so encouraging. In a phase III randomized trial including more than 3,000 patients, sequential A every 2 weeks followed by C every 2 weeks failed to show the pre-planned 30% improvement in DFS as compared with concurrent AC every 3 weeks (Charles et al. 2002). More recently, dense FEC every 2 weeks has been compared to standard FEC every 3 weeks in 1,214 node-positive (less than 10 positive nodes) or high-risk node negative breast cancer patients. At a median follow-up of 10.4 years, no statistically significant difference in the hazard of recurrence or death was observed (Venturini et al. 2005). To date, dose-dense regimens might be a reasonable option for selected high-risk patients.

The role of high-dose chemotherapy in patients with early high-risk disease has been explored for many years, with disappointing results in the majority of the trials. A recently published analysis including 15 randomized trials comparing high-dose chemotherapy and auto-graft (2,535 patients) versus conventional chemotherapy (2,529 patients) has shown a statistically significant benefit in event-free survival for the high-dose group at 3 and at 4 years. However, this benefit is lost at 5 and 6 years, and no differences in terms of overall survival have emerged (Farquhar et al. 2005). High-dose chemotherapy remains an interesting research tool in selected very poor prognosis categories.

19.2.2.6 Trastuzumab

Between 20% and 25% of breast cancers overexpress HER2-neu, a receptor of the EGFR family; HER2-neu signalling plays a crucial role to sustain tumor proliferation, inhibition of apoptosis and chemotherapy resistance. Overexpression is defined as 3+ immunohistochemical staining (IHC 3+) or positive in situ hybridization (FISH positive). The availability of a humanized monoclonal antibody (trastuzumab) directed onto the external portion of this receptor has profoundly changed the treatment and prognosis of these patients. This agent, which has been approved for HER2-positive metastatic breast cancer since 1998, has been recently tested in the adjuvant setting, with exciting results.

Four large randomized trials have been completed and reported. The HERA trial is exploring the efficacy of 1 or 2 years of trastuzumab administered at the completion of adjuvant chemotherapy. To date, only data from the 1-year arm have been presented: at a median follow-up of 2 years, treatment with trastuzumab significantly decreases the risk of relapse (HR 0.64, $P<0.0001$) and death (HR 0.66, $P=0.0115$) (Piccart-Gebhart et al. 2005; Smith et al. 2007).The BCIRG006, the N9831 and the NSABP B31 trials are evaluating the role of trastuzumab administered in combination with chemotherapy. In the BCIRG 006 trial, the addition of trastuzumab to chemotherapy resulted in a significant improvement in DFS (Slamon et al. 2005). The joint analysis of the N9831 and NSABP B31 has shown an absolute benefit in DFS of 12% between the trastuzumab and the control group, with a 33% reduction in the risk of death at 3 years (Romond et al. 2005). More recently, the FinHer trial has evaluated trastuzumab administered in combination with chemotherapy for a very limited period (9 weeks), showing a significant improvement in the 3-year DFS for the trastuzumab arm (Joensuu et al. 2006). Despite the very limited number of HER2-positive patients randomized in this trial, which is a concern, these results raise the debate of the optimal duration of trastuzumab in the adjuvant setting, which is not a secondary issue taking into account the costs of this therapy, and the potential for cardiac toxicity. The results of the 2-year arm of the HERA trial will help to clarify this question. To date, trastuzumab is approved in the US and in the majority of European countries as adjuvant therapy for HER2-neu-positive breast cancer patients.

19.3 Primary Chemotherapy for Operable Breast Cancer

Preoperative systemic treatment was first introduced for locally advanced breast cancer, with the primary aim of achieving operability. In subsequent years, it has become widely accepted also in earlier stages. The up-front utilization of primary systemic therapy can allow for breast conservative surgery when up-front mastectomy would be recommended, or can offer a better cosmetic result in case of unfavorable breast-to-tumor size ratio (Bonadonna et al. 1990; Fisher et al. 1997). Moreover, this strategy permits an in vivo evaluation of treatment efficacy and allows the identification of subgroups of patients with different prognoses: the patients who achieve a pathological complete response (pCR) benefit most from the treatment and have an excellent prognosis, while those with residual breast and/or nodal disease after primary chemotherapy have a worse prognosis (Fisher et al. 1998; Pierga et al. 2000; Hennessy et al. 2005).

To date, several tumor characteristics have been identified as predictors of the probability of pCR: poorly differentiated tumors with a high proliferation rate and without expression of HR are more likely to respond to chemotherapy (Colleoni et al. 2004; Fisher et al. 2002; Guarneri et al. 2006).

Several studies have been performed to improve the rate of breast conservative surgery and of pCR, and to date the more promising results have been obtained with anthracyclines and taxanes, in particular with the sequential schedules (Gianni et al. 2005; Smith et al. 2002; von Minkwitz et al. 2005; Bear et al. 2006). More recently, preoperative endocrine therapy, which has been limited for several years to elderly patients unfit for chemotherapy with locally advanced disease, is becoming increasingly studied also in younger patients and in earlier stages. In fact, it has been clearly demonstrated that the likelihood of obtaining a pathologic complete response to chemotherapy is significantly lower in case of hormone receptor positive tumors. Therefore, endocrine manipulation may represent an attractive therapeutic option for these patients. As compared to tamoxifen, the aromatase inhibitors have shown superiority in both advanced and early disease, and have shown very interesting results in the preoperative setting (Eiermann et al. 2001; Smith et al. 2005).

To date, preoperative hormonal therapy with aromatase inhibitors can be considered a safe option for patients with endocrine-sensitive tumors not suitable for chemotherapy and a reasonable alternative to chemotherapy for aged or unfit patients. In younger postmenopausal patients with hormone receptor-positive tumors, this approach represents an interesting research tool.

It is, however, clear that primary systemic therapy represents the best scenario to test the new targeted agents for several reasons: the molecular target can be measured in the individual tumor at baseline and after treatment; the interactions between the targeted treatment and tumor biomarkers can be evaluated in vivo; the rate of pCR is a validated, early measure of treatment effect. The most remarkable results have been achieved by combining trastuzumab with chemotherapy in HER2-positive patients: as compared to chemotherapy alone, the addition of trastuzumab resulted in a more than doubled pCR rate (66.7% vs. 25%) (Buzdar et al. 2005).

In a randomized trial including patients selected for the expression of EGFR and hormone receptor, gefitinib monotherapy induced a tumor shrinkage in 54% of the patients, while the combination gefitinib+anastrozole vs. gefitinib alone resulted in a higher inhibition of tumor proliferation (Polychronis et al. 2005).

In conclusion, primary systemic therapy can increase the rate of breast-conserving surgery, assuring an outcome as least as good as compared to standard adjuvant therapy. Moreover, the achievement of pCR is a short-term surrogate marker for survival, and the observed response to primary systemic therapy can be helpful in selecting patients still at high risk of relapse, and thus suitable for further therapies. Because of the opportunity to collect tumor samples before and after therapy, and the possibility to observe the treatment effects on tumor biology in a relatively short time, this model represents the ideal model to develop treatment strategy including targeted agents.

19.4 Locally Advanced Breast Cancer

In spite of screening programs, about 10% of breast cancer patients are still diagnosed with a large (>5 cm) tumor size, skin or chest wall infiltration, and fixed axillary node or internal mammary node involvement. The definition of locally advanced breast cancer (LABC) includes disease that is either extensive within the breast and/or ipsilateral lymph nodes. Because the breast cancer staging system has varied over time, the LABC categorization slightly changes across different studies, including in some cases all the AJCC stages > IIB, while according to the EBTCG, the stages IIB-IIIA are considered early breast cancer. Historically, all cases not eligible for radical surgery were considered to be LABC. Inflammatory breast cancer (IBC) is defined clinically by erythema, skin warmth, peau d'orange and ridging in the breast skin, and pathologically by dermal lymphatic invasion. IBC represents a distinct clinical entity with different presentation, natural history and prognosis; however, it is usually included in this category because the therapeutic approach is similar. The management of LABC has evolved from a loco-regional treatment that included radiation therapy surgery to a multimodality approach with chemo-hormonal therapy, surgery and radiation therapy (Brito et al. 2001; Perloff et al. 1988; Bartelink et al. 1997). Even if data from randomized trials are scanty, the general consensus favors a preoperative chemotherapy with anthracycline or anthracycline-taxane combinations, followed by total mastectomy, axillary lymph node dissection and radiation therapy (Ueno et al. 1997). Conservative surgery can be considered for good responders. Postoperative adjuvant therapy includes hormonal therapy in cases of steroid receptor positivity. Further chemotherapy can be considered, taking into account the number of preoperative courses and the response obtained. For elderly patients or patients with significant co-morbidities, preoperative hormonal therapy is an acceptable option in the presence of steroid receptor positivity (Preeca et al. 1982). This multimodality approach has substantially changed the prognosis of these patients, with 5-year survival rates now in the range of 40–60% as compared to less than 10% with loco-regional treatments alone (Zucali et al. 1976; Hortobagy et al. 1988; Baldini et al. 2003). Novel targeted agents such as trastuzumab, lapatinib or bevacizumab in combination with chemotherapy are currently under investigation, showing very promising results (Montemurro and Aglietta 2005; Cristofanilli et al. 2006; Wedam et al. 2006).

19.5 Metastatic Disease

About 25–40% of breast cancer patients develop distant metastases during the course of their disease, while less than 5% of patients have metastases at the time of initial diagnosis. Median survival of metastatic breast cancer patients ranges from 2 to 4 years; the life expectancy is more prolonged for patients with limited metastatic disease (e.g., lymph nodes, skin and isolated lung metastases) or bone disease only, while patients with multiple visceral lesions or CNS metastases have a median survival ranging from 4 to 13 months.

In spite of therapeutic advances, metastatic breast cancer is still an incurable disease; therefore, a careful balance between treatment effects and tolerability must be taken into consideration. At this stage the disease is heterogeneous with respect to patient characteristics such as age, performance status, co-morbidities, prior adjuvant therapies and tumor features such as disease-free interval, site and extension of metastases, hormonal sensitivity and HER2-neu status.

Aims of treatment must therefore be tailored to individual patient needs: from survival prolongation to symptomatic control and maintenance of quality of life. The choice between endocrine treatment and chemotherapy is mainly dictated by the steroid receptor status; however, other factors such as performance status and relapse-free interval are important in the decision-making process. The availability of new active agents has produced a clinically meaningful survival advantage, as demonstrated by a recent analysis performed by the British Columbia Cancer Agency (Chia et al. 2003).

This study evaluated the effect on survival of population-based access to new chemotherapeutic or hormonal agents since 1990. A total of 2,145 patients were assigned to four cohorts based on the dates of introduction of new agents: paclitaxel and vinorelbine, docetaxel and aromatase inhibitors, capecitabine and trastuzumab. There was a statistically significant longer survival for more recent cohorts, showing that the access to new therapeutic agents results in improvement in survival.

19.5.1 Treatment Options for Hormone-Sensitive Metastatic Breast Cancer

Because of its effectiveness and the excellent toxicity profile, endocrine therapy is the treatment of choice in hormone receptor-positive metastatic disease; the possible exception is the case of life-threatening visceral metastases with impending organ failure, where chemotherapy can assure more rapid tumor shrinkage.

Several trials and clinical observations have clarified some important features of hormonal therapies: (1) response to one line of hormonal manipulation predicts the activity of further hormonal therapies, (2) prolonged disease stabilization (>24 weeks) is frequent and is as clinically worthwhile as tumor response and (3) combined hormonal treatments are not superior to their sequential use, with the possible exception of Gn-RH agonists plus tamoxifen for premenopausal patients. For many years the accepted standard sequence of hormonal therapies was tamoxifen followed by progestins and, in patients with prior response and slowly growing disease, a third line with aminoglutethimide, a first-generation aromatase inhibitor.

For premenopausal women, a meta-analysis of randomized trials comparing total estrogen blockade with Gn-RH agonists plus tamoxifen versus Gn-RH agonists alone suggested that the combined approach might result in an improved clinical outcome (Klijn et al. 2001). For postmenopausal women, the third-generation aromatase inhibitors, anastrozole, letrozole and exemestane, have shown a better tolerability and efficacy as compared with megestrol acetate (Buzdar et al. 1998, 2001; Kufmann 2000). More recently, the two non-steroidal aromatase inhibitors anastrozole and letrozole have been compared with tamoxifen as first line hormonal treatment. Overall, the data indicate that aromatase inhibitors are more active in terms of clinical benefit (which includes the objective response rate and the stable disease for longer than 24 weeks) and time to progression (Nabholtz et al. 2000). It is of interest that the steroidal aromatase inhibitor exemestane can still induce prolonged disease stabilization after failure of a non-steroidal aromatase inhibitor (Lonning et al. 2000). A further endocrine option is represented by the estrogen receptor down-regulator fulvestrant. This drug is a pure anti-estrogen and is therefore devoid of the partial agonist activity of tamoxifen on end organs such as the endometrium and vascular system. Two randomized trials have shown that fulvestrant is as active as tamoxifen as first-line treatment, and as anastrozole in postmenopausal patients with disease progression during endocrine treatment (Howell et al. 2004; Osborne et al. 2002). In particular, this agent has shown similar efficacy in patients with or without visceral metastases, and can provide clinical benefit even in heavily pre-treated patients (Howell et al. 2002; Perey et al. 2007). A recently reported study conducted in patients progressing on non-steroidal aromatase inhibitor has shown that both exemestane, a steroidal aromatase inhibitor, and fulvestrant, a pure antiestrogen, are equally effective, providing a clinical benefit in around 30% of patients (Gradishar et al. 2006).

In conclusion, for pre-menopausal patients, the optimal sequence of hormonal treatment is tamoxifen in association with OA until disease progression, followed by aromatase inhibitor, fulvestrant and megestrol acetate. For post-menopausal women the appropriate first-line treatment is an aromatase inhibitor. Upon failure of aromatase inhibitors, the other active endocrine drugs include tamoxifen, fulvestrant and megestrol acetate; however, the optimal sequence has yet to be established.

19.5.2 Treatment Options for Hormone Resistant/Refractory Metastatic Breast Cancer

Chemotherapy represents the treatment of choice for patients with hormone-resistant/refractory metastatic breast cancer; however, it must be considered the first treatment option for patients developing a rapidly progressive and life-threatening disease requiring a rapid reduction of tumor burden. Besides age and performance status, the main determinant of chemotherapy choice is prior exposure to adjuvant chemotherapy. Anthracyclines represent the most active agents, and anthracycline-containing regimens are more effective in terms of response rates, complete remission rates, remission duration and survival (Fossati et al. 1998). However, anthracycline regimens are increasingly used in the adjuvant setting; therefore re-treatment with anthracyclines, even if effective, is limited to patients exposed to low cumulative anthracycline doses and with a relapse-free survival after adjuvant chemotherapy of longer than 12 months (Gennari et al. 2004). The main limitation to anthracyclines is their dose-dependent cardiac toxicity; patients should not exceed the cumulative dose of 450–550 mg/m^2 for doxorubicin and 800–900 mg/m^2 for epirubicin, respectively (Pawan et al. 1998; Gennari et al. 1999). Conventional first-line regimens include two- or three-drug combinations such as doxorubicin and cyclophosphamide, EC, FAC and FEC.

In this context, new formulations of anthracyclines have been studied: for example, pegylated liposomal doxorubicin has provided comparable efficacy to doxorubicin with a significantly reduced incidence of cardiotoxicity in the first-line therapy of metastatic breast cancer (O'Brien et al. 2004). Besides anthracyclines, the taxanes represent the most active agents in the treatment of breast cancer. However, in the first-line setting, the randomized trials comparing anthracycline/taxane combinations versus anthracycline-based regimens have failed to demonstrate a clear advantage of the former: in most of the cases the anthracycline/taxane combination was superior in terms of response rate, but a progression-free or overall survival advantage was observed in only some of the trials (Nabholtz et al. 2003; Mackey et al. 2002; Bonneterre et al. 2004; Bontenbal et al. 2005; Sledge et al. 2003; Luck et al. 2000; Langley et al. 2005; Jassem et al. 2001; Zielinski et al. 2005; Biganzoli et al. 2002). The limited numbers of patients included in many trials, the use of suboptimal doses in combination and the activity of salvage chemotherapy may account for this inconsistency regarding the superiority of more aggressive versus less aggressive combinations or combinations versus single-agent chemotherapy. In order to overcome some of these limitations and to achieve a better estimate of the impact of new drugs/combinations, several meta-analyses have been performed. The results from these analyses clearly indicate that combinations are superior to single agents, that anthracycline regimens are superior to non-anthracycline combinations and, finally, that combinations including taxanes are better than non-taxane treatments (Howell et al. 2004; Ghersi et al. 2006). These results are in line with a retrospective analysis conducted in our institution on 640 patients with metastatic breast cancer enrolled in prospective clinical trials between 1994 and 2001. Multivariate analysis suggested that the epirubicin/paclitaxel (ET) combination was an independent predictor of progression-free survival (HR=0.61; 95% C.I 0.51–0.74; $P<0.0001$) and overall survival (HR=0.59; 95% C.I. 0.47–0.74; $P<0.0001$) and was associated with a 40% reduction in the hazard of progression or death (Gennari et al. 2005).

After anthracycline failure, the taxanes have shown activity, and several trials have demonstrated that single-agent docetaxel or a taxane combined with antimetabolites can produce significant time to progression or survival gain (Nabholtz et al. 1999; Sjostrom et al. 1999; O'Shaughnessy et al. 2002; Albain et al. 2004; Chan et al. 2005). All these studies have, however, shown that combination chemotherapy is significantly more toxic than single agents and cannot be considered the preferred option for all patients with hormone-refractory metastatic breast cancer. Several trials have demonstrated that the weekly administration of single agents such as paclitaxel, docetaxel or vinorelbine can assure an interesting balance between activity and tolerability (Perez et al. 2001; Zelek et al. 2001; Mey et al. 2003). A further advance in palliation comes from the availability of an oral fluoropyrimidine, capecitabine, with activity in anthracycline and taxane pre-treated patients (Blum et al. 2001).

Ixabepilone is a potent inducer of microtubule stabilization and has demonstrated efficacy in taxane-sensitive and taxane-resistant tumors and has also shown synergy with other cytotoxic agents (Lee et al. 2001). Results from phase II studies have shown a tolerable safety profile and evidence of objective responses in pretreated metastatic breast cancer patients (Low et al. 2005). It is clear from all these data that chemotherapy can provide survival prolongation, symptomatic control and maintenance of quality of life. The clinician must identify the most desirable end point of treatment for the individual patient and make the appropriate therapeutic choice accordingly.

19.5.3 Targeted Therapies for Metastatic Breast Cancer

The better understanding of the biology of breast cancer cells has led to the identification of newer potential target for anticancer therapy. So far, trastuzumab for the treatment of HER2 overexpressing tumors represents the most successful example of this strategy. In fact, about 25% of advanced breast cancers overexpress HER2-neu, a receptor of the EGFR family that is associated with poorer outcome. The availability of trastuzumab, the humanized monoclonal antibody directed onto the external portion of this receptor, has profoundly changed the treatment strategy and prognosis of these patients. As a single agent trastuzumab can induce a 30% response rate in HER2-overexpressing tumors and the addition of trastuzumab to chemotherapy as compared with chemotherapy alone is associated with a significant improvement in objective response rate, duration of response and overall survival (Sjostrom et al. 1999; Marty et al. 2005).

Many other new agents targeting receptors in the cancer cells or in the stromal cells are currently under clinical investigation in breast cancer. These include epidermal growth factor receptor (EGFR)-targeted agents and angiogenesis inhibitors.

Lapatinib is an orally administered small-molecule tyrosine kinase inhibitor that targets both EGFR and HER-2 receptors. Studies have demonstrated its activity as single agent and in combination with other agents in HER-2-positive patients whose disease was trastuzumab resistant. A phase III randomized trial evaluating vs. capecitabine alone in patients refractory to trastuzumab has shown a significant improvement in time-to-progression in the patients receiving lapatinib (Geyer et al. 2006).

Bevacizumab is a monoclonal antibody targeting vascular endothelial growth factor (VEGF). A randomized phase III trial comparing the combination of bevacizumab plus capecitabine vs. capecitabine alone in metastatic breast cancer patients previously treated with anthracyclines and taxanes has shown a significantly increased overall response rate without improvement in survival (Miller et al. 2005). On the other hand, the addition of bevacizumab to paclitaxel versus paclitaxel alone as first line therapy resulted in a significantly higher overall response rate and significantly prolonged disease-free survival (Miller et al. 2005).

19.6 Treatment of Skeletal Metastases

The large majority of patients with metastatic breast cancer will develop bone metastases during the course of the disease, with several complications such as pain, hypercalcemia, fractures, spinal cord compression and consequent deterioration in performance status. External radiotherapy, radiometabolic therapy, surgery and pain medications can control symptoms, but these treatments are not devoid of toxicities, and their effects are usually shorter than the disease course. Bisphosphonates, initially developed to treat malignant hypercalcemia, inhibit the osteoclastic recruitment and activation, and can induce apoptosis of cancer cells while interfering with their attachment on bone matrix. Several bisphosphonates have been approved in the United States and Europe for the treatment of breast cancer patients with skeletal metastases.

Pamidronate has been known to be effective since the early 1990s, following the results of two pivotal phase III randomized trials (Hortabagyi et al. 1998; Conte et al. 1996). In these trials, pamidronate significantly reduced the incidence and delayed the onset of skeletal complications as compared to placebo. The more potent bisphosphonate zoledronic acid has been directly compared to pamidronate. The results of this trial have shown that zoledronic acid was at least as effective as pamidronate; furthermore, the multiple events analysis, which accounts for the occurrence of skeletal complications and for time between these events, zoledronic acid was significantly more effective than pamidronate in the subset of breast cancer patients (Rosen et al. 2003).

Ibandronate is a single-nitrogen bisphosphonate available in both intravenous and oral formulation. The efficacy of ibandronate has been assessed in three placebo-controlled phase III randomized trials (Body et al. 2003, 2004a,b). Both the i.v. and oral formulations significantly reduced skeletal complications as compared to placebo and improved bone pain and patient quality of life.

More recently, the Cochrane Collaboration has conducted a review of randomized controlled trials of bisphosphonates in breast cancer. Twenty-one studies were included. Overall, i.v. bisphosphonates reduce the risk of skeletal-related events by 17% as compared to oral bisphosphonates, which reduce the risk by 16%. Zoledronic acid reduces the risk of skeletal-related events by 41%, compared with 33% by pamidronate, 18% by i.v. ibandronate, 14% by oral ibandronate and 16% by oral clodronate (Pavlakis 2005). The last American Society of Clinical Oncology guidelines recommend i.v. pamidronate or zoledronic acid for the treatment of documented skeletal metastases (Hilner et al. 2003).

References

Albain KS, Nag S, Calderillo-Ruiz G, Jordaan JP, Llombart A, Pluzanska A, Pawlicki M, Melemed AS, O'Shaughnessy J, Reyes JM (2004) Global phase III study of gemcitabine plus paclitaxel (GT) vs. paclitaxel (T) as frontline therapy for metastatic breast cancer (MBC): First report of overall survival (abstract). Proc Am Soc Clin Oncol 22:510

Ayers M, Symmans WF, Stec J et al (2004) Gene expression profiles predict complete pathologic response to neoadjuvant paclitaxel and fluorouracil, doxorubicin, and cyclophosphamide chemotherapy in breast cancer. J. Clin. Oncol 22:2284–2293

Baldini E, Gardin G, Giannessi PG, Evangelista G, Roncella M, Prochilo T, Collecchi P, Rosso R, Lionetto R, Bruzzi P, Mosca F, Conte PF (2003) Accelerated versus standard cyclophosphamide, epirubicin and 5-fluorouracil or cyclophosphamide, methotrexate and 5-fluorouracil: a randomized phase III trial in locally advanced breast cancer. Ann Oncol 14:227–232

Bartelink H, Rubens RD, van der Schueren E, Sylvester R (1997) Hormonal therapy prolongs survival in irradiated locally advanced breast cancer: a European Organization for Research and Treatment of Cancer Randomized Phase III Trial. J Clin Oncol 15:207–215

Baum M, Budzar AU, Cuzick J et al (2002) Anastrozole alone or in combination with tamoxifen versus tamoxifen alone for adjuvant treatment of postmenopausal women with early breast cancer: first results of the ATAC randomised trial. Lancet 359:2131–2139

Bear HD, Anderson S, Smith RE et al (2006) Sequential preoperative or postoperative docetaxel added to preoperative doxorubicin plus cyclophosphamide for operable breast cancer. National Surgical Adjuvant Breast and Bowel Project Protocol B-27. J Clin Oncol 24:2019–2027

Beatson GT (1898) On the treatment of inoperable carcinoma of the mamma: suggestions for a new method of treatment, with illustrative cases. Lancet 1898; 2:104–162

Bianco AR, De Matteis A, Manzione L, Boni C, Palazzo S, Di Palma M, Iacono C, De Placido S, Papaldo P, Cognetti F (2006) Sequential Epirubicin-Docetaxel-CMF as adjuvant therapy of early breast cancer: results of the Taxit216 multicenter phase III trial. Proc Am Soc Clin Oncol 24 (abstract LBA520)

Biganzoli L, Cufer T, Bruning P, Coleman R, Duchateau L, Calvert AH, Gamucci T, Twelves C, Fargeot P, Epelbaum R, Lohrisch C, Piccart MJ (2002) Doxorubicin and paclitaxel versus doxorubicin and cyclophosphamide as first-line chemotherapy in metastatic breast cancer: The European Organization for Research and Treatment of Cancer 10961 Multicenter Phase III Trial. J Clin Oncol 20:3114–3121

Blum JL, Dieras V, Lo Russo PM, Horton J, Rutman O, Buzdar A, Osterwalder B (2001) Multicenter, phase II study of capecitabine in taxane-pretreated metastatic breast carcinoma patients. Cancer 92:1759–1768

Boccardo F, Rubagotti A, Puntoni M et al (2005) Switching to anastrozole versus continued tamoxifen treatment of early breast cancer: preliminary results of the Italian tamoxifen anastrozole trial. J Clin Oncol 23:5138–5147

Body JJ, Diel IJ, Lichinitser MR et al (2003) Intravenous ibandronate reduces the incidence of skeletal complications in patients with breast cancer and bone metastases. Ann Oncol 14:1399–1405

Body JJ, Diel IJ, Lichinitser MR et al (2004a) Oral ibandronate reduces the risk of skeletal complications in breast cancer patients with metastatic bone disease: results from two randomised, placebo-controlled phase III studies. Br J Cancer 90:1133–1137

Body JJ, Diel IJ , Bell R et al (2004b) Oral ibandronate improves bone pain and preserves quality of life in patients with skeletal metastases due to breast cancer. Pain 111:306–312

Bonadonna G, Veronesi U, Brambilla C et al (1990) Primary chemotherapy to avoid mastectomy in tumors with diameters of three centimeters or more. J Natl Cancer Inst 82:1539–1545

Bonneterre J, Buzdar A, Nabholtz JM, Robertson JF, Thurlimann B, von Euler M, Sahmoud T, Webster A, Steinberg M (2001) Anastrozole is superior to tamoxifen as first-line therapy in hormone receptor positive advanced breast carcinoma. Cancer 92:2247–2258

Bonneterre J, Dieras V, Tubiana-Hulin M, Bougnoux P, Bonneterre ME, Delozier T,Mayer F, Culine S, Dohoulou N, Bendahmane B (2004) Phase II multicentre randomised study of docetaxel plus epirubicin vs 5-fluorouracil plus epirubicin and cyclophosphamide in metastatic breast cancer. Br J Cancer 91:1466–1471

Bontenbal M, Creemers GJ, Braun HJ, de Boer AC, Janssen JT, Leys RB, Ruit JB, Goey SH, van der Velden PC, Kerkhofs LG, Schothorst KL, Schmitz PI, Bokma HJ,Verweij J, Seynaeve C (2005) Phase II to III study comparing doxorubicin and docetaxel with fluorouracil, doxorubicin, and cyclophosphamide as first-line chemotherapy in patients with metastatic breast cancer: results of a Dutch Community Setting Trial for the Clinical Trial Group of the Comprehensive Cancer Centre. J Clin Oncol 23:7081–7088

Brito RA, Valero V, Buzdar AU, Booser DJ, Ames F, Strom E, Ross M, Theriault RL, Frye D, Kau SW, Asmar L, McNeese M, Singletary SE, Hortobagyi GN (2001) Long-term results of combined-modality therapy for locally advanced breast cancer with ipsilateral supraclavicular metastases: The University of Texas M.D. Anderson Cancer Center experience. J Clin Oncol 19:628–633

Buzdar AU, Jonat W, Howell A et al (1998) Anastrozole versus megestrol acetate in the treatment of postmenopausal women with advanced breast carcinoma: results of a survival update based on a combined analysis of data from two mature phase III trials. Arimidex Study Group Cancer 83:1142–1152

Buzdar A, Douma J, Davidson N, Elledge R, Morgan M, Smith R, Porter L, Nabholtz J, Xiang X, Brady C (2001) Phase III, multicenter, double-blind, randomized study of letrozole, an aromatase inhibitor, for advanced breast cancer versus megestrol acetate. J Clin Oncol 19:3357–3366

Buzdar AU, Singletary SE, Valero V et al (2002) Evaluation of paclitaxel in adjuvant chemotherapy for patients with operable breast cancer: preliminary data of a prospective randomized trial. Clin Cancer Res 8:1073–1079

Buzdar AU, Ibrahim NK, Francis D et al (2005) Significantly higher pathologic complete remission rate after neoadjuvant therapy with trastuzumab, paclitaxel, and epirubicin chemotherapy: results of a randomized trial in human epidermal growth factor receptor 2-positive operable breast cancer. J Clin Oncol 23:3676–3685

Chan S, Romieu G, Huober J, Delozier T, Tubiana-Hulin M, Lluch M, Schneeweiss A, Llombart A, Carrasco E, Fumoleau P (2005) Gemcitabine plus docetaxel (GD) versus capecitabine plus docetaxel (CD) for anthracycline-pretreated metastatic breast cancer (MBC) patients (pts): Results of a European phase III study. Proc Am Soc Clin Oncol 23:581

Chia SKL, Speers C, Kang A, D'Yachkova Y, Malfair Taylor S, Barnett J, Coldman A, Gelmon K, Olivotto I (2003) The impact of new chemotherapeutic and hormonal agents on the survival of women with metastatic breast cancer (MBC) in a population based cohort. Proc Am Soc Clin Oncol 22 (abstract 22)

Colleoni M, Viale G, Zahrieh D et al (2004) Chemotherapy is more effective in patients with breast cancer not expressing steroid hormone receptors: a study of preoperative treatment. Clin Cancer Res 10:6622–6628

Conte PF, Latreille J, Mauriac L, Calabresi F, Santos R, Campos D, Bonneterre J, Francini G, Ford JM (1996) Delay in progression of bone metastases in breast cancer patients treated with intravenous pamidronate: results from a multinational randomized controlled trial. The Aredia Multinational Cooperative Group. J Clin Oncol 14:2552–2559

Coombes RC, Hall E, Gibson LJ et al (2004) A randomized trial of exemestane after 2 to 3 years of tamoxifen therapy in postmenopausal women with primary breast cancer. N Engl J Med 350:1081–1092

Coombes RC, Paridaens R, Jassem J et al (2006) First mature analysis of the Intergroup Exemestane Study. Proc Am Soc Clin Oncol, Part I. Vol 24, No. 18S (abstract LBA527)

Cristofanilli M, Boussen H, Baselga J et al (2006) A phase II combination study of lapatinib and paclitaxel as a neoadjuvant therapy in patients with newly diagnosed inflammatory breast cancer (IBC). Breast Cancer Res Treat 100 (abstract 1)

De Naeyer B, De Meerleer G, Braems S, Vakaet L, Huys J (1999) Collagen vascular diseases and radiation therapy: A critical review. Int J Radiat Oncol Biol Phys 44:975–980

Early Breast Cancer Trialists Collaborative Group (1988) Effects of adjuvant tamoxifen and of cytotoxic therapy on mortality in early breast cancer: an overview of 61 randomised trials among 28,896 women. N Engl J Med 319:1681–1692

Early Breast Cancer Trialists Collaborative Group (1992) Systemic treatment of early breast cancer by hormonal, cytotoxic, or immune therapy: 133 randomised trials involving 31,000 recurrences and 24,000 deaths among 75,000 women. Lancet 339:71–85

Early Breast Cancer Trialists Collaborative Group (1996) Ovarian ablation in early breast cancer: overview of the randomised trials. Lancet 348:1189–1196

Early Breast Cancer Trialists Group (1998a) Polychemotherapy for early breast cancer; an overview of the randomised trials. Lancet 352:930–942

Early Breast Cancer Trialists Group (1998b) Tamoxifen for early breast cancer: an overview of randomised trials. Lancet 351:1451–1467

Early Breast Cancer Trialists' Collaborative Group (EBCTCG) (2005) Effects of chemotherapy and hormonal therapy for early breast cancer on recurrence and 15-year survival: an overview of the randomised trials. Lancet 365:1687–1717

Eiermann W, Paepke S, Appfelstaedt J et al (2001) Preoperative treatment of postmenopausal breast cancer patients with letrozole: a randomized double-blind multicenter study. Ann Oncol 12:1527–1532

Ejlertsen B, Mouridsen HT, Jensen M et al (2006) Similar efficacy for ovarian ablation compared with cyclophosphamide, methotrexate, and fluorouracil: from a randomized comparison of premenopausal patients with node-positive breast cancer. J Clin Oncol 24:4956–4962

Farquhar C, Marjoribanks J, Basser R, Lethaby A (2005) High dose chemotherapy and autologous bone marrow or stem cell transplantation versus conventional chemotherapy for women with early poor prognosis breast cancer (Review). Cochrane Database Syst Rev (3): CD003139

Ferlay J, Bray F, Sankila R, Parkin DM (1999) EUCAN: Cancer incidence, mortality and prevalence in the European Union 1998, version 5.0. IARC Cancer Base No. 4, IARCPress, Lyon

Ferlay J, Bray F, Pisani P, Parkin DM (2004) GLOBOCAN 2002: Cancer incidence, mortality and prevalence worldwide. IARC Cancer Base No. 5. version 2.0, IARCPress, Lyon

Fisher B, Anderson S, Redmond CK, Wolmark N, Wickerham DL, Cronin WM (1995) Reanalysis and results after 12 years of follow-up in a randomized clinical trial comparing total mastectomy with lumpectomy with or without irradiation in the treatment of breast cancer. N Engl J Med 333:1456–1461

Fisher B, Brown A, Mamounas E et al (1997) Effect of preoperative chemotherapy on local-regional disease in women with operable breast cancer: findings from National Surgical Adjuvant Breast and Bowel Project B-18. J Clin Oncol 15:2483–2493

Fisher B, Bryant J, Wolmark N et al (1998) Effect of preoperative chemotherapy on the outcome of women with operable breast cancer. J Clin Oncol 16:2672–2685

Fisher ER, Wang J, Bryant J et al (2002) Pathobiology of preoperative chemotherapy: findings from the National Surgical Adjuvant Breast and Bowel (NSABP) protocol B-18. Cancer 95:681–695

Fossati R, Confalonieri C, Torri V, Ghislandi E, Penna A, Pistotti V, Tinazzi A, Liberati A (1998) Cytotoxic and hormonal treatment for metastatic breast cancer: a systematic review of published randomized trials involving 31,510 women. J Clin Oncol 16:3439–3460

Gennari A, Salvadori B, Donati S, Bengala C, Orlandini C, Danesi R, Del Tacca M, Bruzzi P, Conte PF (1999) Cardiotoxicity of epirubicin/paclitaxel-containing regimens: role of cardiac risk factors. J Clin Oncol 17:3596–3602

Gennari A, Bruzzi P, Orlandini C, Salvadori B, Donati S, Landucci E, Guarneri V, Rondini M, Ricci S, Conte P (2004) Activity of first line epirubicin and paclitaxel in metastatic breast cancer is independent of type of adjuvant therapy. Br J Cancer 90:962–967

Gennari A, Conte P, Rosso R, Orlandini C, Bruzzi P (2005) Survival of metastatic breast carcinoma patients over a 20-year period: a retrospective analysis based on individual patient data from six consecutive studies. Cancer 104:1742–1750

Geyer CE, Forster J, Lindquist D, Chan S, Romieu CG, Pienkowski T, Jagiello-Gruszfeld A, Crown J, Chan A, Kaufman B, Skarlos D, Campone M, Davidson N, Berger M, Oliva C, Rubin SD, Stein S, Cameron D (2006) Lapatinib plus capecitabine for HER2-positive advanced breast cancer. N Engl J Med 355:2733–2743

Ghersi D, Wilcken N, Simes J, Donoghue E (2006) Taxane containing regimens for metastatic breast cancer. The Cochrane Library 2006: issue 3

Gianni L, Baselga J, Eiermann W et al (2005) Feasibility and tolerability of sequential doxorubicin/paclitaxel followed by cyclophosphamide, methotrexate, and fluorouracil and Its effects on tumor response as preoperative therapy. Clin Cancer Res 11:8715–8721

Giuliano AE, Jones RC, Brennan M, Statman R (1997) Sentinel lymphadenectomy in breast cancer. J Clin Oncol 15:2345–2350

Goldhirsch A, Glick JH, Gelber RD, Coates AS, Thurlimann B, Senn HJ; Panel members (2005) Meeting highlights: international expert consensus on the primary therapy of early breast cancer 2005. Ann Oncol 16:1569–1583

Goldstein LJ, O'Neill A, Sparano JA et al (2005) E2197: a phase III of AT vs AC in the adjuvant treatment of node-positive and high-risk node-negative breast cancer. Proc Am Soc Clin Oncol 23 (abstract 512)

Goss PE, Ingle JN, Martino S et al (2003). A randomized trial of letrozole in postmenopausal women after 5 years of tamoxifen therapy for early-stage breast cancer. N Engl J Med 349:1793–1802

Gradishar W, Chia S, Piccart M, on behalf of the EFECT writing committee (2006) Fulvestrant versus exemestane following prior non-steroidal aromatase inhibitor therapy: first results from EFECT, a randomized, phase III trial in postmenopausal women with advanced breast cancer. Breast Cancer Res and Treat 100 (abstract 12)

Guarneri V, Broglio K, Kau SW et al (2006) Prognostic value of pathologic complete response after primary chemotherapy in relation to hormone receptor status and other factors. J Clin Oncol 24:1037–1044

Haskell CM, Green SJ, Sledge GW, Shapiro CL, Ingle JN, Lew D, Martino S, Livingston RB, Osborne C (2002) Phase III comparison of adjuvant high-dose doxorubicin plus cyclophosphamide (AC) versus sequential doxorubicin followed by cyclophosphamide (A->C) in breast cancer patients with 0-3 positive nodes (intergroup 0137). Proc Am Soc Clin Oncol 21 (abstr 142)

Henderson IC, Berry DA, Demetri GD et al (2003) Improved outcomes from adding sequential paclitaxel but not from escalating doxorubicin dose in an adjuvant chemotherapy regimen for patients with node-positive primary breast cancer. J Clin Oncol 21:976–983

Hennessy BT, Hortobagyi GN, Rouzier R et al (2005) Outcome after pathologic complete eradication of cytologically proven breast cancer axillary node metastases following primary chemotherapy. J Clin Oncol 23:9304–9311

Hilner BE, Ingle JN, Chelbowski RT, Gralow J, Yee GC, Janjan NA, Cauley JA, Blumenstein BA, Albain KS, Lipton A, Brown S, American Society of Clinical Oncology (2003) American Society of Clinical Oncology 2003 update on the role of bisphosphonates and bone health issues in women with breast cancer. J Clin Oncol 21:4042–4057

Hortobagyi GN, Ames FC, Budzar AU et al (1988) Management of stage III primary breast cancer with primary chemotherapy, surgery and radiation therapy. Cancer 62:2507–2516

Hortobagyi GN, Theriault RL, Lipton A, Porter L, Blayney D, Sinoff C, Wheeler H, Simeone JF, Seaman JJ, Knight RD, Heffernan M, Mellars K, Reitsma DJ (1998) Long-term prevention of skeletal complications of metastatic breast cancer with pamidronate. Protocol 19 Aredia Breast Cancer Study Group. J Clin Oncol 16:2038–2044

Howell A, Robertson JF, Quaresma Albano J et al (2002) Fulvestrant, formerly ICI 182,780, is as effective as anastrozole in postmenopausal women with advanced breast cancer progressing after prior endocrine treatment. J Clin Oncol 20:3396–3403

Howell A, Robertson JF, Abram P et al (2004) Comparison of fulvestrant versus tamoxifen for the treatment of advanced breast cancer in postmenopausal women previously untreated with endocrine therapy: a multinational, double-blind, randomized trial. J Clin Oncol 22:1605–1613

Howell A, Cuzick J, Baum M et al (2005) Results of the ATAC (arimidex, tamoxifen, alone or in combination) trial after completion of 5 years' adjuvant treatment for breast cancer. Lancet 365:60–62

Hudis C, Citron ML, Berry DA et al (2005) Five-year follow-up of INT C9741: dose-dense (DD) chemotherapy (CRx) is safe and effective. Breast Cancer Res Treat 94 (abstract 41)

Ingle J, Tu D, Shepherd L, Palmer M, Pater J, Goss P (2006) NCIC CTG MA.17: Intent to treat analysis (ITT) of randomized patients after a median follow-up of 54 months. Proc Am Soc Clin Oncol. Part I. Vol 24, No. 18S (abstract 549)

Jacobson JA, Danforth DN, Cowan KH et al (1995) Ten-year results of a comparison of conservation with mastectomy in the treatment of stage I and II breast cancer. N Engl J Med 332:907–911

Jassem J, Pienkowski T, Pluzanska A et al (2001) Doxorubicin and paclitaxel versus fluorouracil, doxorubicin, and cyclophosphamide as first-line therapy for women with metastatic breast cancer: final results of a randomised phase III multicenter trial. J Clin Oncol 19:1707–1715

Joensuu H, Kellokumpu-Lehtinen PL, Bono P et al (2006) Adjuvant docetaxel or vinorelbine with or without trastuzumab for breast cancer. N Engl J Med 354:809–820

Jonat W, Gnant M, Boccardo F, Kaufmann M, Rubagotti A, Zuna I, Greenwood M, Jakesz R (2006) Effectiveness of switching from adjuvant tamoxifen to anastrozole in postmenopausal women with hormone-sensitive early-stage breast cancer: a meta-analysis. Lancet Oncol 7:991–996

Jones SE, Savin MA, Holmes FA, O'Shaughnessy JA, Blum JL, Vukelja SJ, George TK, McIntyre KJ, Pippen JE, Sandbach J, Kirby RL, Bordelon JH, Hyman WJ, Negron AG, Khandelwal P, Richards DA, Anthony S, Nugent JE, Mennel RG, Banerji M, Edelman G, Ruxer RL, Amare M, Kampe CE, Koutrelakos N, Meyer WG, Asmar L (2005) Final analysis: TC (docetaxel/cyclophosphamide, 4 cycles) has a superior disease-free survival compared to standard AC (doxorubicin/cyclophosphamide) in 1,016 women with early stage breast cancer. Breast Cancer Res Treat 94 (abstract 40)

Kaufmann M, Jonat W, Blamey R et al (2003) Survival analyses from the ZEBRA study. Goserelin (Zoladex) versus CMF in premenopausal women with node-positive breast cancer. Eur J Cancer 39:1711–1717

Klijn JG, Blamey RW, Boccardo F, Tominaga T, Duchateau L, Sylvester R, Combined Hormone Agents Trialists' Group and the European Organization for Research and Treatment of Cancer (2001) Combined tamoxifen and luteinizing hormone-releasing hormone (LHRH) agonist versus LHRH agonist alone in premenopausal advanced breast cancer: a meta-analysis of four randomized trials. Clin Oncol 19:343–353

Krag D, Weaver D, Ashikaga T et al (1998) The sentinel node in breast cancer: A multicenter validation study. N Engl J Med 339:941–946

Kufmann M, Bajetta E, Dirix LY, Fein LE, Jones SE, Zilembo N, Dugardyn JL, Nasurdi C, Mennel RG, Cervek J, Fowst C, Polli A, di Salle E, Arkhipov A, Piscitelli G, Miller LL, Massimini G (2000) Exemestane is superior to megestrol acetate after tamoxifen failure in postmenopausal women with advanced breast cancer: results of a phase III randomized double-blind trial. The Exemestane Study Group. J Clin Oncol 18:1399–1411

Kurtz JM, Jacquemier J, Amalric R et al (1990) Breast-conserving therapy for macroscopically multiple cancers. Ann Surg 212:38–44

Langley RE, Carmichael J, Jones AL, Cameron DA, Qian W, Uscinska B, Howell A, Parmar M (2005) Phase III trial of epirubicin plus paclitaxel compared with epirubicin plus cyclophosphamide as first-line chemotherapy for metastatic breast cancer: United Kingdom National Cancer Research Institute trial AB01. J Clin Oncol 23:8322–8330

Lee FY, Borzilleri R, Fairchild CR et al (2001) BMS-247550: a novel epothilone analog with a mode of action similar to paclitaxel but possessing superior antitumor efficacy. Clin Cancer Res 7:1429–1437

Levine MN, Pritchard KI, Bramwell VH, Shepherd LE, Tu D, Paul N (2005) National Cancer Institute of Canada Clinical Trials Group. Randomized trial comparing cyclophosphamide, epirubicin, and fluorouracil with cyclophosphamide, methotrexate, and fluorouracil in premenopausal women with node-positive breast cancer: update of National Cancer Institute of Canada Clinical Trials Group Trial MA5. J Clin Oncol 23:5166–5170

Lindahl T, Landberg G, Ahlgren J et al (2004) Overexpression of cyclin E protein is associated with specific mutation types in the p53 gene and poor survival in human breast cancer. Carcinogenesis 25:375–380

Lonning PE, Bajetta E, Murray R, Tubiana-Hulin M, Eisenberg PD, Mickiewicz E, Celio L, Pitt P, Mita M, Aaronson NK, Fowst C, Arkhipov A, di Salle E, Polli A, Massimini G (2000) Activity of exemestane in metastatic breast cancer after failure of nonsteroidal aromatase inhibitors: a phase II trial. J Clin Oncol 18:2234–2244

Low JA, Wedam SB, Lee JJ et al (2005) Phase II clinical trial of ixabepilone (BMS-247550), an epothilone B analog, in metastatic and locally advanced breast cancer. J Clin Oncol 23:2726–2734

Luck HJ, Thomssen C, Untch M et al (2000) Multicentric phase III study in first line treatment of advanced metastatic breast cancer (ABC): epirubicin/paclitaxel (ET) vs epirubicin/cyclophosphamide (EC): a study of the AGO Breast Cancer Group [abstract]. Proc Am Soc Clin Oncol 19:73

Lyman GH, Giuliano AE, Somerfield MR et al (2005) American Society of Clinical Oncology guideline recommendations for sentinel lymph node biopsy in early-stage breast cancer. J Clin Oncol 23:7703–7720

Mackey JR, Paterson A, Dirix LY, Dewar J, Chap L, Martin M, Chan S, Tang S-C, Dugan W, Gil M, Zaluski J, Russel C, Vogel C, Efremedis A, Appia F, Brunel E, Hatteville L, Azli N, Nabholtz JM (2002) Final results of the phase III randomized trial comparing docetaxel (T), doxorubicin (A) and cyclophosphamide (C) to FAC as first line chemotherapy (CT) for patients (pts) with metastatic breast cancer (MBC). Proc Am Soc Clin Oncol 35 (abstract 137)

Mamounas EP, Bryant J, Lembersky B et al (2005) Paclitaxel after doxorubicin plus cyclophosphamide as adjuvant chemotherapy for node-positive breast cancer: results from NSABP B-28. J Clin Oncol 23:3686–3696

Martin M, Pienkowski T, Mackey J et al (2005a) Breast Cancer International Research Group 001 Investigators. Adjuvant docetaxel for node-positive breast cancer. N Engl J Med 352:2302–2313

Martin M, Rodriguez-Lescure A, Ruiz A et al (2005b) Multicenter, randomized phase III study of adjuvant chemotherapy for node-positive breast cancer comparing 6 cycles of FEC versus 4 cycles of FEC followed by 8 weekly paclitaxel administrations: interim analysis of GEICAM 9906 trial. Breast Cancer Res Treat 94 (abstract 39)

Marty M, Cognetti F, Maraninchi D, Snyder R, Mauriac L, Tubiana-Hulin M, Chan S, Grimes D, Anton A, Lluch A, Kennedy J, O'Byrne K, Conte P, Green M, Ward C, Mayne K, Extra JM (2005) Efficacy and safety of trastuzumab combined with docetaxel in patients with human epidermal growth factor receptor 2-positive metastatic breast cancer given as first-line treatment: results of a randomized phase III trial by the M7701 study group. J Clin Oncol 23:4265–4274

Mey U, Gorschluter M, Ziske C, Kleinschmidt R, Glasmacher A, Schmidt-Wolf IG (2003) Weekly docetaxel in patients with pretreated metastatic breast cancer: a phase II trial. Anticancer Drugs 14:233–238

Miller KD, Chap LI, Holmes FA et al (2005a) Randomized phase III trial of capecitabine compared with bevacizumab in patients with previously treated metastatic breast cancer. J Clin Oncol 23:792–799

Miller KD, Wang M, Gralow J, Dickler M, Cobleigh MA, Perez EA, Shenkier TN, Davidson NE (2005b) A randomized phase III trial of paclitaxel versus paclitaxel plus bevacizumab as first-line therapy for locally recurrent or metastatic breast cancer: a trial coordinated by the Eastern Cooperative Oncology Group (E2100). Breast Cancer Res Treat 94 (abstract 3)

Montemurro F, Aglietta M (2005) Incorporating trastuzumab into the neoadjuvant treatment of HER2-overexpressing breast cancer. Clin Breast Cancer 6:77–80

Mouridsen H, Gershanovich M, Sun Y, Perez-Carrion R, Boni C, Monnier A, Apffelstaedt J, Smith R, Sleeboom HP, Janicke F, Pluzanska A, Dank M, Becquart D, Bapsy PP, Salminen E, Snyder R, Lassus M, Verbeek JA, Staffler B, Chaudri-Ross HA, Dugan M (2001) Superior efficacy of letrozole versus tamoxifen as first-line therapy for postmenopausal women with advanced breast cancer: results of a phase III study of the International Letrozole Breast Cancer Group. J Clin Oncol 19:2596–2606

Nabholtz JM, Senn HJ, Bezwoda WR, Melnychuk D, Deschenes L, Douma J, Vandenberg TA, Rapoport B, Rosso R, Trillet-Lenoir V, Drbal J, Molino A, Nortier JW, Richel DJ, Nagykalnai T, Siedlecki P, Wilking N, Genot JY, Hupperets PS, Pannuti F, Skarlos D, Tomiak EM, Murawsky M, Alakl M, Aapro M (1999) Prospective randomized trial of docetaxel versus mitomycin plus vinblastine in patients with metastatic breast cancer progressing despite previous anthracycline-containing chemotherapy. 304 Study Group. J Clin Oncol 17:1413–1424

Nabholtz JM, Buzdar A, Pollak M, Harwin W, Burton G, Mangalik A, Steinberg M, Webster A, von Euler M (2000) Anastrozole is superior to tamoxifen as first-line therapy for advanced breast cancer in postmenopausal women: results of a North American multicenter randomised trial. Arimidex Study Group. J Clin Oncol 18:3758–3776

Nabholtz JM, Falkson C, Campos D, Szanto J, Martin M, Chan S, Pienkowski T, Zaluski J, Pinter T, Krzakowski M, Vorobiof D, Leonard R, Kennedy I, Azli N, Murawsky M, Riva A, Pouillart P (2003) Docetaxel and doxorubicin compared with doxorubicin and cyclophosphamide as first-line chemotherapy for metastatic breast cancer: results of a randomized, multicenter, phase III trial. J Clin Oncol 21:968–975

O'Brien M, Wigler N, Inbar M et al (2004) Reduced cardiotoxicity and comparable efficacy in a phase III trial of pegylated liposomal doxorubicin HCl (CAELYX/Doxil) versus conventional doxorubicin for first-line treatment of metastatic breast cancer. Ann Oncol 15:440–449

Osborne CK, Pippen J, Jones SE et al (2002) Double-blind, randomized trial comparing the efficacy and tolerability of fulvestrant versus anastrozole in postmenopausal women with advanced breast cancer progressing on prior endocrine therapy: results of a North American trial. J Clin Oncol 20:3386–3395

O'Shaughnessy J, Miles D, Vukelja S, Moiseyenko V, Ayoub JP, Cervantes G, Fumoleau P, Jones S, Lui WY, Mauriac L, Twelves C, Van Hazel G, Verma S, Leonard R (2002) Superior survival with capecitabine plus docetaxel combination therapy in anthracycline-pretreated patients with advanced breast cancer: phase III trial results. J Clin Oncol 20:2812–2823

Park CC, Mitsumori M, Nixon A et al (2000) Outcome at 8 years after breast-conserving surgery and radiation therapy for invasive breast cancer: Influence of margin status and systemic therapy on local recurrence. J Clin Oncol 18:1668–1675

Pavlakis N, Schmidt RL, Stockler M (2005) Bisphosphonates for breast cancer (review). The Cochrane Library 2005, Issue 3

Pawan KS, Iliskovic N (1998) Doxorubicin-induced cardiomiopathy. N Engl J Med 339:900–905

Perey L, Paridaens R, Hawle H, Zaman K, Nole F, Wildiers H, Fiche M, Dietrich D, Clement P, Koberle D, Goldhirsch A, Thurlimann B (2007) Clinical benefit of fulvestrant in postmenopausal women with advanced breast cancer and primary or acquired resistance to aromatase inhibitors: final results of phase II Swiss Group for Clinical Cancer Research Trial (SAKK 21/00). Ann Oncol 18:64–69

Perez EA, Vogel CL, Irwin DH, Kirshner JJ, Patel R (2001) Multicenter phase II trial of weekly paclitaxel in women with metastatic breast cancer. J Clin Oncol 19:4216–4223

Perloff M, Lesnick GJ, Korzun A et al (1988) Combination chemotherapy with mastectomy or radiotherapy for stage III breast carcinoma: a Cancer and Leukemia Group B study. J Clin Oncol 6:261–269

Piccart-Gebhart MJ, Procter M, Leyland-Jones B et al (2005) Trastuzumab after adjuvant chemotherapy in HER2-positive breast cancer. N Engl J Med 353:1659–1672

Pierce LJ, Strawderman M, Narod SA et al (2000) Effect of radiotherapy after breast-conserving treatment in women with breast cancer and germline BRCA1/2 mutations. J Clin Oncol 18:3360–3369

Pierga JY, Mouret E, Dieras V et al (2000) Prognostic value of persistent node involvement after neoadjuvant chemotherapy in patients with operable breast cancer. Br J Cancer 83:1480–1487

Polychronis A, Sinnett HD, Hadjiminas D et al (2005) Preoperative gefitinib versus gefitinib and anastrozole in postmenopausal patients with oestrogen-receptor positive and epidermal-growth-factor-receptor-positive primary breast cancer: a double-blind placebo-controlled phase II randomised trial. Lancet Oncol 6:383–391

Poole CJ, Earl M, Dunn JA et al (2003) NEAT (National Epirubicin Adjuvant Trial) and SCTBG BR9601 (Scottish Cancer Trials Breast Group) phase III adjuvant breast trials show a significant relapse-free and overall survival advantage for sequential ECMF. Proc Am Soc Clin Oncol 22 (abstr 13)

Preece PE, Wood RAB, Mackie CR, Cuschieri A (1982) Tamoxifen as initial sole treatment of localized breast cancer in elderly women: a pilot study. Br Med J 284:869–870

Rivkin S, Green S, O.Sullivan J, Cruz A, Abeloff M, Jewell W, Costanzi J, Farrar W, Osborne C (1996) Adjuvant CMFVP versus adjuvant CMFVP plus ovariectomy for premenopausal, node-positive, and estrogen receptor-positive breast cancer patients: a Southwest Oncology Group study. J Clin Oncol 14:46–51

Roche H, Fumoleau P, Spielman M et al (2004) Five years analysis of the PAC01 trial: 6 cycles of FEC 100 versus 3 cycles of FEC 100 followed by 3 cycles of docetaxel for the adjuvant treatment of node positive breast cancer. Breast Cancer Res Treat 88 (abstract 27)

Romond EH, Perez EA, Bryant J et al (2005) Trastuzumab plus adjuvant chemotherapy for operable HER2-positive breast cancer. N Engl J Med 353:1673–1684

Rosen LS, Gordon D, Kaminski M, Howell A, Belch A, Mackey J, Apffelstaedt J, Hussein MA, Coleman RE, Reitsma DJ, Chen BL, Seaman JJ (2003) Long-term efficacy and safety of zoledronic acid compared with pamidronate disodium in the treatment of skeletal complications in patients with advanced multiple myeloma or breast carcinoma: a randomized, double-blind, multicenter, comparative trial. Cancer 98:1735–1744

Scottish Cancer Trials Breast Group (1993) Adjuvant ovarian ablation versus CMF chemotherapy in premenopausal women with pathological stage II breast carcinoma: the Scottish Trial. Lancet 341:1293–1298

Sjostrom J, Blomqvist C, Mouridsen H, Pluzanska A, Ottosson-Lonn S, Bengtsson NO, Ostenstad B, Mjaaland I, Palm-Sjovall M, Wist E, Valvere V, Anderson H, Bergh J (1999) Docetaxel compared with sequential methotrexate and 5-fluorouracil in patients with advanced breast cancer after anthracycline failure: a randomised phase III study with crossover on progression by the Scandinavian Breast Group. Eur J Cancer 35:1194–1201

Slamon DJ, Leyland-Jones B, Shak S, Fuchs H, Paton V, Bajamonde A, Fleming T, Eiermann W, Wolter J, Pegram M, Baselga J, Norton L (2001) Use of chemotherapy plus a monoclonal antibody against HER2 for metastatic breast cancer that overexpresses HER2. N Engl J Med 344:783–792

Slamon D, Eiermann W, Robert N, Pienkowski T, Martin M, Pawlicki M, Chan M, Smylie M, Liu M, Falkson C, Pinter T, Fornander T, Shiftan T, Valero V, Mackey J, Tabah-Fisch I, Buyse M, Lindsay MA, Riva A, Bee V, Pegram M, Press M, Crown J (2005) Phase III randomized trial comparing doxorubicin and cyclophosphamide followed by docetaxel (ACT) with doxorubicin and cyclophosphamide followed by docetaxel and trastuzumab (ACTH) with docetaxel, carboplatin and trastuzumab (TCH) in HER2 positive early breast cancer patients: BCIRG 006 study. Breast Cancer Res Treat 94 (abstract 1)

Sledge GW, Neuberg D, Bernardo P et al (2003) Phase III trial of doxorubicin, paclitaxel, and the combination of doxorubicin and paclitaxel, as front-line chemotherapy for metastatic breast cancer: an intergroup trial (E1193). J Clin Oncol 21:588–592

Smith IC, Heys SD, Hutcheon AW et al (2002) Neoadjuvant chemotherapy in breast cancer: significantly enhanced response with docetaxel. J Clin Oncol 20:1456–1466

Smith IE, Dowsett M, Ebbs SR et al (2005) Neoadjuvant treatment of postmenopausal breast cancer with anastrozole, tamoxifen, or both in combination: the Immediate Preoperative Anastrozole, Tamoxifen, or Combined with Tamoxifen (IMPACT) multicenter double-blind randomized trial. J Clin Oncol 23:5108–5116

Smith I, Procter M, Gelber RD et al (2007) Two-year follow-up of trastuzumab after adjuvant chemotherapy in HER2-positive breast cancer: a randomised controlled trial. Lancet 369:29–36

Sorlie T, Perou CM, Tibshirani R et al (2001) Gene expression patterns of breast carcinomas distinguish tumor subclasses with clinical implications Proc Natl Acad Sci USA 98:10869–10874

Sparano JA, Wang M, Martino S et al (2005) From the Eastern Cooperative Oncology Group (ECOG), Southwest Oncology Group (SWOG), Cancer and Acute Leukemia Group B (CALBG), and the North Central Cancer Treatment Group (NCCTG). Phase III study of doxorubicin-cyclophosphamide followed by paclitaxel or docetaxel given every 3 weeks or weekly in patients with axillary node-positive or high-risk node-negative breast cancer: results of North American Breast Cancer Intergroup Trial E1199. Breast Cancer Res Treat 94 (abstract 48)

Spyratos F, Bouchet C, Tozlu S et al (2002) Prognostic value of uPA, PAI-1 and PAI-2 mRNA expression in primary breast cancer. Anticancer Res 22:2997–3003

Thurlimann B, Keshaviah A, Coates AS et al (2005) A comparison of letrozole and tamoxifen in postmenopausal women with early breast cancer. N Engl J Med 353:2747–2757

Ueno NT, Buzdar AU, Singletary SE, Ames FC, McNeese MD, Holmes FA, Theriault RL, Strom EA, Wasaff BJ, Asmar L, Frye D, Hortobagyi GN (1997) Combined-modality treatment of inflammatory breast carcinoma: twenty years of experience at M.D. Anderson Cancer Center. Cancer Chemother Pharmacol 40:321–329

Van de Vijver MJ, He YD, van't Veer LJ et al (2002) A gene-expression signature as a predictor of survival in breast cancer A gene-expression signature as a predictor of survival in breast cancer. N Engl J Med 347:1999–2009

Venturini M, Del Mastro L, Aitini E, Baldini E, Caroti C, Contu A, Testore F, Brema F, Pronzato P, Cavazzini G, Sertoli MR, Canavese G, Rosso R, Bruzzi P (2005) Dose-dense adjuvant chemotherapy in early breast cancer patients: results from a randomized trial. J Natl Cancer Inst 97:1712–1714

Veronesi U, Banfi A, Salvadori B et al (1990) Breast conservation is the treatment of choice in small breast cancer: Long-term results of a randomized trial. Eur J Cancer 26:668–670

von Minckwitz G, Blohmer JU, Raab G et al (2005) In vivo chemosensitivity-adapted preoperative chemotherapy in patients with early-stage breast cancer: the GEPARTRIO pilot study. Ann Oncol 16:56–63

von Minckwitz G, Graf E, Geberth M et al (2006) CMF versus goserelin as adjuvant therapy for node-negative, hormone-receptor-positive breast cancer in premenopausal patients: A randomized trial (GABG trial IV-A-93). Eur J Cancer 42:1780–1788

Wedam SB, Low JA, Yang SX, Chow CK, Choyke P, Danforth D, Hewitt SM, Berman A, Steinberg SM, Liewehr DJ, Plehn J, Doshi A, Thomasson D, McCarthy N, Koeppen H, Sherman M, Zujewski J, Camphausen K, Chen H, Swain SM (2006) Antiangiogenic and antitumor effects of bevacizumab in patients with inflammatory and locally advanced breast cancer. J Clin Oncol 24:769–777

Zelek L, Barthier S, Riofrio M, Fizazi K, Rixe O, Delord JP, Le Cesne A, Spielmann M (2001) Weekly vinorelbine is an effective palliative regimen after failure with anthracyclines and taxanes in metastatic breast carcinoma. Cancer 92:2267–2272

Zielinski C, Beslija S, Mrsic-Krmpotic Z, Welnicka-Jaskiewicz M, Wiltschke C, Kahan Z, Grgic M, Tzekova V, Inbar M, Cervek J, Chernozemsky I, Szanto J, Spanik S, Wagnerova M, Ghilezan N, Pawlega J, Vrbanec D, Khamtsov D, Soldatenkova V, Brodowicz T (2005) Gemcitabine, epirubicin, and paclitaxel versus fluorouracil, epirubicin, and cyclophosphamide as first-line chemotherapy in metastatic breast cancer: a Central European Cooperative Oncology Group International, multicenter, prospective, randomized phase III trial. J Clin Oncol 23:1401–1408

Zucali R, Uslenghi C, Kenda R, Bonadonna G (1976) Natural history and survival of inoperable breast cancer treated with radiotherapy and radiotherapy followed radical mastectomy. Cancer 37:1422–1431

^{186}Re-HEDP for Metastatic Bone Pain in Breast Cancer Patients

20

Marnix G. E. H. Lam, John M. H. de Klerk, and Peter P. van Rijk

CONTENTS

Abstract

Metastases in the skeleton are the most common of all bone neoplasms. The ultimate prognosis for patients suffering from bone metastases is poor. Therapy such as hormonal manipulation (for carcinomas of the breast and prostate) and cytotoxic chemotherapy (for breast cancer and lung cancer) may result in control of both the disease and the accompanying pain for months or possibly years, and it may improve the quality of life.

In clinical practice pain caused by bone secondaries is a common cause of cancer pain, because the incidence of patients with bone metastases is very high. Common malignancies including breast, prostate and lung cancer frequently spread to the skeleton. Approximately 65% of patients with bone metastases suffer from bone pain. Two-thirds of patients with breast cancer will develop metastatic bone disease. The average survival time following the appearance of bone metastases varies between 2 and 4 years.

Whereas osteoblastic metastases predominate in prostate cancer, patients with breast cancer usually present with mixed (osteoblastic and osteolytic) bone lesions. Bone metastases are seldom solitary. They most commonly affect the spine, pelvis, ribs, proximal thigh and upper arm bones and skull.

The therapeutic options are rarely (if ever) curative, and at some point in time the vast majority of patients suffering from osseous metastases will develop progressive disease. Patients with progressive disease require palliation for painful bone metastases. Current options for palliation of bone pain in this group of patients include conventional analgesics, external beam radiotherapy, chemotherapy and bisphosphonates.

An alternative approach to the relief of multifocal bone pain is the systemic administration of a radionuclide, which concentrates at sites of increased bone turnover. Bone metastases from breast cancer will excite an osteoblastic response in bone, leading to an increased uptake of the radiopharmaceutical. In this way therapeutic doses of radionuclides may be localized close to the tumor by utilizing uptake mechanisms in adjacent non-tumor tissue. Bone-seeking radiopharmaceuticals have traditionally been used to image tumors in bone, but, depending on the carrier ligand and energy of the radioactive label, these agents can also be used to treat primary or metastatic tumors in bone (Lewington 1993).

20.1 Rhenium-186-HEDP

^{186}Re-hydroxyethylidene diphosphonate (HEDP) was developed at the University of Cincinnati. It is strongly adsorbed on hydroxy-apatite in vitro. HEDP is markedly concentrated in vivo by primary and metastatic bone lesions. In 1979 Mathieu et al. first suggested the possible use of ^{186}Re-HEDP in the treatment of osseous metastases. However, it took until 1986 to generate therapeutically useful bone-seeking compounds, when Deutsch and Maxon were able to purify the ineffective mixture originally reported by Mathieu (Deutsch et al. 1986).

^{186}Re is produced by irradiating enriched ^{185}Re, and it is chemically similar to ^{99m}Tc. It can be readily complexed with HEDP with a high radiochemical purity (>97%). ^{186}Re is a beta-emitting radionuclide with a maximum beta emission of 1.07 MeV. It has a 9% abundant gamma emission of 137 KeV, which makes it suitable for diagnostic imaging. The physical half-life of 89.3 h is short when compared with some other isotopes.

Short-lived radionuclides in therapy for bone metastases could have potential advantages in comparison with longer-lived isotopes. Radionuclides with long half-lives will produce a lower dose rate than those with short lifetimes. At low dose rates (long-lived radionuclides), there is presumably more opportunity to repair radiation-induced damage, unless the repair system itself was inactivated. Fairly rapid delivery of therapeutic radiation is a potential method for obviating the DNA repair mechanism. Short-lived radionuclides provide opportunities for multi-dose deliveries and for bone marrow ablation, by allowing earlier reinfusion of the transplant marrow. Another important factor in the use of short-lived radionuclides is that the onset of pain relief is reported to be more rapid in patients with painful bone metastases after the use of short-lived rather than longer-lived isotopes (Lewington 1993).

20.2 Pharmacokinetics

The pharmacokinetics of ^{186}Re-HEDP was previously investigated by our group in 11 patients (17 treatments) with bone metastases from breast or prostate cancer (de Klerk et al. 1992). Half-life times of ^{186}Re-HEDP in three blood fractions (whole blood, plasma and plasma water) were 40.1±5.0, 41.0±6.0 and 29.5±6.4 h, respectively. This implies that repeated doses may be administered after a theoretical interval of 200 h (elimination of a drug is over 99% after five half-lives). However, the optimal interval time between two doses will also depend on the overall clinical condition of the patient. With respect to the plasma water (free) half-life time, this value is quite different from whole blood and plasma half-life times. This phenomenon is explained by non-constant protein binding. A time-dependent increase in plasma protein binding was observed, probably caused by in vivo decomposition of ^{186}Re-HEDP. Total urinary ^{186}Re-HEDP excretion was 69±15%, of which 71±6% was excreted in the first 24 h after injection. The post-therapy ^{186}Re-HEDP scintigram showed no uptake in organs other than the skeleton and kidneys. The ^{186}Re-HEDP images were identical to the ^{99m}Tc-hydroxymethylene diphosphonate (^{99m}Tc-HDP), showing the same number and localization of the metastases (Fig. 20.1).

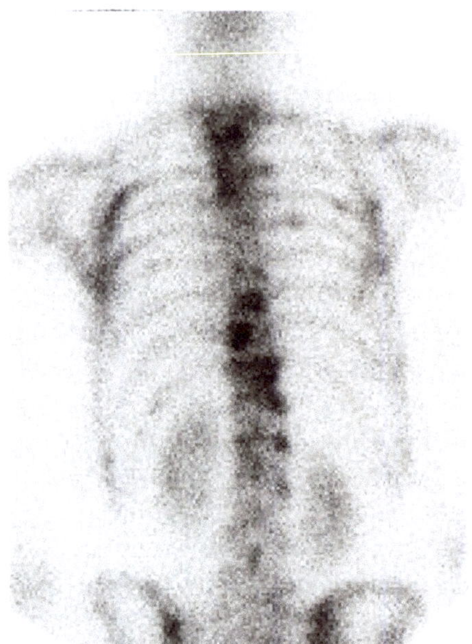

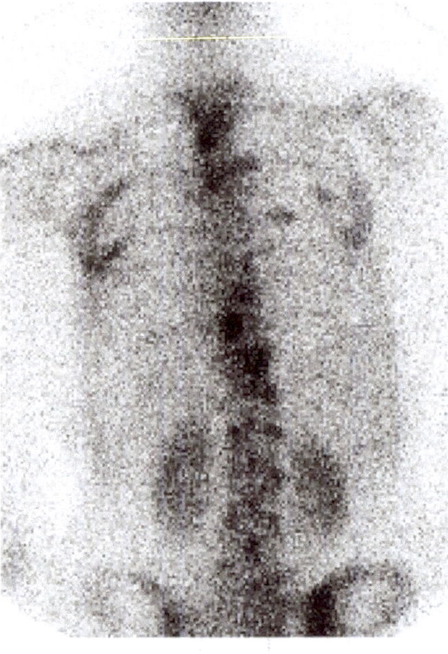

Fig. 20.1. A patient with breast cancer and skeletal metastases. Left: ^{99m}Tc-HDP scintigram 3 h post injection; right ^{186}Re-HEDP scintigram 3 h post injection

The Bone Scan Index (BSI) (i.e., fraction of the skeleton showing scintigraphic evidence of metastatic disease) closely correlated with the fraction of dose nonrenally cleared (R=0.98). This implies that the amount of radioactivity taken up by the skeleton, and hence the bone marrow absorbed dose, can be predicted from a diagnostic pretherapy ^{99m}Tc-HDP scintigram.

20.3 Dosage and Toxicity

In using bone-seeking radiopharmaceuticals as a palliative therapeutic agent for bone metastases, it is important to know the maximum tolerated dosage (MTD). We previously reported our experiences with ^{186}Re-HEDP in escalating dosages in prostatic cancer patients (de Klerk et al. 1994 and 1996). Our dose-escalation study in prostate cancer patients found a maximal tolerated dose (MTD) of 2960 MBq for prostate cancer patients with symptomatic bone metastases. Thrombocytopenia proved to be the dose-limiting factor, with the lowest point in platelet count being at 4 weeks post-treatment. Leucopenia played a minor role.

We also conducted a dose escalation study with ^{186}Re-HEDP in patients suffering from metastatic bone pain originating from breast cancer (de Klerk et al. 1996). Hematological toxicity was limited to thrombocytopenia and leucopenia. The decline in peripheral platelet and leucocyte counts were reversible and returned to normal ranges in most patients. The mean value of platelet and leucocyte count are shown in Figures 20.2 and 20.3. The lowest point in platelet count occurred at week 4 (P<0.01) and in leucocyte count at week 5 (P<0.05). Englaro et al. (1992) reported a sustained decrease in both pain and analgesic intake in two patients treated with repeated sequential administrations of ^{186}Re-HEDP. Therefore, it is not only the grade of toxicity that is an important factor for the clinical use of ^{186}Re-HEDP because of the possibility of carrying

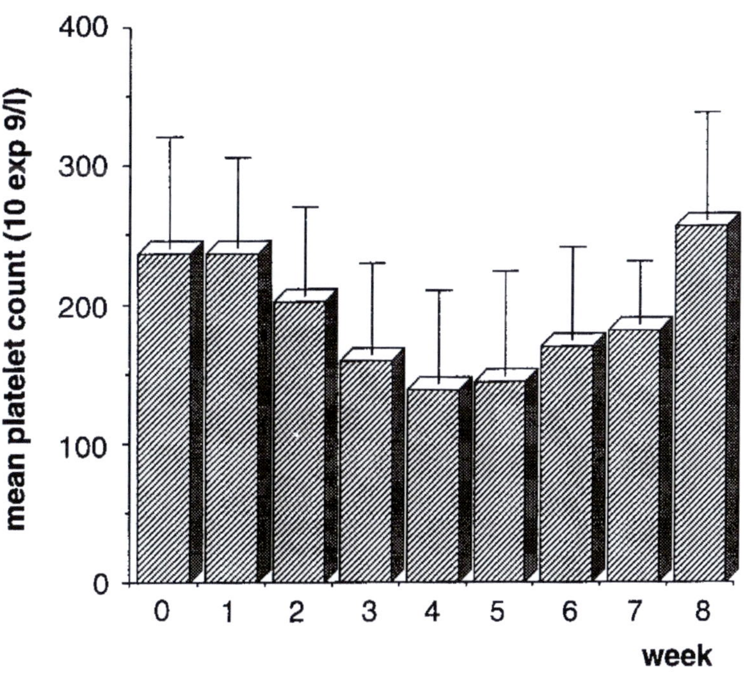

Fig. 20.2. Course of platelet count in breast cancer patients after ^{186}Re-HEDP therapy. Reprinted by permission of the Society of Nuclear Medicine from: de Klerk JM, van het Schip AD, Zonnenberg BA, van Dijk A, Quirijnen JM, Blijham GH et al. Phase 1 study of rhenium-186-HEDP in patients with bone metastases originating from breast cancer. J Nucl Med 1996;37(2):244–249

out repeated administrations of ^{186}Re-HEDP, but also the pattern of the peripheral platelet count recovery is of great importance. Our study indicates that the MTD in breast cancer patients is defined as 2,405 MBq ^{186}Re-HEDP. This value appears to be lower for breast cancer patients than for prostatic cancer patients (2,960 MBq) (de Klerk et al. 1994). However, when the administered dose is normalized to a body surface area of 1.73 m^2 (ADN), the ADNs of the 2,405 MBq group in breast cancer patients (ADN mean: 2,329±234 MBq, range: 2,176 to 2,598 MBq, n=3) and the 2,960 MBq group in prostate cancer patients (ADN mean: 2,509±194 MBq, range: 2,253 to 2,720 MBq, n=6) are of the same order.

Since it is difficult to assess the degree to which hematopoietic reserve has been compromised by prior chemotherapy and radiotherapy, it is of paramount importance to be able to assess toxicity prior to treatment, in order to avoid serious myelotoxic sequelae. The study showed that the percentage of decrease in peripheral platelet count (%DEC) cannot be predicted adequately by the ADN alone, as is the case with prostate cancer patients. In contrast to prostate cancer patients, the prediction of %DEC did not improve when the scintigraphic evidence of the metastatic load in the bone (BSI) was taken into account. In prostate cancer patients, the BSI proved to be a good predictor of the amount of ^{186}Re-HEDP taken up by the skeleton, which explains the impact of the BSI as a parameter of the prediction of platelet toxicity (de Klerk et al. 1994). However, the BSI is not a good indicator of the amount of ^{186}Re-HEDP taken up by the skeleton in breast cancer patients. This may be due to the fact that bone metastases of breast cancer are mostly of a lytic or mixed cell type–osteoblastic plus osteolytic lesions–and rarely purely osteoblastic, such as bone metastases originating from prostate cancer. It is a known fact that bone-seeking radiopharmaceuticals are only taken up by osteoblastic or mixed lesions. This may lead to low BSI values in breast cancer patients and an underestimation of their metastatic load, while the toxicity is in the same order as that in prostate cancer patients. Using the standard recommended dosage of 1,295 MBq ^{186}Re-HEDP, this treatment is safe even for heavily pretreated breast cancer patients, and repeated treatment is possible.

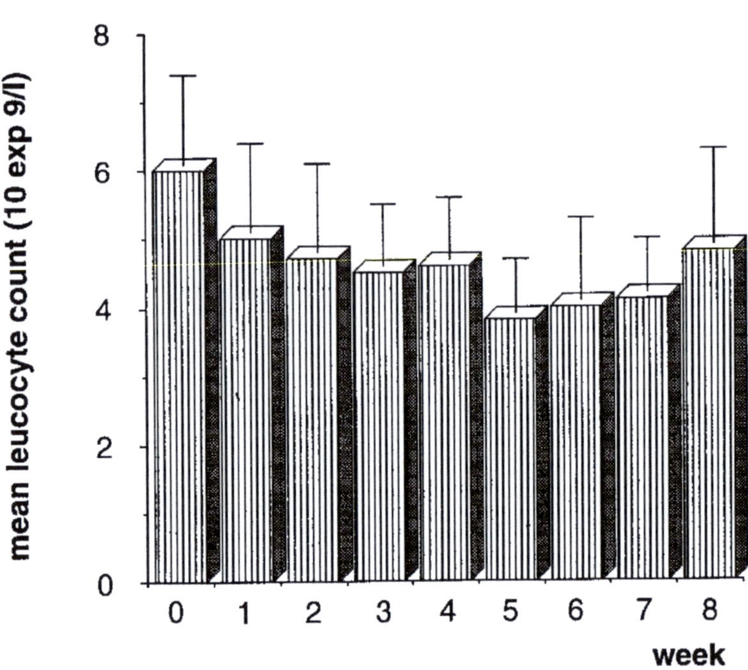

Fig. 20.3. Course of leucocyte count in breast cancer patients after ^{186}Re-HEDP therapy. Reprinted by permission of the Society of Nuclear Medicine from: de Klerk JM, van het Schip AD, Zonnenberg BA, van Dijk A, Quirijnen JM, Blijham GH et al. Phase 1 study of rhenium-186-HEDP in patients with bone metastases originating from breast cancer. J Nucl Med 1996;37(2):244–249

20.4 Dosimetry

Dosimetric studies with an injected dose of 1,295 MBq found a high tumor absorbed dose, with a mean dose to the tumor lesions of 35.3 Gy and a mean marrow dose of 0.92 mGy/MBq (Maxon et al. 1992). We calculated bone marrow absorbed doses using a non-invasive (based on urine collection) and a pharmacokinetic (based on urine and blood data) approach after 19 treatments. The mean bone marrow absorbed doses were 1.137±0.243 mGy/MBq and 1.092±0.247 mGy/MBq, respectively (de Klerk et al. 1996). The tumor-to-non-tumor ratios have a high therapeutic index, with a mean value of 34:1 and a median value of 20:1 (Maxon et al. 1992). Israel et al. (2000) found a good predictive value by measuring the radiation dose using quantitative bone single photon emission computed tomography (SPECT) for the prediction of pain relief. Furthermore, bone SPECT using ^{99m}Tc -MDP predicts radiation doses delivered by ^{186}Re-HEDP.

20.5 Efficacy

Using a computer-aided search of the literature, 21 clinical studies evaluating ^{186}Re-HEDP for the treatment of painful osseous metastases were identified. The studies included patients with painful osseous metastases from predominantly prostate and breast cancer. Table 20.1 gives a summary of the efficacy results of all ^{186}Re-HEDP studies. The overall response rate in these 21 studies was 73% (range 50-92%) after treatment with ^{186}Re-HEDP for painful osseous metastases. In addition to studies that concentrated solely on prostate cancer, many studies that concentrated on breast cancer and other tumors have been published.

Sciuto et al. (2000) studied the efficacy of ^{186}Re-HEDP among different groups of patients with predominantly prostate and breast cancer. She found a global pain relief of 90% for breast cancer patients. In this study a pain assessment was used as proposed by our group, using very strict pain response

Table 20.1. The efficacy results of ^{186}Re-HEDP studies

References	Year	No. of patients	Group diagnosis	Dosage (MBq)	Response rate (%)
Maxon	1990	20	Prostate	1225±152	80
Maxon	1992	44	Prostate, breast, miscellaneous	1,258	77
Quirijne	1996	37	Prostate	1,295–3,515	54
Guerra	1997	5	Breast	1,406	80
Schoeneich	1997	44	Prostate, breast, miscellaneous	1,295	60
Limouris	1997	16	Prostate	1,400±100	81
Limouris	1997	14	Breast	1,400±100	71
Virotta	1997	14	Breast	1,300	80
Holle	1997	15	Prostate	1,810–2,590	87
Hauswirth	1998	17	Breast	1,295	59
Han	1999	24	Breast	1,295–2,960	58
Palmedo	1999	30	Breast	1,295	60
Giannakenas	2000	25	Prostate, breast, miscellaneous	1,300	80
Liepe	2000	13	Prostate, breast	1,336±166	77
Kolesnikov-Gauthier	2000	26	Prostate, breast	1,295	50
Tennvall	2000	14	Prostate	2,590	79
Kucuk	2000	31	Prostate, breast, miscellaneous	1,295	68
Sciuto	2000	60	Prostate, breast, miscellaneous	1,406	80
Sciuto	2001	25	Breast	1,406	92
Dafermou	2001	58	Prostate	1,295	86
Han	2002	43	Prostate	1,295–2,960	65

criteria. We reported our results in breast cancer patients who entered a clinical phase I/II study using these criteria (Han et al. 1999). A total of 30 patients entered this study. All patients had histologically proven breast cancer, had been treated with hormonal therapy, chemotherapy or both, and had bone pain that required the use of analgesics. They had at least four scintigraphically and radiologically proven metastatic bone lesions. Adequate platelet count (>150×10 exp 9/l), leucocyte count (>4.0×10 exp 9/l) and renal function were required for eligibility. Karnofsky performance status was required to be >60% and life expectancy estimated to be at least 3 months. Although no specific recommendations with regard to alteration of the analgesic treatment were made, the patients were requested to keep the analgesic regimen constant if possible. The injected doses ranged from 1,295 to 2,960 MBq (35 to 80 mCi). ^{186}Re-HEDP (total volume 2 ml) was injected as a bolus through a running intravenous saline drip, and patients were hospitalized for 24 h. After ^{186}Re-HEDP administration, patients were seen and examined weekly, usually on an out-patient basis.

For pain assessment, a paper-and-pencil diary was used to assess the patient's pain. The diary contained validated questions for 7 days and was kept twice a day. In order to determine the efficacy of ^{186}Re-HEDP, strict criteria were formulated in which the pain intensity, medication index and daily activities were included as core determinants. Based upon these criteria, a clinically relevant response was reached when (1) pain reduction was >25% for at least 2 consecutive weeks and when the medication index and daily activities remained at least constant or (2) pain reduction was <25% for at least 2 consecutive weeks, and one of the two other factors showed an improvement >25% for at least 2 consecutive weeks, while the remaining factor remained at least constant. The studies were open label, so that the patients functioned as their own controls. For each patient, post-treatment data were compared with pretreatment data (baseline). Because scores fluctuated considerably over the week, median scores for the aforementioned dependent variables were calculated: one median score over the 2-week pre-treatment period (baseline) and weekly median scores for the 6 or 8 weeks after treatment. After the ^{186}Re-HEDP administration, several patients complained of a transient increase in pain intensity, compared with the baseline pain. Typically, this so-called "flare" reaction started within the 1st week post-therapy and lasted for no longer than a week. In this analysis, a "flare" reaction is defined as an increase in pain intensity of more than 25% of the intensity of pre-treatment pain. The independent t-test was used to test the influence of age, dosage and BSI on the response ($P<0.05$ was considered to be statistically significant).

Thirty patients entered the study, of whom 24 proved to be evaluable. The administered dose of ^{186}Re-HEDP was 1,295 MBq (35 mCi) in six patients, 1,850 MBq (50 mCi) in six patients, 2,405 MBq (65 mCi) in nine patients and 2,960 MBq (80 mCi) in three patients. Pain reduction >25% lasting for more than 2 consecutive weeks was achieved in 17 patients (71%) (Fig. 20.4). The maximum follow-up period was 8 weeks. Duration of response ranged from 2 to 8 weeks (mean, 4 weeks). Response rate of pain reduction was not correlated to treatment dosage. Four patients (67%) in the 1,295 MBq (35 mCi) group, four patients (67%) in the 1,850 MBq (50 mCi) group, seven patients (78%) in the 2,405 MBq (65 mCi) group and two patients (67%) in the 2,960 MBq (80 mCi) group had responses. Within this group of 17 patients, 2 patients increased their medication indices simultaneously. Improvement in daily activities was noted in 14 patients (58%). In six patients, daily activities remained constant. Three patients reported worsening of their daily activities, accompanied by progression of their pain and medication indices or both. One patient reported a worsening of her daily activities, despite a period of >25% pain reduction, lasting 6 weeks. Ten of 14 responders showed increases in daily activity combined with reductions of the medication index. Based upon the criteria for determination of the overall efficacy of ^{186}Re-HEDP in 58% ($n=14$) of the patients in the total group, clinically relevant responses were reached. No responders were found with pain reduction of less than 25% in combination with >25% improvement of daily activity or demand for pain medication (Fig. 20.5). All patients had received chemotherapy and/or hormonal therapy before rhenium therapy, but responses were not related to previous chemotherapy and/or hormonal therapy. Transient worsening of bone pain, the so-called "flare" phenomenon, occurred in about 29% of patients. The incidence was similar for both responders and non-responders. The mean BSI of all patients was 37 (range 8–68). The BSI was not correlated to the chance of response, indicating that there was no relationship between the scintigraphic metastatic load and the response. The BSI was not correlated to the chance of flare.

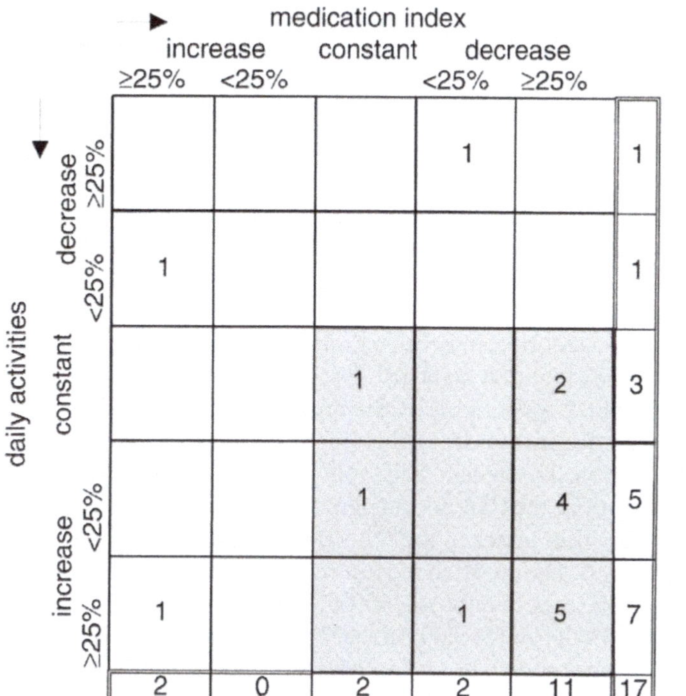

Fig. 20.4. Number of responders in terms of at least 25% pain relief. Reprinted by permission of the Society of Nuclear Medicine from: Han SH, Zonnenberg BA, de Klerk JM, Quirijnen JM, van het Schip AD, van Dijk A et al. 186Re-etidronate in breast cancer patients with metastatic bone pain. J Nucl Med 1999;40(4):639–642

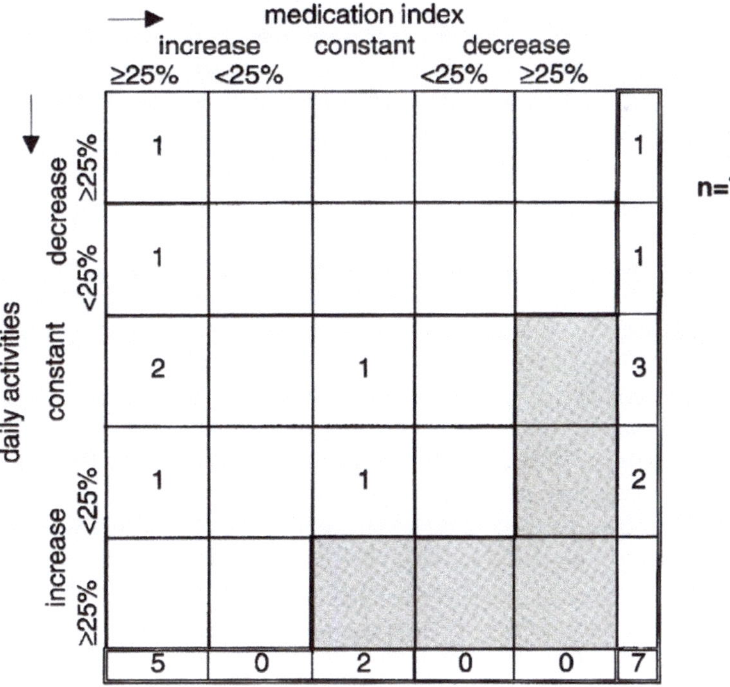

Fig. 20.5. Patients with less than 25% pain reduction. Reprinted by permission of the Society of Nuclear Medicine from: Han SH, Zonnenberg BA, de Klerk JM, Quirijnen JM, van het Schip AD, van Dijk A et al. ^{186}Re-etidronate in breast cancer patients with metastatic bone pain. J Nucl Med 1999;40(4):639–642

This study showed an overall response rate of 58%. Using the same pain response criteria a response rate of 54% in prostate cancer patients was found by our group (Quirijnen et al. 1996). If pain reduction was considered to be the only parameter of response, we would have scored a 71% response rate, instead of the 58%, based upon our more stringent criteria of response.

In another study by Sciuto et al. (2001) concerning 25 patients with breast cancer, a high response rate of 92% was reported, this being the highest response rate found in the literature. This was a comparative study with ^{89}Sr-chloride, in which a group response rate of 84% was found. A standard dosage of 1,400 MBq ^{186}Re-HEDP was used, and the onset of pain relief appeared significantly earlier in this group ($P<0.001$). Clinically evident pain relief occurred within 1 month in the ^{89}Sr-chloride group (median 21 days) and within 1 week in the ^{186}Re-HEDP group (median 4 days). The duration of pain relief ranged from 2 months to 14 months (mean value 125 days with a median value of 120 days) in the ^{89}Sr-chloride group, and from 1 month to 12 months (mean duration of 107 days with a median value of 60 days) in the ^{186}Re-HEDP group. However, the difference in duration was not statistically significant ($p=0.39$). Duration of pain relief showed a significant positive correlation with the degree of response ($P<0.05$) and Karnofsky performance status score ($P<0.05$).

In contrast Kolesnikov-Gauthier et al. (2000) (26 patients: 12 breast, 14 prostate) reported an objective response of only 36% in breast cancer patients (67% response in prostate cancer patients) using a dosage of 1,295 MBq (35 mCi) ^{186}Re-HEDP. All patients in this study were severely ill and had failed traditional treatments. The less favorable results in the breast cancer patients may reflect more severely advanced disease, in comparison with those patients with prostate cancer. The average survival of the breast cancer patients after treatment was only 88 days, with no survivors at 7 months. However, the average survival of all patients (12 men with prostate cancer, 16 women with breast cancer) after the first ^{186}Re-HEDP administration was 114 days, with 3 survivors after 1 year. Life expectancy of the patients is an important criterion to consider when comparing results between different types of cancer or different studies.

Palmedo et al. (1999) found a 60% response rate in breast cancer patients, using a pain assessment through daily documentation of the visual analog scale and analgesic consumption. A significant response to treatment was determined if the visual analog scale or analgesic consumption decreased significantly for at least 2 weeks. A 1,295 MBq dosage of ^{186}Re-HEDP was used. They also found that treatment with ^{186}Re-HEDP resulted in pain reduction if the patient experienced pain in a region where local external beam radiotherapy had previously been applied. Furthermore, after a single or repeated injection of ^{186}Re-HEDP, they did not observe an intolerable toxicity (which was defined as grade 3) in any patient, although most patients had undergone previous chemotherapy. However, the interval between ^{186}Re-HEDP injection and chemotherapy was always at least 3 months. In a study conducted by Limouris et al. (1997) in 14 breast cancer patients using 1295 MBq ^{186}Re-HEDP, two patients became free of pain, 6 experienced marked pain reduction and 2 showed some improvement, resulting in an 71% overall response rate.

Schoeneich et al. (1997) studied 44 patients in total: prostate cancer, $n=17$; breast cancer, $n=24$; others (not specified), $n=3$. Each patient received an injection of 1,295 MBq ^{186}Re-HEDP. Twenty-six of the 44 patients (60%) observed pain reduction. In response to ^{186}Re-HEDP therapy ($n=26$), there was no difference between patients with prostate and with breast cancer. Hauswirth et al. (1998) found a response rate of 59% (treating 17 breast cancer patients) and concluded that ^{186}Re-HEDP can be used in conjunction with analgesics and external beam radiation in patients with painful bone metastases from breast cancer.

On treating 31 patients with various cancers, Kucuk et al. (2000) found an overall response rate of 67.5%. The group consisted of ten prostate cancer, ten breast cancer, four rectum carcinoma, five lung cancer and two nasopharynx cancer. The pain relief was assessed in accordance with the Eastern Cooporative Oncologic Group (ECOG), using the Karnofsky status index. The mean response rate was 87.5% in patients with breast and prostate cancer, 75% in patients with rectum cancer and 20% in patients with lung cancer. It should be stressed that the response rate mentioned in this study is not the percentage of responders, but the mean percentage of response in each group. For example, in the breast cancer and prostate cancer group, all patients showed a response, in breast cancer patients varying from 20% to 100%, with a mean value of 87.5%. In the prostate cancer group the range was 10 to 100, also with a mean of 87.5%. The authors concluded that ^{186}Re-HEDP therapy is highly effective in prostate, breast and rectum cancer, but less effective in lung cancer.

The activity used was approximately 1,295 MBq in the majority of studies. However, in the dose escalating studies from our group, using dosages ranging from 1,295 MBq to 2,405 MBq of ^{186}Re-HEDP, a clear dose-response relationship could not be demonstrated neither by us nor by other studies. Tennvall et al. (2000) used 2,590 MBq ^{186}Re-HEDP (i.e., twice the activity normally used) to evaluate the safety of intravenously administered ^{186}Re-HEDP and to investigate whether the response rates would significantly improve. In their study, pain relief was observed in 11 out of 14 evaluable patients (79%), 4 of whom became completely free from pain.

Repetitive treatments with ^{186}Re-HEDP were used in several studies, in order to prolong the duration of response, and there was a general agreement that further pain relief could be expected if the patient had responded previously to treatment with ^{186}Re-HEDP. Length of response differed in most studies, with a wide range of up to several months in this difficult patient group in their very advanced stage of disease.

A few studies have concentrated on the difference in efficacy of different radionuclides in the treatment of painful osseous metastases. Dafermou et al. (2001) reported a multicenter study, in which from 510 evaluable patients with painful bone metastases of prostate cancer, 453 patients were treated with ^{89}Sr and 58 patients were treated with ^{186}Re-HEDP (one patient was first treated with ^{89}Sr and later with ^{186}Re-HEDP). They found no statistically significant difference in palliative efficacy of the two radiopharmaceuticals. Sciuto et al. (2001) studied the difference in pain palliation of ^{186}Re-HEDP and ^{89}Sr, treating 50 patients with painful osseous metastases of breast cancer with either ^{89}Sr (25 patients) or ^{186}Re-HEDP (25 patients). They found a response rate of 84% for ^{89}Sr and 92% for ^{186}Re-HEDP, which is an insignificant difference (P=0.66). In a group of 44 patients (38 prostate, 6 breast), Liepe et al. (2000) treated 15 patients (11 prostate, 4 breast) with ^{89}Sr, 13 patients (12 prostate, 1 breast) with ^{186}Re-HEDP and 16 patients (15 prostate, 1 breast) with ^{188}Re-HEDP. They recorded response rates of 80%, 77% and 81% for the ^{89}Sr, ^{186}Re-HEDP and ^{188}Re-HEDP group, respectively, which is also insignificant.

In conclusion, the overall response rate in all studies that concentrated solely on breast cancer patients with painful osseous metastases ranged from 58% to 92%. This is comparable with response rates found in studies that concentrated on prostate cancer (range 54% to 87%) and groups of mixed cancers (prostate, breast and miscellaneous; range 50% to 80%). It should be mentioned that the contribution of patients other than prostate or breast cancer patients was very small.

20.6 Discussion

Treatment of metastatic bone pain using bone-seeking radiopharmaceuticals has become an important modality. In particular, patients with multiple painful osseous lesions or patients with recurrent pain in a radiotherapy field may benefit from this systemic treatment. Theoretically, the optimal characteristics of a radiopharmaceutical for metastatic bone pain make ^{186}Re-HEDP a potentially very useful isotope providing: (1) a relatively short physical half-life (90 h), (2) beta emission, (3) imageable gamma emission, (4) selective bone seeking properties, (5) rapid blood clearance and low extra osseous uptake, (6) economical and ready availability and (7) good chemical stability.

The toxicity of ^{186}Re-HEDP is limited and reversible. In breast cancer patients, the overall clinical response of ^{186}Re-HEDP is reported to be up to 92%. Thrombocytopenia is found to be the dose-limiting factor in the treatment of painful bone metastases with bone-seeking radiopharmaceuticals. De Klerk et al. evaluated thrombocytopenia in patients with hormone refractory prostate carcinoma treated with ^{186}Re-HEDP. As an index of the extent of bone involvement, the bone scan index (BSI) was determined from the pre-therapy ^{99m}Tc-HDP scintigram. They described a functional relationship (r=0.78; P<0.001) of the percentage of platelet decrease after treatment with the extent and distribution of skeletal metastases (BSI) and administered activity normalized to standard body surface area. Using this relationship, it is possible to predict thrombocytopenia by pre-treatment bone scintigraphy and to adjust the dosage to each patient in order to avoid unacceptable toxicity. The formula of de Klerk may also be used to calculate an individually based optimized dose (de Klerk et al. 1994).

In the 21 studies analyzed in this paper, the response rate varied from 50% to 92%. No significant differences in the range of response rate between different groups of patients (primarily prostate and breast cancer) exist. The rate of response may depend upon the pretreatment condition of the patient, the etiology of the bone metastases, differences in the population treated, extent of the disease and any previous local or systemic therapy given. In some studies it was not possible to differentiate between whether single or repetitive injections with ^{186}Re-HEDP were given either in order to extend the duration of relief or to enlarge the response of pain relief. However, it is more important to know that treatment with ^{186}Re-HEDP can be repeated several times when needed, due to its limited transient hematological toxicity and short physical half-life.

When using bone-seeking radiopharmaceuticals for metastatic bone pain, pain relief will occur in a high percentage of patients. Unfortunately, numbers of patients achieve incomplete pain resolution, and some patients obtain no pain relief at all. In addition, there is little evidence that this therapy results in improved survival, and relatively few patients exhibit evidence of significant anti-tumor effect. McCready and O'Sullivan (2002) have suggested possibilities for improvement of the therapeutic efficacy. These include: (1) local dose escalation: in a phase I study with dosages of 5,000 MBq ^{186}Re-HEDP using autologous peripheral blood stem cell rescue, O'Sullivan et al. (2002) reported a PSA response >50% lasting at least 4 weeks. (2) Enhancement of radionuclide uptake: an increased uptake of bone-seeking radiopharmaceuticals would appear to occur 4 weeks to 3 months following the start of hormonal therapy. Administering the bone-seeking radiopharmaceutical at the time of this flare-up reaction may increase the tumor-absorbed dose. This is illustrated by the study of Bushnell et al. (1999), who reported an enhanced uptake of ^{99m}Tc-MDP in skeletal metastases from prostate cancer, following initiation of hormone treatment. They found that approximately 3 weeks following initiation of hormone blockade, most skeletal metastases from prostate cancer will demonstrate significantly enhanced ^{99m}Tc-MDP uptake, relative to normal bone. (3) Chemosensitization: Chemotherapeuticals can be used in combination with bone-seeking radiopharmaceuticals in order to enhance the effect of the therapy. In the field of external radiotherapy, chemosensitization is a well recognized, accepted, and widely used method for improving the overall efficacy of treatment. The cytotoxic effect of chemotherapy makes cancer cells more susceptible to radiation damage. In the field of bone-seeking radiopharmaceuticals, chemosensitization may also lead to an overall improved efficacy. Early studies have already suggested a synergistic effect (Mertens et al. 1992). This synergism was shown in vitro by Geldof et al. (1999), who studied the combined effect of ^{186}Re-HEDP and cisplatin in prostate cancer cells. The more than accumulative effect of the combined treatment was also shown in human patients (Akerley et al. 2002; Nilsson et al. 2005; Pagliaro et al. 2003; Sciuto et al. 1996, 1998 and 2002; Tu et al. 2001). (4) Repeated administrations: Repeated administrations with a relatively short interval may lead to an enhanced effect compared to single treatments alone (Kasalicky et al. 1998; Palmedo et al. 2003). It is recognized that the therapeutic effect of radionuclide therapy is increased in patients with a less advanced stage of their disease (Sciuto et al. 2000; Kraeber-Bodere et al. 2000). Repeated dosing may be more effective on larger metastatic lesions in patients with a more advanced stage of disease. (5) Radionuclide "cocktails": The combination of short-lived radionuclides, such as ^{186}Re (or ^{188}Re) and ^{153}Sm-EDTMP, in combination with longer lived radionuclides (^{89}Sr) and alpha emitters, may enhance this effect on larger metastatic lesions. Henriksen et al. (2002) reported the use of the alpha-particle-emitting ^{223}Ra in nude rats with skeletal metastases. A significant antitumor effect was found, while sparing the bone marrow. A combination of different radionuclides with different radiation energies, half-lives and ranges may be more effective for patients with osseous metastases, which are generally of all sizes. Toxicity may be kept low while offering high-dose treatment.

In addition to these suggestions we would like to add (6) combined modality treatment: Due to their tolerability, efficacy and ease of use, bone-seeking radiopharmaceuticals may be administered in combination with other anti-cancer agents or therapy. A combination for example of external beam radiotherapy and bone-seeking radiopharmaceuticals could lead to synergy, with higher efficacy in the radiation field and prevention of new pain sites (Smeland et al. 2003; Porter et al. 1993). Other agents such as bisphosphonates exhibit a proven anti-tumor effect in several tumor cell lines, including carcinomas of the breast and prostate (Lee et al. 2001; Boissier et al. 2000; Oades et al. 2003). Although they are currently indicated for the prevention of skeletal related events, their anti-tumor efficacy needs to be further evaluated. Concomitant administration of bone-seeking radiopharmaceuticals and bisphosphonates in patients with painful osseous metastases may lead to an increased clinical benefit. Furthermore, it is of interest to note that several new anti-cancer agents are under investigation, which may have potential as monotherapy, but which may also be used in combination with bone-seeking radiopharmaceuticals. The process of osseous metastasis offers a broad range of potential intervention (Smith et al. 2005). New anti-cancer agents may be used in combination with bone seeking radiopharmaceuticals with an aim to increase overall efficacy.

20.7 Conclusion

Patients with multiple symptomatic lesions benefit from the systematic approach of targeted radionuclide therapy with ^{186}Re-HEDP. In breast cancer patients with painful bone metastases, ^{186}Re-HEDP is at least as effective as in those with metastatic prostate cancer. It is to be preferred above radiopharmaceuticals with a long physical half-life, which have a more extensive hematological toxicity in this group of patients who have frequently been pretreated with bone marrow suppressive chemotherapy. ^{186}Re-HEDP treatment offers a safe and effective treatment option for patients with painful osseous metastases with an overall reported response rate of ±70%. It is a systemic, simple and well-tolerated single-session procedure that usually achieves good pain palliation and sometimes pain-free periods of several months. It is effective for fast palliation of painful bone metastases, and the effect tends to last longer the earlier patients are treated in the course of their disease. Because of the earlier onset of pain relief and the faster time to hematological recovery, ^{186}Re-HEDP is indicated in patients with unbearable pain and with a lower estimated life expectancy. ^{186}Re-HEDP therapy can also be used safely in patients where pain reoccurs in regions previously treated by local external beam radiotherapy. Repeated treatments are also very effective and safe, with unlimited numbers of repetitions, provided that some safety restrictions are respected such as adequate hematological reserve. These repeated protocols and the use of high activity ^{186}Re-HEDP show promising results, not only for pain relief, but also for tumor control.

References

Akerley W, Butera J, Wehbe T, Noto R, Stein B, Safran H, Cummings F, Sambandam S, Maynard J, Di Rienzo G, Leone L (2002) A multiinstitutional, concurrent chemoradiation trial of strontium-89, estramustine, and vinblastine for hormone refractory prostate carcinoma involving bone. Cancer 94:1654–1660

Boissier S, Ferreras M, Peyruchaud O, Magnetto S, Ebetino FH, Colombel M, Delmas P, Delaisse JM, Clezardin P (2000) Bisphosphonates inhibit breast and prostate carcinoma cell invasion, an early event in the formation of bone metastases. Cancer Res 60:2949–2954

Bushnell DL, Madsen M, Kahn D, Nathan M, Williams RD (1999) Enhanced uptake of 99Tcm-MDP in skeletal metastases from prostate cancer following initiation of hormone treatment: potential for increasing delivery of therapeutic agents. Nucl Med Commun 20:875–881

Dafermou A, Colamussi P, Giganti M, Cittanti C, Bestagno M, Piffanelli A (2001) A multicentre observational study of radionuclide therapy in patients with painful bone metastases of prostate cancer. Eur J Nucl Med 28:788–798

de Klerk JM, van Dijk A, van het Schip AD, Zonnenberg BA, van Rijk PP (1992) Pharmacokinetics of rhenium-186 after administration of rhenium-186-HEDP to patients with bone metastases. J Nucl Med 33:646–651

de Klerk JM, van het Schip AD, Zonnenberg BA, van Dijk A, Stokkel MP, Han SH (1994) Evaluation of thrombocytopenia in patients treated with rhenium-186-HEDP: guidelines for individual dosage recommendations. J Nucl Med 35:1423–1428

de Klerk JM, Zonnenberg BA, van het Schip AD, van Dijk A, Han SH, Quirijnen JM (1994) Dose escalation study of rhenium-186 hydroxyethylidene diphosphonate in patients with metastatic prostate cancer. Eur J Nucl Med 21:1114–1120

de Klerk JM, van het Schip AD, Zonnenberg BA, van Dijk A, Quirijnen JM, Blijham GH (1996) Phase 1 study of rhenium-186-HEDP in patients with bone metastases originating from breast cancer. J Nucl Med 37:244–249

de Klerk JM, van Dieren EB, van het Schip AD, Hoekstra A, Zonnenberg BA, van Dijk A (1996) Bone marrow absorbed dose of rhenium-186-HEDP and the relationship with decreased platelet counts. J Nucl Med 37:38–41

de Klerk JM, Zonnenberg BA, Krouwer HG, Blijham GH, van Dijk A, van het Schip AD (1996) Transient cranial neuropathy in prostatic cancer with bone metastases after rhenium-186-HEDP treatment. J Nucl Med 37:465–467

Deutsch E, Libson K, Vanderheyden JL, Ketring AR, Maxon HR (1986) The chemistry of rhenium and technetium as related to the use of isotopes of these elements in therapeutic and diagnostic nuclear medicine. Int J Rad Appl Instrum B 13:465–477

Englaro EE, Schroder LE, Thomas SR (1992) Safety and efficacy of repeated sequential administrations of Re-186(Sn)HEDP as palliative therapy for painful skeletal metastases. Initial case reports of two patients. Clin Nucl Med 17:41–44

Geldof AA, de Rooij L, Versteegh RT, Newling DW, Teule GJ (1999) Combination ^{186}Re-HEDP and cisplatin supra-additive treatment effects in prostate cancer cells. J Nucl Med 40:667–671

Giannakenas C, Kalofonos HP, Apostolopoulos DJ, Zarakovitis J, Kosmas C, Vassilakos PJ (2000) Preliminary results of the use of Re-186-HEDP for palliation of pain in patients with metastatic bone disease. Am J Clin Oncol 23:83–88

Guerra UP, Englaro E, Cattaruzzi E (1997) Palliative therapy with rhenium-186-HEDP for bone metastases of breast cancer. Tumori 83:560–562

Han SH, Zonnenberg BA, de Klerk JM, Quirijnen JM, van het Schip AD, van Dijk A (1999) ^{186}Re-etidronate in breast cancer patients with metastatic bone pain. J Nucl Med 40:639–642

Han SH, de Klerk JM, Tan S, van het Schip AD, Derksen BH, van Dijk A et al (2002) The PLACORHEN study: a double-blind, placebo-controlled, randomized radionuclide study with (186)Re-etidronate in hormone-resistant prostate cancer patients with painful bone metastases. Placebo Controlled Rhenium Study. J Nucl Med 43:1150–1156

Hauswirth AE, Palmedo H, Dierke-Dzierzon C, Biersack HJ, Krebs D (1998) Pain therapy in multiple bone metastases in breast carcinoma with rhenium 186 HEDP. Zentralbl Gynakol 120:83–86

Henriksen G, Breistol K, Bruland OS, Fodstad O, Larsen RH (2002) Significant antitumor effect from bone-seeking, alpha-particle-emitting (223)Ra demonstrated in an experimental skeletal metastases model. Cancer Res 62:3120–3125

Holle LH, Humke U, Trampert L, Ziegler M, Kirsch CM, Oberhausen E (1997) Palliative treatment for pain in osseous metastasized prostatic carcinoma with osteotropic rhenium-186 hydroxyethylidene diphosphonate (HEDP). Urologe A 36:540–547

Israel O, Keidar Z, Rubinov R, Iosilevski G, Frenkel A, Kuten A (2000) Quantitative bone single-photon emission computed tomography for prediction of pain relief in metastatic bone disease treated with rhenium-186-etidronate. J Clin Oncol 18:2747–2754

Kasalicky J, Krajska V (1998) The effect of repeated strontium-89 chloride therapy on bone pain palliation in patients with skeletal cancer metastases. Eur J Nucl Med 25:1362–1367

Kolesnikov-Gauthier H, Carpentier P, Depreux P, Vennin P, Caty A, Sulman C (2000) Evaluation of toxicity and efficacy of ^{186}Re-hydroxyethylidene diphosphonate in patients with painful bone metastases of prostate or breast cancer. J Nucl Med 41:1689–1694

Kraeber-Bodere F, Campion L, Rousseau C, Bourdin S, Chatal JF, Resche I (2000) Treatment of bone metastases of prostate cancer with strontium-89 chloride: efficacy in relation to the degree of bone involvement. Eur J Nucl Med 27:1487–1493

Kucuk NO, Ibis E, Aras G, Baltaci S, Ozalp G, Beduk Y (2000) Palliative analgesic effect of Re-186 HEDP in various cancer patients with bone metastases. Ann Nucl Med 14:239–245

Lee MV, Fong EM, Singer FR, Guenette RS (2001) Bisphosphonate treatment inhibits the growth of prostate cancer cells. Cancer Res 61:2602–2608

Lewington VJ (1993) Targeted radionuclide therapy for bone metastases. Eur J Nucl Med 20:66–74

Liepe K, Franke WG, Kropp J, Koch R, Runge R, Hliscs R (2000) Comparison of rhenium-188, rhenium-186-HEDP and strontium-89 in palliation of painful bone metastases. Nuklearmedizin 39:146–151

Limouris GS, Shukla SK, Condi-Paphiti A, Gennatas C, Kouvaris I, Vitoratos N (1997) Palliative therapy using rhenium-186-HEDP in painful breast osseous metastases. Anticancer Res 17(3B):1767–1772

Limouris G, Shukla SK, Manetou A, Kouvaris I, Plataniotis G, Triantafyllou N et al (1997) Rhenium-186-HEDP palliative treatment in disseminated bone metastases due to prostate cancer. Anticancer Res 17(3B):1699–1704

Mathieu L, Chevalier P, Galy G, Berger M (1979) Preparation of rhenium-186 labelled EHDP and its possible use in the treatment of osseous neoplasms. Int J Appl Radiat Isot 30:725–727

Maxon HR, III, Schroder LE, Thomas SR, Hertzberg VS, Deutsch EA, Scher HI et al (1990) Re-186(Sn) HEDP for treatment of painful osseous metastases: initial clinical experience in 20 patients with hormone-resistant prostate cancer. Radiology 176:155–159

Maxon HR, III, Thomas SR, Hertzberg VS, Schroder LE, Englaro EE, Samaratunga R (1992) Rhenium-186 hydroxyethylidene diphosphonate for the treatment of painful osseous metastases. Semin Nucl Med 22:33–40

McCready VR, O'Sullivan JM (2002) Future directions for unsealed source radionuclide therapy for bone metastases. Eur J Nucl Med Mol Imaging 29:1271–1275

Mertens WC, Porter AT, Reid RH, Powe JE (1992) Strontium-89 and low-dose infusion cisplatin for patients with hormone refractory prostate carcinoma metastatic to bone: a preliminary report. J Nucl Med 33:1437–1443

Nilsson S, Strang P, Ginman C, Zimmermann R, Edgren M, Nordstrom B, Ryberg M, Kalkner KM, Westlin JE (2005) Palliation of bone pain in prostate cancer using chemotherapy and strontium-89. A randomized phase II study. J Pain Symptom Manag 29:352–357

Oades GM (2003) The use of bisphosphonates in prostate cancer. BJU Int 91:310–311

O'Sullivan JM, McCready VR, Flux G, Norman AR, Buffa FM, Chittenden S (2002) High activity Rhenium-186 HEDP with autologous peripheral blood stem cell rescue: a phase I study in progressive hormone refractory prostate cancer metastatic to bone. Br J Cancer 86:1715–1720

Pagliaro LC, Delpassand ES, Williams D, Millikan RE, Tu SM, Logothetis CJ (2003) A phase I/II study of strontium-89 combined with gemcitabine in the treatment of patients with androgen independent prostate carcinoma and bone metastases. Cancer 97:2988–2994

Palmedo H, Bender H, Dierke-Dzierzon C, Carl UM, Risse J, Krebs D (1999) Pain palliation with rhenium-186 HEDP in breast cancer patients with disseminated bone metastases. Clin Nucl Med 24:643–648

Palmedo H, Manka-Waluch A, Albers P, Schmidt-Wolf IG, Reinhardt M, Ezziddin S, Joe A, Roedel R, Fimmers R, Knapp FF, Jr., Guhlke S, Biersack HJ (2003) Repeated bone-targeted therapy for hormone-refractory prostate carcinoma: tandomized phase II trial with the new, high-energy radiopharmaceutical rhenium-188 hydroxyethylidenediphosphonate. J Clin Oncol 21:2869–2875

Porter AT, McEwan AJ, Powe JE, Reid R, McGowan DG, Lukka H, Sathyanarayana JR, Yakemchuk VN, Thomas GM, Erlich LE (1993) Results of a randomized phase-III trial to evaluate the efficacy of strontium-89 adjuvant to local field external beam irradiation in the management of endocrine resistant metastatic prostate cancer. Int J Radiat Oncol Biol Phys 25:805–813

Quirijnen JM, Han SH, Zonnenberg BA, de Klerk JM, van het Schip AD, van Dijk A (1996) Efficacy of rhenium-186-etidronate in prostate cancer patients with metastatic bone pain. J Nucl Med 37:1511–1515

Schoeneich G, Palmedo H, Dierke-Dzierzon C, Muller SC, Biersack HJ (1997) Rhenium-186 HEDP: palliative radionuclide therapy of painful bone metastases. Preliminary results. Scand J Urol Nephrol 31:445–448

Sciuto R, Maini CL, Tofani A, Fiumara C, Scelsa MG, Broccatelli M (1996) Radiosensitization with low-dose carboplatin enhances pain palliation in radioisotope therapy with strontium-89. Nucl Med Commun 17:799–804

Sciuto R, Festa A, Tofani A, Pasqualoni R, Semprebene A, Cucchi R, Ferraironi A, Rea S, Maini CL (1998) Platinum compounds as radiosensitizers in strontium-89 metabolic radiotherapy. Clin Ter 149:43–47

Sciuto R, Tofani A, Festa A, Giannarelli D, Pasqualoni R, Maini CL (2000) Short- and long-term effects of ^{186}Re-1,1-hydroxyethylidene diphosphonate in the treatment of painful bone metastases. J Nucl Med 41:647–654

Sciuto R, Festa A, Pasqualoni R, Semprebene A, Rea S, Bergomi S (2001) Metastatic bone pain palliation with 89-Sr and 186-Re-HEDP in breast cancer patients. Breast Cancer Res Treat 66:101–109

Sciuto R, Festa A, Rea S, Pasqualoni R, Bergomi S, Petrilli G, Maini CL (2002) Effects of low-dose cisplatin on 89Sr therapy for painful bone metastases from prostate cancer: a randomized clinical trial. J Nucl Med 43:79–86

Smeland S, Erikstein B, Aas M, Skovlund E, Hess SL, Fossa SD (2003) Role of strontium-89 as adjuvant to palliative external beam radiotherapy is questionable: results of a double-blind randomized study. Int J Radiat Oncol Biol Phys 56:1397–1404

Smith MR, Nelson JB (2005) Future therapies in hormone-refractory prostate cancer. Urology 65:9–16

Tennvall J, Abrahamsson PA, Ahlgren G, Darte L, Flodgren P, Garkavij M (2000) Palliative radiation with a radiolabeled diphosphonate (rhenium-186 etidronate) in patients with hormone-refractory disseminated prostate carcinoma. Scand J Urol Nephrol 34:188–193

Tu SM, Millikan RE, Mengistu B, Delpassand ES, Amato RJ, Pagliaro LC, Daliani D, Papandreou CN, Smith TL, Kim J, Podoloff DA, Logothetis CJ (2001) Bone-targeted therapy for advanced androgen-independent carcinoma of the prostate: a randomised phase II trial. Lancet 357:336–341

Virotta G, Medolago G, Arrigoni S, Butti I, Bertocchi C (1997) Rhenium-186 hydroxyethylidene diphosphonate for treatment of painful osseous metastases from mammary carcinoma. Tumori 83:563–565

^{153}Sm-EDTM for Bone Pain Treatment in Skeletal Metastases

21

Carlo Ludovico Maini, Serenella Bergomi, Rosella Pasqualoni, Lidia Strigari, and Rosa Sciuto

CONTENTS

Abstract

Metastases to the skeleton occur in approximately 75% of patients with advanced breast carcinoma, and skeletal metastases are present in >90 % of patients who die from breast carcinoma (Coleman and Rubens 1987; Hortobagyi 1991). Bone disease is most often lytic or mixed lytic/blastic, determining a series of disease-related events that have the most significant impact on quality of life in these relatively long-surviving patients (Kakonen and Mundy 2003). The symptomatic treatment of skeletal pain due to metastases from breast cancer is a complex task that may require administration of drugs, including bisphosphonates and analgesics, and external beam radiotherapy (Lipton 2000; Hoskin 2003). Bisphosphonates target osteoclast-mediated bone resorption and reduce the skeletal complication rate arising from osteolytic metastases in breast cancer (Coleman 2000). External beam radiotherapy allows an effective pain control with a relatively low dose and a low toxicity if the metastatic disease is not extensive, but the toxicity rapidly increases with wide irradiation fields (Hoskin 1995). Systemic radioisotope therapy with radionuclides linked to a bone seeker agent may be the option of choice for the radiation treatment of patients with multiple skeletal localizations due to its efficacy, low cost and low toxicity (Dearnaley et al. 1992). Nonetheless, it still appears to have a low priority among medical oncologists and remain underutilized. Physician education regarding radioisotope therapy should be improved, and clinical trials to evaluate newer treatment paradigms including radionuclides should be strongly encouraged (Damerla et al. 2005).

Radionuclides suitable for systemic metabolic radiotherapy of bone pain, and commercially available, include ^{89}Sr, ^{186}Re chelated by HEDP and ^{153}Sm chelated by EDTMP (Serafini 1994; McEwan 1997; Serafini 2001). The main physical characteristic of the three radionuclides are illustrated in Table 21.1. Beta emitters with short half-lives, such as ^{186}Re and ^{153}Sm, deliver their radiation dose at higher dose rates, which may be more therapeutically effective than equivalent doses given at lower dose rates. The short range of ^{153}Sm beta emission, actually the shortest of the three available radionuclides, may be of advantage limiting red marrow irradiation (Serafini 2000, 2001). ^{153}Sm-EDTMP was developed by Goeckeler at the University of Missouri as a 1:1 chelation complex of radioactive ^{153}Sm and a tetraphosphonate, (ethylenediamine-tetramethylene phosphonate), also known as lexidronam (Goeckeler et al. 1987).

^{153}Sm-EDTMP shows high selective skeletal uptake like conventional ^{99m}Tc bone scanning agents: its bone localization is by chemiabsorption of the tetraphosphate by hydroxyapatite and by the formation of samarium oxide involving oxygen of the hydroxyapatite. The therapeutic effect is due to the irradiation by the short range beta emission of ^{153}Sm.

Table 21.1. Physical characteristics of the three radionuclides

		Physical T ½ (days)	β max energy (MeV)	β max range in soft tissue (mm)	β mean range in bone (mm)	γ Energy (KeV - %)
^{89}Sr	Chloride	50.5	1.46	7–8	3.5	909 (0.02%)
^{186}Re	HEDP	3.7	1.07	4.7	1.0	137 (9%)
^{153}Sm	EDTMP	1.93	0.81 (20%) 0.71 (50%) 0.64 (30%)	3.4	1.7	103 (29%)

Early phase I/II studies were published over 10 years ago (Turner et al. 1989; Podoloff et al. 1991; Eary et al. 1993; Turner and Claringbold 1991), and since then this agent has been clinically used for pain palliation in symptomatic bone metastases from several cancers, mainly prostate and breast carcinoma.

This review will address the characteristics of ^{153}Sm-EDTMP as a radiopharmaceutical and its clinical applications for bone pain palliation in breast carcinoma.

21.1 The Radiopharmaceutical

21.1.1 The Radionuclide

^{153}Sm is a rare earth element, a reactor produced by thermal neutron irradiation of >99% enriched ^{152}Sm in the form of Sm_2O_3. Production is quite efficient as the thermal neutron cross-section is 210 barn and the resonance integral is 3,020 barn.

A1÷2×10^{14} neutrons/cm^2 per second flux applied for 50–60 h typically yields ^{153}Sm with a specific activity up to 1.300 Ci/g; the maximal theoretical specific activity is 3.0 Ci/mg; radionuclide purity is practically 100%. ^{153}Sm has a complex decay scheme with X-rays, gamma-rays and atomic electrons (Auger and conversion) in addition to the dominant beta decay; its physical half-life is 46.3 h. The energy of the beta emissions is relatively low (E_{max} = 640 keV, 30%; 710 keV, 50%; 810 keV, 20%. E_{mean} = 233 keV), resulting in an average penetration range of 0.83 mm in water and a maximum penetration range of 1.7 mm in bone and of 3.1 mm in soft tissue. The main gamma emission (103.2 keV, 29%) is well suited for imaging yielding scans comparable to ^{99m}Tc-MDP bone scans (Fig. 21.1) and for dosimetric estimates.

21.1.2 The Radiopharmaceutical

^{153}Sm is easily complexed with EDTMP (lexidronate) in a single step leading to a percentage of complexed ^{153}Sm exceeding 99%; the preparation is chemically stable and does not undergo any appreciable decomposition for over 48 h (Goeckeler et al. 1987). ^{153}Sm-EDTMP is commercially available (Quadramet®, Schering, Berlin) as monodose vials with a concentration of 1.3 GBq/ml and a specific activity of 28–65 MBq/microg of samarium; the suggested dose is 37 MBq/Kg administered as a slow injection through an i.v. line to avoid extravasation. The registered indication is for pain palliation of osteoblastic skeletal metastases from any cancer provided that a previous ^{99m}Tc-MDP scan is positive for uptake. The radiopharmaceutical is shipped frozen in dry ice and must be thawed just before use.

21.1.3 Biodistribution and Dosimetry

^{153}Sm-EDTMP binds to normal and pathological bone like ^{99m}Tc-MDP and ^{99m}Tc-HDP. In fact, Singh et al. found lesion-to-normal bone ratios for ^{153}Sm-EDTMP and ^{99m}Tc-HDP to be 4.04±2.62 and 4.01±1.97, and lesion-to-soft-tissue ratios to be 5.98±3.18 and 6.87±4.67, respectively (Singh et al. 1989). Eary et al. (1993) reported similar data for ^{99m}Tc-MDP. The total quantity that binds to bone is generally 50% or more of the injected dose depending of course on the extent of metastatic disease, with the rest of the dose being rapidly excreted through the urine by glomerular filtration. Urinary excretion is essentially complete at 6 h, which is of practical interest for radiation safety if the treatment is administered in a day-hospital manner. There is no appreciable metabolism besides bone uptake and urinary excretion.

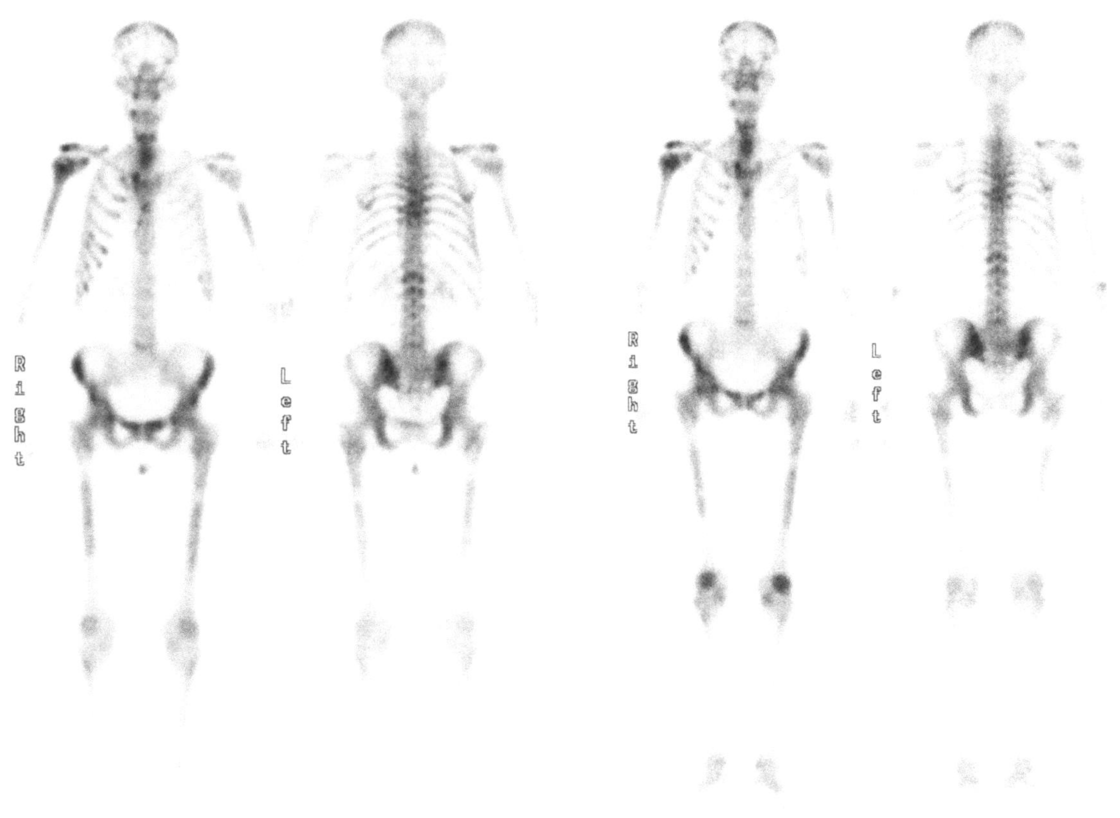

Fig. 21.1a,b. Extensive skeletal disease in breast cancer patient with multiple focal uptakes and a superscan pattern. ^{99m}Tc-MDP image (**a**) and ^{153}Sm-EDTMP image (**b**)

After injection, ^{153}Sm-EDTMP is cleared rapidly from the vascular space to be permanently bound without translocation on bone (Bayouth et al. 1994). The exact site of bone localization is important for red marrow dosimetry; as ^{153}Sm has a short half-life diffusion of radioactivity into the bone mineral, if any, can be neglected, and thus a surface model of deposition is most appropriate (Heggie 1991). Published dosimetric estimates have used the MIRD formalism with different S-factors and animal (Heggie 1991; Logan et al. 1987) or human (Eary et al. 1993; Bayouth et al. 1994) biokinetic data. It is of interest that Heggie has considered contributions from X-rays, gamma-rays, Auger and conversion electrons in addition to the dominant beta-emission (Heggie 1991).

The urinary excretion and the bone uptake clearly identify the bladder wall and the red marrow as the critical organs. The radiation dose to the bladder wall has been reported as 12.5±3.0 cGy/GBq by Bayouth et al. (1994), 964±407 Gy/MBq by Eary et al. (1993), 1.23 mGy/MBq by Logan et al. (1987) and 0.793 mGy/MBq by the package insert. Actual bladder dose is of course inversely related to the extension of bone metastatic disease and critically dependent on the frequency of voiding so that a moderate hyperhydratation of the patient is generally advisable, and a catheter may be used in selected cases. Radiation dose to the red marrow is clearly a critical issue as marrow toxicity is the dose-limiting factor in clinical practice. Published dose estimations are 64.1±18.7 cGy/GBq (Bayouth et al. 1994), 1,514±261 Gy/MBq (Eary et al. 1993), 1.86 mGy/MBq (Heggie 1991), 1.03 mGy/MBq (Logan et al. 1987) and 1.54 mGy/MBq by the package insert. Even if rapid plasma clearance makes the red marrow dose from activity in the blood negligible, actual marrow irradiation is probably not measurable in the individual patient because of: unknown partition of radioactivity between trabecular and cortical bone, heterogeneity of the activity within a given bone and heterogeneity of red marrow distribution. Whatever estimation of the red marrow dose is made, the actual biological response will also be critically dependent on marrow reserve of the single patient. Again from the package insert for an injected dose of 2,590 MBq in a 70-kg patient, radiation doses are reported as follows: red marrow: 4 Gy; bladder wall: 2.5 Gy; effective dose: 796 mSv; metastases: 86.5 Gy. For practical purposes, it is strongly suggested that empirical guidelines are used limiting injected dose to 37 MBq/kg after proper evaluation of platelet and white cells counts. Anticipating up to about a 50% drop, the former should be > 00×10^9/l and the latter >3.5×10^9/l; recent chemotherapy, external beam radiotherapy and in general actual trends in hematological counts also have to be taken into account.

21.2 Clinical Applications in Breast Carcinoma

Available literature reporting clinical applications of ^{153}Sm-EDTMP for bone pain palliation in breast cancer is less extensive than that regarding prostate cancer, and anyway many results of breast cancer have to be extrapolated from studies evaluating different tumors. Approximately only 5%–10% of patients reported in clinical trials on radiopharmaceutical treatment for bone metastases had metastatic breast cancer versus 80%–90% of patients with metastatic hormone-refractory prostate cancer. To date, there is only one study performed specifically on breast cancer, but it is of limited value as it is written in Chinese (Wu et al. 2003). A summary of the published ^{153}Sm-EDTMP clinical studies including evaluation of breast cancer is reported in Table 21.2.

21.2.1 Early Phase I/II Trials

Several early phase I and II studies were performed between the late 1980s and 1990s to evaluate the safety and effectiveness of ^{153}Sm-EDTMP used at doses ranging from 10.36 to 111 MBq/kg (Turner et al. 1989; Farhanghi et al. 1992; Collins et al. 1993). The first clinical reports of efficacy in breast cancer were two phase I studies of Turner et al., both published in 1989 and partially overlapping (Turner et al. 1989a; Turner et al. 1989b). In these studies, using an individual dosimetric approach to provide an estimated red marrow exposure from 100 cGy to 280 cGy, a 75–85% response rate was observed in breast cancer with a similar response to retreatments. The dose-limiting toxicity was delayed thrombocytopenia: the maximum tolerated marrow dose was 280 cGy, corresponding to an administered activity of 24.42–31.08 MBq/kg. No evidence of a dose-response relationship was identified. The same authors further confirmed these preliminary efficacy data in a phase II study where the administered activity of ^{153}Sm-EDTMP was determined fixing the radiation adsorbed dose to bone marrow at 2 Gy (Turner and Claringbold 1991). This study reported also repeated treatment with the aim of prolonging the duration of pain control. Both the median duration of pain control and survival were substantially greater in the re-treated group (24 weeks vs. 8 weeks, and 9 months vs. 4 months, respectively), while additional toxicity in the re-treated patients was confined to anemia, which required blood transfusion in 60% of cases. Another phase I/II study (Alberts et al. 1997) focused on the evaluation of efficacy and toxicity of multiple escalating doses from 27.75- to 111 MBq/kg, again concluding that there is no evidence of a clear dose-response relationship for pain control, tumor response and survival, while toxicity increased using higher doses of ^{153}Sm-EDTMP. Multiple doses can be given with acceptable toxicity and pain control even if duration of pain control in this study resulted in being shorter for subsequent doses (31–35 days in subsequent treatments vs. 56 days in the first treatment).

In conclusion, these preliminary studies, aimed primarily to evaluate the toxicity and the feasibility of the therapy with ^{153}Sm-EDTMP, have shown that doses in the range of 10.36–111 MBq/kg provide rapid pain relief in a majority of patients with breast cancer (Turner et al. 1989a,b; Turner and Claringbold 1991; Alberts et al. 1997; Ahonen et al. 1994). These trials, unfortunately involving a very small number of patients with breast cancer (up to a maximum of 15 patients), substantially confirm the results observed in prostate cancer patients and other tumors (Farhanghi et al. 1992; Collins et al. 1993). The cumulative evidence observed in these early studies can be so summarized: there is no difference in the overall degree of pain palliation at doses ranging from 37 to 111 MBq/kg, while myelotoxicity is clearly dose-dependent; repeated

Table 21.2. Published clinical studies on ^{153}Sm-EDTMP in breast cancer

	Study design	End points	Administered activity	Number of patients		Rate of response		Response measure	Pain relief		Platelet toxicity	
				Total	Br. ca.	Total	Br. ca.		Onset days	Duration weeks	Nadir weeks	Grade
Turner (1989b)	Phase I Dose-escalating	Dosimetry Toxicity MTD	10.36–31.08 MBq/kg calculated to provide a bone marrow dose 100–275 cGy	19	8	84%	75%	VAS[a]	<14	4–35	6	Counts < 100×109/l in 42% of courses with bone marrow dose > 200 cGy
Turner (1989a)	Phase I Dose-escalating	Dosimetry Toxicity MTD	10.36–31.08 MBq/kg calculated to provide a bone marrow dose 100–280 cGy	35	15	65%	85%	VAS[a] Analgesia	<14	4–35	6	Counts < 100×109/l in 42% of courses with bone marrow dose > 200 cGy
Turner (1991)	Phase II Fixed dose	Efficacy Toxicity	Calculated to provide a bone marrow dose of 2 Gy	23	9	61%	n.e.	VAS[a] Analgesia	<14	4–40	4	Median nadir < 133×109/l
Ahonen (1994)	Phase I	Dosimetry Toxicity	4 MBq/kg: 2 patients 8 MBq/kg: 8 patients 19 MBq/kg: 19 patients	35	10	80%	n.e.	VAS[a] Analgesia	<7	2–17	5	WHO[b] case grade III in 1 patient
Alberts (1997)	Phase I/II Dose-escalating	Efficacy Toxicity	27.75–55.55–111 MBq/kg	82	14	78–95%	n.e.	VAS[a]	<2	5.7–8	4	ECOG[c] grade III–IV in: 12% patients with 55.55 MBq/kg 20% pateints with 111 MBq/kg
Resche (1997)	Phase III RCT	Efficacy Toxicity Optimal dose	Gr.1 = 18.5 MBq/kg Gr.2 = 37 MBq/kg	114	36	Gr.1 55% Gr.2 70%	Gr.1 40% Gr.2 80%	VAS[a]-AUPC[d] PGA[e]	<14	4–16	4	NCICTC[f] grade III–IV 12% patients group 1 15% patients group 2
Serafini (1998)	Phase III RCT	Efficacy Toxicity Optimal dose	Gr.1 = placebo Gr.2 = 18.5 MBq/kg Gr.3 = 37 MBq/kg	118	21	Gr 1 20–40% Gr.2 55–60% Gr 3 62–72%	n.e.	VAS[a]-AUPC[d] PGA[e]	<7	4–16	5	NCICTC[f] grade III in 1 patient
Tian (1999)	Phase III RCT	Efficacy Toxicity Optimal dose	Gr.1 = 18.5 MBq/kg Gr.2 = 37 MBq/kg	105	14	83.8%	n.e.	VAS[a]-AUPC[d] PGA[e]	2–26	3–16	3.5 3.3	32% PLT < 100×106
Li (2002)	Phase I	Relationship between bone uptake/efficacy	1.4–2.27 GBq calculated to provide a bone marrow dose of 1.4 Gy	66	18	75%	n.e.	Bone scan KPS[g] Pain relief	7	n.e.	n.e.	n.e.
Dolezaj (2003)	Phase II single fixed dose	Efficacy Toxicity	40 MBq/kg	57	23	75 %	n.e.	n.e.	n.e.	12	4	Counts decrease 50% after 1 month 23% after 3 month
Wu (2003)	Phase II	Efficacy	n.e.	76	76	85.5	85.5	n.e.	n.e.	n.e.	n.e.	WHO[b] grade: I–II–III

Br. Ca. = breast cancer; n.e. = not evaluable; [a]VAS = visual analog scale (Turner et al. 1992); [b]WHO = World Health Organization criteria of toxicity; [c]ECOG = Eastern Cooperative Oncology Group criteria of toxicity; [d]AUPC = area under the curve; [e]PGA = Physician Global Assessment; [f]NCICTC = National Cancer Institute Common Toxicity Criteria; [g]KPS = Karnofsky Performance Score

treatments are feasible and safe provided that the retreatment is deferred until full hemathological recovery from the initial treatment has occurred. Experimental evidence showed the optimum therapeutic dose range for ^{153}Sm-EDTMP to be from 18.5–27.75 MBq to 37 MBq/kg (Holmes 1993). Therefore, subsequent studies were designed as dose-controlled clinical trials employing only 18.5 and 37 MBq/kg doses in larger series of patients to assess the comparative efficacy and safety of these doses in patients with bone metastases from a variety of primary tumors.

21.2.2 Controlled Clinical Studies

To date only three controlled multicenter clinical studies assessing the efficacy of ^{153}Sm-EDTMP in breast cancer have been published in the current literature (Resche et al. 1997; Serafini et al. 1998; Tian et al. 1999). These pivotal studies have been conducted in North America, Europe and Asia and included a variety of tumors among which breast cancer represented only a small sample: a total of 61 patients out of 337 patients.

The first study, called BA-108, is a multicenter single-blind dose-controlled randomized trial (Resche et al. 1997). In this trial 114 patients with different tumors were randomized to receive either 18.5 MBq/kg or 37 MBq/kg ^{153}Sm-EDTMP. Among this cohort of patients, 36 were breast cancers and were randomized as follows: 16 patients received the lower dose and 20 patients the higher dose. The second study, called BA-106/110, is a multicenter double-blind placebo-controlled trial in which 118 patients with painful metastases from a variety of tumors were randomized to receive either placebo, 18.5 MBq/kg or 37 MBq/kg ^{153}Sm-EDTMP (Serafini et al. 1998). In particular, considering only breast cancer (n=21) four patients received placebo, 11 patients 18.5 MBq/kg and 6 patients 37 MBq/kg ^{153}Sm-EDTMP. These two studies can be easily compared because they used the same criteria for data collections and analysis, and all the study procedures were designed in similar manner. Both evaluated efficacy, safety and excretion of the radionuclide during the 16 weeks after the treatment. The methodology used to assess ^{153}Sm-EDTMP efficacy included a double system of pain palliation check: a self- patient evaluation and a physician global assessment (PGA).

The self-patient evaluation was obtained by a pain diary that each patient completed daily specifying several variables: (1) a multi-site pain intensity (rated with the system of the visual analog scale, VAS); (2) the daily analgesic use, subsequently converted to oral morphine equivalent dose; (3) sleep characteristics; (4)– five-point level of discomfort; (5) a weekly statement on the help of a study drug to decrease pain. Finally, to obtain a meaningful overall score, the area under the curve (AUPC) scores for each 7-day period were computed moving from the transformed daily overall scores obtained according the method of Donaldson (1992). The PGA was based on patients' overall conditions (including pain, discomfort and daily activities) evaluated by unblinded (Resche et al. 1997) or blinded (Serafini et al. 1998) investigators and was rated as six categories: much worse, worse, no change, better, much better or completely better. The overall agreement between these two pain assessment methods was attested by the significance (P<0.005) of the correlation coefficients (r>0.402) in the Serafini study. The results of these two studies can be so summarized:

- Efficacy: Efficacy was generally evident with both doses in all patients; a clear superiority of the effect for the higher dose of 37 MBq/kg was confirmed in both studies (a higher percentage of patients presenting a marked or complete response and with their response lasting up to 16 weeks) (Serafini et al. 1998). The 37 MBq/kg dose of ^{153}Sm-EDTMP also showed statistically significant improvements over placebo in both patient self-evaluations (AUPC-VAS) and physician rate (PGA) efficacy measures at each of the first 4-week periods after administration. In contrast, no consistent significant improvement over placebo occurred in patients treated with 18.5 MBq/kg (Serafini et al. 1998). Interestingly enough, dose-related response was apparently higher in breast cancer than other tumors. Breast cancer treated with 37 MBq/kg had thus the most noticeable improvement. In the Resche study 40% of breast cancer treated with 18.5 MBq/kg and 80% of those treated with 37 MBq/kg were considered responders by the PGA evaluation, while in the overall population the corresponding responder fractions were 55% and 70%, respectively. This difference was further confirmed by AUPC results at 4 weeks. In fact, the decrease of AUPC from baseline scores was larger with 37 MBq/kg than with 18.5 MBq/kg in all patients, but the difference between doses was greater for females and particularly for females with breast cancer than for males and males with prostate cancer. This trend was confirmed also by the results of Serafini's study (Serafini et al. 1998).

- Survival: The survival of breast cancer patients who had received 37 MBq/kg was longer than that of patients receiving 18.5 MBq/kg.
- Safety: A predictable level of dose-related marrow suppression was the only toxicity associated with ^{153}Sm-EDTMP. Platelet and white blood cells counts are reduced by approximately 40–50% from baseline with nadirs at 3 to 5 weeks and recovery in 8 weeks. Grade III-IV mielotoxicity was 10–15%. Breast cancer patients presented generally lower platelet and white blood cell baseline values, but also a lower percentage of higher grades of toxicity than males patients. All these results seem to suggest that a 37 MBq/kg dose would be expected to work well even in highly pre-treated patients such as breast cancer patients.

The third study is a multicenter single-blind dose-controlled trial organized in China as a part of an international coordinated research project sponsored by the International Atomic Energy Agency (Tian et al. 1999): 105 patients with a variety of tumors were randomized to receive 18.5 MBq/kg or 37 MBq/kg ^{153}Sm-EDTMP. In particular, breast cancer (n=14) received 18.5 MBq/kg (n=6) or 37 MBq/kg (n=8). The protocol of this study was similar to protocols employed by the two mentioned controlled studies, but the evaluation of therapy efficacy was based on a new measurement system defined "sum of the effect product" (SEP). In this study both the response to ^{153}Sm-EDTMP and the toxicity were suggested to be independent of the dose. Also, no statistically significant differences were observed between SEPs in different primary tumors.

In the last years several minor uncontrolled studies have also been published, often in languages other than English (Wu et al. 2003; Li et al. 2002; Dolezal et al. 2003) confirming the efficacy and safety of the treatment both with individually calculated and standard fixed doses of ^{153}Sm-EDTMP.

21.2.3 Personal Experience

In the period from January 2000 until December 2005 we performed in our Institute over 110 treatments in 80 patients with painful bone metastases from different tumors: the primary histologically proven malignancy was breast cancer (20 patients), prostate cancer (46 patients) and other tumors (14 patients) (Maini et al. 2003). Seventy-five patients received a fixed dose of 37 MB/kg ^{153}Sm-EDTMP once, and 18 patients (4 breast cancers and 14 prostate cancers) were treated twice. All breast cancers had been previously treated by at least three courses of chemotherapy and by at least two cycles of bisphosphonates; eight patients had been also treated by local external beam radiotherapy. A minimum of 1 month from chemo-radiotherapy and of 15 days from bisphosphonate was required before ^{153}Sm-EDTMP therapy; hormonal therapy was not discontinued. This series of patients was evaluated with the same homogeneous and clearly defined criteria for entry into the treatment and for response evaluation according to the protocols widely validated at our Institute (Sciuto et al. 2000, 2001). Clinical follow-up was prolonged until patient's death to evaluate long-term effects. Pain relief was evident within 2 weeks in 86% of breast cancer patients with a mean duration of 18 weeks (range: 9–40 weeks). This pattern of response is quite similar to the pattern observed in the other tumors (83% response rate with mean duration of pain relief of 16 weeks). Neither overall global response rate nor complete response rate (6/20 patients, 30%) showed a significant correlation with any pre-therapy variables, while duration of pain relief showed a significant positive correlation with the Karnofsky performance score (P<0.005) and a negative correlation with bone scan score (P<0.005). No patient showed any clinically evident acute adverse side effect following radionuclide administration, and only one patient experienced a mild increase in pain, i.e., a flare-up response. A good correlation was found between the ^{99m}Tc-MDP images before therapy and the ^{153}Sm images obtained 24 h after therapy. Toxicity was generally mild with a mean decrease from baseline values of 25% for platelet and 20% for white blood cells counts, respectively, reaching the nadir value at 4 weeks. The mean time to recovery after nadir was 21 days and did not correlate with previous chemotherapy cycles. No breast cancer presented severe hematological toxicity (grade III–IV according to WHO criteria), which is at variance with the severe and quite persistent myelotoxicity observed in 12/46 (26%) prostate cancer patients. The four breast cancer patients who received two treatment cycles presented a similar response and toxicity as after the first treatment.

22.3 Conclusions

^{153}Sm-EDTMP radioisotope therapy for breast cancer bone metastases is indeed effective, but clinical experience is still limited, and many issues still remain unresolved. To date, fewer than 250 breast cancer patients treated are partially evaluable in the 11 published clinical trial compared with 730 patients enrolled in the same studies. This low percentage observed with ^{153}Sm-EDTMP (34%) reflects the general limited availability of clinical databases concerning all radioionuclide treatments in bone metastases from breast cancer as previously reported also for ^{89}Sr and ^{186}Re-HEDP (Sciuto et al. 2001). Additionally, the relatively short follow-up (up to 16 weeks only in controlled studies), the small number of patients completing the study (only 30% and 48% in Serafini's and Resche's studies, respectively) and the overall limited number of patients evaluable for efficacy limit the validity of generalization of the reported results. Also, survival or bone progression issues have never been specifically addressed in breast cancer. All these criticisms could determine the lower priority assigned to radionuclide treatments in oncological algorithms for treatment of breast cancer bone metastases.

An intriguing result showed by available data is the more pronounced dose-response relationship evidenced in breast cancer in controlled studies. Doses tailored for prostate cancer may be not adequate for breast cancer. In fact, pain palliation in breast cancer metastases shows peculiar features that could be justified by a different biological response. The radiation dose delivered to skeletal metastases has been demonstrated to be influenced by bone lesion density (Samaratunga et al. 1995), and bone metastases' microenvironment is different from prostate cancer with a prevalence of lytic or mixed lesions in breast cancer. Moreover, breast cancer radiosensitivity could be higher than prostate cancer (Mauch 1993). These issues could suggest the need of specifically targeted higher dose escalating studies in breast cancer to identify the "best dose." Future clinical trial designs in breast cancer have to incorporate prospective whole-body and tumor dosimetry to tailor a patient-specific activity in order to enhance response rates within predictable toxicity.

A number of possible improvements can be also explored to improve disease control and survival prolongation in breast cancer using ^{153}Sm-EDTMP such as the radio-chemosensitization enhancement effect (Sciuto et al. 1996; Sciuto et al. 1998; Sciuto et al. 2002; Turner et al. 1992), interaction with cold bisphosphonates, earlier treatment/prophylaxis of subclinical micrometastes and different schedules with higher activities (McCready and O'Sullivan 2002). A comprehensive and multidisciplinary clinical approach could help to optimize radiopharmaceutical therapy for pain palliation in breast cancer and increase its awareness among oncologist.

In conclusion, summarizing the evidence drawn from available data on ^{153}Sm-EDTMP treatment in breast cancer bone metastases, the state of the art can be synthesized as follows:

- A dose of 37 MBq/kg has a better therapeutic ratio than 18.5 MBq/kg;
- the mean pain palliation rate after a single treatment of ^{153}Sm-EDTMP in breast cancer is about 80%, and it is not significantly different from that observed in other tumors;
- toxicity is generally mild and transitory and again not different from other tumors despite usually worse basal hematological baseline function;
- retreatments are effective and safe provided that hematological values have fully recovered;
- efficacy is probably directly correlated to the intensity of uptake, while duration of palliation is inversely correlated to disease extension as evaluated by ^{99m}Tc-MDP bone scan;
- more well-designed controlled studies enrolling larger series of breast cancer patients are undoubtedly needed to fully characterize the role of ^{153}Sm-EDTMP in the short- and long-term follow-up and management of breast cancer.

Evidence-based and cost-effectiveness studies are also necessary to identify operative guidelines for systemic therapy with different radionuclides used alone and in combination with the more traditional treatment options.

References

Ahonen A, Joensuu H, Hiltunen J et al (1994) Samarium-153-EDTMP in bone metastases. J Nucl Biol Med 38 (suppl I):123–127

Alberts AS, Smit BJ, Louw WKA et al (1997) Dose response relationship and multiple dose efficacy and toxicity of samarium-153-EDTMP in metastatic cancer to bone. Radiother Oncol 43:175–179

Bayouth JE, Macey DJ, Kasi LP et al (1994) Dosimetry and toxicity of samarium-153-EDTMP administered for bone pain due to skeletal metastases. J Nucl Med 35:63–69

Coleman RE (2000) Optimizing treatment of bone metastases by Aredia and Zometa. Breast Cancer 7:361–369

Coleman RE, Rubens RD (1987) The clinical course of bone metastases from breast cancer. Br J Cancer 55:61–66

Collins C, Eary JF, Donaldson G et al (1993) Samarium-153-EDTMP in bone metastases of hormone refractory prostate carcinoma: a phase I/II trial. J Nucl Med 34:1839–1844

Damerla V, Packianathan S, Boerner PS et al (2005) Recent developments in nuclear medicine in the management of bone metastases: a review and perspective. Am J Clin Oncol 28: 513–520

Dearnaley DP, Bayly RJ, A'Hern RP et al (1992) Palliation of bone metastases in prostate cancer. Hemibody irradiation or strontium-89? Clin Oncol 4:101–107

Dolezal J, Vizd'a J, Cermakova E (2003) Myelotoxicity after systemic radionuclide therapy of painful bone metastases with 153Samarium-EDTMP. Vnitr Lek 49:189–193

Donaldson G (1992) A new approach to calculating pain measurements for cancer patients. Sci Comput Automation 1:45–48

Eary JF, Collins C, Stabin M et al (1993) Samarium-153-EDTMP biodistribution and dosimetry estimation. J Nucl Med 34:1031–1036

Farhanghi M, Homes RA, Volkert WA et al (1992) Samarium-153-EDTMP: pharmacokinetic, toxicity and pain response using an escalating dose schedule in treatment of metastatic bone cancer. J Nucl Med 33:1451–1458

Goeckeler WF, Edwards B, Volkert WA et al (1987) Skeletal localization of samarium-153 chelates: potential therapeutic bone agents. J Nucl Med 28:495–504

Heggie JC (1991) Radiation absorbed dose calculations for samarium-153-EDTMP localized in bone. J Nucl Med 32:840–844

Holmes RA (1993) Radiopharmaceuticals in clinical trials. Semin Oncol 20 (suppl 2):22–26

Hortobagyi GN (1991) Bone metastases in breast cancer patients. Semin Oncol 18:11–15

Hoskin PJ (1995) Radiotherapy for bone pain. Pain 63:137–139

Hoskin PJ (2003) Bisphosphonates and radiation therapy for palliation of metastatic bone disease. Cancer Treat Rev 29:321–327

Kakonen SM, Mundy GR (2003) Mechanisms of osteolytic bone metastases in breast carcinoma. Cancer 97 (suppl):834–839

Li L, Liang Z, Deng H et al (2002) Samarium-153-EDTMP bone uptake rate and its relation to therapeutic effect. Chin Med J 115:1096–1098

Lipton A (2000) Bisphosphonates and breast carcinoma: present and future. Cancer 88 (suppl):3033–3037

Logan KW, Volkert WA, Holmes RA (1987) Radiation dose calculations in persons receiving injection of samarium-153-EDTMP. J Nucl Med 28:505–509

Maini CL, Sciuto R, Romano L et al (2003) Radionuclide therapy with bone seeking radionuclides in palliation of painful bone metastases. J Exp Clin Cancer Res 22:71–74

Mauch PM (1993) Treatment of metastatic cancer to bone. In: De Vita VT Jr, Hellman S, Rosenberg Sam (eds) Cancer. Principles and practice of oncology. JB Lippincott, Philadelphia, pp 1564–1579

McCready VR, O'Sullivan JM (2002) Future directions for unsealed source radionuclide therapy for bone metastases. Eur J Nucl Med 29:1271–1275

McEwan AJ (1997) Unsealed source therapy of painful bone metastases: an update. Semin Nucl Med 27:165–182

Podoloff DA, Kasi LP, Kim EE et al (1991) Evaluation of Sm-153-EDTMP as a bone imaging agent during a therapeutical trial. J Nucl Med 32:A918

Resche I, Chatal JF, Pecking A et al (1997) A dose-controlled study of 153-Sm-ethylenediaminetetramethylenephosphonate (EDTMP) in the treatment of patients with painful bone metastases. Eur J Cancer 33:1583–1591

Samaratunga RC, Thomas SR, Hinnefeld JD et al (1995) A Monte Carlo simulation model for radiation dose to metastatic skeletal tumor from Rhenium-186(Sn)-HEDP. J Nucl Med 36:336–350

Sciuto R, Maini CL, Tofani A et al (1996) Radiosensitization with low-dose carboplatin enhances pain palliation in radioisotope therapy with strontium-89. Nuc Med Commun 17:799–804

Sciuto R, Festa A, Tofani A et al (1998) Platinum compounds as radiosensitizers in strontium-89 metabolic radiotherapy. Clin Ther 149:43–47

Sciuto R, Tofani A, Festa A et al (2000) Short- and long-term effects of 186 Re-1,1-hydroxyethylidene diphophonate in the treatment of painful bone metastases. J Nucl Med 41:647– 654

Sciuto R, Festa A, Pasqualoni R et al (2001) Metastatic bone pain palliation with 89-Sr and 186-Re-HEDP in breast cancer patients. Breast Cancer Res Treat 66:101– 109

Sciuto R, Festa A, Rea S et al (2002) Effects of low-dose cisplatin on ^{89}Sr therapy for painful bone metastases from prostate cancer: a randomized clinical trial. J Nucl Med 43:79–86

Serafini AN (1994) Current status of systemic intravenous radiopharmaceuticals for the treatment of painful metastatic bone disease. Int J Radiat Oncol Biol Phys 30:1187–1194

Serafini AN (2000) Samarium Sm-153 lexidronam for the palliation of bone pain associated with metastases. Cancer 88 (suppl):2934– 2939

Serafini AN (2001a) Therapy of metastatic bone pain. J Nucl Med 42:895-906

Serafini AN (2001b) Systemic metabolic radiotherapy with samarium-153 EDTMP for the treatment of painful bone metastases. Q J Nucl Med 45:91–99

Serafini AN, Houston SJ, Resche I et al (1998) Palliation of pain associated with metastatic bone cancer using samarium-153 Lexidronam: a double-blind placebo-controlled clinical trial. J Clin Oncol 16:1574–1581

Singh A, Holmes RA, Farhangi M et al (1989) Human pharmacokinetics of samarium-153 EDTMP in metastatic cancer. J Nucl Med 30:1814–1818

Tian JH, Zhang JM, Hou QT et al (1999) Multicentre trial on the efficacy and toxicity of single-dose samarium-153-ethylene diamine tetramethylene phosphonate as a palliative treatment for painful skeletal metastases in China. Eur J Nucl Med 26:2–7

Turner JH, Claringbold PG (1991) A phase II study of treatment of painful multifocal skeletal metastases with single and repeated dose of samarium-153 ethylenediaminetetramethylene phosphonate. Eur J Cancer 27:1084–1086

Turner JH, Claringbold PG, Hetherington EL et al (1989a) A phase I study of samarium-153 ethylenediaminetetramethylene phosphonate therapy for disseminated skeletal metastases. J Clin Oncol 7:1926–1931

Turner JH, Martindale AA, Sorby P et al (1989b) Samarium-153 EDTMP therapy of disseminated skeletal metastasis. Eur J Nucl Med 15:784–795

Turner JH, Claringbold PG, Martindale AA (1992) Samarium-153- EDTMP and radiosensitizing chemotherapy for treatment of disseminated skeletal metastases. Eur J Nucl Med 16:s125

Wu H, Tan T, Fang L et al (2003) Evaluation of efficacy of ^{153}Sm-EDTMP in patients with painful bone metastases of breast cancer. Sichuan Da Xue Xue Bao Yi Xue Ban 34:716–718

The Choice of the Correct Imaging Modality in Breast Cancer Management

22

Paola Mariani and Luca Gianni

CONTENTS

Abstract

Substantial progress has been made in the diagnosis and treatment of primary and metastatic breast cancer in the last 20 years. New technical instruments and laboratory tools have emerged in recent years that expand the options for the study of breast cancer at different stages. Such an improved platform requires a departure from standard approaches and prompts testing of the innovative tools in the workup of women with breast cancer, with the aim of investigating at which stage, in the natural history of breast cancer, they should be applied to optimize clinical management.

It is known that the widespread use of routine mammography has led to an increase in the early detection of primary breast lesions that significantly contributes to the decrease of mortality from breast cancer that is now measurable in Europe and North America. The dramatic shift in the stage of breast cancer at diagnosis has been associated with the successful application of less mutilating surgical procedures, with the widespread resort to breast-conserving surgery and, more recently, with avoidance of useless surgical staging of the axillary lymph node status through the use of sentinel node biopsy. In addition, adjuvant and preoperative systemic therapy has been optimized in terms of drug availability and activity and refinement of the criteria for administration, thus significantly contributing to prolongation of survival in women with early breast cancer. The challenge at this time is to define procedures and tools that allow easy characterization of the tumor, its aggressiveness and its pattern of sensitivity/resistance to drug therapy, so that treatment can be tailored to individual needs rather than to the average risk of the average patient.

The technological development of the diagnostic imaging has been impressive in the field of radiology and nuclear medicine allowing for the dependable detection of small lesions. These tools have generated new approaches permitting the successful differential diagnosis of doubtful lesions and the rapid identification of systemic metastases, and are providing a means for the non-invasive characterization of biology of cancer tissue. It is likely that these advances will provide further contributions to the optimization of therapeutic strategies, considering that the metabolic information offered by nuclear medicine procedures, combined with the anatomical data provided by conventional radiological techniques, should find a place in predicting tumor response and monitoring the outcome of patients. It is difficult to formulate conclusive diagnostic guidelines for application in the workup of breast cancer, since while the role of some examinations, such as mammography and US, is well established, that of others, such as MRI and PET, is still a matter of investigations.

New technical instruments and laboratory tools have emerged in recent years that expand the options for the study of breast cancer at different stages. Such an improved platform requires a departure from standard approaches and prompts testing of the innovative tools in the workup of women with breast cancer, with the aim of investigating at which stage, in the natural history of breast cancer, they should be applied to optimize clinical management.

Assessment may be simplified by evaluating their role: (1) in screening for and in diagnosing of breast cancer; (2) for loco-regional staging; (3) for extensive staging and follow-up; (4) for better characterization of the tumor; (5) for monitoring/predicting patterns of sensitivity or resistance to therapy.

Clinical observation is the mainstay of evaluation in each phase of the patient's management, and histopathological analysis is the gold standard for diagnosis, but laboratory tests, radiological imaging and nuclear medicine imaging are assuming a growing role in the workup of patients with breast cancer (Table 22.1).

22.1 Screening and Diagnosis of Breast Cancer

Early detection of breast cancer is important to improve the prognosis and survival of patients, allowing for the timely identification of lesions at a curable stage. So an accurate screening and a correct diagnosis represent the most important outcome. Imaging in breast cancer has an important role at all stages of the disease, from initial screening of the women who are unaware they may have the disease, to the application in symptomatic women who present a lump or other symptoms of breast disease or established breast cancer (Elmore et al. 2005; Liang et al. 2003; Gotzsche and Nielsen 2006).

Mammography remains the main screening tool and the most extensively studied screening modality that can be associated with clinical breast evaluation and breast self-examination (Gotzsche and Nielsen 2006). Many randomized clinical trials show that screening mammography reduces breast cancer mortality, especially in women aged 50 to 69 years. Thus mammography represents the most sensitive and specific screening test, and it is recommended annually for women aged 50 through 70 years. Recent trial results have indicated the possible beneficial effects of screening mammography beginning at the age of 40 years (Moss et al. 2006). On the basis of these considerations, there is a general consensus that women should undergo to periodic test from the age of 45 years, every 2 years.

The principal predictors of mammography's accuracy are the breast density and the age of the woman. So mammography may be less sensitive or not optimal in women with a dense breast or in young women at high risk for breast cancer (BRCA1 and BRCA2 mutation) (Warner et al. 2004). In these cases other imaging modalities, such as magnetic resonance imaging (RMI) and ultrasound (US), are being studied as screening tests. In particular in women at high risk for breast cancer many clinical trials have reported a higher sensitivity for breast RMI than for ultrasound, mammography or both. Moreover, MRI can detect otherwise occult breast cancer in this subgroup of women (Kuhl et al. 2005; Kuhl 2006; Lehman 2006).

In women with dense breast, ultrasound is usually performed as adjuvant of screening mammography (Crystal et al. 2003). This imaging test has some limitations as a screening tool because it requires a well-trained operator and it cannot detect microcalcifi-

Table 22.1. Options for breast cancer imaging

Study of a breast mass	Mammography–digital mammography Ultrasounds Magnetic resonance (MRI) Nuclear medicine imaging : - Lymphoscintigraphy (with ^{99}mTc-colloids) and sentinel node - Breast scintigraphy (scintimammography with ^{99m}Tc-sestamibi) - PET or PET/CT with ^{18}F-FD
Study of distant metastases	Thorax X-rays Bone scintigraphy (with ^{99}mTc-phosphonates) Ultrasounds of upper abdomen Computed tomography (CT) Nuclear medicine imaging - Bone scintgraphy (with ^{99}mTc-phosphonates) - Whole body PET or PET/CT with ^{18}F-FDG

cations. Therefore, in clinical practice ultrasound is better used as a targeted diagnostic examination with the purpose of characterizing lesions that are palpable or detected by mammography, and of discriminating cystic from solid lesions.

The guidelines for breast cancer screening vary according to the age of the women. In women younger than 40 years who are symptom-free, no particular recommendation exists with respect to the need for preventive check-up, except for those women at high risk who should be involved in particular programs of diagnostic surveillance (RMI and mammography) (Lehman et al. 2005).

In women over 45 years of age, mammography is considered the standard screening examination that preferentially should be integrated with US, especially in women with dense breasts. The frequency suggested for such procedures is every 1–2 years. In this subgroup nuclear medicine techniques (breast scintigraphy or positron emission tomography PET) could contribute to solving some diagnostic problems unsolved with other radiological modalities (mammography or US).

The identification of new breast symptoms or a suspicious mass requires a timely clinical examination by a well-trained physician, a careful examination of the patient's history including the evaluation of risk factors, and an adequate diagnostic assessment (Hackshaw and Paul 2003; Cuzick 2003; Kolb et al. 2002).

Mammography represents the principal diagnostic examination, and its limitation can be overcome by combining it with RMI and US (Leconte et al. 2003; Bedrosian et al. 2003; Kuhl et al. 2005). In this area, nuclear medicine imaging (breast scintigraphy or PET) can provide additional information on the presence of hyper-metabolic lesions (Liberman et al. 2003; McDonough et al. 2004; Czernin 2002).

The diagnostic procedures suggested for the assessment of breast cancer vary according to age and symptoms (Mehta 2003; Prats et al. 2001; Adler et al. 2003; De Gery et al. 2003). In women with symptoms and younger than 40 years of age, after a clinical examination, US and fine needle aspiration (FNA) are usually adequate to rule out or confirm malignancy (Hall 2003).

If clinical doubt about the nature of the breast lesion remains, the diagnostic workup should continue with RMI and mammography or other nuclear medicine tests. Here again, MRI and nuclear medicine approaches can supply additional and discriminating information. Several studies have demonstrated the potential of MRI in the detection of multicentric and multifocal disease not seen at mammography and the capacity to map the extension of the tumor (Schnall et al. 2006; Irwing et al 2004). Furthermore, MRI can better identify ductal carcinoma in situ (DCIS), particularly in a dense breast, and allows for dependably evaluating the breast tissue after prior radiation or surgery.

For the detection of primary breast cancer, the role of PET with ^{18}F-fluoro-2-deoxy-D-glucose (FDG-PET) does not appear comparable with the standard imaging. In particular several studies showed that the sensitivity of PET for primary breast cancer was modest especially for detecting small tumors (<0.6 cm), well-differentiating histological subtype (tubular carcinoma and DCIS) and lobular carcinoma (Schoder et al. 2007). In the same way scintimammography with ^{99m}Tc sestamibi, after a large clinical evaluation, did not show a sufficient diagnostic sensitivity to be proposed as the test of first choice to study a breast mass. Some dedicated gamma cameras for breast imaging are under study, but until now this modality did not enter the clinical routine.

The results of imaging procedures are key in determining whether further tests such as biopsy are needed. Histological assessment is always suggested whenever doubtful finding or elements of suspicion persist in order to confirm the malignancy and to characterize the tumor's biology. Whether this will involve cytological examination of FNA or histological investigation of core biopsy (CB) depends on a combination of factors such as the type and size of the lesion, local expertise and operator's choice (Liberman 2000). Guidelines usually recommend FNA for nodules smaller than 1 cm, and core biopsy in all other cases whenever possible. In case of an impalpable lesion identified by radiological tests or lesions requiring more accurate sampling, the use of image-guided biopsy is recommended.

22.2 Loco-Regional Staging

Staging after the diagnosis of breast cancer is obligatory. At a loco- regional level, axillary lymph node involvement is still considered the single most important factor associated with prognosis and treatment selection. Current practice requires that all women with invasive breast cancer undergo a staging of axillary nodal status. Considering the large proportion of women with early breast cancer without nodal metastasis, the role of routine axillary lymph node dissection (ALND) has been challenged. In the last 10 years, a new surgical technique, the sentinel lymph node biopsy (SLNBB) has progressively gained the role of a minimally invasive and dependable procedure for staging axillary lymph node status in women with early breast cancer. This conservative surgical approach has a high level of accuracy in the identification of axillary lymph node involvement that allows the selection of patients who will be candidates for ALND. Moreover, SLNBB biopsy is associated with a lower risk of morbidity than full axillary dissection (lymphedema, sensory arm changes and wound complication) (Silberman et al. 2004). After adequate learning and with the appropriate experience, SLNBB biopsy has such a reliable negative predictive value that it allows sparing full axillary dissection in most cases with negative findings (Jakub et al. 2003; Veronesi et al. 2006b).

The imaging approach also has been used to perform the loco regional staging. Particularly FDG-PET has been proposed as an adequate radiological tool for the study of the axillary lymph node status (Schwarz et al. 2005). Different clinical trials reached conflicting conclusions as to the reliability of this imaging approach because the diagnostic sensitivity ranged from 60 to over 90%. Some authors reported data almost as good as those expected from SLNB biopsy when performed by a well-trained surgeon in a well-equipped hospital (Greco et al. 2001; Smith et al. 1998; Kuehn et al. 2004; Veronesi et al. 2006a). There is no doubt that the added value of PET consists of the possibility of also imaging supraclavicular or internal mammary lymph node regions. In addition PET is a non-invasive technique that concomitantly allows staging of the entire body with high sensitivity. The hybrid systems PET/CT combining the detection of metabolic imaging (PET) and morphological imaging (CT) are under evaluation. Some very recent clinical evidence on the usefulness of PET in loco-regional staging concluded that on the basis of the good specificity of PET and its high positive predictive value, this test should not be considered as an alternative diagnostic tool instead of SLNB, but in patients with clinically negative axilla can select cases eligible for ALND (those with FDG positive axillary uptake) from those who should go previously to SLNB (those with FDG negative axillary uptake).

These considerations justify the investigation of PET for axillary staging in women with breast cancer. Where PET is not available, single-photon emission computed tomography (SPECT) could be a valid alternative. SPECT, especially if performed with special collimators and according to ad hoc protocols, can provide better anatomical information of the breast than planar scintigraphy and results in more accurate detection of axillary lymph nodes (Spanu et al. 2001; Mankoff et al. 2006).

Finally, MRI is the focus of great interest for loco-regional staging. Final conclusions and recommendations were not as yet reached about its use as a routine test. However, a growing body of evidence suggests the value of MRI prior to breast-conserving surgical intervention (Walter et al. 2003). MRI is indeed capable of defining the size and the number of lesions and of assessing the possible presence of multifocal and multi-centric disease and of controlateral lesions that may escape over standard imaging approaches.

22.3 Systemic Staging

The clinical evaluation of breast cancer and the systemic staging are necessary in order to define the disease clinical stage and consequently the correct approach, surgery or systemic treatment for primary breast cancer or metastatic disease.

Systemic staging usually requires a set of different imaging strategies than those applied to loco-regional staging. Currently, it is performed using chest X-ray, bone scintigraphy with phosphonates and liver US or abdominal CT (Newman and Sabel 2003; Kubota et al. 2003). CT may be preferred, especially in those patients who are considered for clinical trials. The other radiological exams (PET, PET/CT, RMI) may be used to better evaluate a doubtful lesion detected by conventional imaging.

The utility of systemic staging for women with small tumors without clinical evidence of axillary involvement and in the absence of symptoms is not universally considered worth the cost of performing such examinations. For this reason it does not appear in the recommendations found in many guidelines developed by scientific societies in Europe (Mille et al. 2000; Williams 1994).

In particular the value of bone scintigraphy in detecting bone metastasis has been challenged, and the conclusions from different study groups are controversial. There is general agreement that the application of the above diagnostic approaches at baseline depends on the individual risk of developing metastatic spread, which is related to several prognostic factors, including clinical stage.

The availability of new prognostic tools based on the molecular characterization of the tumor will eventually lead to a better definition of risk and a more refined set of criteria for the application of instrumental systemic staging.

22.4 Breast Cancer Follow-up

The optimal strategy for planning follow-up of breast cancer patients is also the subject of diverging opinions (Emens and Davidson 2003; Collins et al. 2004). The main goals of follow up are: (1) early diagnosis of metastases, (2) diagnosis of loco regional relapse and (3) diagnosis of controlateral breast cancer.

The measure of the impact of any successful strategy should consist in the improvement of overall survival, disease-free survival or in the achievement of measurable changes in quality of life. There is no clear evidence that the early diagnosis of metastases affects survival, although the early identification of solitary metastases has recently been proposed as a means to increase the proportion of metastatic patients (almost 10%) who are potentially curable with multimodality approaches including surgery, irradiation and drugs (Hortobagyi 2002).

Similarly, the early diagnosis of local relapse does not affect mortality, although this conclusion is in contrast with findings suggesting that better locoregional control with irradiation after mastectomy may influence survival, and with claims that ipsilateral breast cancer recurrence may adversely affect long-term outcome after breast-conserving procedures (Mamounas 2001). In such a controversial scenario, early detection of metastases and accurate restaging of recurrent breast cancer are clearly important for the selection of the most appropriate treatment and for early identification of patients with limited disease who could benefit from the multiple treatments with curative intent.

Different consensus conferences have proposed specific guidelines for the follow-up of breast cancer patients, and the American Society of Clinical Oncology (ASCO) published a recent update in 2006 (Khatcheressian et al. 2006). The recommendations have been based on balancing the potential benefits for the health of patients against the psychological stress of undergoing serial assessments and the cost of the diagnostic procedures.

Careful history and physical examination are considered the first modality for a correct follow-up that should be repeated every 3 to 6 months for the first 3 years after primary therapy and every 6 months for the next 2 years, and then annually. Every physician should research signs or symptoms related to local or distant recurrence such as new lumps, bone pain, chest pain, dyspnea or abdominal pain considering that more than half of breast cancer recurrence is symptomatic.

During the follow-up, mammography is considered the only relevant radiological examination for the detection of recurrence in the residual breast for patients who underwent breast-conserving surgery, and in the controlateral breast (Grunfeld et al. 2002). It is recommended alone or, when necessary, in combination with US every year. All other laboratory, radiological and nuclear medicine tests should not be carried out in patients without symptoms and/or at low risk of metastatic tumor spread. Therefore, they are not recommended for the routine breast cancer follow-up.

The ASCO guidelines summarized above propose a minimalist breast cancer surveillance with physical examination and mammography, taking into account the results of clinical trials mostly published before 1998 as retrospective studies that showed no significant survival advantage between intensive (conventional radiological exams and chemistry panel) and routine follow-up (physical examination and mammography) (Joseph et al. 1998; Palli et al. 1999). Concurrently the authors underlined the need to conduct new prospective clinical trials in order to evaluate the main role of new radiological imaging modalities such as CT, RMI and nuclear medicine tests (PET and PET-CT) in the follow-up of breast cancer.

In the current clinical practice the approach adopted as first choice for the surveillance consists in the performance of abdominal US for hepatic involvement, thoracic X-rays for lung spread and bone scintigraphy for skeletal metastases, while other instrumental exams, such has CT, MRI and PET, are not considered for routine use. Such examinations should always be taken into account to help in solving diagnostic uncertainties originating from conventional imaging and may be of value when included in the follow-up during clinical trials. The advantage of PET over conventional imaging is the ability to provide functional and metabolic features of the tumor. Such a limitation in spatial localization has been overcome by integrating the PET and CT systems (PET/CT), thus allowing collecting at the same time topographical and metabolic information's of lesions (Fueger et al. 2005). FDG-PET and/or FDG-PET/CT have really increased and evolved their role in all stages of the disease for staging purposes, for monitoring response to therapy and for defining the loco-regional and distant recurrence both in the clinical practice and in research setting (Esserman 2005; Weir et al. 2005).

So PET is today considered a powerful technique capable of exploring the whole body and has great potential for staging the tumor with a single procedure detecting both the primary tumor and axillary lymph node involvement and providing the presence of distant metastases (Isasi et al. 2005). Many clinical studies have shown that FDG-PET is often superior to conventional imaging modalities in localizing tumor lesions and in the evaluation of anatomical regions that have been previously treated by radiation or surgery and which could be problematic in the discrimination between tumour relapse and scar tissue (Bombarieri and Crippa 2002). In this case, the variability of tumor cells results in active uptake of radiopharmaceuticals, and therefore the scan depicts positive foci, while tissues with low metabolism or dying cells produce a faint or negative uptake

It is well known that PET is reliable in assessing soft tissue and visceral lesions (liver, lung, distant lymph nodes), whereas also providing information on possible bone metastases (Lind et al. 2004).

There is evidence in the literature that FDG-PET detects more osteolytic lesions than bone scan, although bone scan is more sensitive than PET for imaging of osteoblastic lesions. Studies comparing the two methods have shown a high level of concordance and a minor number of discordant findings (Peterson et al. 2003; Nakamoto et al. 2003; Quon and Gambhir 2005). The difference between the bone scintigraphy and FDG-PET in detecting skeletal metastases is obviously related to the different mechanisms of scintigraphy detection. Bone scintigraphy visualizes the osteoblastic response to bone destruction by cancer cells, while FDG-PET visualizes metabolic activity of the tumor cells. Both processes are important, and the two techniques could theoretically be combined in view of the complementary information that they provide. Nevertheless, the real plus of FDG-PET is a high efficacy in evaluating soft tissue and visceral lesions (liver, lung, distant lymph nodes) and in detecting tumor recurrence from scar tissue due to radiation or surgery.

With the limitation we have highlighted for bone detection, FDG-PET therefore provides a single instrumental examination allowing complete tumor staging and re-staging and having the capability to detect metastases, which would have been missed or incorrectly diagnosed by CT, US, MRI or bone scintigraphy.

The future role of whole body PET or PET-CT as a tool for comprehensive assessment of disease status in breast cancer at different times during the course of the disease will depend to a large extent on its availability, as costs will likely decrease. The examination may offer a rapid, non-invasive, sensitive and whole body approach to confirmed metastases when they are suspected on the basis either symptoms or progressive increase in serum tumor markers in an otherwise healthy and well patient during follow-up.

22.5 Tumor Characterization

In the past few years there has been a growing body of evidence indicating the possible advantage deriving from appropriate molecular characterization of breast cancer (Hanahan and Weinberg 2000). Much is expected from new tools allowing for the most refined characterization of gene expression in parallel with a potentially even more informative definition of patterns of protein function abnormalities associated with the tumor.

Overall these new molecular tools will likely contribute to a new classification of breast cancer, to the redefinition of prognosis and eventually to the a priori prediction of sensitivity or resistance to commonly prescribed drug therapies. Conventional laboratory and pathology tests have already contributed to a significant revision of many aspects of breast tumor characterization. In the last years, the imaging technique has demonstrated that it can play an increasingly important role also in this setting.

The information provided by MRI is based on contrast enhancement dynamics after the administration of paramagnetic contrast medium. The enhancement is closely related to the volume and the permeability of the vessels, and to the width of the interstitial space.

US is also able to characterize some biological aspects because the imaging does not depend only on morphology and structure, but also on the vascularization and the peri-lesional reaction. The use of color power Doppler and new bubble contrast agents provide additional information on the vascular flow (Tuncbilek et al. 2003; Maidment 2003).

Nuclear medicine imaging is based on the metabolism of the tumor, so it may have special application in the study of the biological factors that influence prognosis. The radiopharmaceuticals mainly used for breast scintigraphy are lipophilic cations such as ^{99m}Tc-sestamibi or ^{99m}Tc-tetrafosmin. The tumor's accumulation of these traces depends on specific mechanisms. The uptake of these cations is inversely correlated with the expression of the P-glycoprotein (Pgp), which is encoded by the multi-drug resistance gene (MDR-1) (Moretti et al. 1996; Kostakoglu et al. 1997). Investigation has indicated that tumors with high uptake tend to respond better to specific pharmacological therapies. It is also of interest that dynamic acquisitions in untreated breast cancer patients after injection of ^{99m}Tc-sestamibi have demonstrated that the tumor release of the radiopharmaceutical seems directly correlated with the concentration of Pgp measured in the biopsy specimen. Such functional tests could be applied to differentiate between tumor phenotypes that are resistant to chemotherapy and those that are sensitive to it (Del Vecchio et al. 1997; Ciarmiello et al. 1998).

PET particularly is indicated for the study of the biological aggressiveness of the neoplastic tissue, especially if intense cellular proliferation is present with an associated increase in metabolic requirements. It should be remembered that radiopharmaceuticals labeled with positron emitters allow for the evaluation of a series of different biological parameters: glucose and protein metabolism, oxygen perfusion and/or consumption, persistence of integral blood brain barrier, proliferate activity and synthesis of cell structures (Avril et al. 1999).

Established and validated radiopharmaceuticals are now available to explore various metabolic pathways of the cancer cell, such as amino acid uptake and metabolism (^{11}C-methionine, ^{11}C-aminoisobutyric acid), membrane synthesis (^{11}C-choline, ^{18}F-fluoro-choline), nucleic acid synthesis (^{11}C-thymidine), dopamine synthesis (^{18}F-fluorodopa), cancer cell hypoxia (^{11}C-fluoromisonidazole) and hormone receptor expression (^{18}F-16α-fluorestradiol) (Linden et al. 2006; Aboagye and Price 2003). Furthermore these new tracers could allow the monitoring of different biological tumor processes, such as cell proliferation, apoptosis and neoagiogenesis, or the assessment of therapeutic target expression as estrogen receptor or HER2 receptor.

The clinical experience of PET in oncology is primarily based on FDG for glucose metabolism and on ^{11}C-methionine for amino acid uptake. PET allocations in metabolic studies require measurement of the uptake radiopharmaceutical in the tumor with semi-quantitative or quantitative approaches (Crippa et al. 1998; Maisey 2002). The correlation between FDG uptake and tumor histology, microscopic tumor growth patterns and tumor cell proliferation is constant probably because metabolic changes after malignant transformation depend on so many and complex interactions between the cellular energy requirements and the peri-tumoral microenvironment. The lack of correlation may in part explain why published results are heterogeneous and discordant. However, all studies show very clearly that FDG-PET can provide important information in vivo that could have prognostic interest and that findings can sometimes be correlated with overall survival and disease-free survival. The promise is there, but for the time being the application of PET is still investigational and cannot be recommended outside a research project.

22.6 Monitoring Response

Tumor response can be revealed measuring morphological changes by means of radiological imaging such as X-ray, MRI, CT and other techniques (Knopp et al. 2003; Pondero et al. 2004; Morakkabati et al. 2003). The decrease in tumor size is currently the common way to evaluate the response to therapy in solid tumors according to the RECIST criteria.

The use of morphological and metabolic imaging has revealed the possibility to provide an early and more accurate assessment of response than changes in tumor size associated with additional and relevant information about tumor biology.

It is well known that metabolic tumor response to therapy always precedes the dimensional changes measurable with standard imaging. This is because the effects of anticancer treatment primarily influence the tumor metabolism, which only in a second time is followed by a decrease in tumor mass. This information has relevance in measuring early response of the tumor in order to predict the degree of clinical response.

PET has demonstrated an early reduction in tissue uptake of FDG in the course of treatment after the first cycles of therapy that correlates with the response to treatment and to a subsequent morphological decrease in tumor diameter (Shelling et al. 2000). On the other hand, unchanged or enhanced FDG uptake indicates tumor progression or resistance to the delivered therapy.

The early assessment of response or resistance has immediate application not only in the metastatic setting, but also in women with operable breast cancer who are undergoing primary systemic treatment before surgery (Mariani et al. 1999; Schwarz et al. 2005; Biersack et al. 2004). In the neoadjuvant setting, PET could be applied to identify those patients in whom pathological tumor eradication will eventually be achieved (Smith et al. 2000; Rousseau et al. 2006). It has already been reported that response on PET represents an independent variable associated with the likelihood of favorable long-term outcome in terms of disease-free and overall survival (Krak et al. 2003; Donckier et al. 2003; Inoue et al. 2004).

Future application of PET and PET/CT using new tracers in addition to FDG could allow a better characterization of tumor biology and a better evaluation of response to therapy in all the stages of the disease.

22.7 Conclusions

Substantial progress has been made in the diagnosis and treatment of primary and metastatic breast cancer in the last 20 years. The widespread use of routine mammography has led to an increase in the early detection of primary breast lesions that significantly contributes to the decrease of mortality from breast cancer that is now measurable in Europe and North America. The dramatic shift in the stage of breast cancer at diagnosis has been associated with the successful application of less mutilating surgical procedures, with the widespread resort to breast-conserving surgery and, more recently, with avoidance of useless surgical staging of the axillary lymph node status through the use of sentinel node biopsy. In addition, adjuvant and preoperative systemic therapy has been optimized in terms of drug availability and activity and refinement of the criteria for administration, thus significantly contributing to prolongation of survival in women with early breast cancer. The challenge at this time is to define procedures and tools that allow easy characterization of the tumor, its aggressiveness and its pattern of sensitivity/resistance to drug therapy, so that treatment can be tailored to individual needs rather than to the average risk of the average patient. Such a challenge can today be met.

The technological development of imaging tools has been impressive in the field of diagnostic radiology and nuclear medicine allowing for the dependable detection of small lesions. These tools have generated new approaches permitting the successful differential diagnosis of doubtful lesions and the rapid identification of systemic metastases, and are providing a means for the non-invasive characterization of the biology of cancer tissue.

Several proposals for a diagnostic workup in breast cancer patients have been examined on the occasion of many interdisciplinary meetings, where the positions of different diagnostic modalities have been discussed and defined at the different steps of patient management. These indications can be considered only as possible choices that of course can change over time according to the resources, the facilities, the clinical situations and the evolution of knowledge about oncology (Table 22.2).

All the studies in this field are the basis of the continuous advances that will lead to the optimization of therapeutic strategies, considering that the metabolic information offered by nuclear medicine procedures, combined with the anatomical data provided by conventional radiological techniques should find a place in predicting tumor response and monitoring the outcome of patients. It is difficult to formulate conclusive diagnostic guidelines for application in the workup of breast cancer, since while the role of some examinations, such as mammography and US, is well established, that of others, such as MRI and PET, is still a matter of debate. There is a need for further and larger prospective evaluations with appropriate clinical trials in order to establish the impact of these approaches in improving survival and quality of life.

Table 22.2. Choice of diagnostic procedures for breast cancer patient workup (*)

Diagnosis of primary tumor	Staging	Biological characterization	Follow-up treated patients (clinically free from disease)	Recurrence and restaging	Monitoring of treatment response
Firstline: patient history, clinical examination, mammography/US **Complementary:** PET or scintimammography (only in selected patients)	**All patients:** chest X-ray, hepatic US, (CT) **Patients at high risk of metastases** (poor prognostic factors: T2N1, T3, T4): bone scan (CT or PET, or PET/CT) **Patients low risk stage T1-2N0:** sentinel node biopsy and/or PET (to select or exclude patients for ALND)	**In vitro:** pathology, tumor markers **In vivo:** PET or scintimammography (to check MDR)	Physical examination, mammography **Symptomatic patients or high risk of relapses** (poor prognostic factors: T2N1, T3, T4): chest X-ray, hepatic US, bone scan (CT), tumor markers. If doubtful results: PET7CT Note: PET/CT and tumor markers could substitute for all the examinations proposed for high risk	***Ipsilateral breast:*** **First choice:** mammography, US. **Complementary** PET or scintimammography (only in selected patients) ***Controlateral breast:*** **First choice:** mammography, US **Complementary:** PET or scintimammography, MRI Patients staged T1-2N0: PET ***Bone and soft tissues:*** Chest X-ray, CT; hepatic US, CT or MRI; bone scan or PET/CT Note PET/CT could substitute for any other morphological imaging for whole-body studies	**Early response:** tumor markers, PET **Delayed response:** *Breast*: mammography, US, scintimammography, MRI. *Skeleton*: bone scan Liver: US and CT Or: whole body PET/CT

Consensus conference of the EANM oncology Committee, May 2001, Milan, Italy modified 2004

References

Aboagye EO, Price PM (2003) Use of positron emission tomography in anticancer drug development. Invest New Drug 21:169–181

Adler LP, Weinberg IN, Bradbury MS, Levine EA, Lesko NM, Geisinger KR, Berg WA, Freimanis RI (2003) Method for combined FDG-PET and radiographic imaging of primary breast cancer. Breast J 9:163–166

Avril N, Schelling M, Dose J, Weber WA, Schwaiger M (1999) Utility of PET in breast cancer. Clin Positron Imaging 2:261–271

Bedrosian I, Mick R, Orel SG, Schnall M, Reynolds C, Spitz FR, Callans LS, Buzby GP, Rosato EF, Fraker DL, Czerniecki BJ (2003) Changes in the surgical management of patients with breast carcinoma based on preoperative magnetic resonance imaging. Cancer 98:468–473

Biersack HJ, Bender H, Palmedo H (2004) FDG-PET in monitoring therapy of breast cancer. Eur J Nucl Med Mol Imaging 31(suppl 1):s112–117

Bombardieri E, Crippa F (2002) The increasing impact of PET in the diagnostic work-up of cancer patients. In: Freeman LM, ed. Nuclear medicine annual 2002. Philadelphia: Lippincott Williams & Wilkins, p 75–121

Ciarmiello A, Del Vecchio S, Silvestro P, Potena MI, Carriero MV, Thomas R, Botti G, DAiuto G, Salvatore M (1998) Tumor clearance of technetium-99m-sestamibi as a predictor of response to neoadjuvant chemotherapy for locally advanced breast cancer. J Clin Oncol 16:1677–1683

Collins RF, Bekker HL, Dodwell DJ (2004) Follow-up care of patients treated for breast cancer: a structured review. Cancer Treat Rev 30:19–35

Crippa F, Seregni E, Agresti R, Chiesa C, Pascali C, Bogni A, Decise D, De Sanctis V, Greco M, Daidone MG, Bombardieri E (1998) Association between [18F]fluorodeoxyglucose uptake and postoperative histopathology, hormone receptor status, thymidine labelling index and p53 in primary breast cancer: a preliminary observation. Eur J Nucl Med 25:1429–1434

Crystal P, Strano SD, Shcharynski S, Koretz MJ (2003) Using sonography to screen women with mammographically dense breasts. AJR Am J Roentgenol 181:177–182

Cuzick J (2003) Epidemiology of breast cancer-selected highlights. Breast 12:405–411

Czernin J (2002) FDG-PET in breast cancer: a different view of its clinical usefulness. Mol Imaging Biol 4:35–45

De Gery S, Perret F, Espie M, Frija J (2003) Breast imaging and biopsy procedures in the diagnosis of breast cancer. Presse Med 25:125–133

Del Vecchio S, Ciarmiello A, Potena MI, Carriero MV, Mainolfi C, Botti G, Thomas R, Cerra M, Daiuto G, Tsuruo T, Salvatore M (1997) In vivo detection of multidrug-resistant (MDR1) phenotype by technetium-99m-sestamibi scan in untreated breast cancer patients. Eur J Nucl Med 24:150–159

Donckier V, Van Laethem JL, Goldman S, Van Gansbeke D, Feron P, Ickx B, Wikler D, Gelin M (2003) F-18 fluorodeoxyglucose positron emission tomography as a tool for early recognition of incomplete tumor destruction after radiofrequency ablation for liver metastases. J Surg Oncol 84:215–223

Elmore JG, Armstrong K, Lehman CD, Fletcher SW (2005) Screening for breast cancer. JAMA 293:1245–1256

Emens LA, Davidson NE (2003) The follow-up of breast cancer. Semin Oncol 30:338–348

Esserman L (2005) Integration of imaging in the management of breast cancer. J Clin Oncol 23:1601–1602

Fueger BJ, Weber WA, Quon A et al (2005) Performance of 2-deoxy-2-F18fluoro-D-glucose positron emission tomography and integrated PET/CT in restaged breast cancer patient Mol Imaging Biol 7:369–376

Gotzsche PC, Nielsen M (2006) Screening for breast cancer with mammography. Cochrane Database Syst Rev, 4: CD001877

Greco M, Crippa F, Agresti R, Seregni E, Gerali A, Giovanazzi R, Micheli A, Asero S, Ferrarsi C, Genaro M, Bombardieri E, Cascinelli N (2001) Axillary lymph node staging in breast cancer by 2-fluoro-2-deoxy-d-glucose positron emission tomography: clinical evaluation and alternative management. J Natl Cancer Inst 93:635–650

Grunfeld E, Noorani H, McGahan L et al (2002) Surveillance mammography after treatment of primary breast cancer: A systemic review. Breast 11:228–235

Hackshaw AK, Paul EA (2003) Breast self-examination and death from breast cancer: a meta-analysis. Br J Cancer 88:1047–1053

Hall FM (2003) Mammography and sonography in young symptomatic women. AJR Am J Roentgenol 181:1424–1425

Hanahan D, Weinberg RA (2000) The hallmarks of cancer. Cell 100:57–70

Hortobagyi GN (2002) Can we cure limited metastatic breast cancer? J Clin Oncol 20:620–623

Inoue T, Butani K, Taguchi T, Tamaki Y, Shiba E, Noguchi S (2004) Preoperative evaluation of prognosis in breast cancer patients with (18F)2-Deoxy-2-fluoro-D-glucose-positron emission tomography. J Cancer Res Clin Oncol 130:273–278

Irwing L, Houssami N, Vanvliet C (2004) New techonologies in screening for breast cancer: a systematic review of their accuracy. Br J Cancer 90:2118–2122

Isasi CR, Moadel RM, Blaufox MD (2005) A meta analysis of FDG-PET for the evaluation of breast cancer recurrence and metastases. Breast Cancer Res Treat 90:105–112

Jakub JW, Pendas S, Reintgen DS (2003) Current status of sentinel lymph node mapping and biopsy: facts and controversies. Oncologist 8:59–68

Joseph E, Hyacinthe M, Lyman GH et al (1998) Evaluation of an intensive strategy for follow-up and surveillance of primary breast cancer. Ann Surg Oncol 5:522–528

Khatcheressian JL, Wolff AC, Smith TJ, Grunfeld E, Muss HB, Vogel VG, Halberg F, Somerfild MR, Davidson NE (2006) American Society of Clinical Oncology 2006 update of the breast cancer follow-up and management guidelines in the adjuvant setting. J Clin Oncol24:1–7

Knopp MV, von Tengg-Kobligk H, Choyke PL (2003) Functional magnetic resonance imaging in oncology for diagnosis and therapy monitoring. Mol Cancer Ther 2:419–426

Kolb TM, Lichy J, Newhouse JH (2002) Comparison of the performance of screening mammography, physical examination, and breast US and evolution of factors that influence them: an analysis of 27,825 patient evaluations. Radiology 225:165–175

Kostakoglu L, Elahi N, Kiratli P, Ruacan S, Sayek I, Baltali E, Sungur A, Hayran M, Bekdik CF (1997) Clinical validation of the influence of P-glycoprotein on technetium-99m-sestamibi uptake in malignant tumors. J Nucl Med 38:1003–1008

Krak NC, Van Der Hoeven JJ, Hoekstra OS, Twisk JW, Van Der Wall EE, Lammertsma AA (2003) Measuring 18F-FDG uptake in breast cancer during chemotherapy: comparison of analytical methods. Eur J Nucl Med Mol Imaging 30:674–681

Kubota M, Inoue K, Koh S, Sato T, Sugita T (2003) Role of ultrasonography in treatment selection. Breast Cancer 10:188–197

Kuehn T, Vougle FD, Helms G et al (2004) Sentinel node biopsy for axillary staging in breast cancer: results from a large prospective German multi-institutional trial. Eur J Surg Oncol 30:252–259

Kuhl CK, Schrading S, Leutner CC, Morakkabati-Spitz N, Wardelmann E, Fimmers R, Kuhn W, Schild HH (2005) Mammography, breast ultrasound, and magnetic resonance imaging for surveillance of women at high familial risk for breast cancer. J Clin Oncol 23:8469–8476

Kuhl CK (2006) MR imaging for surveillance of women at high familial risk for breast cancer. Magn Reson Imaging Clin N Am 14:391–402

Leconte I, Feger C, Galant C, Berliere M, Berg BV, Dohore W, Maldague B (2003) Mammography and subsequent whole-breast sonography of non palpable breast cancers: the importance of radiologic breast density. AJR Am J Roentgenol 180:1675–1679

Lehman CD (2006) Role of MRI in screening women at high risk for breast cancer. J Magn Reson Imaging 24:964–970

Lehman CD, Blume JD, Weatherall P, Thickman D, Hylton N, Warner E, Pisano E, Schnitt SJ, Gatsonis C, Schnall M, DeAngelis GA, Stomper P, Rosen EL, O'Loughlin M, Harms S, Bluemke DA; International Breast MRI Consortium Working Group (2005) Screening women at high risk for breast cancer with mammography and magnetic resonance imaging. Cancer 103:1898–1905

Liang W, Lawrence WF, Burnett CB, Hwang YT, Freedman M, Trock BJ, Mandelblatt JS, Lippman ME (2003) Acceptability of diagnostic tests for breast cancer. Breast Cancer Res Treat 79:199–206

Liberman L (2000) Clinical management issues in percutaneos core breast biopsy. Radiol Clin North Am 38:791–807

Liberman M, Sampalis F, Mulder DS, Sampalis JS (2003) Breast cancer diagnosis by scintimammography: a meta-analysis and review of the literature. Breast Cancer Res Treat 80:115–126

Lind P, Igerc I, Beyer T, Reinprecht P, Hausegger K (2004) Advantages and limitations of FDG PET in the follow up of breast cancer. Eur J Nucl Med Mol Imaging 31(suppl 1): s125–134

Linden HM, Stekhova SA, Link JM et al (2006) Quantitative fluoroestradiol positron emission tomography imaging predicts response to endocrine treatment. J Clin Ocol 24:2793–2799

Maidment AD (2003) Digital mammography. Semin Roentgenol 38:216–230

Maisey MN (2002) Overview of clinical PET. Br J Radiol 2002; 75:S1–S5

Mamounas EP (2001) Ipsilateral breast tumor recurrence after lumpectomy: is it time to take the bull by the horns? J Clin Oncol 19:3798–3800

Mankoff DA, Eubank WB (2006) Current and future use of positron emission tomography SPECT in breast cancer. J Mam Gland Biol neoplasia 11:125–136

Mariani G, Gennai A, Giorgetti A, Donati S, Puccini G, Nista N, Dani D, Bengala C, Conte PF, Salvatori PA (1999) Early assessment by PET with FDG of response to first-line chemotherapy of metastatic breast cancer. Clin Positron Imaging 2:342

McDonough MD, De Peri ER, Mincey BA (2004) The role of positron emission tomography imaging in breast cancer. Curr Oncol Rep 6:62–68

Mehta TS (2003) Current uses of ultrasound in the evaluation of the breast. Radiol Clin North Am 41:841–856

Mille D, Roy T, Carre MO, Ray I, Ferdjaoui N, Spath HM, Chauvin F, Philip T (2000) Economic impact of harmonizing medical practices: compliance with clinical practice guidelines in the follow-up of breast cancer in a French comprehensive cancer center. J Clin Oncol 18:1718–1724

Morakkabati N, Leutner CC, Schmiedel A, Schild HH, Kuhl CK (2003) Breast MR imaging during or soon after radiation therapy. Radiology 229:893–901

Moretti JL, Azaloux H, Boisseron D, Kouyoumdjian JC, Vilcoq J (1996) Primary breast cancer imaging with technetium-99m sestamibi and its relation with P-glycoprotein overexpression. Eur J Nucl Med 23:980–986

Moss SM, Cuckle H, Evans A, Johns L, Waller M, Bobrow L; Trial Management Group (2006) Effect of mammographic screening from age 4 years on breast cancer mortality at 10 years' follow-up: a randomised controlled trial. Lancet 368:2053–2060

Nakamoto Y, OSman M, Wahl RL (2003) Prelevance and patterns of bone metastases detected with positron emission tomography using F-18 FDG. Clin Nucl Med 28:302–307

Newman LA, Sabel M (2003) Advances in breast cancer detection and management. Med Clin North Am 87:997–1028

Palli D, Russo A, Sapeva C et al (1999) Intensive vs clinical follow up after treatment of primary breast cancer: 10 year update of a randomized trial-National Research Council Project on Breast Cancer Follow-Up. JAMA 281:15896

Peterson JJ, Kransdorf MJ, OConnor MI (2003) Diagnosis of occult bone metastases: positron emission tomography. Clin Orthop 415:S120–S128

Pondero V, Mazzocchi M, Del Frate C, Pugliesi F, Di Loreto C, Francescutti G, Zuiani C (2004) Locally advanced breast cancer: comparison of mammography sonography and MR imaging in evaluation of residual disease women receiving neoadjuvant chemotherapy. Eur Radiol 14:1371–1379

Prats E, Banzo J, Merono E, Herranz R, Carril JM (2001) ^{99m}Tc-MIBI scintimammography as a complement of the mammography in patients with suspected breast cancer. A multicentre experience. Breast 10:109–116

Quon A, Gambhir S (2005) FDG-PET and beyond: molecular breast cancer imaging. J Clin Oncol 23:1664–1673

Rousseau C, Devillers A, Sagan C et al (2006) Monitoring of early response to neoadjuvant chemotherapy in stage II and III breast cancer by fluorodeoxyglucose positron emission tomography. J Clin Oncol 24:5366–5372

Schnall M, Orel S (2006) Breast MR imaging in the diagnostic setting. Magn Reson Imaging Clin N Am 14:329–337

Schoder H, Gonen M (2007) Screening for cancer with PET and PET/CT: potential and limitations. J Nuc Med 48:4–17

Schwarz JD, Bader M, Jenicke L, Hemminger G, Janicke F, Avril N (2005) Early prediction of response to chemotherapy in metastatic breast cancer using sequential F-FDG PET. J Nucl Med 46:1144–1150

Silberman AW, MecVay C, Cohen JS et al (2004) Comparative morbidity of axillary lymph node dissection and the sentinel lymph node technique. Ann Surg 240:1–6

Smith IC, Ogston KN, Whitford P et al (1998) Staging of the axilla in breast cancer: accurate in vivo assessment using positron emission tomography with 2-fluorine-18-fluoro-2-deoxy-d-glucose. Ann Surg 228:220–227

Smith IC, Welch AE, Hutcheon AW et al (2000) Positron emission tomography using ^{18}F-fluorodeoxy-D-glucose to predict the pathologic response of breast cancer to primary chemotherapy. J Clin Oncol 18:1676–1688

Spanu A, Dettori G, Chessa F, Porcu A, Cottu P, Solinas P, Falchi A, Solinas ME, Scanu AM, Nuvoli S, Madeddu G (2001) ^{99m}Tc-tetrofosmin pinhole-SPECT (P-SPECT) and radioguided sentinel node (SN) biopsy and in breast cancer axillary lymph node staging. Cancer Biother Radiopharm 16:501–513

Shelling M, Avril N, Nahrig J et al (2000) Positron emission tomography using ^{18}F-fluorodeoxy-D-glucose for monitoring primary chemotherapy in breast cancer. J Clin Oncol 18:1689–1695

Tuncbilek N, Unlu E, Karakas HM, Cakir B, Ozylmaz F (2003) Evaluation of tumor angiogenesis with contrast-enhanced dynamic magnetic resonance mammography. Breast J 9:403–408

Veronesi U, De Cicco C, Galimberti VE, Fernandez JR, Rotmensz N, Viale G, Sapno G, Luini A, Intra M, Veronesi P, Berettini A, Paganelli G (2006a) A comparative study on the value of FDG-PET and sentinel node biopsy to identify occult axillary metastasis. Ann Oncol 12:1–6

Veronesi U, Paganelli G, Viale G, Luini A, Zurrida S, Galimberti V, Intra M, Veronesi P, Maisonneuve P, Gatti G, Mazzorol G, De Cicco C, Manfredi G, Fernadez JR (2006b) Sentinel-lymph-node biopsy as a staging procedure in breast cancer: update of a randomized controlled study. Lancet Oncol 7:983–990

Walter C, Scheidhauer K, Scharl A, Goering UJ, Theissen P, Kugel H, Krahe T, Pietrzyk U (2003) Clinical and diagnostic value of preoperative MR mammography and FDG-PET in suspicious breast lesions. Eur Radiol 13:1651–1656

Warner E, Pleves DB, Hill KA et al (2004) Surveillance Of BRCA1 and BRCA2 mutation carriers with magnetic resonance imaging, ultrasound, mammography, and clinical breast examination. JAMA 292:1317–1325

Weir L, Worsley D, Bernstein V (2005) The value of FDG positron emission tomography in the management of patients with breast cancer. Breast J 11:204–209

Williams A (1994) How should information on cost effectiveness influence clinical practice. In: Delamothe T, ed. Outcomes into clinical practice. London: BMJ Publishing Group, p 99–107

Subject Index

A

B

C

D

K

L

M

N

T

U

V

W

X

Z